An Invitation to Health

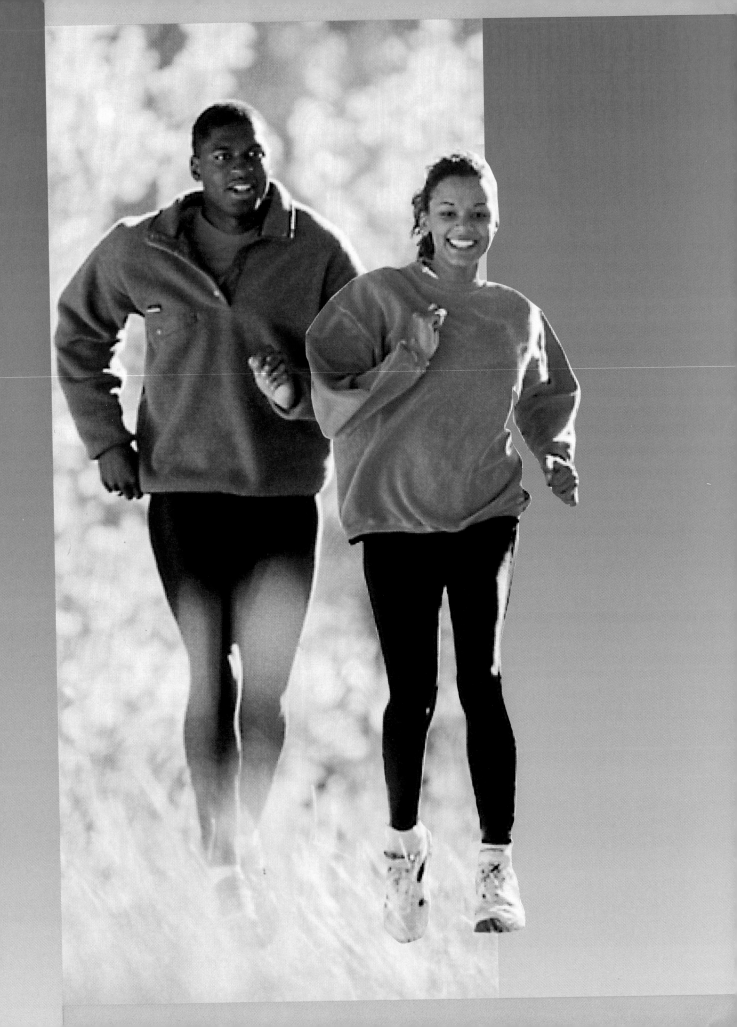

An Invitation to Health

Brief Edition

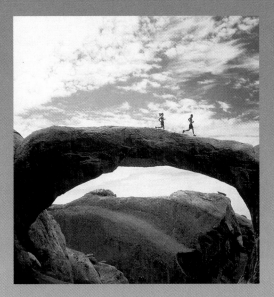

The Power of Prevention

Dianne Hales

Wadsworth Publishing Company
ITP® An International Thomson Publishing Company

Belmont, CA • Albany, NY • Boston • Cincinnati • Johannesburg • London • Madrid • Melbourne
Mexico City • New York • Pacific Grove, CA • Scottsdale, AZ • Singapore • Tokyo • Toronto

Health Editors: *Vicki Knight and Peter Marshall*
Development Editors: *Jim Strandberg and Megan Rundel*
Editorial Assistant: *Stephanie Andersen*
Marketing Manager: *Lori Braumberger*
Production Coordinator: *Mary Anne Shahidi*
Print Buyer: *Vena Dyer*
Permissions Editor: *Lillian Campobasso*

Production Services: *Pre-Press Company, Inc.*
Interior Design: *Pre-Press Company, Inc.*
Cover Design: *E. Kelly Shoemaker*
Cover Photo: *John Terence Turner,*
   FPG International
Compositor: *Pre-Press Company, Inc.*
Printer: *World Color–Versailles*

Printed in the United States of America
3 4 5 6 7 8 9 10

For more information, contact Wadsworth Publishing Company, 10 Davis Drive, Belmont, CA 94002, or
electronically at http://www.wadsworth.com

International Thomson Publishing Europe
Berkshire House
168-173 High Holborn
London, WC1V 7AA, United Kingdom

Nelson ITP, Australia
102 Dodds Street
South Melbourne
Victoria 3205 Australia

Nelson Canada
1120 Birchmount Road
Scarborough, Ontario
Canada M1K 5G4

International Thomson Publishing Southern Africa
Building 18, Constantia Square
138 Sixteenth Road, P.O. Box 2459
Halfway House, 1685 South Africa

International Thomson Editores
Seneca, 53
Colonia Polanco
11560 México D.F. México

International Thomson Publishing Asia
60 Albert Street
#15-01 Albert Complex
Singapore 189969

International Thomson Publishing Japan
Hirakawa-cho Kyowa Building, 3F
2-2-1 Hirakawa-cho, Chiyoda-ku
Tokyo 102, Japan

Library of Congress Cataloging-in-Publication Data
Hales, Dianne R.
   An invitation to health : the power of prevention / Dianne Hales.
   — Brief 8th ed.
      p. cm.
   Includes bibliographical references and index.
   ISBN 0-534-36478-0
   1. Health. 2. Self-care, Health.   I. Title.
RA776.H148   1999b
613—DC21   99-11140

To my husband, Bob, and my daughter, Julia, who make every day an invitation to joy.

Preface

To the Student

An Invitation to Health, Brief Edition, is an invitation to you. What you learn from this book can have a direct impact on how you look, feel, and act—now and for decades to come. Whatever stage of life you are at as you begin this course, I hope you will find much of personal value in these pages.

Perhaps you are in good health and think that you know all that you need to know about how to take care of yourself. If so, take a minute and ask yourself some questions:

- How well do you understand yourself? Are you able to cope with emotional upsets and crises? Do you often feel stressed out?

- How nutritiously do you eat? Are you always going on—and off—diets? Do you exercise regularly?

- How solid and supportive are your relationships with others? If you are sexually active, are you conscientious about birth control and safer-sex practices?

- Are you caught up in any compulsive behaviors? Do you get drunk or high occasionally? Do you smoke?

- What do you know about your risk for infectious diseases, heart problems, cancer, or other serious illnesses?

- Have you taken steps to insure your personal safety at home, on campus, or on the streets? Have you confronted your own feelings about the processes of aging and dying?

As you consider these questions, chances are that there are some aspects of health you've never considered before—and others that you feel you don't have to worry about for years. Yet the choices you make and the actions you take now will have a dramatic impact on your future.

Your health is your personal responsibility. Over time, your priorities and needs will inevitably change, but the connections between various dimensions of your well-being will remain the same: The state of your mind will affect the state of your body, and vice versa. The values that guide you through today can keep you mentally, physically, and spiritually healthy throughout your lifetime. Your ability to cope with stress will influence your decisions about alcohol and drug use. Your commitment to honest, respectful relationships will affect the nature of your sexual involvements. Your eating and exercise habits will determine whether you develop a host of medical problems.

An Invitation to Health, Brief Edition, is based on extensive health research and is packed with information, advice, and recommendations. This book provides the first step in taking full charge of your own well-being. An important theme of this book is prevention. Ultimately, the power of prevention belongs to you—and it's a lot easier than you might think. You might simply add a walk or workout to your daily routine. You might snack on fruit instead of high-fat foods. You might cut back on alcohol. You might use a condom each and every time you have sex. You might buckle your seat belt whenever you get in a car. These things may not seem like a big deal now, yet they may well make a crucial difference in determining how active and fulfilling the rest of your life will be.

Packaged with every copy of the *Brief Edition* is a collection of Health Assessment tools to assist you in making positive changes in your life. A Wellness Inventory and a set of Self-Surveys will help you to evaluate the current state of your health and, I hope, prompt you to consider changes where improvements are needed. Health Monitor worksheets encourage you to take a weekly measure of how you are faring in making positive strides toward a more healthy lifestyle. Also packaged with every text is a set of practice quizzes for every chapter of the *Brief Edition.* These sample quizzes focus on the essential points and key terms in each chapter and will help you prepare for objective tests.

Keep in mind, however, that a personal health class is unlike any other course you'll take in college. You can't simply read the text, do your assignments, and pass the exams; you have to live what you learn. To help you on your way, *Personal Health Interactive,* a CD-ROM, is available for sale through your bookstore. Besides providing enhancement activities and chapter key term reviews specific to the *Brief Edition, Personal Health Interactive* features a Wellness Clinic. Visiting the Wellness Clinic, you have the opportunity to set personal health goals and assess your daily progress toward achieving those goals.

This textbook is an invitation—an invitation to health in its broadest sense, to personal fulfillment, to life itself. Its pages provide the practical tools you need to work toward achieving your full potential. I hope that you keep this book and use it often as your personal health manual. I also hope that you accept this invitation in another sense—that you live what you learn and make the most of your life—now and through all the years and adventures the future may bring you.

May you live long and prosper.
Dianne Hales

To the Instructor

We have entered a new era in health care, and its hallmark is prevention. ***An Invitation to Health, Brief Edition,*** introduces students to this way of thinking about their health and their future. This book, an abridgment of my best-selling introductory health text, outlines the keys to preventing the major killers of Americans—heart disease, cancer, and accidents—and to preparing for a life of health in the fullest sense of the word.

In this text, health is defined in the broadest possible way—not as an entity in itself but as a process of discovering, using, and protecting all the resources within the individual, family, and community. I emphasize how health is a subject that encompasses body, mind, and spirit, and the *Brief Edition* brings this vision more fully to life by providing students with the information and inspiration they need to make healthful decisions and changes.

I have tried to "invite" students in new ways, to entice and excite them by making the content as relevant to their lives as possible. I place a strong emphasis on personal responsibility, a commitment to prevention, practical applications of knowledge, and a focus on behavioral change. These concepts are fundamental for any health course and do not change from year to year.

Because the field of health science is so broad and changes so rapidly, keeping up with the most recent developments provides an enormous challenge. In preparing *An Invitation to Health, Brief Edition,* I have had the same goal in mind as I aspired to in the past: creating the best health textbook on the market. The response from students and instructors to past editions of *An Invitation to Health* has been enthusiastic and gratifying. But that positive feedback is due to the tradition of keeping the textbook *extraordinarily current* and responding to input from reviewers who teach this course.

An Invitation to Health, Brief Edition, includes hundreds of citations from 1996 to 1998 references. The majority are from primary sources, including professional books; medical, health, and mental health journals; health education periodicals; scientific meetings; federal agencies; publications from research laboratories and universities; and personal interviews with specialists in a number of fields. For those who have come to expect the very latest in the best available health information in *An Invitation to Health,* you won't be disappointed in the *Brief Edition.*

The *Brief Edition* includes the goals of Healthy People 2010, recent research findings on the effects of different types of fat in the diet, the phenomenon of sexual communication and fantasy in cyberspace, 1998 cancer incidence estimates, the health risks associated with cigar smoking, the latest drug therapies for treating AIDS, and much, much more. Every chapter contains up-to-date coverage, offering the best available information to students seeking to ascertain and implement healthy choices.

Packaged with every copy of the text—*at no additional charge*—is a set of health assessments to help students take stock of their current attitudes and behaviors in regard to a host of health issues. These assessments include a Wellness Inventory and a series of Self-Surveys related to each major health topic in the text.

Special Features and Pedagogy in the Brief Edition

An Invitation to Health, Brief Edition, consists of fifteen chapters, covering the essential core topics of a college-level introductory health course. The book's organization is flexible, so you can use the chapters in any order that suits your needs. The chapters present key concepts in health in a comprehensive manner and cover the most current, as well as most controversial, issues in the field.

To enliven the text and to assist students in getting the most out of the material, *An Invitation to Health, Brief Edition,* contains a wealth of features and pedagogy. First, the special features:

Campus Focus. How much vigorous exercise do college students get? How many have contemplated suicide? How many are eating nutritious meals? How many are using contraception if they engage in sexual intercourse? How many smoke, drink alcohol, and/or take drugs? How many have carried a weapon? These and other questions were the focus of a 1995 study, the National College Health Risk Behavior Survey. The results of this survey, published in a September 1997 article in the *Journal of American College Health,* are displayed in new pie charts and bar graphs prepared for this edition. Starting in Chapter 1 with a description of this study and a graph depicting the demographic breakdown of the 4,600 students who filled out the questionnaire, graphic illustrations of the results of this study appear in relevant chapters. For example, in Chapter 6, a Campus Focus graphic depicts the numbers of students who had dieted, and the number of those who had vomited or had taken laxatives to lose or keep from gaining weight.

Health Online. With the use of the Internet soaring over the past few years, the potential for using the Web to attain practical, up-to-date, and vital health information is phenomenal. Each chapter of the *Brief Edition* includes a Health Online feature box, focusing on one informative Web site pertaining to material covered in that chapter, which the student is encouraged to visit. The Web sites chosen are dynamic ones, offering on-line assessments, interesting animations, or especially practical advice. For example, in Chapter 3, mental health screening tests at NYU's Department of Psychiatry Web site are highlighted. The value of good Web sites on the Internet is brought home, and practical health information is conveyed in yet another format to enhance each chapter. Moreover, this feature offers an additional resource: critical thinking questions appear at the end of Health Online, asking students to evaluate what they have seen at the Web site.

Pulsepoints. This popular feature, appearing in every chapter, offers a snappy list of relevant, practical health tips. For example, in Chapter 5, the Pulsepoints lists and describes the "Top Ten Ways to Cut Fat" or, in Chapter 9, "Ten Ways to Prevent Sexually Transmitted Diseases."

Strategies for Prevention. The power of prevention is a major focus throughout the book. To help bring that theme home, bulleted lists of Strategies for Prevention appear in every chapter. These offer practical strategies for preventing health problems and reducing health risks—from something as basic as "Preventing Test Stress" in Chapter 2 to "Scanning Your Skin" for signs of cancer in Chapter 10.

Strategies for Change. To offer guidance for taking charge of every facet of healthful living, *An Invitation to Health, Brief Edition,* incorporates behavioral strategies within the text of every chapter, and emphasizes these strategies with this special feature. Like Strategies for Prevention, these bulleted lists are meant to offer practical advice on how to make the changes needed to achieve better health, such as "Safe Stretching" in Chapter 4 or "If Someone Close to You Drinks Too Much" in Chapter 12.

Spotlight on Diversity. This feature highlights issues of cross-cultural or multicultural diversity pertinent to specific chapters, such as "Cultural Variations in Sexual Arousal" in Chapter 7.

Pedagogy. The *Brief Edition* contains a wealth of pedagogical assistance to help students master the essential material.

■ *Learning Objectives.* Each chapter opens with a set of learning objectives, outlining the most essential information on which students should focus while reading the chapter.

■ *Key Terms.* Key terms are boldfaced when they first appear in the chapter, are listed (with page references) at the back of each chapter, and are defined in the Glossary at the end of the book.

■ *Making This Chapter Work for You.* Each chapter ends with a bulleted, detailed summary titled "Making This Chapter Work for You," which lists the key points covered in the chapter.

■ *Review Questions.* A set of review questions appears at the back of each chapter, helping students to assess whether or not they have mastered the most important information.

■ *Critical Thinking Questions.* Moving beyond just a review, a number of questions are also included at the end of the chapter, which ask students to consider some applications of the chapter's coverage or weigh in on some health-related controversy.

■ *Connections to Personal Health Interactive.* Also listed at the end of each chapter is a list of pertinent study aids on Wadsworth's newly revised CD-ROM for health, *Personal Health Interactive.* Produced by Arthur and Wendy Kohn of Kwamba Multimedia Productions, this CD includes a Wellness Clinic, providing a variety of assessment tools to help students monitor their own health on a daily basis. It also features a selection of study aids, including a chapter-by-chapter review of key terms tied directly to the book, and 10 Online Research Activities on core health topics. *Personal Health Interactive* is sold separately.

Ancillary Package

Instructors adopting *An Invitation to Health, Brief Edition,* receive an extraordinary package of complimentary support materials to use with the textbook.

Instructor's Guide. The IG includes chapter outlines and summaries, learning objectives, discussion questions, ideas for guest speakers, self-assessment exercises, references, readings, resources, and transparency masters.

Test Bank. An outstanding test bank is available, including multiple choice, short answer, and essay questions. Correct answers are referenced to the pages in the text, and multiple choice questions are categorized as factual, applied, or conceptual. In addition to the printed test bank, the questions are available on computer disks in Windows or Macintosh format, and Tele-Testing is also available.

Full-Color Transparency Acetates. Instructors adopting *An Invitation to Health, Brief Edition,* may request a set of Transparency Acetates, containing full-color acetates taken from main text figures. The set of transparencies will also be available on CD-ROM.

Health Study Center on Wadsworth's Web Site. Wadsworth's Health Study Center is located at **http:// healthstudy.wadsworth.com** and features a variety of resources for the health instructor as well as the student. Adopters of *An Invitation to Health, Brief Edition,* will be given the passwords to make full use of the site. Students will be able to visit the Health Study Center online and take practice quizzes for each chapter.

Wadsworth Video Library for Health. Adopting departments may select from the Wadsworth Video Library an evolving list of documentary-style videos dealing with such subjects as weight control and fitness, AIDS and sex, sexual communication, peer pressure, compulsive and addictive behavior, and the relationship between alcohol and violence. Most of these videos, including several offered exclusively by Wadsworth, use interviews with students, professors, and experts to make the subject more real and personal. Contact your Wadsworth-ITP representative for details and eligibility.

"Trigger" Video Series. These video complements—one on stress, the other on fitness—to *An Invitation to Health, Brief Edition,* are designed to promote or "trigger" class discussion on a variety of important topics related to stress and fitness. These 60-minute videos contain five 8-10 minute clips, followed by questions for discussion. Each segment is keyed to material in the text.

***Dine Healthy* Software (Windows and Macintosh).** *Dine Healthy* teaches you how to eat sensibly, eliminating the need for crash diets. Clear, concise bar charts show how well you eat, with recommendations for food-choice changes. An exercise section enables you to track caloric expenditures and calculate ideal caloric intakes. A recipe analysis feature suggests how your favorite recipes can be improved nutritionally. An expandable database lets you add new food products as they come into the marketplace. Each adopting department is eligible to receive one copy of this powerful personal trainer for nutrition and fitness.

***Diet Analysis Plus* Software (Windows and Macintosh).** This user-friendly software program helps simplify the process of diet analysis. It contains comprehensive information on nutrients in foods and energy expenditures from exercise. *Diet Analysis Plus* calculates the Recommended Dietary Allowances, analyzes daily intakes, identifies diet deficiencies and excesses, calculates comparisons and ratios, helps locate alternative foods, and helps plan an exercise program, as well as a weight-gain or -loss program. The database has been updated to include more foods common to college students as well as a comprehensive list of microwaveable foods.

The University of California at Berkeley Wellness Newsletter. Instructors who adopt *An Invitation to Health, Brief Edition,* will receive a complimentary one-year subscription to the *University of California at Berkeley Wellness Newsletter.* Adopters should contact their local Wadsworth-ITP representative.

In addition, the following items are available for sale.

Chapter Quizzes. A set of chapter quizzes with twenty multiple choice items per chapter is available to bundle with the text.

Personal Health Interactive Integrator Online CD-ROM. Produced by Arthur J. Kohn and Wendy Kohn of Kwamba Multimedia Productions, this newly revised CD-ROM contains a Wellness Clinic and a set of activities most appropriate for use with this text. In the Wellness Clinic, a variety of interactive tools are offered to help students assess their own health and monitor progress towards wellness goals. An interactive study guide built around the chapter organization of *An Invitation to Health, Brief Edition,* includes a variety of innovative study aids including ten Online Research Activities on core health topics. At the end of each chapter, *Personal Health Interactive* offers review sections to test on the key terms included in each chapter. For instructors, an important benefit of *Personal Health Interactive* is its innovative CourseWeaver program, which allows professors to prepare lectures quickly and easily and to export multimedia elements to popular presentation packages, such as PowerPoint, Persuasion, and Astound. The built-in "LecturePresenter" program enables instructors to present professional-quality multimedia lectures.

To Order

To adopt *An Invitation to Health, Brief Edition,* contact your local ITP representative. To receive a review copy of this book, send your request on department letterhead to:

Wadsworth Publishing Company
Dept. Hales 001
10 Davis Drive
Belmont, CA 94002

Or visit the Wadsworth Web site at
http://healthstudy.wadsworth.com or e-mail us at
info@wadsworth.com.

Acknowledgments

I am deeply indebted to the many instructors and students, reviewers, editors, and others without whom *An Invitation to Health* would never have enjoyed so many years of success.

For the *Brief Edition,* I was fortunate to work with a great team at Brooks/Cole and Wadsworth. A warm thanks to Vicki Knight, Jim Strandberg, Mary Anne Shahidi, Vernon Boes, Faith Stoddard, Lori Braumberger, Peter Marshall, and Stephanie Andersen for all your hard work. My thanks, as well, to Megan Rundel, freelance developmental editor, and Lillian Campobasso, freelance permissions editor.

Finally, let me express my appreciation to the reviewers whose input has been so valuable in completing the *Brief Edition.* For their great help with this edition, I thank the following for their timely assistance:

Judy Baker, East Carolina University
Dianne Bartley, Middle Tennessee State University
Lynn Bloomberg, Worcester State College
Diane Foster-Burke, Westminster College
Pat Hanson, California State University-Monterey Bay
Pamela Hoalt, Malone College
Robert Huff, California State University-Northridge
Richard Kaye, Kingsborough Community College
Becky Kennedy-Koch, Ohio State University
Shawn Ladda, Manhattan College
Sandra Mull, Northwest Missouri State University
Fred Randolph, Western Illinois University

For their recent help with the eighth edition of the longer book—and suggestions which influenced the *Brief Edition* as well—I offer my gratitude to:

Rick Barnes, East Carolina University
Lois Beach , SUNY-Plattsburgh
James Brik, Willamette University
Stephen Haynie, College of William and Mary
Becky Kennedy-Koch, Ohio State University
Darlene Kluka, University of Central Oklahoma
Sabina White, University of California-Santa Barbara
Roy Wohl, Washburn University

Please R.S.V.P.

This book is an invitation to good health in its broadest sense—to personal fulfillment, to life itself. Its pages provide the practical tools students need to achieve their full potential. I also hope that your students accept this invitation in another sense: that they *live* what they learn and make the most of their health and of their lives.

I also have another invitation for you—a request to tell us what you think. *An Invitation to Health, Brief Edition,* was created for your students and for you. I would like to know what I'm doing right, what I could do better, and what I might include or drop in future editions. Your opinions and ideas matter a great deal to me. I look forward to hearing from you.

Dianne Hales
c/o Wadsworth Publishing Company
10 Davis Drive
Belmont, CA 94002

About the Author

Dianne Hales, one of the most widely published freelance writers in the country, is the author of *Just Like a Woman: How Gender Science is Redefining What Makes Us Female* and numerous other trade and reference books. She also is a contributing editor for *Ladies Home Journal* and *Working Mother* and has written more than 1,000 articles for national consumer and health publications.

Dianne Hales was the 1998 recipient of the EMMA (Exceptional Media Merit Award) for health reporting from the National Women's Political Caucus and Radcliffe College. She is one of the few journalists to be honored with national magazine-writing awards by both the American Psychiatric Association and the American Psychological Association and has won other writing awards from various organizations, including the Council for the Advancement of Scientific Education, National Easter Seal Society, and the New York City Public Library.

Brief Contents

Contents

15 Taking Charge of Your Health   304

Features

■ Pulsepoints

■ Health Online

Chapter 1

An Invitation to Health for the 21st Century

After studying the material in this chapter, you should be able to:

■ **Identify** and **explain** the dimensions of health and how they relate to total wellness.

■ **Explain** the principles of health promotion.

■ **Discuss** the relationship between culture, economics, and health care.

■ **Describe** the factors that influence the development of health behavior.

■ **Create** a complete plan to change or develop a health behavior.

■ **Explain** the principles and goals of prevention and **differentiate** prevention from protection.

Health involves more than physical well-being. It is a state of body, mind, and spirit that must be viewed within the context of community, society, and environment. By providing the information and understanding you need to take care of your own health, *An Invitation to Health* can help you live more fully, more happily, and more healthfully. It also goes beyond the basics of health maintenance. Its primary themes—prevention of health problems, protection from health threats, and promotion of the health of others—can establish the basis for good health now and in the future.

The invitation to health that we extend to every reader is one offer you literally cannot afford to refuse: The quality of your life depends on it.

The Dimensions of Health

By simplest definition, **health** means being sound in body, mind, and spirit. The World Health Organization defines health as "not merely the absence of disease or infirmity," but "a state of complete physical, mental, and social well-being."[1] Health is the process of discovering, using, and protecting all the resources within our bodies, minds, spirits, families, communities, and environment.

Health has many components: physical, psychological, spiritual, social, intellectual, and environmental. This book takes a *holistic* approach that looks at health and the individual as a whole, rather than part by part. Your own definition of health may include different elements, but chances are that you and your classmates would agree that it includes at least some of the following:

- A positive, optimistic outlook.
- A sense of control over stress and worries; time to relax.
- Energy and vitality; freedom from pain or serious illness.
- Supportive friends and family and a nurturing intimate relationship with someone you love.
- A personally satisfying job.
- A clean environment.

Increasingly, Americans are striving to achieve the state of optimal health known as **wellness**. Wellness has been defined as purposeful, enjoyable living or, more specifically, a deliberate lifestyle choice characterized by personal responsibility and optimal enhancement of physical, mental, and spiritual health. Wellness means more than not being sick; it means taking steps to prevent illness and to lead a richer, more balanced, and more satisfying life. (See Pulsepoints: "Ten Simple Changes to Improve Your Health.")

While physical well-being is essential to health, the term *wellness*, as used by health professionals, has a broader meaning. To understand how the concepts of wellness and health fit together, think of an automobile transmission: Having a disease (illness) is like being in reverse; absence of disease (health) puts you in neutral; but positive health changes (wellness) push you into drive—forward motion. When your entire lifestyle is based on health-enhancing behaviors, you're in high gear and going at top speed—and you've achieved total wellness. In wellness, health, and sickness, there's considerable overlap in the functions of the mind, body, and spirit. Understanding the various dimensions of health can help you appreciate these complex interactions.

Physical Health

The various states of good and ill physical health can be viewed as points on a continuum (see Figure 1-1). At

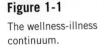

Figure 1-1
The wellness-illness continuum.

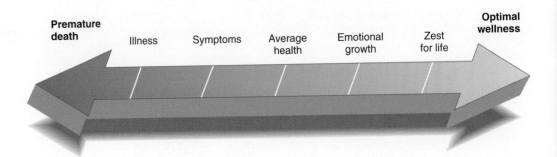

Premature death · Illness · Symptoms · Average health · Emotional growth · Zest for life · Optimal wellness

Pulsepoints

Ten Simple Changes to Improve Your Health

1. Use seat belts. In the last decade seat belts have saved more than 40,000 lives and prevented millions of injuries.

2. Eat an extra fruit or vegetable every day. Adding more fruit and vegetables to your diet can improve your digestion and lower your risk of several cancers.

3. Get enough sleep. A good night's rest provides the energy you need to make it through the following day.

4. Take regular stress breaks. A few quiet minutes spent stretching, looking out the window, or simply letting yourself unwind are good for body and soul.

5. Lose a pound. If you're overweight, you may not think a pound will make a difference, but it's a step in the right direction.

6. If you're a woman, examine your breasts regularly. Get in the habit of performing a breast self-examination every month after your period (when breasts are least swollen or tender).

7. If you're a man, examine your testicles regularly. These simple self-exams can spot the early signs of cancer when they're most likely to be cured.

8. Get physical. Just a little exercise will do some good. A regular workout schedule will be good for your heart, lungs, muscles, bones—even your mood.

9. Drink more water. Eight glasses a day are what you need to replenish lost fluids, prevent constipation, and keep your digestive system working efficiently.

10. Do a good deed. Caring for others is a wonderful way to care for your own soul and connect with others.

---

one end is early and needless death; at the other is optimal wellness, in which you feel and perform at your very best. In the middle, individuals are neither sick enough to need medical attention nor well enough to live each day with zest and vigor. For the sake of optimal physical health, we must take positive steps away from illness and toward well-being. We must feed our bodies nutritiously, exercise them regularly, avoid harmful behaviors and substances, watch out for early signs of sickness, and protect ourselves from accidents.

Psychological Health

Like physical well-being, psychological health is more than the absence of problems or illness. Psychological health refers to both our emotional and mental states—that is, our feelings and thoughts. It involves awareness and acceptance of a wide range of feelings in oneself and others, the ability to express emotions, to function independently, and to cope with the challenges of daily stressors. (Chapter 3 provides more information on psychological health.)

Spiritual Health

Being *spiritual* doesn't always mean belonging to a formal religion. Its essential component is a belief in some

meaning or order in the universe, a higher power that gives greater significance to individual life. Spiritually healthy individuals identify their own basic purpose in life; learn how to experience love, joy, peace, and fulfillment; and help themselves and others achieve their full potential. They concern themselves with "giving, forgiving, and attending to others' needs before one's own," says psychiatrist Roger Smith, M.D., of Michigan State University. Smith notes that spiritual development "produces a new meaning in one's life through a connectedness to something greater and mysterious."[2]

Social Health

Social health refers to the ability to interact effectively with other people and the social environment, to develop satisfying interpersonal relationships, and to fulfill social roles. It involves participating in and contributing to your community, living in harmony with fellow human beings, developing positive interdependent relationships with others, and practicing healthy sexual behaviors.

Intellectual Health

The brain is the only organ capable of self-awareness. Every day you use your mind to gather, process, and act on information; to think through your values; to make decisions, set goals, and figure out how to handle a problem or challenge. Intellectual health refers to your ability to think and learn from life experience, your openness to new ideas, and your capacity to question and evaluate information. Throughout your life, you'll use your critical thinking skills, including your ability to evaluate health information to safeguard your well-being.

Environmental Health

You live in a physical and social setting that can affect every aspect of your health. Environmental health refers to the impact that your world has on your well-being. It means protecting yourself from dangers in the air, water, soil, and products you use—and also working to preserve the environment itself.

Health for the 21st Century

At the eve of the 20th century, the average American could expect to live for about 50 years. Infectious diseases, such as smallpox and tuberculosis, claimed tens of thousands of lives, particularly among the young and the poor. A high percentage of women died during childbirth or shortly afterward. By 1900, the average American woman could expect to live to an age of 50.9 years, compared with 47.9 years for a man. By 1950, women's projected lifespan had grown to 71.1 years and men's to 65.6.[3]

We have come a very long way. According to the National Center for Health Statistics, life expectancy in 1996 reached an all-time high: 76.1 years. The projected lifespans of both white and black males are longer than ever: 73.8 years and 66.1 years, respectively. The race differential has narrowed more than in the past, as has the gender gap. American women are expected to outlive men by 6 years, compared with a difference of 6.4 years in 1995.[4]

Infant mortality has reached another all-time low of 7.2 deaths per 1000 live births. The white infant mortality rate declined 5% in 1996 from the previous year (from 6.3 to 6), while the black rate dropped 6% (from 15.1 to 14.2). An estimated 15% decline in mortality rates stems from a decline in Sudden Infant Death Syndrome (SIDS).

The top killers of Americans remain the same as the previous year (see Table 1-1), but there has been a dramatic decline in mortality related to Human Immunodeficiency Virus (HIV) infection and Acquired Immune Deficiency Syndrome (AIDS). In 1995, HIV/AIDS was

TABLE 1-1 THE TOP TEN KILLERS	
	Number of Victims in the U.S.
Heart diseases	737,563
Cancer	538,455
Stroke	157,991
Chronic lung diseases	102,899
Accidents	93,320
Pneumonia and flu	82,923
Diabetes	59,254
HIV infection	43,115
Suicide	31,284
Chronic liver disease and cirrhosis	25,222

SOURCE: National Center for Health Statistics.

the leading cause of death among 25- to 44-year-olds. In a single year, mortality declined 26% and slipped into second place behind accidents and injuries. HIV/AIDS mortality had increased an average of 16% per year between 1987 and 1994 before leveling off in 1995.

Homicide and suicide declined as causes of death in 1996 for the total population, but among young persons 15 to 24 years of age, they remain, respectively, the second and third leading causes of death. Accidents are the number-one cause of death in this age group.

According to the Women's Research and Education Institute, gender is the single most important factor in predicting a person's life expectancy—more important than race, income, education, or lifestyle. Throughout the industrialized world, the gender that lives longer—by an average of 5% to 10%—is female. Insurance industry statistics indicate that every year, for every 100,000 Americans, 803 men and just 447 women die. The gender difference in mortality rates emerges before birth. From the moment of conception, baby girls are less likely to die in the womb or after delivery than baby boys. Once past age 30, women consistently outnumber and outlive men. By age 85, there are three women for every man. By the year 2020, according to current projections, the average woman's life may increase by 10 years—and the average man's by just 6.[5]

Healthy People 2000 and 2010

Ever since 1990, the U.S. Public Health Service, state health departments, and professional and voluntary organizations have been working to meet national health goals first outlined in a publication called *Healthy People 2000*. By 1995, this program had met 8% of its target goals and was moving in the direction of accomplishing 40% of the others. Progress has continued in many areas. According to a 1997 update, disparities in health services have declined for several minority groups. Infant mortality rates have dropped among Hispanic Americans, for instance, although they are still higher than for the U.S. population as a whole. The percentage of Hispanic women receiving prenatal care, regular Pap smears, and mammograms (for women over 50) has increased. However, other health problems, including obesity and diabetes, remain more prevalent among Hispanic Americans than the population as a whole. Of all ethnic and racial groups in the United States, Hispanic Americans and Asian Americans and Pacific Islanders (AAPIs) are the least likely to have health insurance and are less likely to have regular sources of primary care than other Americans.

The campaign for better health for all Americans will not end with the 20th century. Plans have been proposed for a new *Healthy People 2010*. Its two overarching goals are increasing years of healthy life and eliminating health disparities. In addition, policymakers have suggested four enabling goals: promoting healthy behaviors, protecting health, achieving access to quality health care, and strengthening community prevention. New areas of focus include the needs of the disabled, people with low incomes, and the chronically ill.[6]

Diversity and Health

We live in the most diverse nation on Earth. Look around your classroom or campus: Your fellow students come from dozens of different ethnic, racial, religious, and cultural groups. Minority students, who represented about 6% of undergraduates in 1960, now make up 25%.[7]

Your own family background may be woven of threads reaching back to several other countries and cultures. For society, this variety can be both enriching and divisive. Tolerance and acceptance of others have always been part of the American creed. By working together, Americans have created a country that remains a symbol of opportunity around the world. Yet members of different ethnic groups still struggle against discrimination. Today, in this country's third century, all Americans still aren't equal in every way, including their health and health care. Poverty remains the single greatest barrier to better health for minorities in the United States. Without adequate insurance or ability to pay,

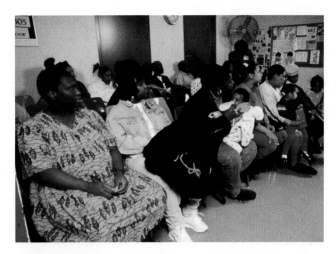

Neighborhood clinics can provide medical care that is sensitive to language differences and culturally diverse attitudes about health and medicine.

many cannot afford the tests and treatments that could prevent illness or overcome it at the earliest possible stages. Some groups, particularly African Americans, also rate the health services in their communities as lower than those available to white Americans and have more negative opinions of the health care they receive.[8]

Can Race Be Hazardous to Health?

Different racial and ethnic groups often face different health risks. Consider the following statistics:

- The infant mortality rate for African-American babies remains higher than that of white babies.[9]

- Life expectancy for African Americans, though increasing, is 6.5 years lower than that for whites.[10]

- African Americans have higher rates of high blood pressure (hypertension), develop this problem earlier in life, suffer more severe hypertension, and have higher rates of hypertension-related deaths than whites.

- The death rate for heart disease among middle-aged black women is 150% higher than among white women the same age; among those with diabetes, their death rate is 134% higher than white female diabetics. Twice as many black as white women die of strokes and more than twice as many of diabetes.[11]

- Among young African-American women, breast cancer is a special threat. Of all black women diagnosed with breast cancer, 37% are younger than 50—compared with 22% of white women.[12]

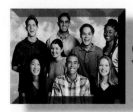

Spotlight on Diversity
Closing the Minority Health Gap

How long can you expect to live? Are you at a higher-than-average risk for potentially deadly diseases? Do you have access to health services? If you are ill or injured, can you expect to receive the best possible care?

To some extent, your answer to these questions depends on your racial and ethnic background. As a growing number of studies indicate, many minority groups in the United States have shorter life expectancies, higher risks of illness, more limited access to services, and more negative expectations of and experiences with the health-care system than the population as a whole.

But race itself isn't the primary reason for the health problems faced by minorities in the United States. Poverty is. Without adequate insurance or ability to pay, many cannot make the lifestyle choices or afford the tests and treatments that could prevent illness or overcome it at the earliest possible stages. According to public health experts, low income may account for one-third of the racial differences in death rates for middle-

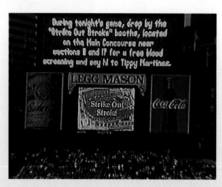

The "Strike Out Stroke" campaign in the Southern United States features prevention messages and offers free blood pressure screenings in ballparks. Such community-based campaigns increase awareness of hypertension.

aged African-American adults. High blood pressure, high cholesterol, obesity, diabetes, and smoking are responsible for another third. The final third has been blamed on "unexplained factors," which may include poor access to health care and the stress of living in a society in which skin color remains a major barrier to equality. As the American Medical Association's Council on Ethical and Judicial Affairs has reported, many minorities "are likely to require health care but are less likely to receive health services."

The National Institutes of Health (NIH) have established an Office of Research on Minority Health (ORMH) with the goal of "closing the gap that currently exists between the health of minorities and the majority population." Since 1992, ORMH has provided funds for research and prevention efforts aimed at improving minority health. Some focus on prenatal care to improve survival rates. Others are educating minority youths about HIV infection and AIDS.

- Native Americans have the highest rates of diabetes in the world. Among the Pima Indians, half of all adults have diabetes.[13]

- Southeast Asian men have a higher incidence of lung and liver cancer than the population as a whole.[14]

- Native Americans, including those indigenous to Alaska, are more likely to die young, primarily as the result of accidental injuries, cirrhosis of the liver, homicide, suicide, pneumonia, and the complications of diabetes than the population as a whole.[15]

Are these increased susceptibilities the result of racial or ethnic background, the stress of living with discrimination, an unhealthy lifestyle, lack of access to health services, or poverty? It is hard to say precisely. Certainly, poverty presents the greatest barrier to making healthy lifestyle choices, seeking preventive care, and getting timely and effective treatment.

Health-care providers often fail to recognize racial or ethnic factors in part because the discussion of race and ethnicity in health is politically controversial. Some fear that it could lead to misconceptions about genetic superiority or inferiority. Yet recognition of different health needs and risks is the first step toward overcoming the health problems of many Americans. (See Spotlight on Diversity: "Closing the Minority Health Gap.")

The Health of College Students

As one of the nation's 12 million full- or part-time college students, you belong to one of the most diverse groups in America. Although more than half of all young people ages 20 to 24 years have attended college, little is known about the health of college students nationwide. Some studies have focused on drinking, drug use, and sexual activity, but none have assessed the health behaviors of students. To correct this information gap, in

1995 the National College Health Risk Behavior Survey surveyed the health behaviors of more than 4600 students at 136 institutions. The findings—featured throughout this edition of *Invitation to Health* in our new "Campus Focus" feature—represent a snapshot of the state of college students' health.

The primary finding from the mass of data collected was that many college students in the United States engage in behaviors that put them at risk for serious health problems.[16] The survey findings are important because they reveal a gap between what students know they should be doing to ensure good health and what they actually do. And college may be an ideal time to make permanent life-enhancing changes.

Whether you're still in your teens or well into middle age, college can represent a turning point in your life. If you're a young adult, college offers the opportunity to shape your identity, define your goals, forge strong relationships, and prepare yourself for the future.

If you've returned to school or are starting college at midlife or later, you may already know what you need and want from school. If you're taking courses solely to enrich yourself, you can savor the opportunity to make your mind a more interesting place to live for the rest of your life. Whatever your age or stage of life, knowing how to prevent health problems can help you reach your goals.

Becoming All You Can Be

Many external factors often affect us—from the weather, which can temporarily dampen or brighten our mood, to genetic predispositions, which can result in certain health conditions. In addition, those who are poor, disabled, or discriminated against have fewer options for preventing illness or promoting health. But even if you can't control all your life circumstances, you are

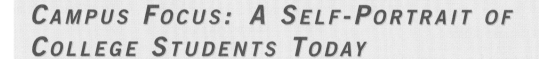

CAMPUS FOCUS: A SELF-PORTRAIT OF COLLEGE STUDENTS TODAY

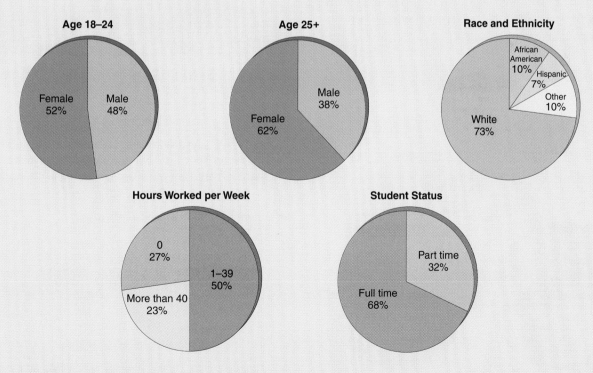

SOURCE: Douglas, Kathy, et al., "Results from the 1995 National College Health Risk Behavior Study," *Journal of American College Health*, Vol. 46, September 1997.

responsible for making the most of those circumstances. The first step is understanding that your own behaviors and choices can pose threats to your health.

Understanding Health Behavior

Behaviors that affect your health include exercising regularly, eating a balanced, nutritious diet, seeking care for symptoms, and taking necessary steps to overcome illness and restore well-being. If there is one health behavior that you would like to improve, you have to realize that change isn't easy. Between 40% and 80% of those people who try to kick bad health habits lapse back into their unhealthy ways within 6 weeks. To make lasting beneficial changes, you have to understand the three types of influences that shape behavior: predisposing, enabling, and reinforcing factors (Figure 1-2).

Predisposing Factors

Predisposing factors include:

- *Knowledge* about the effects of health-related behaviors.

- *Attitudes*—that is, likes and dislikes.

- *Beliefs* that you are at risk for the negative consequences of your behavior, that these consequences may be severe, and that you will experience benefits if you change your behavior.

- *Values* or importance you give to health and related issues such as appearance or productivity.

- *Perception* that the benefits of making health changes are worth the sacrifices.

Enabling Factors

Enabling factors include skills, resources, accessible facilities, and physical and mental capacities. Before you initiate a change, assess the means available to reach your goal. No matter how motivated you are, you'll become frustrated if you keep encountering obstacles. That's why breaking a task or goal down into step-by-step strategies is so important in behavioral change.

Reinforcing Factors

Reinforcing factors may be praise from family and friends, rewards from teachers or parents, or encouragement and recognition for meeting a goal. Although these help a great deal in the short run, lasting change depends not on external rewards, but on an internal commitment and sense of achievement. To make a difference, reinforcement must come from within.

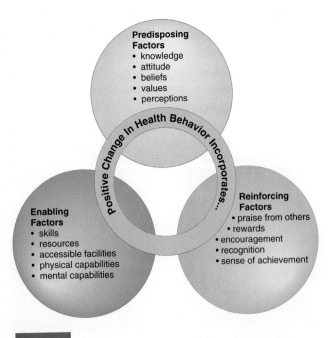

Figure 1-2

Factors that shape positive behavior.

Strategies for Change

Setting Realistic Goals

Here's a framework for setting goals and objectives, the crucial preliminary step for making changes:

✔ Determine your goal or objective. Define it in words and on paper. Then test your definition against your own value system. Can you attain your goal and still be the person you want to be?

✔ Think in terms of evolution, not revolution.

✔ Identify your resources. Do you have the knowledge, skills, finances, time—whatever it takes? Find out from others who know. Be sure you're ready for the next step.

✔ Systematically analyze barriers. How can you acquire missing resources? Identify and select alternative plans. List solutions for any obstacles you foresee.

✔ Choose a plan. Think it through step by step and try to anticipate what might go wrong and why.

Making Decisions

Every day you make decisions that have immediate and long-term effects on your health. You decide what to eat, whether to drink or smoke, when to exercise, and how to cope with a sudden crisis. Beyond these daily matters, you decide when to see a doctor, what kind of doctor, and with what sense of urgency. You decide what to tell your doctor and whether to follow the advice given, whether to keep up your immunizations, whether to have a prescription filled and comply with the medication instructions, and whether to seek further help or a second opinion. The entire process of maintaining or restoring health depends on your decisions.

The small decisions of everyday life—what to eat, where to go, when to study—are straightforward choices. Larger decisions—which major to choose, what to do about a dead-end relationship, how to handle an awkward work situation—are more challenging. However, if you think of decision making as a process, you can break down even the most difficult choices into manageable steps:

- *Set priorities.* Rather than getting bogged down in details, step back and look at the big picture. What matters most to you? What would you like to accomplish in the next week, month, year? Look at the decision you're about to make in the context of your values and goals (both discussed in Chapter 3).

- *Inform yourself.* The more you know—about a person, a position, a place, a project—the better you'll be able to evaluate it. Gathering information may involve formal research, such as an online or library search for relevant data or informal conversations with teachers, counselors, family members, or friends.

- *Consider all your options.* Most complex decisions don't involve simple either-or alternatives. List as many options as you can think of, along with the advantages and disadvantages of each.

- *Tune in to your gut feelings.* After you've gotten the facts and analyzed them, listen to your intuition. While it's not infallible, your "sixth sense" can provide valuable feedback. If something just doesn't feel right, try to figure out why. Are there any fears you haven't dealt with? Do you have doubts about taking a certain path?

- *Consider a "worst case" scenario.* When you've pretty much come to a final decision, imagine what will happen if everything goes wrong—the workload becomes overwhelming, your partner betrays your trust, your expectations turn out to be unrealistic. If you can live with the worst consequences of a decision, you're probably making the right choice.

Changing Health Behavior

Change is never easy, even if it's done for the best possible reasons. When you decide to change a behavior, you have to give up something familiar and easy for something new and challenging. Change always involves risk and the prospect of rewards.

Before they reach the stage where they can and do take action to change, most people go through a process comparable to religious conversion. First, they reach a level of accumulated unhappiness that makes them ready for change. Then they have a moment of truth that makes them want to change. One pregnant woman, for instance, felt her unborn baby quiver when she drank a beer and swore never to drink again. As people change their behavior, they change their lifestyles and identities as well. Ex-smokers, for instance, may start an aggressive exercise program, make new friends at the track or gym, and participate in new types of activities, like racquetball games or fun runs.

Social and cultural **norms**—behaviors that are expected, accepted, or supported by a group—can make change much harder if they're constantly working against a person's best intentions. You may resolve to eat less, for instance, yet your mother may keep offering you homemade fudge and brownies because your family's norm is to show love by making and offering delicious treats. Or you might decide to drink less, yet your friends' norm may be to equate drinking with having a good time.

Large decisions may seem overwhelming, but they can be broken down into manageable steps to help you gather information and focus on what's best for you.

If you're aware of the norms that influence your behavior, you can devise strategies either to change them (by encouraging your friends to dance more and drink less at parties, for example) or adapt to them (having just a bite of your mother's sweets). Another option is to develop relationships with people who share your goals and whose norms can reinforce your behavior.

The Keys to Successful Change

Awareness of a negative behavior is always the first step toward changing it. Once you identify what you'd like to change, keep a diary for 1 or 2 weeks, noting what you do, when, where, and what you're feeling at the time. If you'd like, enlist the help of friends or family to call attention to your behavior. Sometimes self-observation in itself proves therapeutic: Just the act of keeping a diary can be enough to help you lose weight or kick the smoking habit.

Once you've identified the situations, moods, thoughts, or people that act as cues for a behavior, identify the most powerful ones and develop a plan to avoid them. For instance, if you snack continuously when studying in your room, try working in the library, where food is forbidden.

Planning ahead is a crucial part of successful change. If you can't avoid certain situations, anticipate how you might cope with the temptation to return to your old behavior. Develop alternatives. Visualize yourself walking past the desserts in the cafeteria or chewing gum instead of lighting a cigarette.

Some people find it helpful to sign a "contract," a written agreement in which they make a commitment to change, with their partner, parent, or health educator. Spelling out what they intend to do and why underscores the seriousness of what they're trying to accomplish (see Figure 1-3).

Above all else, change depends on the belief that you can and will succeed. In his research on **self-efficacy**, psychologist Albert Bandura of Stanford University found that the individuals most likely to reach a goal are those who believe they can. The more strongly they feel that they can and will change their behavior, the more energy and persistence they put into making the change.[17] Other researchers have linked positive health change with optimism. Individuals who see themselves as optimists may underestimate their susceptibility to problems, such as hypertension, because they always expect things to turn out well. Individuals who perceive themselves as susceptible—that is, who anticipate potentially negative consequences—may be more cautious.[18]

Another crucial factor is **locus of control**. If you believe that your actions will make a difference in your health, your locus of control is internal. If you believe that external forces or factors play a greater role, your locus of control is external. Individuals with an external locus of control for health are less likely to seek preventive health care, are less optimistic about early treatment, rate their own health as poorer, and spend more time in bed because of illness than those with an internal locus of control.[19]

Reinforcements—either positive or negative—also can play a role. If you decide to set up a regular exercise program, for instance, you might reward yourself with a new sweat suit if you stick to it for 3 months or you might punish yourself for skipping a day by doing 10 extra minutes of exercises the following day.

Your **self-talk**—the messages you send yourself—also can play a role. In recent decades, mental health professionals have recognized the conscious use of positive self-talk as a powerful force for changing the way individuals think, feel, and behave.

A New Era in Health Education

In the past, health education focused on individual change. Today many educators are using a new framework in which behavior change occurs within the context of the entire environment of a person's life. The primary themes that bring together personal health,

---

Strategies for Change

How to Make a Change

✔ Get support from friends, but don't expect them to supply all the reinforcement you need.

✔ Focus on the immediate rewards of your new behavior.

✔ To boost your self-confidence, remind yourself of past successes you've had in making changes. Give yourself pep talks, commending yourself on how well you've done so far and how well you'll continue to do.

✔ Reward yourself regularly. Small, regular rewards are more effective in keeping up motivation than one big reward that won't come for many months.

✔ Expect and accept some relapses.

My Contract for Change

Date: _____

Personal Goal: _____

_____

Motivating Factors: _____

_____

Change(s) I Promise to Make to Reach This Goal: _____

_____

Plan for Making This Change: _____

_____

_____

Start Date: _____

Assessment Plan: _____

_____

_____

_____

If I Need Help: _____

_____

_____

Target Date for Reaching Goal: _____

Reward for Achieving Goal: _____

Penalty for Failing to Achieve Goal: _____

_____

Signed: _____

Witnessed by: _____

Figure 1-3

A sample health-change contract.

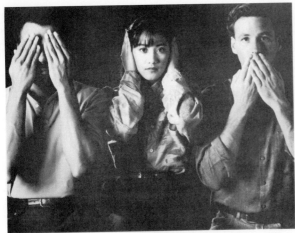

This is the way many people deal with HIV.

A lot of people don't think they have to worry about HIV. But the truth is, anyone can get HIV infection if they are sharing drug needles and syringes or having sex with an infected person. Call your State or local AIDS hotline. Or call the National AIDS Hotline at 1-800-342-AIDS. Call 1-800-243-7889 (TTY) for deaf access.

U.S. DEPARTMENT OF HEALTH & HUMAN SERVICES   CDC   **HIV is the virus that causes AIDS.**   AMERICA RESPONDS TO AIDS

Prevention includes education and training that empowers us and enhances our well-being.

social context, and a community focus are prevention and protection.

The Power of Prevention

No medical treatment, however successful or sophisticated, can compare with the power of **prevention**. Two of every three deaths and one in three hospitalizations in the United States could be prevented by changes in six main risk factors: tobacco use, alcohol abuse, accidents, high blood pressure, obesity, and gaps in screening and primary health care. Preventive efforts have already proved helpful in increasing physical activity, quitting smoking, reducing dietary fat, preventing sexually transmitted diseases (STDs) and unwanted pregnancy, reducing intolerance and violence, and avoiding alcohol and drug abuse.

The Potential of Protection

There is a great deal of overlap between prevention and **protection**. Some people might think of immunizations (discussed in Chapter 9) as a way of preventing illness; others see them as a form of protection against dangerous diseases. In many ways, protection picks up where prevention leaves off. You can prevent STDs or unwant-

ed pregnancy by abstaining from sex. But if you decide to engage in potentially risky sexual activities, you can protect yourself by means of condoms and spermicides (discussed in Chapter 8).

The very concept of protection implies some degree of risk—immediate and direct (for instance, the risk of intentional injury from an assailant or unintentional harm from a fire) or long-term and indirect (such as the risk of heart disease and cancer as a result of smoking). To know how best to protect yourself, you have to be able to assess risks realistically.

Hereditary Risks

In all, more than 4000 diseases have been traced to flaws in the basic genetic blueprints for life. According to the American Society of Human Genetics, about 5% of adults under age 25 have a genetically linked disease; among adults over 25, 60% develop a genetically influenced disorder.

In addition to rare genetic syndromes, hereditary diseases include common problems such as certain types of cataracts, glaucoma, gallbladder disease, hypertension, nearsightedness, ulcers, and dyslexia. "The general perception is that all hereditary diseases are

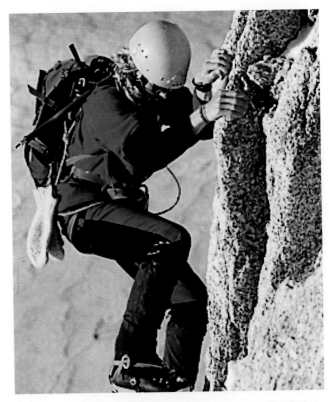

Wearing a helmet is a health choice that diminishes your risk of serious injury during a potentially dangerous activity.

Education about health choices is a major aspect of health promotion.

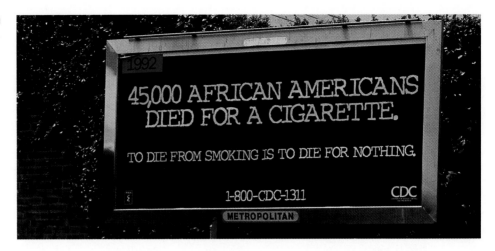

unalterable and deadly, but that's not the case," observes geneticist Reed Pyeritz, M.D. of Johns Hopkins School of Medicine in Baltimore. "The vast majority don't necessarily shorten life, although they can cause pain and suffering."[20] Most adult-onset illnesses, such as cancer, heart disease, and alcoholism, are caused by the interaction of multiple genes and environmental factors.

Assessing Risks

At this point, you cannot change your genes or the risks they carry, but this isn't true of all health risks. The risk of head injury is very real every time you get on your mountain bike; however, it diminishes greatly when you put on a helmet. While the world can be a dangerous place, the greatest health threats stem from high-risk behaviors—smoking, excessive drinking, not getting enough exercise, eating too many high-fat foods, and not getting regular medical checkups, to name just a few. That's why changing unhealthy habits is the best way to reduce risks and prevent health problems. Yet how do we know whether or not alleged health risks are acceptable? Some key factors to consider are:

- *Possible benefits.* Advantages or payoffs—such as the high salary paid for working with toxic chemicals or radioactive materials—may make some risks seem worthwhile.

- *Whether the risk is voluntary.* All of us tend to accept risks that we freely choose, such as playing a sport that could lead to injuries, as opposed to risks imposed on us, such as pollution from a nearby factory.

- *Is it fair?* The risk of skin cancer, which is increasing because of ozone depletion, affects us all. We may worry about it and take action to protect our-

selves and our planet, but we don't resent it the way we resent living with the risk of violent crime because the only housing we can afford is in a high-crime area.

- *Are there alternatives?* As consumers, we may become upset about cancer-causing pesticides or food additives when we learn about safer chemicals or methods of preservation.

- *"Framing."* Our thinking about risks often depends on how they're presented or framed—for instance, if we're told that a new drug may kill 1 out of every 100 people, instead of that it may save the lives of 99% of those who use it.

Making This Book Work for You
Taking Charge of Your Future

Through every chapter of this book, you'll recognize some familiar themes and messages that apply to every aspect of your health. Among the most important are:

- You're not simply a creature of mind, body, or spirit, but of all three. Physical, psychological, spiritual, social, intellectual, and environmental factors are interrelated in complex and crucial ways that affect your health.

- Prevention has the power to enhance the quality and duration of your life. Rather than waiting for bad health habits to take their toll, you can delay or eliminate many problems by adopting healthful behaviors now.

- Positive lifestyle changes—the basics of health promotion—enhance your health and enrich your well-being.

Health Online

New York Online Access to Health (NOAH)
http://www.noah.cuny.edu:8080/about.html

NOAH, created by the City University of New York, Metropolitan New York Library Council, New York Academy of Medicine, and New York Public Library, is a responsible and authoritative bilingual (English and Spanish) site providing health information on many topics, including mental health, birth control, AIDS and HIV, alternative medicine, nutrition, cancer, pregnancy, sexuality, heart disease, and aging.

Think about it . . .

- The most commonly accessed pages on NOAH are related to pregnancy, contraception, abortion, and birth. What would be the topic you'd look up first? Why? Where else would you turn for information on this subject?

- NOAH's site includes the following disclaimer: "NOAH offers this information to you with the understanding that it not be interpreted as medical or professional advice. All medical information needs to be carefully reviewed with your health care provider." How would you go about evaluating any information you find on this or other health-related sites?

- NOAH, which uses various experts to check medical information, has received many commendations for accuracy. What do you think makes some Web sites more credible than others? Are there certain sites or types of information that do not seem credible or authoritative to you? Why?

■ You can take charge of your health and prevent illness by changing your health behaviors. The keys to success are motivation, accurate information, workable strategies, and a belief in your ability to change.

■ You are not alone. Your ties to the people around you and to the environment in which you live give richness and meaning to your life.

■ You face undeniable risks in life, but you can do a great deal to avoid or minimize their impact on your well-being.

To help safeguard your health, you need to understand basic theories about human health and life and to have up-to-date information about health practices. With the aid of your health instructors, *An Invitation to Health* can provide the basic knowledge and skills you need for a lifetime of well-being. But knowledge isn't enough; action is the key. The habits you form now, the decisions you make, and the ways in which you live day by day all shape your health and your future.

This book can give you the understanding you'll need to make good decisions and establish a healthy lifestyle, but you can't simply read and study health the way you study French or chemistry—you must decide to live it.

This is our invitation to you.

Key Terms

The terms listed here are used within the chapter. Page numbers are included for each term.
A definition of each term is given in the green Glossary pages at the end of this book.

health *2*	**prevention** *12*	**self-efficacy** *10*
locus of control *10*	**protection** *12*	**self-talk** *10*
norms *9*	**reinforcements** *10*	**wellness** *2*

Review Questions

1. What are the dimensions of health? How do they relate to total wellness?
2. How does lifestyle affect health prevention?
3. What strategies can promote wellness? What are some possible benefits of practicing these strategies?
4. What kinds of factors shape the development of health behavior? How so?
5. What should health-care providers know about cultural and gender differences? Why?
6. What are some overall strengths and weaknesses of the health of college students?
7. What could you do to change or develop a health behavior on your own? What kinds of strategies might you use? What could be the benefits?

Critical Thinking Questions

1. What is the definition of health according to the textbook? Does your personal definition differ from this, and if so, in what ways? How would you have defined health before reading this chapter?
2. Where do you lie on the wellness-illness continuum? What variables might affect your place on the scale? What do you consider your optimum state of health to be?
3. In what ways would you like to change your present lifestyle? What steps could you take to make those changes?

Connections to Personal Health Interactive

To enhance your understanding of the material covered in this chapter, check out the following study aids on the *Personal Health Interactive CD-ROM*.

- Ethics in Research
- Personal Insights: How Healthy Are You?
- Glossary & Key Term Review

References

1. "Constitution of the World Health Organization." *Chronicle of the World Health Organization*. Geneva, Switzerland: WHO, 1947.
2. Cunningham, Alastair. "Pies, Levels and Languages: Why the Contribution of Mind to Health Has Been Underestimated." *Advances: The Journal of Mind-Body Health*, Vol. 11, No. 2, Spring 1995. Smith, Roger. "Does Spirit Matter?" *Advances: The Journal of Mind-Body Health*, Winter 1992.
3. "Births and Deaths, United States: 1996." National Center for Health Statistics, released September 11, 1997.
4. Ibid.
5. Crose, Royda. *Why Women Live Longer Than Men*. San Francisco: Jossey-Bass, 1997.
6. *Healthy People 2000 Midcourse Review* and *Development of Healthy People 2010 Objectives*. Office of Disease Prevention and Health Promotion, Department of Health and Human Services.
7. Voelker, Rebecca. "Speaking the Languages of Medicine and Culture." *Journal of the American Medical Association*, Vol. 273, No. 21, June 7, 1995.
8. Beckham, Edgar. "Diversity Opens Doors to All." *New York Times Education Supplement*, January 5, 1997.
9. "Births and Deaths, United States: 1996."
10. Ibid.
11. Ibid.
12. Ibid.
13. Marchand, Lorraine. "Minorities Benefit from Diabetes Research." *NIH News & Features*, Spring 1995.
14. "Study Details Health of Chinese-Americans." *American Medical News*, May 18, 1992.
15. Department of Health and Human Services.
16. Douglas, Kathy, et al. "Results from the 1995 National College Health Risk Behavior Study." *Journal of American College Health*, Vol. 46, September 1997.
17. Bandura, Albert. *Self-Efficacy in Changing Societies*. Cambridge, Eng.: Cambridge University Press, 1995.
18. O'Brien, William, et al. "Predicting Health Behaviors Using Measures of Optimism and Perceived Risk." *Health Values*, Vol. 19, No. 1, January–February 1995.
19. Chen, William. "Enhancement of Health Locus of Control Through Biofeedback Training." *Perceptual & Motor Skills*, Vol. 80, No. 2, April 1995.
20. Pyeritz, Reed. Personal interview.

Chapter 2

Managing Stress

After studying the material in this chapter, you should be able to:

- **Define** stress and stressors and **use** the general adaptation syndrome to explain how stress relates to health.

- **List** some personal causes of stress, especially those felt by students, and **discuss** how their effects can be prevented or minimized.

- **List** the major social stressors and **explain** how these can cause stress.

- **Describe** the symptoms of stress-related adjustment disorders.

- **Explain** the relationship of stress to heart disease, high blood pressure, the immune system, and digestive disorders.

- **Explain** how you can improve your resistance to stress and **describe** some techniques to help manage stress.

You know about stress. You live with it every day: the stress of passing exams, preparing for a career, meeting people, facing new experiences. Everyone, regardless of age, gender, race, or income, has to deal with stress—as an individual and as a member of society.

By learning to anticipate stressful events, to manage day-to-day stress, and to prevent stress overload, you can find alternatives to running endlessly on a treadmill of alarm, panic, and exhaustion. The stress-management skills in this chapter provide a good start. As you organize your time, release tension, and build up internal resources, you begin to experience the sense of control and confidence that makes stress a challenge rather than an ordeal.

What Is Stress?

People use the word "stress" in different ways: as an external force that causes a person to become tense or upset, as the internal state of arousal, and as the physical response of the body to various demands. Dr. Hans Selye, a pioneer in studying physiological responses to challenge, defined **stress** as "the nonspecific response of the body to any demand made upon it." In other words, the body reacts to **stressors**—the things that upset or excite us—in the same way, regardless of whether they are positive or negative. A stressor may be a bomb threat in a crowded stadium, a pop quiz, or a parent's announcement of a divorce or remarriage, but the body's response is always the same.

Some of life's happiest moments—births, reunions, weddings—are enormously stressful. We weep with the stress of frustration or loss; we weep, too, with the stress of love and joy. Selye coined the term **eustress** for positive stress in our lives (*eu* is a Greek prefix meaning "good"). Eustress challenges us to grow, adapt, and find creative solutions in our lives. **Distress** refers to the negative effects of stress that can deplete or even destroy life energy. Ideally, the level of stress in our lives should be just high enough to motivate us to satisfy our needs and not so high that it interferes with our ability to reach our fullest potential.

The key to coping with stress is realizing that your *perception* and *response* to a stressor are crucial. Changing the way you interpret events or situations—a skill called *reframing*—makes all the difference. An event, such as a move to a new city, is not stressful in itself. A move becomes stressful if you see it as a traumatic upheaval rather than an exciting beginning of a new chapter in your life.

To get a sense of your own stress level, ask yourself the following questions about the preceding week of your life:

- How often have you felt out of control?

- How often have you felt confident that you'd be able to handle personal problems?

- How often have you felt things were generally going your way?

- How often have you felt that things were piling up so high you'd never be able to catch up?

Think through your answers. If the experiences of being out of control or overwhelmed outnumbered those of confidence and control, it's time to develop a stress-management plan and put it into action.

A Theory of Stress

There are many biological theories of stress. The best known may be the **general adaptation syndrome (GAS),** developed by Hans Selye, who postulated that our bodies constantly strive to maintain a stable and consistent physiological state called **homeostasis.** Stressors, whether in the form of physical illness or a demanding job, disturb this state and trigger a nonspecific physiological response. The body attempts to restore homeostasis by means of an **adaptive response.**

Selye's general adaptation syndrome, which describes the body's response to a stressor—whether threatening or exhilarating—consists of three distinct stages:

1. *Alarm.* When a stressor first occurs, the body responds with changes that temporarily lower resistance. Levels of certain hormones may rise; blood pressure may increase (see Figure 2-1). The body quickly makes internal adjustments so it can cope with the stressor and return to normal activity.

2. *Resistance.* If the stressor continues, the body mobilizes its internal resources to sustain homeostasis. For example, if a loved one is seriously hurt in an accident, we initially respond very intensely and

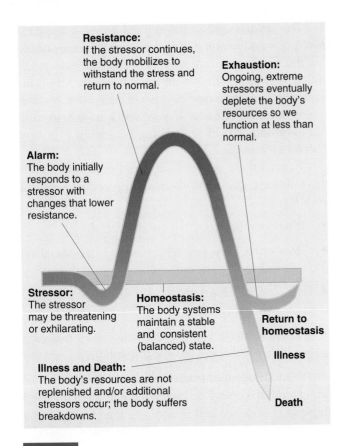

Figure 2-1
The three stages of Selye's general adaptation syndrome: alarm, resistance, exhaustion.

feel great anxiety. During the subsequent stressful period of recuperation, we struggle to carry on as normally as possible, but this requires considerable effort.

3. *Exhaustion*. If the stress continues long enough, we cannot keep up our normal functioning. Even a small amount of additional stress at this point can cause a breakdown.

Stress and the Student

You've probably heard that these are the best years of your life, but being a student—full-time or part-time, in your late teens, early twenties, or later in life—can be extremely stressful. One thing is certain: You're not alone.[1]

According to surveys of students at colleges and universities around the country and the world, stress levels are consistently high and stressors are remarkably similar.[2] Among the most common are:

- Test pressures.
- Financial problems.
- Frustrations, such as delays in reaching goals.
- Problems in friendships and dating relationships.
- Daily hassles.
- Academic failure.
- Pressures as a result of competition, deadlines, and the like.
- Changes, which may be unpleasant, disruptive, or too frequent.
- Losses, whether caused by the breakup of a relationship or the death of a loved one.

During their first year at school, the self-esteem of college freshmen typically falls, but students recover their self-confidence in their second year. They become more positive, introspective, and independent and have a stronger sense of their own intellectual ability. It may be that as students acclimate to college, they experience less stress and therefore view themselves more positively.[3]

Strategies for Prevention

Putting Stress in Perspective

In *Stress Without Distress*, Hans Selye offers these guidelines:

✔ Admit that there is no perfection, but in each category of achievement, something is tops. Be satisfied to strive for that.

✔ Do not underestimate the delight of real simplicity.

✔ Whatever situation you meet in life, consider first whether it is really worth fighting for.

✔ Try to keep your mind on the pleasant aspects of life and on actions that improve your situation. Nothing paralyzes your efficiency more than frustration; nothing helps it more than success.

✔ Even after the greatest defeats, combat the depressing thought of being a failure by taking stock of all your past achievements, which no one can deny you.

✔ When faced with a task that is very painful yet indispensable to achieve your aim, don't procrastinate.

✔ Do not forget that there is no ready-made success formula that suits everybody.

In some studies, certain groups of students, such as women and Asian Americans, report higher levels of stress and more intense reactions to stressors.[4] Students say they react to stress in various ways: physiologically (by sweating, stuttering, trembling, or developing physical symptoms); emotionally (by becoming anxious, fearful, angry, guilty, or depressed); behaviorally (by crying, eating, smoking, being irritable or abusive); or cognitively (by thinking about and analyzing stressful situations and strategies that might be useful in dealing with them). Social support makes a big difference.[5] Students with a truly supportive network of friends and family report greater satisfaction and less psychological distress. This is particularly true of certain cultures, such as Hispanic, that place great value on the family.[6]

Test Stress

For many students, midterms and final exams are the most stressful times of the year. Studies at various colleges and universities found that the incidence of colds and flu soared during finals. The reason seems to be that stress depresses the levels of the protective immune cells that ward off viruses. Students who don't come down with infections during exams often feel the impact of test stress in other ways. Many suffer headaches, upset stomachs, skin flareups, or insomnia.[7]

Test stress affects different people in different ways. Sometimes students become so preoccupied with the possibility of failing that they can't concentrate on studying. Others, including many of the best and brightest students, freeze up during tests and can't comprehend multiple-choice questions or write essay answers, even if they know the material.

Can you do anything to reduce test stress and feel more in control? Absolutely. One way is to defuse stress through relaxation. In a study by researchers Janice Kiecolt-Glaser and Ron Glaser of Ohio State University, one group of students was taught relaxation techniques—such as controlled breathing, meditation, progressive relaxation, and guided imagery (visualization)—a month before finals. The more the students used these "stress busters," the higher were their levels of immune cells during the exam period. The extra payoff was that they felt

Pulsepoints   Top Ten Stress Busters

1. Strive for balance. Review your commitments and plans, and if necessary, scale down.

2. Get the facts. When faced with a change or challenge, seek accurate information, which can bring vague fears down to earth.

3. Talk with someone you trust. A friend or a health professional can offer valuable perspective as well as psychological support.

4. Sweat away stress. Even when your schedule gets jammed, carve out 20 or 30 minutes several times a week to walk, swim, bicycle, jog, or work out at the gym.

5. Express yourself in writing. Keeping a journal is one of the best ways to put your problems into perspective.

6. Take care of yourself. Get enough sleep. Eat a balanced diet. Limit your use of sugar, salt, and caffeine, which can compound stress by leading to fatigue and irritability. Watch your alcohol intake. Drinking can cut down on your ability to cope.

7. Set priorities. Making a list of things you need to do and ranking their impor-tance helps direct your energies so you're more efficient and less stressed.

8. Help others. One of the most effective ways of dealing with stress is to find people in a worse situation and do something positive for them.

9. Cultivate hobbies. Pursuing a personal pleasure can distract you from the stressors in your life and help you relax.

10. Master a form of relaxation. Whether you choose meditation, yoga, mindfulness, or another technique, practice it regularly.

---

calmer and in better control during their tests.[8] (See Pulse-points: "Top Ten Stress Busters.")

Community Stressors

Regardless of your race or ethnic background, college may bring culture shock. You may never have encountered such a degree of diversity in one setting. You probably will meet students with different values, unfamiliar customs, and entirely new ways of looking at the world—experiences you may find both stimulating and stressful.

A stretch break and a few deep breaths help make your studying more effective and help keep your stress level down.

If you're a minority student, you may feel a double burden. In addition to academic demands, financial worries, and the usual campus stressors, many students from racial and cultural minority groups report extra stressors that can be, as one researcher put it, "both the cause and the effect of academic difficulty."[9] Various reports have shown that African-American and non-Asian minority students at predominantly white colleges have lower grade point averages, experience higher attrition rates, and are less likely to graduate within 5 years or to enter graduate programs than are white students or minority students at institutions that are not predominantly white. They also experience college as more stressful and report greater feelings of not belonging.[10]

Other Personal Stressors

At every stage of life, you will encounter challenges and stressors. Among the most common are those related to work: overwork, illness, and disability.

Job Stress

More than ever, many people find that they are working more and enjoying it less. The technological wizardry that was supposed to make life easier—cellular phones, modems, faxes, laptop computers—has simply extended the boundaries of where and when we work. As a result, more people are caught up in an exhausting cycle of overwork, which causes stress, which makes work harder, which leads to more stress.[11]

Workaholism and Burnout

People who become obsessed by their work and careers can turn into *workaholics*, so caught up in racing toward the top that they forget what they're racing toward and why. In some cases they throw themselves into their work to mask or avoid painful feelings or difficulties in their own lives. One consequence is **burnout**, a state of physical, emotional, and mental exhaustion brought on by constant or repeated emotional pressure. Particularly in the helping professions, such as social work and nursing, men and women who've dedicated themselves to others may realize they have nothing left in themselves to give.[12]

Illness and Disability

Just as the mind can have profound effects on the body, the body can have an enormous impact on our emotions. Whenever we come down with the flu or pull a muscle, we feel under par. When the problem is more serious or persistent—a chronic disease like diabetes, for instance, or a lifelong hearing impairment—the emotional stress of constantly coping with it is even greater.

Societal Stressors

Not all stressors are personal. Centuries ago the poet John Donne observed that no man is an island. Today, on an increasingly crowded and troubled planet, these words seem truer than ever. Problems such as discrimination and violence can no longer be viewed only as economic or political issues. Directly or indirectly, they affect the well-being of all who inhabit the earth—now and in the future.

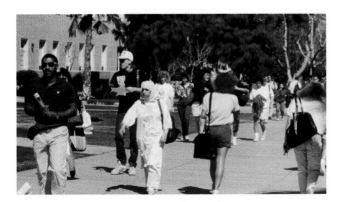

On campus, minority students often feel the stresses of college life as well as the stress of discrimination, however subtle.

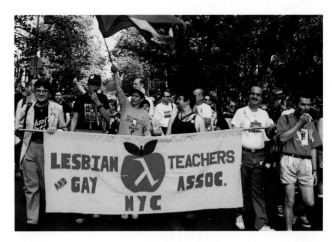

Community action can challenge the hateful assumptions that lead to discrimination, a stressor in its blatant and its subtle forms.

Discrimination can take many forms—some as subtle as not being included in a conversation or joke, some as blatant as threats scrawled on a wall, some as violent as brutal beatings. Because it can be hard to deal with individually, discrimination is a particularly sinister form of stress. By banding together, however, those who experience discrimination can take action to protect themselves, challenge the ignorance and hateful assumptions that fuel bigotry, and promote a healthier environment for all.

The deliberate use of physical force to abuse or injure is a leading killer of young people in the United States and a potential source of stress in all our lives. Chances are that you or someone you know has been the victim of a violent crime, and awareness of our own vulnerability adds to the stress of daily living. As studies have documented, the increased crime rate in inner-city communities results in stress, which leads to various health and mental problems among minority Americans.[13] (Chapter 13 discusses violence, abuse, and other threats to personal safety.)

A Personal Stress Survival Guide

Although stress is a very real threat to emotional and physical well-being, its impact depends not just on what happens to you, but on how you handle it. Some individuals are particularly prone to worry and constantly dwell on the negative aspects of what's happening or what may happen. The inability to feel in control of stress, rather than stress itself, is often the most harmful.

In studying individuals who manage stress so well that they seem "stress-resistant," researchers have observed many of the following traits:

- They respond actively to challenges. If a problem comes up, they look for resources, do some reading or research, and try to find a solution rather than giving up and feeling helpless.

- They have personal goals, such as getting a college degree or becoming a better parent.

- They rely on a combination of planning, goal setting, problem solving, and risk taking to control stress.

- They use a minimum of substances such as nicotine, caffeine, alcohol, or drugs.

- They regularly engage in some form of relaxation, from meditation to exercise to knitting, at least 15 minutes a day.

- They tend to seek out other people and become involved with them.

To achieve greater control over the stress in your life, start with some self-analysis. If you're feeling overwhelmed, ask yourself: Are you taking an extra course that's draining your last ounce of energy? Are you staying up late studying every night and missing morning classes? Are you living on black coffee and jelly doughnuts? While you may think that you don't have time to reduce the stress in your life, some simple changes can often ease the pressure you're under and help you achieve your long-term goals.

Strategies for Change

How to Cope with Stress

✔ Recognize your stress signals. Is your back bothering you more? Do you find yourself speeding or misplacing things? Force yourself to stop whenever you see these early warnings and say, "I'm under stress; I need to do something about it."

✔ Keep a stress journal. Focus on intense emotional experiences and "autopsy" them to try to understand why they affected you the way they did. Rereading and thinking about your notes may reveal the underlying reasons for your response.

✔ Try "stress-inoculation." Rehearse everyday situations that you find stressful, such as speaking in class. Think of how you might handle the situation, perhaps by breathing deeply before you talk.

✔ Put things in proper perspective. Ask yourself: Will I remember what's made me so upset a month from now? If you had to rank this problem on a scale of 1 to 10, with worldwide catastrophe as 10, where would it rate?

One of the simplest, yet most effective, ways to work through stress is by putting your feelings into words that only you will read. The more honest and open you are as you write, the better. In studies at Southern Methodist University, psychologist James Pennebaker, Ph.D., found that college students who wrote in their journals about traumatic events felt much better afterward than those who wrote about superficial topics. Recording your experiences and feelings on paper or audiotape may help decrease stress and enhance well-being.[14]

Since the small ups and downs of daily life have an enormous impact on psychological and physical well-being, getting a handle on daily hassles will reduce your stress load. The positive strategies described in Chapter 3 can help.

Positive Coping Mechanisms

After a perfectly miserable, aggravating day, a teacher comes home and yells at her children for making too much noise. Another individual, after an equally stressful day, jokes about what went wrong during the all-time most miserable moment of the month. Both of these people are using defense mechanisms—actions or

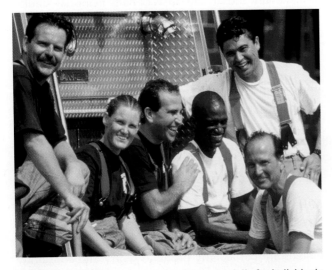

Humor is a positive coping mechanism, especially for individuals in high-stress professions.

behaviors that help protect their sense of self-worth. The first is displacing anger onto other people; the second uses humor to vent frustration.

Under great stress, we all may turn to negative defense mechanisms to alleviate anxiety and eliminate conflict. These can lead to maladaptive behavior, such as rationalizing overeating by explaining to yourself that you need the extra calories to cope with the extra stress in your life. **Coping mechanisms** are healthier, more mature, and adaptive ways of dealing with stressful situations. While they also ward off unpleasant emotions, they usually are helpful rather than harmful. The most common are:

- Sublimation, the redirection of any drives considered unacceptable into socially acceptable channels. For example, someone who is furious with a friend or relative may go for a long run to sublimate anger.

- Religiosity, in which one comes to terms with a painful experience, such as a child's death, by experiencing it as being in accord with God's will.

- Humor, which counters stress by focusing on comic aspects. Medical students, for instance, often make jokes in anatomy lab as a way of dealing with their anxieties about working with cadavers.

- Altruism, which takes a negative experience and turns it into a positive one. For example, an HIV-positive individual may talk to teenagers about AIDS prevention.

Managing Time

The choices you make about how to use your time directly affect your stress level. How can you tell if you've lost control of your time? The following are tell-tale symptoms of poor time management:

- Rushing.

- Chronic inability to make choices or decisions.

- Fatigue or listlessness.

- Constantly missed deadlines.

- Not enough time for rest or personal relationships.

- A sense of being overwhelmed by demands and details and having to do what you don't want to do most of the time.

One of the hard lessons of being on your own is that your choices and actions have consequences. Stress is just one of them. But by thinking ahead, being realis-

tic about your workload, and sticking to your plans, you can gain better control over your time and stress levels.

Overcoming Procrastination

Putting off until tomorrow what should be done today is a habit that creates a great deal of stress for many students. The three most common types of procrastination are: putting off unpleasant things, putting off difficult tasks, and putting off tough decisions. Procrastinators are most likely to delay by wishing they didn't have to do what they must or by telling themselves they "just can't get started," which means they never do.

To get out of a time trap, keep track of the tasks you're most likely to put off and try to figure out why you don't want to tackle them. Think of alternative ways to get tasks done. If you put off library readings, for instance, figure out if the problem is getting to the library or the reading itself. If it's the trip to the library, arrange to walk over with a friend whose company you enjoy.

Develop daily time-management techniques, such as a "To Do" list. Rank items according to priorities—A, B, C—and schedule your days to make sure the A's get accomplished. Try not to fixate on half-completed projects. Divide large tasks, such as a term paper, into smaller ones and reward yourself when you complete a part.

Do what you like least first. Once you have it out of the way, you can concentrate on the tasks you do enjoy. You also should build time into your schedule for interruptions, unforeseen problems, unexpected events, and so on, so you aren't constantly racing around. Establish ground rules for meeting your own needs (including getting enough sleep and making time for friends) before saying yes to any activity. Learn to live according to a three-word motto: Just do it!

Relaxation Techniques

Relaxation is the physical and mental state opposite that of stress. Rather than gearing up for fight or flight, our bodies and minds grow calmer and work more smoothly. We're less likely to become frazzled and more capable of staying in control. The most effective relaxation techniques include progressive relaxation, visualization, meditation, mindfulness, and biofeedback.

Progressive relaxation works by intentionally increasing and then decreasing tension in the muscles. While sitting or lying down in a quiet, comfortable setting, you tense and release various muscles, beginning with those of the hand, for instance, and then proceed to the arms, shoulders, neck, face, scalp, chest, stomach, buttocks, genitals, and so on, down each leg to the toes. Relaxing the muscles can quiet the mind and restore internal balance.[15]

Visualization, or **guided imagery**, involves creating mental pictures that calm you down and focus your mind. As we note in Chapter 15, some people use this technique to promote healing when they are ill. The Glaser study showed that elderly residents of retirement homes in Ohio who learned progressive relaxation and guided imagery enhanced their immune function and reported better health than did the other residents. Visualization skills require practice and, in some cases, instruction by qualified health professionals.[16]

Meditation has been practiced in many forms over the ages, from the yogic techniques of the Far East to the Quaker silence of more modern times. Meditation helps a person reach a state of relaxation, but with the goal of achieving inner peace and harmony. There is no one right way to meditate, and many people have discovered how to meditate on their own, without even knowing what it is they are doing. Among college students, meditation has proven especially effective in increasing relaxation.[17] Most forms of meditation have common elements: sitting quietly for 15 to 20 minutes once or twice a day, concentrating on a word or image, and breathing slowly and rhythmically. If you wish to try meditation, it often helps to have someone guide you through your first sessions. Or try tape recording your own voice (with or without favorite music in the background) and playing it back to yourself, freeing yourself to concentrate on the goal of turning the attention within.

Mindfulness is a modern-day form of an ancient Asian technique that involves maintaining awareness in the present moment. You tune in to each part of your body, scanning from head to toe, noting the slightest sensation. You allow whatever you experience—an itch, an ache, a feeling of warmth—to enter your awareness. Then you open yourself to focus on all the thoughts, sensations, sounds, and feelings that enter your awareness. Mindfulness keeps you in the here and now, thinking about "what is" rather than about "what if" or "if only."

Biofeedback, discussed in Chapter 15, is a method of obtaining feedback, or information, about some physiological activity occurring in the body. An electronic monitoring device attached to a person's body detects a change in an internal function and communicates it back to the person through a tone, light, or meter. By paying attention to this feedback, most people can gain some control over functions previously thought to be beyond conscious control, such as body temperature, heart rate, muscle tension, and brain waves.

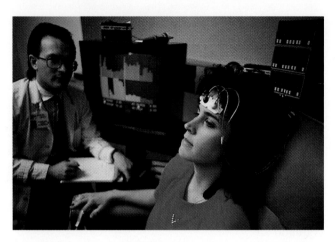

Biofeedback training uses electronic monitoring devices to teach conscious control over heart rate, body temperature, and muscle tension. Once the technique is learned, the electronic feedback is unnecessary.

Stress Overload

Excessive, unmanaged stress can affect every aspect of your life, jeopardizing your physical well-being, your psychological health, your behavior, and your performance at school or work. Monitor yourself for any of the following clues that your body, mind, and behavior may provide—and don't ignore them.

The Toll on the Mind

Life happens: Cars crash. Loved ones leave. Money runs out. Such stressors always take a toll on an individual, and it's normal to feel sad, tense, overwhelmed, angry, or incapable of coping with the ordinary demands of daily living. Usually such feelings and behaviors subside with time. The stressful event fades into the past, and those whose lives it has touched adapt to its lasting impact. But sometimes individuals remain extremely distressed and unable to function as they once did.

Adjustment Disorders

The term **adjustment disorder** refers to an out-of-the-ordinary response to a stressful event or situation. Any event or combination of circumstances can lead to an adjustment disorder. The stressor does not have to be extreme; even a seemingly minor event, such as learning that an ex-boyfriend or ex-girlfriend has married, may cause great psychological pain.[18]

The problem for individuals reeling from the impact of a life crisis is trying to figure out which feelings are normal and which are not. The two key signs of an adjustment disorder are distress and impairment: Individuals feel extremely upset or cannot work or relate to others the way they once did, and their symptoms persist for more than 3 to 6 months after a stressful event.[19]

There is no specific remedy for an adjustment disorder, although the goal is always the same: improving an individual's ability to adapt. Ordinarily, time helps ease the pain or difficulty of coping with a stressful situation. When the impact of a crisis is more intense, supportive counseling or brief psychotherapy (described in Chapter 3) can help an individual understand the significance of what has happened, put it into perspective, and deal with it in a healthier way.

Posttraumatic Stress Disorder

In the past, **posttraumatic stress disorder (PTSD)** was viewed as a psychological response to out-of-the-ordinary stressors, such as captivity or combat. However, these are hardly the only experiences that can forever change the way people view themselves and their world. With the recent surge in violent crime and in natural disasters, thousands of individuals have experienced or witnessed traumatic events.[20] Children, in particular, are likely to develop PTSD symptoms when they live through a traumatic event or witness a loved one or friend being assaulted.

In PTSD, individuals often reexperience their terror and helplessness in their dreams or intrusive thoughts.

Strategies for Prevention

Recognize the Warning Signals of Stress Overload

✔ Experiencing physical symptoms, including chronic fatigue, headaches, indigestion, diarrhea, and sleep problems.

✔ Having frequent illness or worrying about illness.

✔ Self-medicating, including nonprescription drugs.

✔ Having problems concentrating on studies or work.

✔ Feeling irritable, anxious, or apathetic.

✔ Working or studying longer and harder than usual.

✔ Becoming accident-prone.

✔ Breaking rules, whether it's a curfew at home or a speed limit on the highway.

✔ Going to extremes, such as drinking too much, overspending, or gambling.

To avoid this psychic pain, they may try to avoid anything associated with the trauma. Some enter a state of emotional numbness and no longer can respond to people and experiences the way they once did, especially when it comes to showing tenderness or affection. Those who've been mugged or raped may be afraid to venture out by themselves.

The sooner trauma survivors receive psychological help, the better they are likely to fare. Often talking about what happened with an empathic person or someone who's shared the experience as soon as possible—preferably before going to sleep on the day of the event—can help an individual begin to deal with what has occurred. Group sessions, ideally beginning soon after the trauma, allow individuals to share views and experiences. Behavioral, cognitive, and psychodynamic therapy (described in Chapter 3) can help individuals suffering PTSD.

The Toll on the Body

While stress can sometimes be the spice of life, it also can be the kiss of death. Just as it can undermine psychological contentment, it can erode physical well-being. Many medical researchers believe that stress may be the greatest single contributor to disease (see Figure 2-2). According to the American Institute of Stress, 75% to 90% of all visits to physicians involve stress-related complaints.

The Cardiovascular System

In the 1970s, cardiologists Meyer Friedman, M.D., and Ray Rosenman, M.D., suggested that excess stress may be the most important factor in the development of heart disease. They compared their patients to individuals of the same age with healthy hearts and developed two general categories: Type A and Type B.

Hardworking, aggressive, and competitive, Type A's never have time for all they want to accomplish, even though they usually try to do several tasks at once. Type B's are more relaxed, though not necessarily less ambitious or successful. (Of course, people who are extremely Type B may never accomplish anything.) Type-A behavior has been found to be the major contributing factor in the early development of heart disease.

Stress reduction, including biofeedback and relaxation techniques, can help reduce the risk. Social support also helps lower cardiovascular reactivity. In a study of ninety college students, students given support from a confederate before and during the time they gave a speech showed smaller increases in systolic blood pressure than those who faced the stress of public speaking without support.[21]

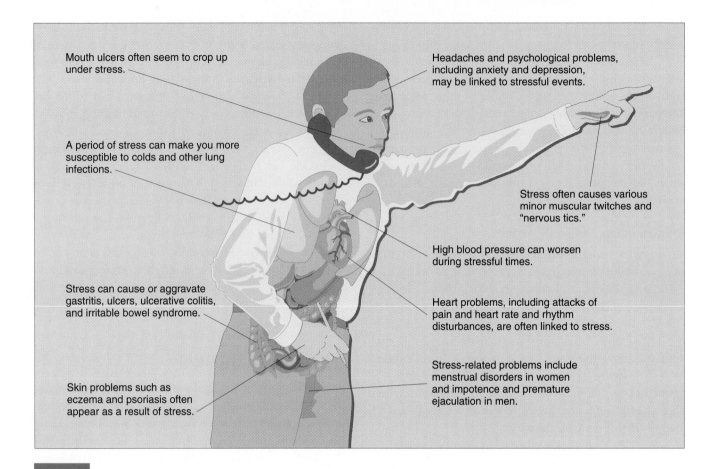

Mouth ulcers often seem to crop up under stress.

A period of stress can make you more susceptible to colds and other lung infections.

Stress can cause or aggravate gastritis, ulcers, ulcerative colitis, and irritable bowel syndrome.

Skin problems such as eczema and psoriasis often appear as a result of stress.

Headaches and psychological problems, including anxiety and depression, may be linked to stressful events.

Stress often causes various minor muscular twitches and "nervous tics."

High blood pressure can worsen during stressful times.

Heart problems, including attacks of pain and heart rate and rhythm disturbances, are often linked to stress.

Stress-related problems include menstrual disorders in women and impotence and premature ejaculation in men.

Figure 2-2

Long-term unmanaged stress can affect any and every part of the body and result in chronic, often serious, disease.

The Immune System

The powerful chemicals triggered by stress dampen or suppress the immune system—the network of organs, tissues, and white blood cells that defend against disease. Impaired immunity makes the body more susceptible to many diseases, including infections (from the common cold to tuberculosis) and disorders of the immune system itself.

The Digestive System

Do you ever get butterflies in your stomach before giving a speech in class or before a big game? The digestive system is, as one psychologist quips, "an important stop on the tension trail." To avoid problems, pay attention to how you eat: Eating on the run, gulping food, or overeating results in poorly chewed foods, an overworked stomach, and increased abdominal pressure. The combination of poor eating habits and stress can add up to real pain in the stomach.

Other Stress Symptoms

Stress can affect any organ system in the body, causing painful symptoms or a flareup of chronic conditions such as asthma. By interfering with our alertness and ability to concentrate, stress also increases the risk of accidents at home, at work, and on the road.

Headaches are one of the most common stress-related conditions. The most common type, tension headache, is caused by involuntary contractions of the scalp, head, and neck muscles. **Migraine headache** is the result of constriction (narrowing) and then dilation (widening) of blood vessels within the brain; chemicals leak through the vessel walls, inflame nearby tissues, and send pain signals to the brain. Surveys of college women show that Type-A behavior can trigger both types of headache.

Stress also is closely linked to skin conditions. If you break out the week before an exam, you know firsthand that skin can be extremely sensitive to stress. Among the other skin conditions worsened by stress are acne, psoriasis, herpes, hives, and eczema. With acne, increased touching of the face, perhaps while cramming for a test, may be partly responsible. Other factors, such as temperature, humidity, and cosmetics and toiletries, may also play a role.

Making This Chapter Work for You
Meeting the Challenge of Stress

■ Stress is the physiological and psychological response to any demand placed on us or our bodies, whether positive or negative.

■ Eustress, or positive stress, challenges us to grow, adapt, and find creative solutions in our lives. Distress refers to the negative effects of stress that can deplete or even destroy life energy.

■ Theories of stress include Hans Selye's general adaptation syndrome, which consists of three distinct stages: alarm, resistance, and exhaustion.

■ Common student stressors on campus include test pressures, financial problems, personal frustrations, problems in friendships and dating relationships, daily hassles, academic failure, competitive pressure, unpleasant or disruptive changes, and personal losses. Adjusting to college life is stressful in itself.

■ Minority students encounter additional stressors, including a hostile or unfriendly social climate, interpersonal tensions between themselves and nonminority students and faculty, experiences of actual or perceived racism, and more subtle racist attitudes and discrimination.

■ Jobs are a major source of stress for Americans. Two problems related to job stress are workaholism, characterized by excessive devotion to work, and burnout, a state of physical, emotional, and mental exhaustion brought on by constant or repeated emotional pressure.

■ Chronic illness and disability, including learning disabilities, can be major sources of stress in an individual's life.

■ Social stressors—such as discrimination and violence—also are a threat to physical and psychological well-being.

■ Stress-management techniques, which include better time management, overcoming procrastination, and increased appreciation of leisure time, can help reduce distress and enhance feelings of control over daily stress.

■ Techniques such as progressive relaxation, visualization, meditation, mindfulness, and biofeedback can help soothe both body and mind and reduce the harmful effects of stress.

Health Online

Biobehavioral Institute of Boston's Stress Audit
http://www.bbinst.org/stressaudit/stress3.cgi

The Biobehavioral Institute of Boston's Stress Audit is a comprehensive assessment of your stress levels in many areas of life, including job, family, social, financial, and emotional stress. After you take the survey, the Stress Audit tells you how you compare with the general population in each area of stress. It also analyzes your general susceptibility to stress, the sources of stress in your life, and the symptoms of stress you now show. You also get some advice on how to lower your vulnerability to stress.

Think about it ...

• According to the Stress Audit, how does your stress level compare with that of the general population? What might you do to reduce your stress in areas where it is especially high?

• Why do you think the things in the Susceptibility to Stress inventory are especially important?

• If you were to design a new inventory for this site on School Stress, what might you include?

■ Stress can affect psychological well-being and cause adjustment disorders and posttraumatic stress disorder. Prompt recognition and treatment can help overcome these problems.

■ Stress overload can contribute to heart disease, high blood pressure, immune disorders, digestive problems, and other ailments.

College is a perfect time to learn and practice the art of stress reduction. You can start applying the techniques and concepts outlined in this chapter immediately. You may want to begin by doing some relaxation or awareness exercises. They can give you the peace of mind you need to focus more effectively on larger issues, goals, and decisions.

You needn't see stress as a problem to solve on your own. Reach out to others. As you build friendships and intimate relationships, you may find that some irritating problems are easier to put into perspective. Don't be afraid to laugh at yourself and to look for the comic or absurd aspects of a situation. In addition, you might try some simple approaches that can help boost your stress resistance and resilience, including the following:

■ *Focusing.* Take a strain inventory of your body every day to determine where things aren't feeling quite right. Ask yourself, "What's keeping me from feeling terrific today?" Focusing on problem spots, such as stomach knots or neck tightness, increases your sense of control over stress.

■ *Reconstructing stressful situations.* Think about a recent episode of distress; then write down three ways it could have gone better and three ways it could have gone worse. This should help you see that the situation wasn't as disastrous as it might have been and help you find ways to cope better in the future.

■ *Self-improvement.* When your life feels out of control, turn to a new challenge. You might try volunteering at a nursing home, taking a long-distance bike trip, or learning a foreign language. As you work toward your new goal, you'll realize that you still can cope and achieve.

■ *Exercise.* Regular physical activity can relieve stress, boost energy, lift mood, and keep stress under control.

If stress continues to be a problem in your life, you may be able to find help through support groups or counseling. Your school may provide counseling services or referrals to mental health professionals; ask your health instructor or the campus health department for this information. Remember that each day of distress robs you of energy, distracts you from life's pleasures, and interferes with achieving your full potential.

▶ Key Terms

The terms listed here are used within the chapter. Page numbers are included for each term.
A definition of each term is given in the green Glossary pages at the end of this book.

adaptive response *17*	**general adaptation syndrome (GAS)** *17*	**posttraumatic stress disorder (PTSD)** *25*
adjustment disorder *24*	**guided imagery** *24*	**progressive relaxation** *23*
biofeedback *24*	**homeostasis** *17*	**stress** *17*
burnout *21*	**meditation** *24*	**stressor** *17*
coping mechanisms *23*	**migraine headache** *26*	**visualization** *24*
distress *17*	**mindfulness** *24*	
eustress *17*		

Review Questions

1. What is stress? What causes stress? What is the general adaptation syndrome?
2. How are stress and heart disease related? Stress and the immune system? Stress and the digestive system?
3. What are the characteristics of a stress-resistant personality?
4. Name some social stressors. How can the effects of these be minimized or prevented?
5. Differentiate between Type-A and Type-B behaviors. What type of behavior do you exhibit? How do these behaviors affect your health?
6. How can you manage stress in your life more effectively?

Critical Thinking Questions

1. Studies have shown that meditation and relaxation techniques can have a positive impact on health. In fact, some insurance companies now pay for medical care that includes these techniques. Critics condemn these practices as unsound, or at least as lacking sufficient scientific proof to warrant their use. Others consider meditation to be too "self-indulgent." What do you think? How valuable are these techniques and for whom?
2. Identify three stressful situations in your life and describe how you might attempt to decrease or eliminate the stressors associated with them. Identify three examples of eustress.
3. Can you think of any ways in which your behavior or attitudes might create stress for others? What changes could you make to avoid doing so?
4. What advice might you give an incoming freshman at your school about managing stress in college? What techniques have been most helpful for you in dealing with stress?

Connections to Personal Health Interactive

*To enhance your understanding of the material covered in this chapter, check out the following study aids on the **Personal Health Interactive CD-ROM**.*

- **Online Research:** Stress and Mental Wellness
- Personal Insights: How Stressed Are You?
- Stress and Health in College Students
- Glossary & Key Term Review

References

1. Wagner, Betsy. "Living on the Edge." *Life Management.* 3rd ed. Guilford, CT: Dushkin Publishing Group, 1995.
2. Gerdes, Eugenia, and Guo Ping. "Coping Differences Between College Women and Men in China and the United States." *Genetic, Social and General Psychology Monographs,* Vol. 120, No. 2, May 1994. Puccio, Gerard, et al. "Person-Environment Fit: Using Commensurate Scales to Predict Student Stress." *British Journal of Educational Psychology,* Vol. 63, No. 3, November 1993.
3. Goldman, Cristin, and Eugene Wong. "Stress and the College Student." *Education,* Vol. 117, No. 4, Summer 1997.
4. Demakis, George, and Dan McAdams. "Personality, Social Support, and Well-Being Among First-Year College Students." *College Health Journal,* Vol. 28, No. 2, June 1994.
5. Neville, Helen, et al. "Relations Among Racial Identity Attitudes, Perceived Stressors, and Coping Styles in African American College Students." *Journal of Counseling and Development,* Vol. 75, No. 4, March–April 1997.
6. Solberg, V. Scott, and Pete Villarreal. "Examination of Self-Efficacy, Social Support and Stress As Predictors of Psychological and Physical Distress Among Hispanic College Students." *Hispanic Journal of Behavioral Sciences,* Vol. 19, No. 2, May 1997.
7. "College-Age Freedom Can Trigger Illness." *USA Today Magazine,* Vol. 125, No. 2610, December 1996.
8. Glaser, Ronald, and Janice Kiecolt-Glaser. *Handbook of Human Stress and Immunity.* San Diego: Academic Press, 1994. Hornig-Rohan, Mary. "Stress, Immune-Mediators, and Immune-Mediated Disease." *Advances: The Journal of Mind-Body Health,* Vol. 11, No. 2, Spring 1995.
9. Saldana, Delia. "Acculturative Stress: Minority Status and Distress." *Hispanic Journal of Behavioral Sciences,* Vol. 16, No. 2, May 1994.
10. Ibid.
11. Kline, Marsha, and David Snow. "Effects of a Worksite Coping Skills Intervention on the Stress, Social Support

and Health Outcomes of Working Mothers." *Journal of Primary Prevention,* Vol. 15, No. 2, Winter 1994.

12. Davis, Susan. "Burnout." *American Health,* December 1994.

13. Wakhisi, Tsitis. "Crime: A Leading Health Hazard for Minorities." *Crisis,* Vol. 101, No. 8, November–December 1994.

14. Pennebaker, James. "Putting Stress into Words: Health, Linguistic and Therapeutic Implications." *Behavioral Research,* Vol. 31, No. 6, 1993. Pitariua, Horia, and Frank Landy. "Some Personality Correlates of Time Urgency." *Revue Roumaine de Psychologie,* Vol. 37, No. 1, January–June 1993.

15. Benson, Herbert, and Michael McKee. "Relaxation and Other Alternative Therapies." *Patient Care,* Vol. 27, No. 20, December 15, 1993.

16. Kiecolt-Glaser, Janice, and Ronald Glaser. "Stress and the Immune System: Human Studies." *Review of Psychiatry* (Vol. 11). Washington, DC: American Psychiatric Press, 1992.

17. Janowiak, John. "The Effects of Meditation on College Students' Self-Actualization and Stress Management." *Dissertation Abstracts International,* Vol. 53, No. 10, April 1993.

18. Greenberg, William, et al. "Adjustment Disorder As an Admission Diagnosis." *American Journal of Psychiatry,* Vol. 152, No. 3, March 1995.

19. Hales, Dianne, and Robert E. Hales. *Caring for the Mind: The Comprehensive Guide to Mental Health.* New York: Bantam Books, 1995.

20. Breslau, Naomi, et al. "Risk Factors for PTSD-Related Traumatic Events: A Prospective Analysis." *American Journal of Psychiatry,* Vol. 152, No. 4, April 1995.

21. Lepore, Stephen, et al. "Social Support Lowers Cardiovascular Reactivity to an Acute Stressor." *Psychosomatic Medicine,* Vol. 55, No. 6, November–December 1993.

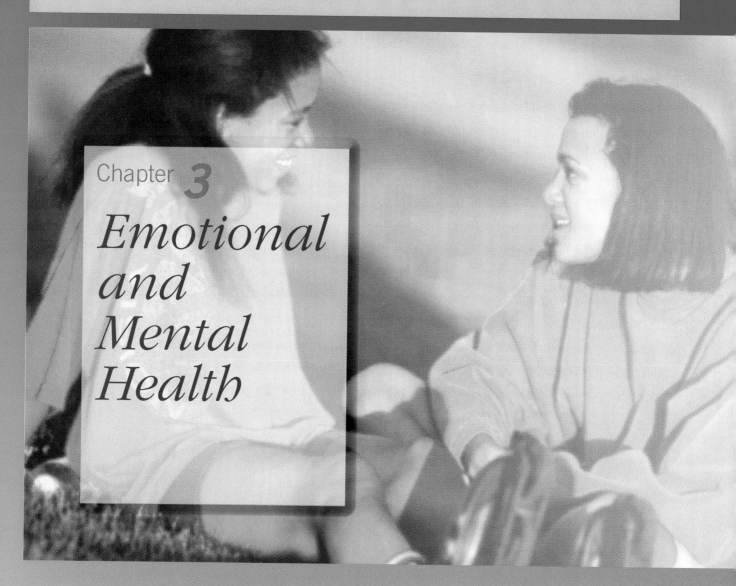

Chapter 3
Emotional and Mental Health

After studying the material in this chapter, you should be able to:

■ **Explain** the goal of psychological health and **list** some strategies for enhancing psychological well-being.

■ **Describe** the roles of autonomy and assertiveness in psychological health.

■ **Identify** the major psychological problems experienced by members of our society.

■ **Describe** the symptoms of and treatments for anxiety disorders, depression, and attention disorders.

■ **Discuss** behaviors indicating the need for professional help and how to find such help.

■ **List** and briefly **explain** a variety of modern approaches used by professional therapists.

*I*n every culture, psychologically healthy men and women generally share certain characteristics: They value themselves and strive toward happiness and fulfillment. They establish and maintain close relationships with others. They accept the limitations as well as the possibilities that life has to offer. And they feel a sense of meaning and purpose that make life worth living.

Yet optimal psychological health isn't always possible for everyone; each year 30% of Americans suffer from at least one mental disorder.[1] Young adulthood—the years from the late teens to the mid-twenties—are a time when many serious mental disorders develop. The good news is that 80% to 90% of those treated for psychological problems recover, most within a few months.[2]

What Is Psychological Health?

"A sound mind in a sound body is a short but full description of a happy state in this world," the philosopher John Locke wrote in 1693. More than 300 years later his statement still rings true. Both physical and psychological well-being are essential to total wellness.

Psychological health encompasses both our emotional and mental states—that is, our feelings and our thoughts. **Emotional health** generally refers to feelings and moods, both of which are discussed later in this chapter. Characteristics of emotionally healthy persons that psychologist Deane Shapiro identified in an analysis of major studies of emotional wellness include the following:

- Determination and effort to be healthy.

- Flexibility and adaptability to a variety of circumstances.

- Development of a sense of meaning and affirmation of life.

- An understanding that the self is not the center of the universe.

- Compassion for others.

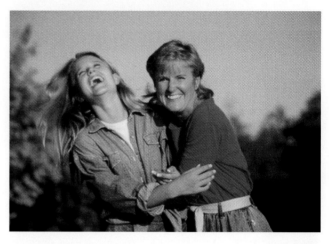

Peak psychological health. Psychologically healthy people value themselves, find meaning and purpose in life, and build close relationships with others.

- The ability to be unselfish in serving or relating to others.

- Increased depth and satisfaction in intimate relationships.

- A sense of control over the mind and body that enables the person to make health-enhancing choices and decisions.[3]

Mental health describes our ability to perceive reality as it is, to respond to its challenges, and to develop rational strategies for living. The mentally healthy person doesn't try to avoid conflicts and distress but can cope with life's transitions, traumas, and losses in a way

Strategies for Prevention

Tips for Psychological Fitness

✔ Recognize and express your feelings. Pent-up emotions tend to fester inside, building into anger or depression.

✔ Don't brood. Rather than merely mulling over a problem, try to find solutions that are positive and useful.

✔ Take one step at a time. As long as you're taking some action to solve a problem, you can take pride in your ability to cope.

✔ Get involved with others. Reach out and communicate your feelings to someone you trust, either a friend or, if necessary, a professional.

that allows for emotional stability and growth. There is considerable overlap between psychological and **spiritual health**, which involves our ability to identify our basic purpose in life and to experience the fulfillment of achieving our full potential.

Pursuing Happiness and Meaning

Psychologist David Myers, author of *The Pursuit of Happiness: Who Is Happy—and Why,* defines happiness as "a sense of well-being, a feeling that life as a whole is going well."[4] This state depends not on big achievements, but on little pleasures. As recent studies have shown, happiness tends to be highest when people combine frequent good experiences—the daily joys of having a caring partner, a productive job, or enjoyable hobbies—with occasional very intense pleasures, such as a special vacation or a promotion.[5]

There is no one route to happiness, nor are there any barriers to achieving it. "Happiness doesn't depend on how old you are or how much money you make, whether you're male or female, or what race you belong to," says Myers. "It does depend on certain personality traits, whether your work suits your skills, whether you have close relationships and an active religious faith."

Happiness also depends on cultural contexts. In studies comparing Western and Chinese views of happiness, individuals in the West define happiness as an internal state, one that relies on internal contentment, whereas the Chinese place greater emphasis on interpersonal or external satisfaction.[6] Age, gender, and personality factors, such as extroversion, dutifulness, and achievement, also affect an individual's sense of happiness.[7]

The best predictors of happiness are the characteristics of good psychological health: high self-esteem, optimism, extroversion, and a sense of being in control. In addition to these four key traits, happy people are more likely to have healthy and fit bodies; realistic goals and expectations; supportive friendships; an intimate, sexually warm marriage; and a faith that provides support, purpose, and acceptance.

Becoming Optimistic

Optimism is an inclination to anticipate the best possible outcome. In *Healthy Pleasures*, Robert Ornstein and David Sobel redefine it psychologically as "the ten-

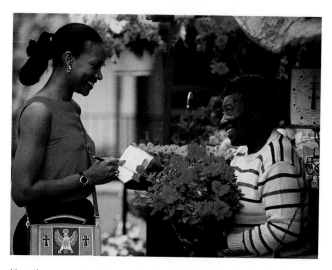

Happiness and optimism go hand in hand. Small rewards can keep your spirits high and remind you that you are special.

dency to seek out, remember, and expect pleasurable experiences. It is an active priority of the person, not merely a reflex that prompts us to look on the sunny side."[8]

For various reasons—because they believe in themselves, because they trust in a higher power, because they feel lucky—optimists expect positive experiences from life. When bad things happen, they tend to see setbacks or losses as specific, temporary incidents. In their eyes, a disappointment is "one of those things" that happens every once in a while, rather than the latest in a long string of disasters. And rather than blaming themselves ("I always screw things up," pessimists might say), optimists look at all the different factors that may have caused the problem.

Savoring Pleasures

"Treating yourself is one of the best ways to cheer yourself up," says psychologist Randy Larsen of the University of Michigan. "A night out is fun in itself, but it also imparts an important message: You're worth it. As adults we all need occasional reminders that we are special and deserve some special things."

This doesn't mean you have to break the bank. When you're feeling low, even simple indulgences, like sleeping in a few extra minutes or eating your lunch out in the sun, can make you feel better. If you're feeling down, plan a reward for yourself every day and make it a habit to include small pleasures, such as sharing a joke with a friend or taking time to watch a splendid sunset, in your daily routine.[9]

Pulsepoints

Ten Ways to Pull Yourself Out of a Bad Mood

1. Accentuate the positive. Think of the parts of your life that are going well rather than mulling over what's not.

2. Review past successes. Remind yourself of what you've already accomplished to motivate yourself to accomplish more in the future.

3. Pray. In a Gallup poll of 1007 Americans, religious practices rated as the most effective way of relieving depression.

4. Listen to music. While many forms of distraction help, at least temporarily, music is one of the most popular and effective mood boosters.

5. Treat yourself. Indulgences—big or small, expensive or not—can bring you up when you're feeling down. The reason: They make you feel special.

6. Volunteer. A third of Americans—some 89 million people—give of themselves through volunteer work. By doing the same, you may feel better too.

7. Exercise. In various studies around the world, physical exertion ranks as one of the best ways to change a bad mood, raise energy, and reduce tension.

8. Act happy. Putting on a happy face doesn't make problems disappear, but it does improve mood.

9. Focus on the future. Although you can't rewrite the past, you can learn from it. Resolve to try harder and do better the next time around.

10. Set a limit on self-pity. Tell yourself, "I'm going to feel sorry for myself this morning, but this afternoon, I've got to get on with my life."

Caring for the Soul

As discussed in Chapter 1, spiritual development is part of total health. "The soul needs an intense, full-bodied spiritual life as much as and in the same way that the body needs food," observes psychologist Thomas Moore in *Care of the Soul*. "Just as the mind digests ideas and produces intelligence, the soul feeds on life and digests it, creating wisdom and character out of the fodder of experience."[10]

Strategies for Prevention

How to Be Happy

✔ Make time for yourself. It's impossible to meet the needs of others without fulfilling your own.

✔ Invest yourself in closeness. Give your loved ones the gift of your time and caring.

✔ Work hard at what you like. Search for challenges that satisfy your need to do something meaningful.

✔ Be upbeat. If you always look for what's wrong about yourself or your life, you'll find it and feel even worse.

✔ Organize but stay loose. Be ready to seize an unexpected opportunity to try something different.

For years, spiritual matters were rarely recognized or discussed by mental health professionals. Until 1982, fewer than 3% of the articles published in leading psychiatry journals focused on spirituality or religiosity. Since then dozens of scientific studies have found that spiritual beliefs and activities, such as prayer or meditation, positively affect psychological well-being and may even speed recovery from medical illness.[11] How? "Faith provides a support community, a sense of life's meaning, a reason to focus beyond self, and a timeless perspective on life's temporary ups and downs," observes psychologist David Myers.

Doing Good

Altruism—helping or giving to others—enhances self-esteem, relieves physical and mental stress, and protects psychological well-being. Hans Selye, the father of stress research, described cooperation with others for the self's sake as altruistic egotism, whereby we satisfy our own needs while helping others satisfy theirs. This concept is essentially an updated version of the golden rule: Do unto others as you would have them do unto you. The important difference is that you earn your neighbors' love and help by offering them love and help.

Giving helps those who give as well as those who receive. People involved in community organizations, for instance, consistently report a surge of well-being called *helper's high*, which they describe as a unique sense of calmness, warmth, and enhanced self-worth.[12] College students who provided community service as part of a semester-long course reported changes in attitude (including a decreased tendency to blame people for their misfortunes), self-esteem (primarily a belief that they can make a difference), and behavior (a greater commitment to do more volunteer work).[13]

Feeling in Control

Although no one has absolute control over destiny, there is a great deal that we can do to control how we think, feel, and behave. By assessing our life situations realistically, we can make plans and preparations that allow us to make the most of our circumstances. By doing so, we gain a sense of mastery. In nationwide surveys, Americans who feel in control of their lives report greater psychological well-being than those who do not, as well as "extraordinarily positive feelings of happiness."[14]

Developing Autonomy

One goal that many people strive for is **autonomy**, or independence. Both family and society influence our ability to grow toward independence. Autonomous individuals are true to themselves. As they weigh the pros and cons of any decision, whether it's using or refusing drugs or choosing a major or career, they base their judgment

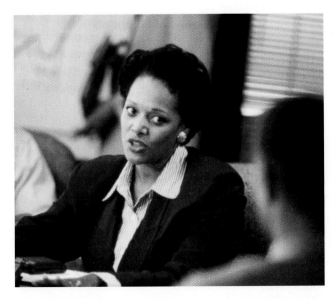

Practicing assertiveness allows you to express yourself actively and without aggression in order to accomplish your goals.

on their own values, not those of others. Their ability to draw on internal resources and cope with challenges has a positive impact on both their psychological well-being and their physical health, including recovery from illness.[15] Those who've achieved autonomy may seek the opinions of others, but they do not allow their decisions to be dictated by external influences. Because of this, it is said that their **locus of control**—that is, where they view control as originating—is *internal* (from within themselves) rather than *external* (from others).

Becoming Assertive

Being **assertive** means recognizing your feelings and making your needs and desires clear to others. Unlike aggression, which is a far less healthy means of expression, assertiveness usually works. You can change a situation you don't like by communicating your feelings and thoughts in nonprovocative words, by focusing on specifics, and by making sure you're talking with the person(s) directly responsible.

Becoming assertive isn't always easy. Many people have learned to cope by being passive and not communicating their feelings or opinions. Sooner or later they become so irritated, frustrated, or overwhelmed that they explode in an outburst, which they think of as being assertive. However, such behavior is so distasteful to them that they'd rather be passive.

Assertiveness doesn't mean screaming or telling someone off. You can communicate your wishes calmly and clearly. Even at its mildest, assertiveness can make you feel better about yourself and your life. The reason: When you speak up or take action, you're in the pilot seat. And that's always much less stressful than taking a back seat and trying to hang on for dear life.

Connecting with Others

At every age, people who feel connected to others tend to be healthier physically and psychologically. College students are no exception: Those who have a supportive, readily available network of relationships are less psychologically distressed and more satisfied with life.[16]

The opposite of *connectedness* is **social isolation**, a major risk factor for illness and early death. Individuals with few social contacts face two to four times the mortality rate of others. The reason may be that their social isolation weakens the body's ability to ward off disease. Medical students with higher-than-average scores on a loneliness scale had lower levels of protective immune cells. The end of a long-term relationship—through separation, divorce, or death—also dampens immunity.[17]

It is part of our nature as mammals and as human beings to crave relationships. But invariably we end up alone at times. Solitude is not without its own quiet joys—time for introspection, self-assessment, learning from the past, and looking toward the future. Each of us can cultivate the joy of our company, of being alone without crossing the line and becoming lonely.[18]

Overcoming Loneliness

More than many other countries, we are a nation of loners. Recent trends—longer work hours, busy family schedules, frequent moves, high divorce rates—have

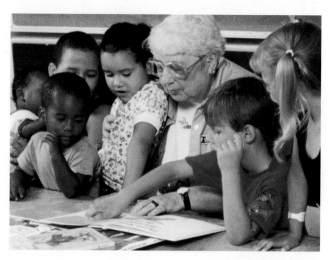

Volunteering is a rewarding way of connecting with others, giving of yourself, and feeling connected to your community.

created even lonelier people. Only 23% of Americans say they're never lonely. Loneliest of all are those who are divorced, separated, or widowed and those who live alone or solely with children. Among single adults who have never been married, 42% feel lonely at least sometimes. However, loneliness is most likely to cause emotional distress when it is a chronic rather than an episodic condition.[19]

To combat loneliness, people may join groups, fling themselves into projects and activities, or surround themselves with superficial acquaintances.[20] Others avoid the effort of trying to connect, sometimes limiting most of their personal interactions to chat groups on the Internet. But the true keys to overcoming loneliness are developing resources to fulfill our own potential and learning to reach out to others. In this way, loneliness can become a means to personal growth and discovery.[21]

Facing Social Anxieties

Many people are uncomfortable meeting strangers or speaking or performing in public. In some surveys, as many as 40% of people describe themselves as shy, or *socially anxious*.[22] Some shy people—an estimated 10% to 15% of children—are born with a predisposition to social anxieties.[23] Others become shy because they don't learn proper social responses or because they experience rejection or shame. As a result, normal apprehension intensifies when they might be watched or criticized by others. They feel extremely self-conscious, embarrassed, and nervous. When attention is on them alone, they may tremble, breathe very rapidly (hyperventilate), sweat, or develop a dry mouth or nausea.

Strategies for Prevention

How to Avoid Feeling Lonely

✔ Learn to be by yourself. Enjoying your own company helps make you the sort of person others enjoy.

✔ Pursue some interests on your own—hiking in the woods, perhaps, or joining a singing group.

✔ Keep in touch with old friends, even when miles or years may separate you.

✔ Give of yourself as a volunteer. Nothing warms the spirit more than reaching out to those who need you.

Strategies for Change
●●●●●●●●●●●●●●●●●●
Developing Social Skills

✔ If you want to get to know someone you see on campus or at work, write down what you want to say and rehearse on your own or with a friend.

✔ Observe and copy the behavior of people who handle social situations well, perhaps those who make clear what they want without being obnoxious.

✔ Every 2 weeks, invite someone to accompany you on an inexpensive outing, such as a visit to a museum.

✔ When you're with others, focus on them and what they're saying. Try not to think about how you look or what you're saying.

If you're shy, you can overcome much of your social apprehensiveness on your own in much the same way as you might set out to stop smoking or lose weight. For example, you can improve your social skills by pushing yourself to introduce yourself to a stranger at a party or to chat about the weather or the food selections with the person next to you in a cafeteria line. Gradually you'll acquire a sense of social timing and a verbal ease that will take the worry out of close encounters with others.

Those with more disabling social anxiety may do best with professional guidance, which has proven highly effective. One common technique used by experts is role playing, in which individuals act out situations that normally produce butterflies in the stomach, such as returning a defective product to a store or calling for a date.[24] With practice and time, most individuals are able to emerge from the walls that shyness has built around them and take pleasure in interacting with others.

What Is a Mental Disorder?

The borders between mental health and illness are not well marked (see Figure 3-1). Where does eccentricity end and abnormality begin? When does sadness deepen into depression? When does stress intensify into endless **anxiety**? How does fantasy lose touch completely with reality? Where is the line between everyday ups and downs and serious problems that urgently need attention?

While laypeople may speak of "nervous breakdowns" or "insanity," these are not scientific terms. The U.S. government's official definition states that a serious mental illness is "a diagnosable mental, behavioral, or emotional disorder that interferes with one or more major activities in life, like dressing, eating, or working."[25]

The mental health profession's standard for diagnosing a mental disorder is the pattern of symptoms, or diagnostic criteria, spelled out for the almost 300 disorders in the American Psychiatric Association's *Diagnostic*

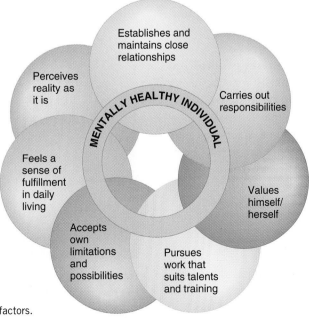

Figure 3-1

Mental well-being is a combination of factors.

and Statistical Manual, 4th edition *(DSM-IV).* It defines a **mental disorder** as "a clinically significant behavioral or psychological syndrome or pattern that occurs in an individual and that is associated with present distress (a painful symptom) or disability (impairment in one or more important areas of functioning) or with a significantly increased risk of suffering death, pain, disability, or an important loss of freedom."[26]

How Mental Health Affects Physical Health

Mental disorders affect not just the mind, but also the body. Depression can have an impact on treatment and recovery from many physical conditions, including asthma, stroke, heart disease, and cancer. Individuals recovering from heart attacks, for example, have a much greater risk of dying if they develop major depression. Anxiety can lead to intensified asthmatic reactions, skin conditions, and digestive disorders. As discussed in Chapter 2, stress can play a role in hypertension, heart attacks, and sudden cardiac death. Research into the relationship between the mind, the central nervous system, and the immune system has spawned a new scientific field, **psychoneuroimmunology**, which explores the intricate connections between the mind and the body. Not acknowledging and addressing psychological distress can contribute to major health problems, including high blood pressure, heart disease, cancer, and immune-related disorders.

Anxiety Disorders

The most common type of mental illness, anxiety disorders may involve inordinate fears of certain objects or situations (**phobias**), episodes of sudden, inexplicable terror (**panic attacks**), chronic distress (**generalized anxiety disorder**, or **GAD**), or persistent, disturbing thoughts and behaviors (**obsessive-compulsive disorder**). Over a lifetime, according to the National Comorbidity Survey, as many as one in four Americans may experience an **anxiety disorder**. Only one of every four of these individuals is ever correctly diagnosed and treated. Yet most who do get treatment, even for severe and disabling problems, improve dramatically.

Phobias

Phobias—the most prevalent type of anxiety disorder— are out-of-the-ordinary, irrational, intense, persistent fears of certain objects or situations. In the course of a lifetime, about 11% of adults develop such acute terror that they go to extremes to avoid whatever it is that they fear, even though they realize that these feelings are excessive or unreasonable. The most common phobias involve animals, particularly dogs, snakes, insects, and mice; the sight of blood; closed spaces (*claustrophobia*); heights (*acrophobia*); air travel and being in places or situations from which they perceive it would be difficult or embarrassing to escape (*agoraphobia*).

Although various medications have been tried, none is effective by itself in relieving phobias. The best approach is behavior therapy, which consists of gradual, systematic exposure to the feared object (a process called *systematic desensitization*). Numerous studies have proven that exposure—especially in vivo exposure, in which individuals are exposed to the actual source of their fear rather than simply imagining it—is highly effective; medical hypnosis—the use of induction of an altered state of consciousness—also can help.[27]

Panic Attacks and Panic Disorder

Individuals who have had panic attacks describe them as the most frightening experiences of their lives. Without reason or warning, their hearts race wildly. They may become lightheaded or dizzy. Because they can't catch their breath, they may start breathing rapidly and hyperventilate. Parts of their bodies, such as their fingers or toes, may tingle or feel numb. Worst of all is the terrible sense that something horrible is about to happen: that they will die, lose their minds, or have a heart

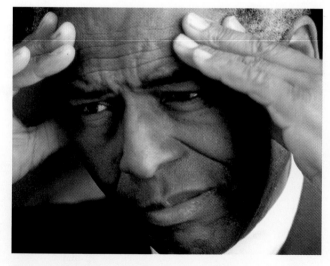

Mental distress may be difficult to see from the outside but can be extremely painful.

attack. Most attacks reach peak intensity within 10 minutes. Afterward individuals live in dread of another one. **Panic disorder** develops when attacks recur or apprehension about them becomes so intense that individuals cannot function normally.

The two primary treatments for panic disorder are cognitive-behavioral therapy, which teaches specific strategies for coping with symptoms like rapid breathing, and medication. Treatment helps as many as 90% of those with panic disorder either improve significantly or recover completely, usually within 6 to 8 weeks. Individuals who receive cognitive-behavioral therapy as well as medication are less likely to suffer relapses than those taking medication alone.[28]

Generalized Anxiety Disorder

The hallmark of a generalized anxiety disorder (GAD) is excessive or unrealistic apprehension that causes physical symptoms and lasts for 6 months or longer. Unlike fear, which helps us recognize and avoid real danger, GAD is an irrational or unwarranted response to harmless objects or situations of exaggerated danger. The most common symptoms are faster heart rate, sweating, increased blood pressure, muscle aches, intestinal pains, irritability, sleep problems, and difficulty concentrating.

Chronically anxious individuals worry not just some of the time, and not just about the stresses and strains of ordinary life, but constantly, about almost everything: their health, families, finances, marriages, potential dangers. Treatment for GAD may consist of a combination of psychotherapy, behavioral therapy, and antianxiety drugs.[29]

Obsessive-Compulsive Disorder

As many as one in forty Americans has a type of anxiety called obsessive-compulsive disorder (OCD). Some of these individuals suffer only from an *obsession*, a recurring idea, thought, or image that they realize, at least initially, is senseless. The most common obsessions are repetitive thoughts of violence (for example, killing a child), contamination (becoming infected by shaking hands), and doubt (wondering whether one has performed some act, such as having hurt someone in a traffic accident). Most people with OCD also suffer from a *compulsion*, repetitive behavior performed according to certain rules or in a stereotyped fashion. The most common compulsions involve handwashing, cleaning, hoarding useless items, counting, or checking (for instance, making sure a door is locked dozens of times).[30]

Individuals with OCD realize that their thoughts or behaviors are bizarre, but they cannot resist or control them. Eventually, the obsessions or compulsions consume a great deal of time and significantly interfere with normal routine, job functioning, or usual social activities or relationships with others.

OCD is believed to have biological roots. It may be a result of gene abnormalities, head injury, or even an autoimmune reaction after childhood infection with strep bacteria.[31] Treatment may consist of cognitive therapy to correct irrational assumptions, behavioral techniques (such as progressively limiting the amount of time someone obsessed with cleanliness can spend washing and scrubbing), and medication. About 70% to 80% of those with OCD improve with treatment.[32]

Depressive Disorders

Comparing everyday "blues" to a **depressive disorder** is like comparing a cold to pneumonia. Major depression can destroy a person's joy for living. Food, friends, sex, or any form of pleasure no longer appeals. It is impossible to concentrate on work and responsibilities. Unable to escape a sense of utter hopelessness, depressed individuals may fight back tears throughout the day and toss and turn through long, empty nights. Thoughts of death or suicide may push into their minds.

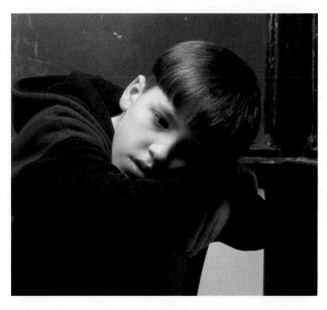

An increasing number of children suffer from bouts of depression, experiencing feelings of overwhelming hopelessness, helplessness, and sadness.

But there is good news: Depression is a treatable disease. Psychotherapy is remarkably effective for mild depression. In more serious cases, antidepressant medication can lead to dramatic improvement in 75% to 80% of depressed patients.[33]

Major Depression

The simplest definition of **major depression** is sadness that does not end. The incidence of major depression has soared over the last two decades, especially among young adults. The National Comorbidity Survey found that major depression is the most widespread mental disorder, affecting 10.3% of Americans in any given year. Unfortunately, fewer than one of three depressed people ever seeks treatment.

Most cases of major depression can be treated successfully, usually with psychotherapy, medication, or both. Psychotherapy alone works in more than half of mild-to-moderate episodes of major depression. Two specific psychotherapies—cognitive-behavioral therapy and interpersonal therapy (described later in this chapter)—have proved as helpful as antidepressant drugs in treating mild cases of depression, although they take longer than medication to achieve results.[34]

Antidepressant medications work for more than half of those with moderate-to-severe depression and may be useful in treating mild depression in individuals who do not improve with psychotherapy alone (see the section on psychiatric drug therapy later in this chapter). These prescription drugs generally take 3 or 4 weeks to produce significant benefits and may not have their full impact for up to 8 weeks. Combined treatment with psychotherapy and medication helps individuals with severe chronic or recurrent major depression as well as those who do not fully improve with medication or psychotherapy alone.

Bipolar Disorder (Manic Depression)

Bipolar disorder, or manic depression, consists of mood swings that may take individuals from *manic* states of feeling euphoric and energetic to depressive states of utter despair. In episodes of full mania, they may become so impulsive and out of touch with reality that they endanger their careers, relationships, health, or even survival.

The characteristic symptoms of bipolar disorder include mood swings (from happy to miserable, optimistic to despairing, etc.); changes in thinking (thoughts speeding through one's mind, unrealistic self-confidence, difficulty concentrating, delusions, hallucinations); changes in behavior (sudden immersion in plans and projects, talking very rapidly and much more than usual, excessive spending, impaired judgment, impulsive sexual involvement); and changes in physical condition (less need for sleep, increased energy, fewer health complaints than usual). During manic periods, individuals may make grandiose plans or take dangerous risks.[35] But they often plunge from this highest of highs to a horribly low depressive episode, in which they may feel sad, hopeless, helpless, and develop other symptoms of major depression. The risk of suicide is very real.

Professional therapy is essential in treating bipolar disorder. Medication—lithium carbonate or an anticonvulsant drug—is the keystone of treatment, although psychotherapy plays a critical role in helping individuals understand their illness and rebuild their lives. Most individuals continue taking medication indefinitely after remission of their symptoms because the risk of recurrence is high.

Strategies for Change

Recognizing Major Depression

The characteristic symptoms of major depression include:

✔ Feeling depressed, sad, empty, discouraged, tearful.

✔ Loss of interest or pleasure in once-enjoyable activities.

✔ Eating more or less than usual and either gaining or losing weight.

✔ Having trouble sleeping or sleeping much more than usual.

✔ Feeling slowed down or restless and unable to sit still.

✔ Lack of energy.

✔ Feeling helpless, hopeless, worthless, inadequate.

✔ Difficulty concentrating, forgetfulness.

✔ Difficulty thinking clearly or making decisions.

✔ Persistent thoughts of death or suicide.

✔ Withdrawal from others, lack of interest in sex.

✔ Physical symptoms (headaches, digestive problems, aches and pains).

Suicide

Suicide is not in itself a psychiatric disorder, but it can be the tragic consequence of emotional and psychological problems. Every year 30,000 Americans—among them many young people who seem to have "everything to live for"—commit suicide. Ten times this many individuals attempt to take their own lives.

In the last 30 years, reported suicides among young adults between the ages of 15 and 24 have tripled. According to a 1995 report by the Centers for Disease Control and Prevention, suicide has become an increasingly serious problem among the nation's youth, with big increases among children between the ages of 10 and 14 and among young African-American men. College students commit suicide at about half the rate of young people their age who are not in school. Suicide rates at highly competitive schools are not significantly

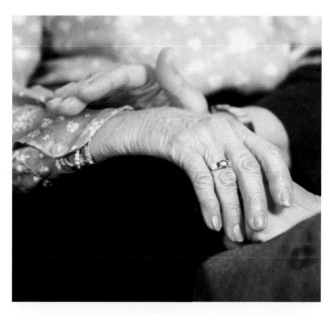

Depression and suicidal thoughts are closely linked. Educating close friends and relatives about depression prepares them to offer help and comfort during difficult times.

Strategies for Prevention

Helping to Prevent Suicide

If someone you know has talked about suicide, behaved unpredictably, or suddenly emerged from a severe depression into a calm, settled state of mind, don't rule out the possibility that he or she may attempt suicide.

✔ Encourage your friend to talk. Ask concerned questions. Listen attentively. Show that you take the person's feelings seriously and truly care.

✔ Suggest solutions or alternatives to problems. Make plans. Encourage positive action, such as getting away for a while to gain a better perspective on a problem.

✔ Don't be afraid to ask whether your friend has considered suicide. The opportunity to talk about thoughts of suicide may be an enormous relief and, contrary to a longstanding myth, will not fix the idea of suicide more firmly in a person's mind.

✔ If you feel that you aren't making any headway, suggest that both you and your friend talk to an expert.

✔ Stay close until you can get help. If you must leave your friend alone, negotiate first. Have your friend promise not to harm himself or herself without first calling you. If your friend does call, get to him or her as soon as possible. Call for help immediately.

different from those at less rigorous ones. However, college students do think about suicide and, in smaller numbers, make specific plans for taking their own lives (see Campus Focus: "College Students and Suicide").

But suicide is not inevitable. Appropriate treatment can help as many as 70% to 80% of those at risk for suicide. Among young people, early recognition and treatment for depressive disorders and alcohol and drug use could save thousands of lives each year.[36]

What Leads to Suicide?

Researchers have looked for explanations of suicide by studying everything from phases of the moon to seasons (suicides peak in the spring in most young people and adults) to birth order in the family. They have found no conclusive answers. A constellation of influences—mental disorders, personality traits, biologic and genetic vulnerability, medical illness, and psychosocial stressors—may combine in ways that lower an individual's threshold of vulnerability. No one factor in itself may ever explain fully why a person chooses death.

Mental Disorders

As many as 95% of those who commit suicide have a mental disorder. Two in particular—depression and alcoholism—account for two-thirds of all suicides. Suicide also is a risk for those with other disorders, including schizophrenia and personality disorders.

CAMPUS FOCUS: COLLEGE STUDENTS AND SUICIDE

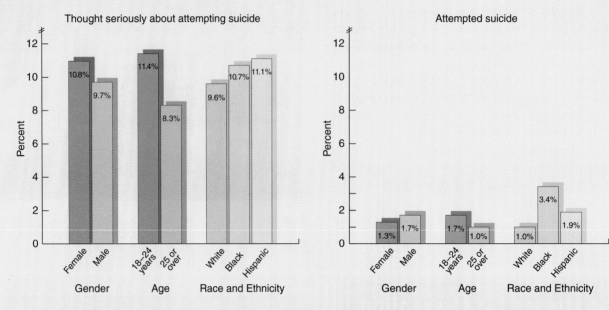

SOURCE: Douglas, Kathy, et al. "Results from the 1995 National College Health Risk Behavior Survey." *Journal of American College Health*, Vol. 46, September 1997.

Substance Abuse

Many of those who commit suicide drink beforehand, and their use of alcohol may lower their inhibitions. Since alcohol itself is a depressant, it can intensify the despondency suicidal individuals are already feeling. Alcoholics who attempt suicide often have other risk factors, including major depression, poor social support, serious medical illness, and unemployment. Drugs of abuse also can alter thinking and lower inhibitions against suicide.

Hopelessness

The sense of utter hopelessness and helplessness may be the most common contributing factors in suicide. When hope dies, individuals view every experience in negative terms and come to expect the worst possible outcomes for their problems. Given this way of thinking, suicide often seems a reasonable response to a life seen as not worth living.

Family History

One of every four people who attempt suicide has a family member who also tried to commit suicide. While a family history of suicide is not in itself considered a predictor of suicide, two mental disorders that can lead to suicide—depression and bipolar disorder (manic depression)—do run in families.

Physical Illness

People who commit suicide are likely to be ill or to believe that they are. About 5% actually have a serious physical disorder, such as AIDS or cancer. While suicide may seem to be a decision rationally arrived at in persons with serious or fatal illness, this may not in fact be the case. Depression, not uncommon in such instances, can warp judgment. When the depression is treated, the person may no longer have suicidal intentions.

More than 80% of those who commit suicide have seen a physician about a medical complaint within the 6 months preceding suicide. To help general physicians identify people at risk of suicide, researchers at Johns Hopkins University developed a set of four crucial questions:

- Have you ever had a period of 2 weeks or more when you had trouble falling asleep, staying asleep, waking up too early, or sleeping too much?

- Have you ever had 2 weeks or more during which you felt sad, blue, depressed, or when you lost interest and pleasure in things you usually cared about or enjoyed?

- Has there been a period of 2 weeks or more when you felt worthless, sinful, or guilty?

- Has there ever been a period of time when you felt that life was hopeless?

Anyone who answers yes to these questions should be referred immediately to a mental health professional.

Brain Chemistry

Investigators have found abnormalities in the brain chemistry of individuals who complete suicide, especially low levels of a metabolite of the neurotransmitter serotonin. There are indications that individuals with a deficiency in this substance may have as much as a ten times greater risk of committing suicide than those with higher levels.[37]

Access to Guns

For individuals already facing a combination of predisposing factors, access to a means of committing suicide, particularly guns, can add to the risk. Unlike other methods of suicide, guns almost always hit their mark. States with strict gun-control laws have much lower rates of suicides than states with more lenient laws.

Other Factors

Individuals who kill themselves often have gone through more major life crises—job changes, births, financial reversals, divorce, retirement—in the previous 6 months compared with others. Longstanding, intense conflict with family members or other important people may add to the danger. In some cases, suicide may be an act of revenge that offers the person a sense of control—however temporary or illusory. For example, a husband whose wife has had an affair may rationalize that he can get back at her, and have the final word, by killing himself. Others may feel that, by rejecting life, they are rejecting a partner or parent who abandoned or betrayed them.

Attention Disorders

A little more than a decade ago, mental health professionals assumed that what is now termed **attention deficit/hyperactivity disorder (ADHD)**, the most

---

Strategies for Prevention

If You Start Thinking About Suicide

At some point, the thought of ending it all—the disappointments, problems, bad feelings—may cross your mind. This experience isn't unusual. But if the idea of taking your life persists or intensifies, you should respond as you would to other warnings of potential threats to your health by getting the help you need:

✔ Talk to a mental health professional. If you have a therapist, call immediately. If not, call a suicide hot line.

✔ Find someone you can trust and talk with honesty about what you're feeling. If you suffer from depression or another mental disorder, educate trusted friends or relatives about your condition so they are prepared if called upon to help.

✔ Write down your more uplifting thoughts. Even if you are despondent, you can help yourself by taking the time to retrieve some more positive thoughts or memories. A simple record of your hopes for the future and the people you value in your life can remind you of why your own life is worth continuing.

✔ Avoid drugs and alcohol. Most suicides are the result of sudden, uncontrolled impulses, and drugs and alcohol can make it harder to resist these destructive urges.

✔ Go to the hospital. Hospitalization can sometimes be the best way to protect your health and safety.

---

common psychiatric diagnosis in childhood, was strictly kids' stuff. They were wrong. A half to two-thirds of youngsters with ADHD do not outgrow their restless, reckless ways at puberty. In all, 1% to 2% of adult men and women—at least 5 million Americans—have problems sustaining attention or controlling their movements and impulses.[38]

ADHD, which has replaced the terms *minimal brain dysfunction* and *hyperactivity,* refers to a spectrum of difficulties in controlling motion and sustaining attention. Adults with ADHD have one or more of three primary symptoms: hyperactivity, impulsivity, and distractibility. Rather than scooting around a room, they may tap their fingers or jiggle their feet. Some appear calm and organized but cannot concentrate long enough to finish reading a paragraph or follow a list of directions. Others, on a whim, go on buying sprees or take wild dares.

Strategies for Change

Recognizing an Attention Disorder

Recognizing ADHD can be the first step in getting help for a person with this disorder, who may have no idea that this is a treatable condition. The characteristic symptoms of ADHD in adults are:

✔ Feelings of restlessness, fidgeting, squirming; difficulty waiting.

✔ Extreme distractibility, forgetfulness, absent-mindedness, irritation when stuck in traffic.

✔ Disorganization, inability to finish tasks, switching from task to task haphazardly; inability to remain still or engage in a focused activity such as reading.

✔ Difficulty in solving problems or managing time.

✔ Hot temper, explosive outbursts, constant irritation; low tolerance of stress, easily overwhelmed by ordinary hassles; frequent mood swings.

✔ Impulsiveness, making decisions with little reflection or information, abruptly beginning and ending relationships, recklessness.

✔ Clumsiness, poor body image, poor sense of direction.

✔ Immaturity.

There is no specific test for detecting attention disorders, and diagnosis based on the patient's history and a therapist's interview can be difficult. Adults with ADHD receive the same medications that children do—stimulant drugs that, paradoxically, can aid concentration and reduce restlessness. Medication often makes it possible for adults with ADHD to benefit from other treatments, such as psychotherapy, general counseling, vocational rehabilitation, and academic tutoring.[39]

Schizophrenia

Schizophrenia, one of the most debilitating mental disorders, profoundly impairs an individual's sense of reality. Individuals with schizophrenia may hear, see, or feel things that do not exist—a voice telling them to jump from a bridge, a statue crying tears of blood, a spaceship beaming a light upon them. Frightened and vulnerable,

they may devote all their energy to warding off the demons within. Unable to take care of themselves, they may look messy and disheveled. They often move in unusual ways, such as rocking or pacing, or repeat certain gestures again and again.

Schizophrenia is most likely to occur between the ages of 17 and 24. One-half to one percent of the population—about 1 in every 150 people—suffers from this disorder. According to the National Institutes of Mental Health's (NIMH) epidemiological data, the total lifetime prevalence for schizophrenia in the United States ranges from 1% to 1.9%. This means that between 2.5 million and 4.75 million Americans may have schizophrenia at any one time.

Today, for the vast majority of individuals with schizophrenia, antipsychotic drugs are the foundation of treatment. They make most people with schizophrenia feel more comfortable and in control of themselves, help organize chaotic thinking, and reduce or eliminate delusions or hallucinations, allowing fuller participation in normal activities. Those who do not improve significantly on medication almost invariably do even worse without it.

Overcoming Problems of the Mind

An estimated 34 million Americans currently receive professional psychotherapy or counseling; millions more need such help. Yet many people do not seek treatment because they see psychological problems as a

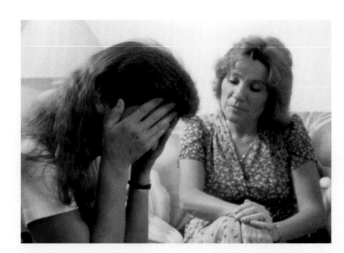

Therapists' educations, titles, and qualifications may vary. The qualities of compassion and caring are important in choosing the right therapist.

sign of weakness rather than illness. They also may not realize that scientifically proven therapies can bring relief, often in a matter of weeks or months.

Where to Turn

As a student, your best contact for identifying local services may be your health education instructor or department. The health instructors can tell you about general and mental health counseling available on campus, school-based support groups, community-based programs, and special emergency services. On campus, you can also turn to the student health services or the office of the dean of student services or student affairs.

Within the community, you may be able to get help through the city or county health department and neighborhood health centers. Local hospitals often have special clinics and services, and there are usually local branches of national service organizations (such as United Way or Alcoholics Anonymous), other twelve-step programs, and various support groups. (Check the telephone directory for listings.) Your primary physician may also be able to help.

Types of Therapists

Many people refer to anyone in the mental health field as a "psychotherapist," but this is not an official designation, and anyone can advertise as one. Only professionally trained individuals who have met state licensing requirements are certified as psychiatrists, psychologists, or social workers. Before selecting any of these mental health professionals, be sure to check the person's background and credentials.

- **Psychiatrists** are licensed medical doctors (M.D.s) who complete medical school; a year-long internship (including at least 4 months of internal medicine and usually 2 months of neurology); and a 3-year residency that provides training in various forms of psychotherapy, psychopharmacology (the study of drugs that affect the mind), and both outpatient and inpatient treatment of mental disorders. They can prescribe medications and make medical decisions.

- **Psychologists** complete a graduate program (including clinical training and internships) in human psychology but do not study medicine and cannot prescribe medication. They must be licensed in most states to practice independently.

Strategies for Change

Choosing a Therapist

In making your final choice of a therapist, here are some considerations and questions to keep in mind:

✔ Do you feel the therapist shows genuine concern, takes you seriously, treats you with respect, and shares or accepts your values? Regardless of his or her qualifications or reputation, a therapist who is not understanding and caring probably is not the right choice.

✔ Is your therapist willing to explore all treatment options to find what works best for you? Will this include medication as well as specific psychotherapeutic techniques?

✔ Remember that you are choosing someone in whom you may confide your most intimate secrets and fears. Of course, you want a competent therapist with the right training, knowledge, skills, and experience. But you also must choose someone you can trust.

- **Certified social workers** or **licensed clinical social workers (LCSWs)** usually complete a 2-year graduate program and have specialized training in helping people with mental problems in addition to conventional social work.

- **Psychiatric nurses** have nursing degrees and have passed a state examination. They usually have special training and experience in mental health care, although no specialty licensing or certification is required.

- **Marriage and family therapists**, licensed in some but not all states, usually have a graduate degree, often in psychology, and at least 2 years of supervised clinical training in dealing with relationship problems.

Options for Treatment

Psychotherapy refers to any type of counseling based on the exchange of words in the context of the unique relationship that develops between a mental health professional and a person seeking help. The process of talking and listening can lead to new insight, relief from distressing psychological symptoms, changes in unhealthy or maladaptive behaviors, and more effective ways of dealing with the world.

Psychodynamic Psychotherapy

For the most part, today's mental health professionals base their assessment of individuals on a **psychodynamic** understanding that takes into account the role of early experiences and unconscious influences in *actively* shaping behavior. (This is the *dynamic* in psychodynamic.) Psychodynamic treatments work toward the goal of providing greater insight into problems and bringing about behavioral change. Therapy may be brief, consisting of twelve to twenty-five sessions, or it may continue for several years.

Interpersonal Therapy (IPT)

Interpersonal therapy (IPT), originally developed for research into the treatment of major depression, focuses on relationships to help individuals deal with unrecognized feelings and needs and improve their communication skills. IPT does not deal with the psychological origins of symptoms but rather concentrates on current problems of getting along with others. IPT usually consists of twelve to sixteen sessions.

Cognitive-Behavioral Therapy

This approach, which focuses on inappropriate or inaccurate thoughts or beliefs, aims to help individuals break out of a distorted way of thinking. The techniques of **cognitive therapy** include identification of an individual's beliefs and attitudes, recognition of negative thought patterns, and education in alternative ways of thinking. Individuals with major depression or anxiety disorders are most likely to benefit, usually in fifteen to twenty-five sessions.

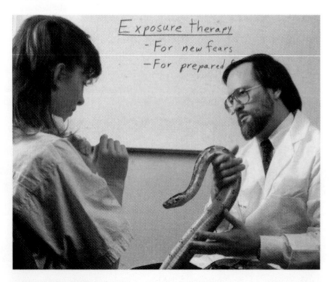

Systematic desensitization is one of the behavior therapies used to treat phobias.

Behavior therapy strives to substitute healthier ways of behaving for maladaptive patterns used in the past. Its premise is that distressing psychological symptoms, like all behaviors, are learned responses that can be modified or unlearned. Behavior therapies work best for disorders characterized by specific abnormal patterns of acting—such as alcohol and drug abuse, anxiety disorders, and phobias—and for individuals who want to change bad habits.

Psychiatric Drug Therapy

Medications that alter brain chemistry and relieve psychiatric symptoms have brought great hope and help to millions of people. Thanks to the recent development of a new generation of more precise and effective **psychiatric drugs**, success rates for treating many common and disabling disorders have soared. Often used in conjunction with psychotherapy, sometimes used as the primary treatment, these medications have revolutionized mental health care.

Strategies for Prevention

What You Need to Know About Psychiatric Drugs

These are some of the questions consumers should ask prior to beginning drug therapy:

✔ Why is it necessary to take this medication? What specific symptoms will it relieve? Are there other possible benefits?

✔ What are the possible side effects and risks? Do I have to take it before or after eating? Will it affect my ability to drive, operate machinery, or work?

✔ How long will it be before the medication begins to help? How can I tell if the drug is working?

✔ Is there any danger from skipping a dose? What are the risks of overdosing? Does this medicine interact with any other medications? Can I drink alcohol while taking this medication? Are there any foods or substances I should avoid?

✔ How long will I have to take this medication? Is there a danger that I'll become addicted? What are the odds that this medicine will help me? What if this drug doesn't work?

Health Online

New York University Department of Psychiatry Online Screening
http://www.med.nyu.edu/Psych/public.html

This site features online screening tests for depression, anxiety, male and female sexual disorders, attention deficit disorder, and personality disorders. There is also information on the diagnosis of psychological problems, their treatment, and self-help options. While it certainly can't take the place of evaluation by a mental health professional, the screening tests at this site may give you a sense of whether or not you should seek professional help for a problem.

Think about it ...

• According to these tests, do you have any warning signs of possible psychological problems? Are these in areas you have felt you had problems with in the past?

• Do you think online screening tests like this might help people with symptoms of psychological problems seek professional help?

• If you were to design a screening test for mental wellness instead of illness, what criteria might you include?

Making This Chapter Work for You

Promoting Psychological Wellness and Understanding Psychological Problems

■ Emotional health and mental health are both components of psychological health, our ability to be in touch with our feelings, to perceive reality as it is, and to work toward personal fulfillment.

■ Happiness is a sense of subjective well-being that tends to be highest when people combine frequent good experiences with occasional very intense pleasures. It is not based on wealth, beauty, or fame, but on characteristics such as high self-esteem, optimism, and the ability to form close relationships.

■ Optimism involves the conscious decision to seek out and expect positive experiences from life. It is a key to maintaining good psychological health.

■ We find meaning and fulfillment in life in various ways, including by loving and being loved, by developing our own spirituality, and by reaching out to help others.

■ Autonomy (a sense of independence) and assertiveness (making your needs and desires clear to others)

are keys to a feeling of mastery and being in control of your life.

■ A mental disorder is "a clinically significant behavioral or psychological syndrome or pattern that occurs in an individual and that is associated with present distress or disability or with a significantly increased risk of suffering death, pain, disability, or an important loss of freedom."

■ The most common type of mental disorders, anxiety disorders may involve episodes of sudden, inexplicable terror (panic attacks), inordinate fears of certain objects or situations (phobias), chronic distress (generalized anxiety disorder), or persistent, disturbing thoughts and behaviors (obsessive-compulsive disorder).

■ Major depression is the most widespread mental disorder. Symptoms include a sense of helplessness or hopelessness, lack of energy, sleep disturbances, and loss of interest in food, sex, and work. Depression can be successfully treated with psychotherapy, drug therapy, or a combination. Bipolar disorder is another form of depression, characterized by extreme mood swings.

■ The number of suicides is growing, especially among young people. As many as 50% of college students say they think about suicide, while 8% to 15% act on these thoughts.

■ Attention disorders are common among adults. Their primary symptoms are hyperactivity, impulsivity, and distractibility. Medication is often very effective.

■ There are many types of mental health professionals, including psychiatrists, psychologists, licensed social workers, psychiatric nurses, and marriage and family therapists. Options for treatment include psychodynamic psychotherapy, interpersonal therapy, cognitive-behavioral therapy, and psychiatric drugs.

Like physical health, psychological well-being is not a fixed state, but a process. The way you live every day affects how you feel about yourself and your world.

Here are some guidelines for making the most of the process of living:

■ **Accept yourself.** As a human being, you are, by definition, imperfect. Come to terms with the fact that you are a worthwhile person despite your mistakes.

■ **Trust yourself.** Learn to listen to the voice within you and let your intuition be your guide.

■ **Stretch yourself.** Be willing to change and grow, to try something new, and dare to be vulnerable.

■ **Think of who and where you want to be a decade from now.** The goals you set, the decisions you make, and the values you adopt now will determine how you feel about yourself and your life in the future.

 ## Key Terms

The terms listed here are used within the chapter. Page numbers are included for each term. A definition of each term is given in the green Glossary pages at the end of this book.

altruism *34*
anxiety *37*
anxiety disorder *38*
assertive *35*
attention deficit/hyperactivity disorder (ADHD) *43*
autonomy *35*
behavior therapy *46*
bipolar disorder *40*
certified social worker *45*
cognitive therapy *46*
depressive disorder *39*
emotional health *32*
generalized anxiety disorder (GAD) *38*

interpersonal therapy (IPT) *46*
licensed clinical social worker (LCSW) *45*
locus of control *35*
major depression *40*
marriage and family therapist *45*
mental disorder *38*
mental health *32*
obsessive-compulsive disorder *38*
optimism *38*
panic attack *38*
panic disorder *39*
phobia *38*

psychiatric drugs *46*
psychiatric nurse *45*
psychiatrist *45*
psychodynamic *46*
psychologist *45*
psychoneuroimmunology *38*
psychotherapy *45*
schizophrenia *44*
social isolation *36*
spiritual health *33*

Review Questions

1. What are the characteristics of an emotionally healthy person?
2. What are some strategies you can use to enhance your psychological well-being?
3. What is mental health? What is a mental disorder?
4. Define and give examples of the following disorders: anxiety, depression, attention disorder. How can individuals with these types of disorders be helped?
5. How can you tell if you need professional help in overcoming a psychological problem? Who can help and what types of therapy might you try?

Critical Thinking Questions

1. Are you aware of your ability to view life positively or negatively? Which way do you most often describe your life? What could you do to become psychologically healthier?

2. Paula went to a therapist when she was feeling depressed and was given a prescription for an anti-depressant called fluoxetine (trade name Prozac). She has heard different things about Prozac in the media and is uncertain about taking the medication. What should she do? How would you weigh the risks and benefits of taking a psychiatric drug?

3. Research has indicated that many of the homeless suffer from chronic mental illness or alcoholism. Yet government funding for the mentally ill is inadequate, and homelessness itself can make it difficult for people to gain access to the care they need. How do you feel when you pass homeless people who seem disoriented or out of touch with reality? Who should take responsibility for their welfare? Should they be forced to undergo psychiatric treatment even if it is against their will?

 ## Connections to Personal Health Interactive

*To enhance your understanding of the material covered in this chapter, check out the following study aids on the **Personal Health Interactive CD-ROM**.*

- Personal Insights: How Good Do You Feel?
- Personal Insights: How Healthy Is Your Mind?
- Dream Diary
- Suicide Notes
- Recovery from Mental Illness

- Your Ideal Self
- Study Page: Applied Psychologists
- Personal Voices: Psychological Disorders—Schizophrenia
- Glossary & Key Term Review

 ## References

1. Kessler, Ronald, et al. "Lifetime and 12-Month Prevalence of *DSM-III-R* Psychiatric Disorders in the United States: Results from the National Comorbidity Study." *Archives of General Psychiatry,* Vol. 51, No. 1, January 1994.
2. Hales, Robert, and Stuart Yudofsky. *The American Psychiatric Press Textbook of Psychiatry.* 3rd ed. Washington, DC: American Psychiatric Press, 1998.
3. Shapiro, Deane, and Roger Walsh. *Beyond Health and Normalcy.* New York: Van Nostrand Reinhold, 1983.
4. Myers, David. *The Pursuit of Happiness: Who Is Happy—and Why.* New York: William Morrow, 1992.
5. Reich, John, et al. "The Road to Happiness." *Psychology Today,* July–August 1994.
6. Lu, Luo, and Jian Bin Shih. "Sources of Happiness: A Qualitative Approach." *Journal of Social Psychology,* Vol. 137, No. 2, April 1997.
7. Furnham, Adrian, and Helen Cheng. "Personality and Happiness." *Psychological Reports,* Vol. 80, No. 3, June 1997. Lu, Luo, et al. "Personal and Environmental Correlates of Happiness." *Personality & Individual Differences,* September 1997.
8. Ornstein, Robert, and David Sobel. *Healthy Pleasures.* Reading, MA: Addison-Wesley, 1990.
9. Brami, Elisabeth, and Philippe Bertran. *Little Moments of Happiness.* New York: Stewart Tabori & Chang, 1997.
10. Moore, Thomas. *Care of the Soul.* New York: Harper Perennial, 1994.
11. Benson, Herbert. *Timeless Healing.* New York: Scribner's, 1996.
12. George, Jennifer, and Arthur Brief. "Feeling Good-Doing Good: A Conceptual Analysis of the Mood at Work—Organizational Spontaneity Relationship." *Psychological Bulletin,* Vol. 112, No. 2, 1992.
13. Giles, Dwight, and Janet Eyler. "The Impact of a College Community Service Laboratory on Students' Personal, Social and Cognitive Outcomes." *Journal of Adolescence,* Vol. 17, No. 4, August 1994.
14. Larsen, Randy. Personal interview.
15. Stone, Arthur, et al. "Psychological Coping: Its Importance for Treating Medical Problems." *Mind/Body Medicine,* Vol. 1. No. 1, March 1995.
16. Demakis, George, and Dan McAdams. "Personality, Social Support and Well-Being Among First-Year College Students." *College Student Journal,* Vol. 28, No. 4, June 1994. Liange, Belle, and Anne Bogat. "Culture, Control and Coping: New Perspectives on Social Support." *American Journal of Community Psychology,* Vol. 22, No. 1, February 1994. Forgas, Joseph. "Sad and Guilty? Affective Influences on the Explanation of Conflict in Close Relationships." *Journal of Personality & Social Psychology,* Vol. 66, No. 1, 1994.
17. Schwartz, Richard. "Loneliness." *Harvard Review of Psychiatry,* Vol. 5, No. 2, July–August 1997.
18. Bucholz, Ester. *The Call of Solitude: Alonetime in a World of Attachment.* New York: Simon & Schuster, 1997.

19. Rokach, Ami, and Heather Brock. "Loneliness and the Effects of Life Changes." *Journal of Psychology,* Vol. 131, No. 3, May 1997.

20. Nurmi, Jari-Erik, and Katarina Salmela-Aro. "Social Strategies and Loneliness." *Personality & Individual Differences,* Vol. 23, No. 2, August 1997.

21. Rokach, Ami. "Relations of Perceived Causes and the Experience of Loneliness." *Psychological Reports,* Vol. 80, No. 3, June 1997.

22. Mannuzza, Salvatore, et al. "Generalized Social Phobia." *Archives of General Psychiatry,* Vol. 52, No. 3, March 1995.

23. Potts, Nicholas, and Jonathan Davidson. "Epidemiology and Pharmacotherapy of Social Phobia." *Psychiatric Times,* February 1995. Morris, Lois. "Social Anxiety." *American Health,* January–February 1995.

24. Ross, Jerilyn. *Triumph over Fear.* New York: Bantam Books, 1994.

25. Hales, Dianne, and Robert Hales. *Caring for the Mind: The Comprehensive Guide to Mental Health.* New York: Bantam Books, 1995.

26. American Psychiatric Association. *Diagnostic and Statistical Manual of Mental Disorders.* 4th ed. Washington, DC: American Psychiatric Association, 1994. Andreasen, Nancy. "The Validation of Psychiatric Diagnosis: New Models and Approaches." *American Journal of Psychiatry,* Vol. 152, No. 2, February 1995.

27. "Hypnosis: More Than a Suggestion," *Harvard Health Letter,* Vol. 22, No. 12, October 1997.

28. Sanderson, William. "Cognitive Behavior Therapy." *American Journal of Psychotherapy,* Vol. 51, No. 2, Spring 1997.

29. Wickelgren, Ingrid. "When Worry Rules Your Life: Can Simple Anxiety Be a Mental Illness?" *Health,* Vol. 11, No. 8, November–December 1997.

30. Leckman, James, et al. "Symptoms of Obsessive-Compulsive Disorder." *American Journal of Psychiatry,* Vol. 35, No. 7, July 1997.

31. Brown, Phyllida. "Over and Over and Over ..." *New Scientist,* Vol. 155, No. 2093, August 2, 1997.

32. Jones, Mairwen K., et al. "The Cognitive Mediation of Obsessive-Compulsive Handwashing." *Behaviour Research & Therapy,* Vol. 35, No. 9, September 1997. Amir, Naden, et al. "Strategies of Thought Control in Obsessive-Compulsive Disorder." *Behaviour Research & Therapy,* Vol. 35, No. 9, September 1997.

33. Klien, Donald, and Michael Thase. "Medication vs. Psychotherapy for Depression." *American Society for Clinical Psychopharmacology,* Vol. 8, No. 2, Fall 1997.

34. Wood, Alison, et al. "Controlled Trial of Brief Cognitive-Behavioral Intervention in Adolescent Patients with Depressive Disorders." *Journal of Child Psychology & Psychiatry & Allied Disciplines,* Vol. 37, No. 6, September 1996.

35. Daly, Ian. "Mania." *Lancet,* Vol. 349, No. 9059, April 19, 1997.

36. Leutwyler, Kristin. "Suicide Prevention." *Scientific American,* Vol. 276, No. 3, March 1997.

37. Cooper-Patrick, Lisa, et al. "Preventing Suicide by Asking the Right Questions." *Journal of the American Medical Association,* December 13, 1994.

38. Biederman, Joseph, et al. "High Risk for Attention Deficit Hyperactivity Disorder Among Children of Parents with Childhood Onset of the Disorder." *American Journal of Psychiatry,* Vol. 152, No. 3, March 1995. Faigel, Harris. "Attention Deficit Disorder in College Students." *Journal of American College Health,* Vol. 43, No. 4, January 1995. Heiligenstein, Eric, and Richard Keeling. "Presentation of Unrecognized Attention Deficit Hyperactivity Disorder in College Students." *Journal of American College Health,* Vol. 43, No. 5, March 1995.

39. Farley, Dixie. "Attention Disorder: Overcoming the Deficit." *FDA Consumer,* Vol. 31, No. 5, July–August 1997.

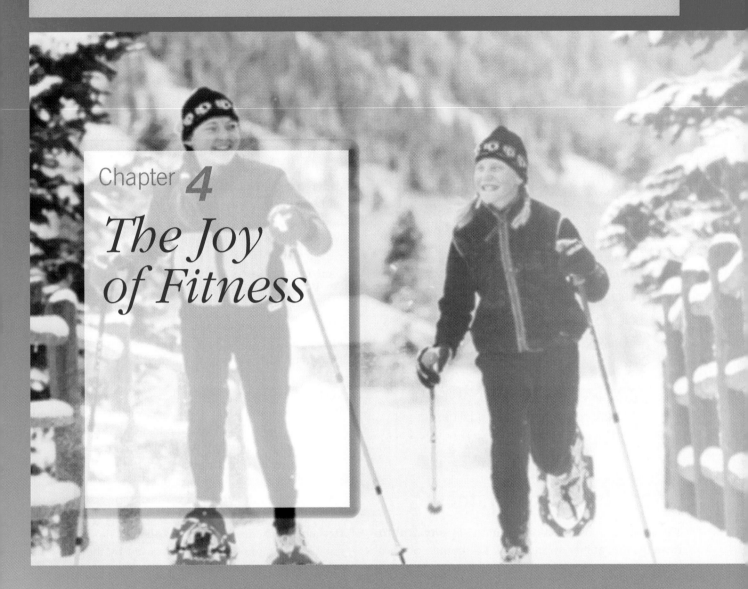

Chapter 4
The Joy of Fitness

After studying the material in this chapter, you should be able to:

- **List** and **explain** the components of physical fitness.
- **Explain** the benefits of exercise as a strategy for health prevention.
- **Compare** and **contrast** aerobic exercises and strength or muscular exercises.
- **Plan** a personal exercise program and **list** safety strategies.

*D*on't just sit there: Do something! This is the latest message from fitness experts to a nation of couch potatoes.[1] Don't worry about fancy equipment, special clothes, personal trainers: Just get moving. Walk rather than ride. Take the stairs, not the elevator. Bend. Twist. Reach. Wherever you go, whenever you can, put your body to use. You might just save your life.

To protect your health, you don't have to turn into a jock or a fitness fanatic. All you have to do is become more active. This chapter can help. It presents current exercise recommendations, explores common barriers to active lifestyles, describes types of exercise, and provides guidelines for getting into shape and exercising safely.

What Is Physical Fitness?

The simplest, most practical definition of **physical fitness** is the ability to respond to routine physical demands with enough reserve energy to cope with a sudden challenge. You can consider yourself fit if you meet your daily energy needs, can handle unexpected extra demands, have a realistic but positive self-image, and are protecting yourself against potential health problems, such as heart disease.

Fitness consists of three basic components: flexibility, cardiovascular or aerobic fitness, and muscular strength and endurance. Other factors, such as body composition and agility, also may be considered in assessing overall fitness. However, if you focus on the three basic components of physical fitness, your body will operate at maximum capacity for as many years as you live.

Flexibility is the range of motion around specific joints—for example, the stretching you do to touch your toes or twist your torso. Flexibility depends on many factors: your age, gender, and posture; bone spurs; and how fat or muscular you are. As children develop, their flexibility increases until adolescence. Then a gradual loss of joint mobility begins and continues throughout adult life. Both muscles and connective tissue, such as tendons and ligaments, shorten and become tighter if not used at all or not used through their full range of motion.

Cardiovascular fitness refers to the ability of the heart to pump blood through the body efficiently. It is achieved through **aerobic exercise**—any activity, such as brisk walking or swimming, in which the amount of oxygen taken into the body is slightly more than, or equal to, the amount of oxygen used by the body. In other words, aerobic exercise involves working out

The three basic components of physical fitness: (a) flexibility, (b) cardiovascular or aerobic fitness, (c) muscular strength and endurance.

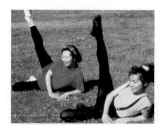

(a)

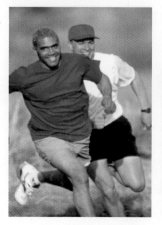

(b)

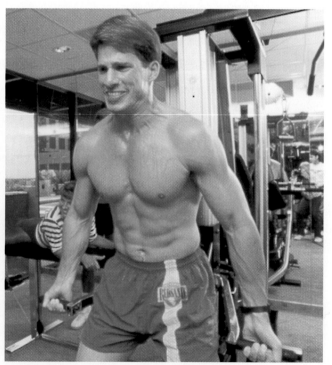

(c)

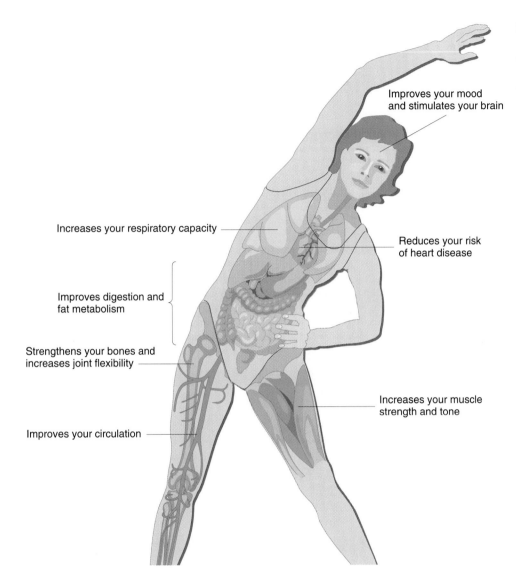

Improves your mood
and stimulates your brain

Increases your respiratory capacity

Improves digestion and
fat metabolism

Strengthens your bones and
increases joint flexibility

Improves your circulation

Reduces your risk
of heart disease

Increases your muscle
strength and tone

Figure 4-1
The benefits of exercise. Exercise
improves your body and mind more
than you might expect.

strenuously without pushing to the point of breathlessness. **Anaerobic exercise** is any activity in which the amount of oxygen taken in by the body cannot meet the demands of the activity; there is thus an oxygen deficit that must be made up later. An example of an anaerobic exercise is sprinting the quarter-mile, which leaves even the best-trained athletes gasping for air. In *nonaerobic exercise*, there is frequent rest between activities, as happens in bowling, softball, and doubles tennis. The body easily takes in all the oxygen needed for these activities, so your heart and lungs don't really get a workout.

Strength—the absolute maximum weight that we can lift, push, or press in one effort—is what most of us equate with muscular fitness. However, **endurance**—the ability to keep lifting, pushing, or pressing—is just as important. It's not enough to be able to hoist a shovelful of snow; you've got to be able to keep shoveling until the entire driveway is clear.

Physical **conditioning** (or training) refers to the gradual building up of the body to enhance one or more of the three main components of physical fitness: flexibility, cardiovascular or aerobic fitness, and muscular strength and endurance.

What Exercise Can Do for You

If exercise could be packed into a pill, it would be the single most widely prescribed and beneficial medicine in the nation. Why? Because nothing can do more to help your body function at its best (Figure 4-1). With regular activity, your heart muscles become stronger and pump blood more efficiently. Your heart rate and resting pulse slow down. Your blood pressure may drop slightly from its normal level.

Pulsepoints

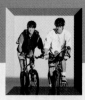

Ten Reasons to Work Out

1. Improve cardiovascular fitness. Regular activity strengthens the heart so it pumps blood more efficiently.

2. Tone muscles. With exercise, muscles become firmer, function more smoothly, and are capable of withstanding much more strain.

3. Reduce stress. Working out releases tensions and enhances your ability to deal with daily challenges.

4. Improve mood. Exercise may be the single most effective strategy for changing a bad mood. It also works wonders for reducing anxiety and depression.

5. Burn calories. Exercise speeds up metabolism, so the body uses more calories during and after a workout.

6. Increase flexibility. Exercise stretches and lengthens muscles and increases flexibility in the joints.

7. Enhance strength and stamina. Muscle workouts improve the circulation of blood in the tissues and increase the body's ability to do sustained work.

8. Keep bones strong. Regular physical activity (especially weight-bearing activities) thickens the bones, possibly

preventing the slow loss of calcium that normally occurs with age.

9. Lower the risk of disease. Exercise helps prevent many serious health problems, including high blood pressure, strokes, heart attacks, and certain cancers.

10. Put more life in your years—and possibly more years in your life. Physical activity slows the aging process, so you remain healthier and more active for a longer time. And if you work out often and vigorously enough, you can actually extend your lifespan.

Regular physical activity thickens the bones and can slow the loss of calcium that normally occurs with age. Exercise increases flexibility in the joints and improves digestion and elimination. It speeds up metabolism, so the body burns up more calories and body fat decreases. It heightens sensitivity to insulin (a great benefit for diabetics) and may lower the risk of developing diabetes. In addition, exercise enhances clot-dissolving substances in the blood, helping to prevent strokes, heart attacks, and pulmonary embolisms (clots in the lungs). Regular, vigorous exercise can actually extend the lifespan. (See Pulsepoints: "Ten Reasons to Work Out.")

A Hardier Heart and Stronger Lungs

Officials at the Centers for Disease Control and Prevention (CDC) have identified insufficient exercise as one of the leading preventable causes of coronary death in this country. Sedentary people are about twice as likely to die of a heart attack as people who are physically active.[2] In addition to its effects on the heart, exercise makes the lungs more efficient. They take in more oxygen, and their vital capacity (ability to take in and expel air) is increased, providing more energy for you to use.

Better Bones

Weak and brittle bones are common among people who don't exercise. **Osteoporosis**, a condition in which bones lose their mineral density and become increasingly soft and susceptible to injury, affects a great many older people. Women, in particular, are more vulnerable because their bones are less dense to begin with.

Brighter Mood

Exercise makes people feel good from the inside out. It boosts mood, increases energy, reduces anxiety, improves concentration and alertness, and enables people to handle stress better.[3] During long workouts, some people experience what is called "runner's high," which may be the result of increased levels of mood-elevating brain chemicals called **endorphins**.

Protection Against Certain Cancers

Exercise reduces the risk of colon and rectal cancers, possibly by enhancing digestion and elimination. In women, exercise also may help reduce the risk of cancer of the breast and reproductive organs.[4]

Less Fat, More Muscle

Aerobic exercise burns off calories during your workout, because as your body responds to the increased demand from your muscles for nutrients, your metabolic rate rises. Moreover, this surge persists for as long as 12 hours after exercise, so you continue to use up more calories than usual even after you've stopped sweating. In addition, aerobic exercise suppresses appetite, so you aren't as tempted to eat. It also helps dieters lose fat rather than lean muscle tissue when they cut back on calories.[5]

A More Active Old Age

Exercise slows the changes that are associated with advancing age: loss of lean muscle tissue, increase in body fat, and decrease in work capacity. In addition to lowering the risk of heart disease and stroke, exercise also helps older men and women retain the strength and mobility needed to live independently. Male and female runners over age 50 have much lower rates of disability and much lower health-care costs than less active seniors.[6]

How Much Exercise Do You Need?

Whatever your age, gender, or health status, you can benefit from exercise. As large, long-term studies have

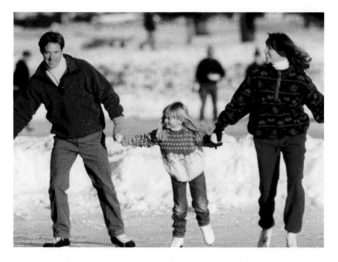

Encouraging children to be physically active gives them an advantage in aerobic fitness and endurance—and establishes the fitness habit for life.

shown, increasing activity, even in middle age, can reduce the danger of dying before one's expected time.[7] Even light exercise (any activity that increases oxygen consumption less than three times the level burned by the body at rest) can improve physical and emotional well-being. The more active you are, the more benefits you gain.

Moderate Exercise

The CDC and the American College of Sports Medicine currently call for a minimum of 30 minutes a day of moderate physical activity at least five times a week.[8] "Moderate" refers to any activity that increases oxygen consumption to three to six times the amount used by the body at rest.

In terms of health benefits, 30 minutes of moderate-intensity exercise, either in one sustained period or in shorter bursts of activity, is the equivalent of a brisk 2-mile walk. Almost any form of exertion—gardening, dancing, housework, playing actively with children—can help lower your risk of many chronic health problems, including heart disease, high blood pressure, diabetes, osteoporosis, colon cancer, anxiety, and depression.

Vigorous Exercise: Adding Years to Your Life

Although becoming more active can improve your overall health, it won't necessarily make you physically fit. To achieve your optimal fitness level—to function at your physiological best—you should follow the

CAMPUS FOCUS: COLLEGE STUDENTS AND EXERCISE

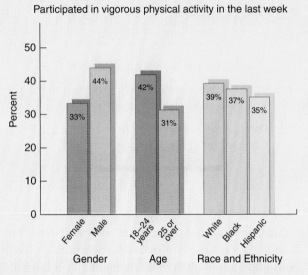

Participated in vigorous physical activity in the last week

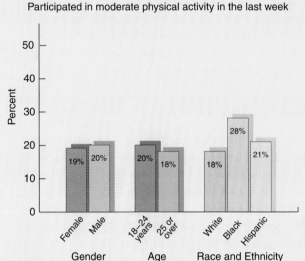

Participated in moderate physical activity in the last week

SOURCE: National College Health Risk Behavior Study, 1995.

recommendations of the American College of Sports Medicine and regularly engage in both aerobic activities for the cardiovascular system and strength-training exercises for the muscles. Aerobic activities should be performed for 20 to 60 minutes three to five times a week; strength workouts, two to three times a week.

Strategies for Prevention

How to Add Years to Your Life

To exercise at a vigorous enough level to burn up 1500 calories a week, you could:

✔ Walk at a rate of 3 to 4 miles an hour five times a week.

✔ Jog at a rate of 6 to 7 miles an hour for 3 hours a week.

✔ Cycle for an hour four times a week.

✔ Swim laps for 3 hours a week.

In addition to producing more health benefits, only vigorous exercise (defined as any activity that raises metabolic rate to six times or more above the resting rate) offers an added reward: a longer life. In a 1995 study that followed 17,300 men for more than 20 years, those who burned up 1500 calories in vigorous exercise—the equivalent of walking briskly or jogging for about 15 miles a week—had a 25% lower death rate than those who expended fewer than 150 calories a week.[9] The more active the men were—up to an activity level of 3000 calories a week—the longer they were likely to live. Smoking history, body weight, and age did not affect the relationship between physical activity and risk of death.

Flexibility

By simplest definition, *flexibility* refers to your ability to go through the complete range of motion that your joints allow in a comfortable, fluid fashion. Some people seem to be born more flexible than others. Other factors that affect flexibility include age, gender, posture, and how fat or muscular you are.

Of all the components of fitness, flexibility is the one most likely to be overlooked—until problems start. Unused muscles hold more tension, which can lead to muscle strain. And muscles shorten and tighten if they aren't used. If you spend a lot of time sitting in front of a computer, for instance, the hamstring muscles in your legs get shorter, and that can lead to lower back pain.

Everyone needs to work on overall flexibility, regardless of general fitness or activity level. But if you exercise, flexibility can be critical. Stiffness in one area (the shoulders, for instance) can increase the risk of injury in others (such as the knees and ankles during a run).

Keep in mind that warming up and stretching are not the same thing. A warmup involves getting the heart beating, breaking a sweat, and readying the body for more vigorous activity. Stretching, on the other hand, is a specific activity intended to elongate muscles and keep joints limber, not simply a prelude to some other activity, such as a game of tennis or a 3-mile run.

Stretching and warming up can prevent the soreness that occurs in surrounding connective tissue when muscle fibers are injured. Stretching actually may be more important after your workout. It helps move lactic acid out of your muscles, increases your range of motion, decreases soreness, and helps get blood, oxygen, and other nutrients to the muscle tissues.[10]

An extra benefit of stretching is that, like a body yawn, it loosens you up and relieves tension. Even a brief stretch break during the day can be relaxing. However, although stretching is one of the safest activities, it's important that you do it properly so you don't end up hurting instead of helping yourself. Always practice *static,* or passive, stretching—moving gradually into a stretch that you hold for a short time (6 to 60 seconds). An example of such a stretch is letting your hands slowly slide down the front of your legs (keeping your knees in a soft, unlocked position) until you reach your toes and holding this final position for several seconds before slowly straightening up.

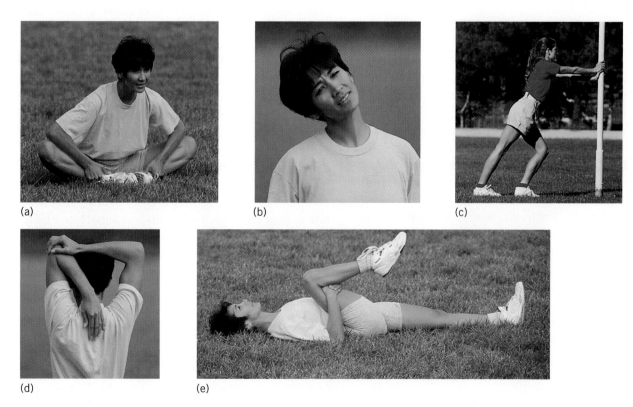

(a) (b) (c)

(d) (e)

Some simple stretching exercises. (a) *Foot pull for the groin and thigh muscles.* Sit on the ground and bend your legs so that the soles of your feet touch. Pull your feet closer as you press on your knees with your elbows. Hold for 10 seconds; repeat. (b) *Lateral head tilt.* Gently tilt your head to each side. Repeat several times. (c) *Wall stretch for the Achilles tendon.* Stand 3 feet from a wall or post with your feet slightly apart. Keeping your heels on the ground, lean into the wall. Hold for 10 seconds; repeat. (d) *Triceps stretch for the upper arm and shoulder.* Place your right hand behind your neck and grasp it above the elbow with your left hand. Gently pull the elbow back. Repeat with the left elbow. (e) *Knee-chest pull for lower back muscles.* Lying on your back, clasp one knee and pull it toward your chest. Hold for 15 to 30 seconds; repeat with the other knee.

Strategies for Change

Safe Stretching

Before you begin, increase your body temperature by slowly marching or running in place. Sweating signals that you're ready to start stretching.

✔ Don't force body parts beyond their normal range of motion. Stretch to the point of tension, back off, and hold for 10 seconds to a minute.

✔ Do a minimum of five repetitions of each stretch, with equal repetitions on each side.

✔ Don't hold your breath. Continue breathing slowly and rhythmically throughout your stretching routine. To strengthen muscles, tighten the muscles opposite the ones you're stretching.

✔ Don't do any stretches that require deep knee bends or full squats. These positions can harm your knees and lower back.

Ballistic stretching, by comparison, is characterized by rapid bouncing or jerking movements, such as a series of up-and-down bobs as you try again and again to touch your toes with your hands. These bounces can stretch muscle fibers too far, causing the muscle to contract rather than stretch; they can also tear ligaments and weaken or rupture tendons, the strong fibrous cords connecting muscles to bones.

Always move slowly into a stretch position. You should never feel pain, although you will feel a slight tugging as you extend your stretch. Reach to this point of discomfort and then back off slightly, relaxing and allowing your muscles to adjust. You should hold this stretch until the feeling of tension diminishes. Concentrate on the feeling of the stretch itself, not on the flexibility you want to attain. Perform stretching exercises regularly. "Use it or lose it" is the motto to keep in mind when it comes to flexibility.

Cardiovascular or Aerobic Fitness

Your heart and lungs need regular work to reach peak efficiency. If you haven't been exercising regularly, even mild forms of exertion, such as climbing stairs, can seem rigorous. As you get in shape, however, your body will be able to handle greater challenges with ease.

Your Target Heart Rate

The best way you can be sure you're working hard enough to condition your heart and lungs but not overdoing it is to use your pulse, or heart rate, as a guide. One of the easiest places to feel your pulse is in the carotid artery on either side of your neck. Tilt your head back slightly and to one side. Use your middle finger or forefinger, or both, to feel for your pulse. (Do not use your thumb; it has a beat of its own.) To determine your heart rate, count the number of pulses you feel for 10 seconds and multiply that number by six, or count for 30 seconds and multiply that number by two. Learn to recognize the pulsing of your heart when you're lying or sitting down. On your fitness record, make note of your **resting heart rate**.

Start taking your pulse during, or immediately after, exercise, when it's much more pronounced than when you're at rest. Three minutes after heavy exercise, take your pulse again. The closer that reading is to your resting heart rate, the better your condition. If it takes a long time for your pulse to recover and return to its resting level, your body's ability to handle physical stress is poor. As you continue working out, however, your pulse will return to normal much more quickly.

You don't want to push yourself to your maximum heart rate; yet you must exercise at about 60% to 85% of that maximum to get cardiovascular benefits from your training. This range is called your **target heart rate**. If you don't exercise intensely enough to raise your heart rate at least this high, your heart and lungs won't benefit from the workout. If you push too hard, on the other hand, and exercise at or near your absolute maximum heart rate, you run the risk of placing too great a burden on your heart.

Table 4-1 lists target heart rates for various ages. The following formulas can also be used to calculate your maximum and target heart rates (in beats per minute). For men, the formula is as follows:

	Maximum		(Target	Target
$220 - \text{Age} =$	Heart	$\times .60$	Zone for	$=$ Heart
	Rate		Beginners)	Rate

Example for a 20-year-old man:

	Maximum		Target
$220 - 20 = 200$	Heart	$\times .60 = 120$	Heart
	Rate		Rate

TABLE 4-1 TARGET HEART RATE

Age	Men Average Maximum Heart Rate (100%)	Men Target Heart Rate (60–85%)		Women Average Maximum Heart Rate (100%)	Women Target Heart Rate (60–85%)	
20	200	120	170	205	123	174
25	195	117	166	200	120	170
30	190	114	162	195	117	166
35	185	111	157	190	114	162
40	180	108	153	185	111	157
45	175	105	149	180	108	153
50	170	102	145	175	105	149
55	165	99	140	170	102	145
60	160	96	136	165	99	140
65	155	93	132	160	96	136
70	150	90	128	155	93	132

For women, the formula is as follows:

| 225 − Age = | Maximum Heart Rate | × .60 | (Target Zone for Beginners) | = | Target Heart Rate |

Example for a 20-year-old woman:

| 225 − 20 = 205 | Maximum Heart Rate | × .60 = 123 | Target Heart Rate |

In the initial stages of training, aim for the lower end of your target zone (the 60% just calculated) and gradually build up to 75% of your maximum heart rate. After 6 months or more of regular exercise, you can push up to 85% of your maximum heart rate if you wish, though you don't have to work that hard just to stay in shape. As long as you use your target heart rate as your guide, your exercise intensity should be just right.

Walking

According to recent studies, walking at an easy to moderate pace for 40 to 60 minutes is actually better than exercising hard for just 20 minutes. While both approaches enhance fitness, walking is less likely to lead to injuries.[11] Walking develops cardiovascular fitness, builds up endurance, burns fat, and strengthens muscles in the lower body. Another bonus is stress reduction. Since you can do it during a break or at lunchtime, walking builds relaxation into your day.[12]

If you're an exercise novice, start with a 10-minute walk every other day. As you get into better condition,

Strategies for Change

Putting Your Best Foot Forward

✔ Walk very slowly for 5 minutes and then do some simple stretches.

✔ Maintain good posture. Focus your eyes ahead of you, stand erect, and pull in your stomach.

✔ Use the heel-to-toe method of walking. The heel of your leading foot should touch the ground before the ball or toes of that foot do. When you push off with your trailing foot, bend your knee as you raise your heel. You should be able to feel the action in your calf muscles.

✔ Pump your arms back and forth to burn 5 to 10% more calories and get an upper-body workout as well.

✔ End your walk the way you started it—let your pace become more leisurely for the last 5 minutes.

you'll go further. In about 4 to 6 weeks, you should be able to manage a mile in 20 minutes. For maximum cardiovascular benefits, the American College of Sports Medicine suggests walking at least 20 to 30 minutes three or four times a week.

Treadmills are a good alternative to outdoor walks—and not just in bad weather. They keep you moving at a certain pace, they're easier on the knees, and they allow you to exercise in a climate-controlled, pollution-free environment—a definite plus for many city dwellers.

Jogging and Running

The difference between jogging and running is speed. You should be able to carry on a conversation with someone on a long jog or run; if you're too breathless to talk, you're pushing too hard.

If you have been sedentary, it's best to launch a walking program before attempting to jog or run. Start by walking for 15 to 20 minutes three times a week at a comfortable pace. Continue at this same level until you no longer feel sore or unduly fatigued the day after exercising. Then increase your walking time to 20 to 25 minutes, speeding up your pace as well.

When you can handle a brisk-minute walk, alternate fast walking with slow jogging. Begin each session walking and gradually increase the amount of time you spend jogging. If you feel breathless while jogging, slow down and walk. Continue to alternate in this manner until you can jog for 10 minutes without stopping. If you gradually increase your jogging time by 1 or 2 minutes with each workout, you'll slowly build up from 10 to 20 or 25 minutes per session. For optimal fitness, you should jog at least three times a week.

Strategies for Change

Running Right

- ✔ As you run, keep your back straight and your head up. Run tall, with your buttocks tucked in. Look straight ahead. Hold your arms slightly away from your body. Your elbows should be bent slightly so that your forearms are almost parallel to the ground. Move your arms rhythmically to propel yourself along.
- ✔ Have your heels hit the ground first. Land on your heel, rock forward, and push off the ball of your foot. If this is difficult, try a more flat-footed style.
- ✔ Avoid running on the balls of your feet; this produces soreness in the calves because the muscles must contract for a longer time. To avoid shin splints (a dull ache in the lower shins), stretch regularly to strengthen the shin muscles and to develop greater flexibility in your ankles.
- ✔ Avoid running on hard surfaces and making sudden stops or turns.
- ✔ Breathe through your nose and mouth to get more volume. Learn to "belly breathe": When you breathe in, your belly should expand; when you breathe out, it should flatten.

Other Aerobic Activities

Because variety is the spice of life, many people prefer different forms of aerobic exercise. All can provide many health benefits. Among the popular options:

- *Swimming.* More than 100 million Americans dive into the water every year. What matters for our heart's health, however, is getting a good workout, not just getting wet. Swimming is an excellent exercise for cardiovascular fitness and also rates fairly high for weight control, muscular function, and flexibility. However, it's not as effective as activities such as walking and running for building strong bones and preventing osteoporosis.

  For aerobic conditioning, you have to swim laps using a freestyle, butterfly, breast-, or backstroke. (The sidestroke is too easy.) You've also got to be a good enough swimmer to keep churning through the water for at least 20 minutes. Your heart will beat more slowly in water than on land, so your heart rate while swimming is not an accurate guide to exercise intensity. You should try to keep up a steady pace that's fast enough to make you feel pleasantly tired, but not completely exhausted, by the time you get out of the pool.
- *Cycling.* Bicycling, indoors and out, can be an excellent cardiovascular conditioner, as well as an effective way to control weight—provided you aren't just along for the ride. To gain aerobic benefits, mountain bikers have to work hard enough to raise their heart rates to their target zone and keep up that intensity for at least 20 minutes.
- *Crosscountry Skiing.* One of the most effective forms of aerobic exercise, crosscountry or Nordic

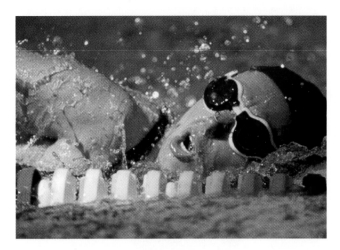

Swimming is good exercise for people of all ages, particularly for cardiovascular fitness and flexibility.

skiing has become an increasingly popular winter sport. Thanks to machines that simulate the moves of Nordic skiing, it's now possible to "ski" in any season. Because almost every muscle in the body gets a workout, crosscountry skiing is excellent for all-around conditioning.

- *Aerobic dancing.* This activity combines music with kicking, bending, and jumping. A typical class (you can also dance at home to a video or TV program) consists of stretching exercises and sit-ups, followed by aerobic dances and cool-down exercises. A particular benefit of aerobic dance is that people get enjoyment and stimulation from the music; they're also able to move their bodies without worrying about skill and technique. "Soft," or low-impact, aerobic dancing doesn't put as much strain on the joints as "hard," or high-impact, routines.

- *Step training or bench aerobics.* This low-impact workout combines step, or bench, climbing with music and choreographed movements. Basic equipment consists of a bench 4 to 12 inches high. The fitter you are, the higher the bench—but the higher the bench, the greater the risk of knee injury. A 40-minute step workout is equivalent to running at 7 miles an hour in terms of oxygen uptake and calories burned.

- *Rollerblading.* In-line skating can increase aerobic endurance and muscular strength and is less stressful on joints and bones than running or high-impact aerobics. Rollerbladers can adjust the intensity of their workout by varying the terrains. (Obviously, they'll have to work harder while

going up hills and less so on the slide down.) They can also buy special training wheels and weights to increase resistance and make muscles work harder. One caution: Protective gear, including a helmet, knee and elbow pads, and wrist guards, is essential.

Muscular Strength and Endurance

Although aerobic workouts condition your insides (heart, blood vessels, and lungs), they don't exercise many of the muscles that shape your outsides and provide power when you need it. Strength workouts are important because they enable muscles to work efficiently and reliably. Conditioned muscles function more smoothly and contract somewhat more vigorously and with less effort. With exercise, muscle tissue becomes firmer and can withstand much more strain—the result of toughening the sheath protecting the muscle and developing more connective tissue within it (see Figure 4-2).

The latest research on fat-burning shows that the best way to reduce your body fat is to add muscle-strengthening exercise to your workouts.[13] Muscle tissue is your very best calorie-burning tissue, and the more you have, the more calories you burn, even when you are resting. You don't have to become a serious body builder. Using handheld weights (also called free weights) two or three times a week is enough. Just be sure you learn how to use them properly because you can tear or strain muscles if you don't practice the proper weightlifting techniques.

A balanced workout regimen of muscle-building and aerobic exercise does more for you than just burn fat. It gives you more endurance by promoting better distribution of oxygen to your tissues and increasing the blood flow to your heart.

Exercise and Muscles

Your muscles never stay the same. If you don't use them, they atrophy, weaken, or break down. If you use them rigorously and regularly, they grow stronger. The only way to develop muscles is by demanding more of them than you usually do. This is called **overloading**. As you train, you have to increase the number of repetitions or the amount of resistance gradually and work the muscle to temporary fatigue. That's why it's important

Strength workouts increase circulation

The heart's right half pumps oxygen-poor blood to capillary beds in lungs. There, O_2 diffuses into blood and CO_2 diffuses out. The oxygenated blood flows into the heart's left half where it is then pumped to capillary beds throughout the body

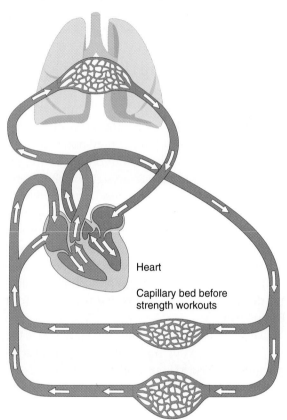

Heart

Capillary bed before strength workouts

Capillary bed after 8–12 weeks of strength workouts (extra capillaries develop, circulation increases)

Strength workouts build muscles

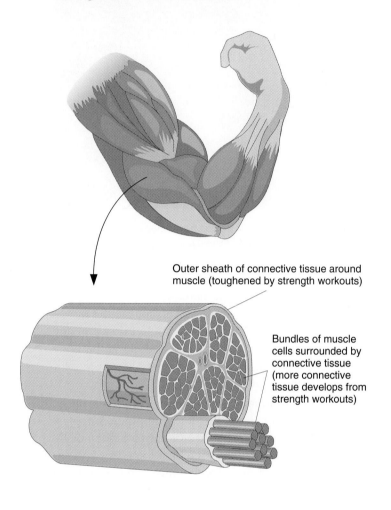

Outer sheath of connective tissue around muscle (toughened by strength workouts)

Bundles of muscle cells surrounded by connective tissue (more connective tissue develops from strength workouts)

Figure 4-2

Strength training in combination with aerobic exercise develops muscles, burns fat, and increases blood circulation and oxygen supply to body tissues.

not to quit when your muscles start to tire. Some exercise enthusiasts believe that the experience of pain—the "burn"—signals that exercise is paying off; however, others contend that it means you're pushing too hard and risking injury.

Muscular training is highly specific, which means that you have to exercise certain muscles for certain results. If you want to build up your leg muscles to run a marathon, push-ups won't help—just as running a marathon won't develop your upper body. If you're training with specific goals in mind, you have to tailor your exercise program to make sure you meet them.

Designing a Muscle Workout

A workout with weights should exercise your body's primary muscle groups: the *deltoids* (shoulders), *pectorals* (chest), *triceps* and *biceps* (back and front of upper arms), *quadriceps* and *hamstrings* (front and back of thighs), *gluteus maximus* (buttocks), and *abdomen* (see Figure 4-3). Various machines and free-weight routines focus on each muscle group, but the principle is always the same: Muscles contract as you raise and lower a weight, and you repeat the lift-and-lower routine until the muscle group is tired.

A weight-training program is made up of both **sets** (set numbers of repetitions of the same movement) and **reps** (the single performance of exercises, such as lifting 75 pounds once). You should allow your breath to return to normal before moving on to each new set. Pushing yourself to the limit builds strength.

Maintaining proper breathing techniques during weight training is crucial. To breathe correctly, inhale when muscles are relaxed, and exhale when you push or lift. Don't ever hold your breath because oxygen flow helps prevent muscle fatigue and injury.

Remember that your muscles need sufficient time to recover from a weight-training session. Allow no less than 48 hours, but no more than 96 hours, between training sessions, so that your body can recover from the workout and so that you'll avoid overtraining. Workouts on consecutive days do more harm than good, because the body can't recover that quickly. Two or three 30-minute training sessions a week should be sufficient for building strength and endurance. Indeed, you can obtain 70% to 80% as much improvement by strength training twice a week as three times a week. However, your muscles will begin to atrophy if you let more than 3 or 4 days pass without exercising them. For total fitness, you may want to schedule aerobic workouts for your days off from weight training.[14]

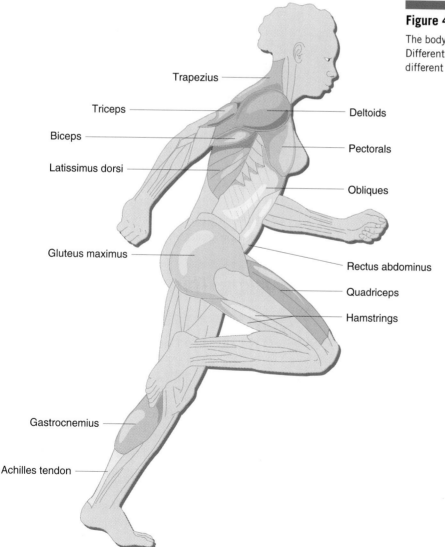

Figure 4-3

The body's primary muscle groups. Different exercises can strengthen and stretch different muscle groups.

Trapezius

Triceps

Biceps

Latissimus dorsi

Gluteus maximus

Gastrocnemius

Achilles tendon

Deltoids

Pectorals

Obliques

Rectus abdominus

Quadriceps

Hamstrings

Strategies for Prevention

Working with Weights

If you plan to work with free weights, here are some guidelines for using them safely and effectively:

✔ Don't train alone—for safety's sake. Work with a partner so you can serve as spotters for each other and help motivate each other as well.

✔ Always warm up and stretch before weight training and be sure to stretch after training.

✔ Begin with relatively light weights (50% of the maximum you can lift) and increase the load slowly until you find the weight that will cause muscle failure at anywhere from eight to twelve repetitions.

✔ In the beginning, don't work at maximum intensity. Increase your level of exertion gradually over 2 to 6 weeks to allow your body to adapt to new stress without soreness.

✔ Always train your entire body, starting with the larger muscle groups.

✔ Always use proper form. Unnecessary twisting, lurching, lunging, or arching can cause serious injury.

Sports Safety

Whenever you work out, you don't want to risk becoming sore or injured. Starting slowly when you begin any new fitness activity is the smartest strategy. Keep a simple diary to record the time and duration of each workout. Get accustomed to an activity first and then begin to work harder or longer. In this way, you strengthen your musculoskeletal system so you're less likely to be injured, you lower the cardiovascular risk, and you build the exercise habit into your schedule.

Even seasoned athletes should "listen to their bodies." If you develop aches and pains beyond what you might expect from an activity, stop. Never push to the point of fatigue. If you do, you could end up with sprained or torn muscles.

Preventing Injuries

According to the American Physical Therapy Association, the most common exercise-related injury sites are the knees, feet, back, and shoulders, followed by the ankles and hips. **Acute injuries**—sprains, bruises, and pulled muscles—are the result of sudden trauma, such as a fall or collision. **Overuse injuries**, on the other hand, are the result of overdoing a repetitive activity, such as running. When one particular joint is overstressed—such as a tennis player's elbow or a swimmer's shoulder—tendinitis, an inflammation at the point where the tendon meets the bone, can develop. Other overuse injuries include muscle strains and aches and stress fractures, which are hairline breaks in a bone, usually in the leg or foot.

To prevent injuries and other exercise-related problems before they happen, use common sense and take appropriate precautions.

Overtraining

About half of all people who start an exercise program drop out within 6 months. One common reason is that they **overtrain**, pushing themselves to work too intensely too frequently. Signs of overdoing it include persistent muscle soreness, frequent injuries, unintended weight loss, nervousness, and an inability to relax. If you're pushing too hard, you may find yourself unable to complete a normal workout or have difficulty recovering afterward.

If you develop any of the symptoms of overtraining, reduce or stop your workout sessions temporarily. Make gradual increases in the intensity of your workouts. Allow 24 to 48 hours for recovery between workouts. Make sure you get adequate rest. Check with a physical education instructor, coach, or trainer to make sure your exercise program fits your individual needs.

Making This Chapter Work for You
Shaping Up

■ A physically fit person has enough energy to meet routine physical demands, with enough reserve energy to cope with unexpected challenges. Fitness itself has three basic components: flexibility, cardiovascular or aerobic fitness, and muscular strength and endurance.

■ The preventive benefits of physical activity include a healthier heart, greater lung capacity, increased metabolism, stronger bones, better mood and mental health, protection against certain forms of cancer, lower weight, and a more active old age.

■ The CDC and the American College of Sports Medicine currently recommend a minimum of 30 minutes

Health Online

Cool Tools http://www.healthcalc.net/hcn/tools.htm

This site helps you with your fitness program by calculating your target heart rate and your energy expenditure during exercise. You can also take the Rockport One Mile Walking Test and calculate your results here. In addition, there are tips for those who would like to start a fitness program but don't know how to begin.

Think about it ...

- How might the information you get from this site help you plan your personal fitness program? How might it help a dedicated athlete?

- This site is maintained by E2 Consulting, a health and fitness software company. Does that information detract from or enhance your impression of the reliability of this site in any way?

a day of moderate physical activity at least 5 days a week. This can take almost any form—gardening, walking, dancing, housework, playing actively with children—and can help lower the risk of many chronic health problems, including heart disease, high blood pressure, diabetes, osteoporosis, colon cancer, anxiety, and depression.

- To achieve optimal fitness and function at your physiological best, the American College of Sports Medicine recommends a regular program of both aerobic activities for the cardiovascular system and strength-training exercises for the muscles. Aerobic activities should be performed for 20 to 60 minutes three to five times a week; strength workouts, two to three times a week.

- Different types of exercise produce different benefits. Stretching can improve flexibility. Aerobic exercises, which cause the heart and lungs to work harder and more efficiently, improve cardiovascular fitness. Building up strength and endurance through strength workouts ensures muscular fitness. A complete fitness program should include exercises for flexibility, aerobic fitness, and muscular strength.

- Among the many options for aerobic exercise are brisk walking, jogging or running, swimming, indoor and outdoor cycling, crosscountry skiing, aerobic dancing, rollerblading, and step training.

- To get the most out of physical activity, you need to eat a balanced diet, use common sense to prevent injuries, and avoid potential risks—such as overtraining.

Even though fitness products and facilities can make exercise more appealing, getting physical doesn't mean joining a health club, buying designer sportswear, or working out on expensive bodybuilding equipment. All you need, other than some good shoes, is a genuine desire to make the most of your body and a strategy for getting started.

Becoming more active is, above all else, a matter of making a commitment to make more of your body. Here are some guidelines to get you going:

- Add a new sport or physical activity you genuinely enjoy to your schedule.

- Carve out time for this activity. Write "Running" or "Tennis" (or whatever) on your calendar.

- Always try to exercise at the same time of day. For instance, you could jog in the morning before breakfast or in the evening before dinner.

- Get someone to go out with you, if that helps.

- As you aim for optimal fitness, start out slowly, proceed gradually, and be aware that there will be plateaus in your progress. Some days you'll exercise more slowly than others; that's okay. Some days you may not be able to exercise at all because of illness or bad weather; that, too, is okay. Just keep in mind that when you start exercising regularly again, you should build up slowly to reach your prior fitness level.

■ Be sure you don't overwork your body so that it becomes fatigued or injured. If your muscles persistently feel sore and stiff, if you have headaches, continuing fatigue, loss of appetite or weight, or cessation of menstruation, or if you develop emotional symptoms, such as depression or a lack of interest in your sport, you may be exercising too hard.

After a few months of leading a more active life, stop and take stock. Think of how much more energy you have at the end of the day. Ask if you're feeling any less stressed, despite the push and pull of daily pressures. Focus on the unanticipated rewards of exercise. Savor the exhilaration of an autumn morning's walk, the thrill of feeling newly toughened muscles bend to your will, or the satisfaction of a long, smooth stretch after a stressful day. Enjoy the pure pleasure of living in the body you deserve.

Key Terms

The terms listed here are used within the chapter. Page numbers are included for each term. A definition of each term is given in the green Glossary pages at the end of this book.

acute injuries *64*

aerobic exercise *52*

anaerobic exercise *53*

cardiovascular fitness *52*

conditioning *53*

endorphins *54*

endurance *53*

flexibility *52*

osteoporosis *54*

overloading *61*

overtrain *64*

overuse injuries *64*

physical fitness *52*

reps (or **repetitions**) *63*

resting heart rate *58*

sets *63*

strength *53*

target heart rate *58*

Review Questions

1. Why should you exercise? What are some of the benefits of exercise?

2. Define physical fitness. What are the three basic components of physical fitness, and how does each contribute to good health?

3. How does exercise help prevent heart disease? Cancer? Osteoporosis? Weight gain?

4. How do you calculate your target heart rate? What kinds of activities should you engage in to reach and maintain that rate?

5. What are some of the elements to consider in designing an exercise program? Design an exercise program for yourself. What are your goals, and how will you stick to them?

Critical Thinking Questions

1. Some exercise advocates have called for mandatory physical fitness training in schools and fitness requirements that students would have to meet to be promoted or graduate. Do you agree? Should schools focus solely on educating students' brains, or should physical fitness be a significant part of their education as well? Do you feel that your education has provided you with the information you need to stay fit throughout your life? Why or why not?

2. Shelley knows that exercise is good for her health, but figures that she can keep her weight down by dieting and worry about her heart and health when she gets older. "I look good. I feel okay. Why should I bother exercising?" she asks. What would you say in reply?

3. When he started working out, Jeff simply wanted to stay in shape. But he felt so pleased with the way his body looked and responded that he kept doing more. Now he runs 10 miles a day (longer on weekends), lifts weights, works out on Nautilus equipment almost every day, and plays racquetball or squash whenever he gets a chance. Is Jeff getting too much of a good thing? Is there any danger in his fitness program? What would be a more reasonable approach?

Connections to Personal Health Interactive

*To enhance your understanding of the material covered in this chapter, check out the following study aids on the **Personal Health Interactive CD-ROM**.*

■ Personal Insights: How Fit Are You?
■ Improving Fitness Through Stretching
■ **Online Research:** Physical Fitness

■ Study Page: Reflex Arc
■ Glossary & Key Term Review

 ## References

1. Pate, Russell, et al. "Physical Activity and Public Health: A Recommendation from the Centers for Disease Control and Prevention and the American College of Sports Medicine." *Journal of the American Medical Association,* Vol. 273, No. 5, February 1, 1995.

2. Franklin, Barry, and James Wappes. "Heart Health for a Lifetime." *Physician & Sports Medicine*, Vol. 28, No. 11, November 1997.

3. Martinsen, Egil, and Thoms Stephens. "Exercise and Mental Health in Clinical and Free-Living Populations." *Advances in Exercise Adherence*. Champaign, IL: Human Kinetics Publishers, 1994. Chollar, Susan. "The Psychological Benefits of Exercise." *American Health*, June 1995. Grabmeier, Jeff. "Exercise to Beat the Blahs." *American Health*, May 1995.

4. Brown, Harriet. "The Other Reward of Exercise; to a Better Mood and Leaner Limbs You Can Add a Lower Cancer Risk." *Health,* Vol. 8, No. 4, July–August 1994.

5. Pinkowish, Mary. "Exercising to Keep Weight Off." *Patient Care*, Vol. 31, No. 19, November 30, 1997.

6. Fries, James, et al. "Older Runners." *Annals of Internal Medicine*, October 1994. Welty, Ellen. "Fitness Through the Ages: Stay in Shape—in Your 20s, 30s, 40s and Beyond." *American Health*, July–August 1994. "Inactivity Increases Chance of Stroke in Older Men." *American Journal of Epidemiology*, Vol. 28, No. 9, November 1994.

7. Blair, Steven, et al. "Changes in Physical Fitness and All-Cause Mortality: A Prospective Study of Healthy and Unhealthy Men." *Journal of the American Medical Association*, Vol. 273, No. 14, April 12, 1995. Paffenbarger, Ralph, et al. "The Association of Changes in Physical-Activity Level and Other Lifestyle Characteristics with Mortality Among Men." *New England Journal of Medicine,* Vol. 328, No. 8, February 25, 1993.

8. Pate, et al., "Physical Activity and Public Health."

9. Lee, I-Min, et al. "Exercise Intensity and Longevity in Men: The Harvard Alumni Health Study." *Journal of the American Medical Association*, Vol. 273, No. 14, April 19, 1995.

10. "To Stretch or Not Stretch?" *Tufts University Health & Nutrition Letter*, Vol. 15, No. 18, December 1997.

11. Dolgener, Forrest, et al. "Validation of the Rockport Fitness Walking Test in College Males and Females." *Research Quarterly for Exercise & Sport,* Vol. 65, No. 2, June 1994.

12. "Improving Your Walking Workout." *University of California, Berkeley Wellness Letter*, Vol. 13, No. 3, December 1997. Early, Tracy. "Test Your Walking I.Q." *Current Health*, Vol. 24, No. 3, November 1997.

13. Artunian, Judy. "Burning Body Fat." *Current Health*, Vol. 21, No. 3, November 1994.

14. Stanten, Michele. "Weights or Aerobics: Which Comes First?" *Prevention*, Vol. 49, No. 12, December 1997.

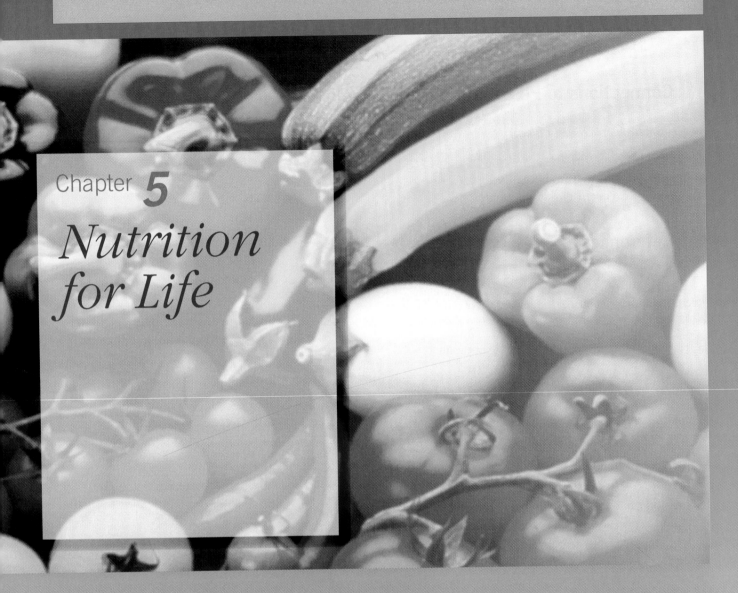

Chapter 5
Nutrition for Life

After studying the material in this chapter, you should be able to:

■ **List** and **define** the basic nutrients necessary for a healthy body.

■ **Explain** current recommendations for healthy eating and **use** the nutritional information provided on the new food labels to make healthy choices.

■ **Describe** the Food Guide Pyramid and **explain** its significance for nutrition.

■ **Explain** the importance of food safety to personal health.

■ **Develop** a personal plan for nutritional choices that promotes good health.

This chapter translates the latest information on good **nutrition** into specific advice that you can use to eat well and to feel well. Even small changes in the food choices you make can have a big payoff. For example, reducing saturated fat intake by an average of just 8 grams a day—the equivalent of two pats of margarine or butter—could prevent 2 million cases of heart disease and cut health-care costs by as much as $17 billion a year.[1]

Eating Right

We are faced with more choices than our great-great-grandparents could ever have imagined. We must figure out how much of which foods we need every day.

We all need the same essential **nutrients** to form muscles, bones, and other tissues and to provide energy for work and play. These nutrients include:

- *Proteins*, the building blocks of the body needed for growth, maintenance, and replacement of body cells.

- *Carbohydrates*, organic compounds that provide our bodies and brains with glucose—their basic fuel. Simple carbohydrates are often referred to as sugars; complex carbohydrates as starches.

- *Fats*, which provide energy and serve as carriers for certain vitamins.

- *Vitamins*, organic substances needed in very small amounts by the body to perform a variety of functions.

- *Minerals*, naturally occurring inorganic substances that are needed in small amounts for certain essential functions in the body.

- *Water*, the often-forgotten but essential substance that helps in digestion, elimination, and maintenance of bodily fluids and temperature.

Nutrients reach our body's structures through the process of digestion (see Figure 5-1). Each of the organs of the digestive system contributes to the process by either mechanically or chemically breaking down foods into small molecules capable of being absorbed into body cells.

Figure 5-1

Digestive system. The organs of the digestive system break down food into nutrients the body can use.

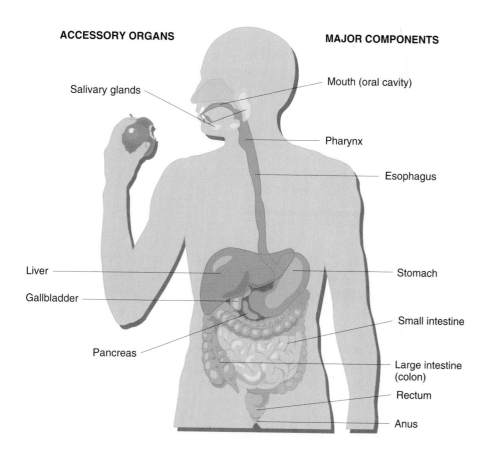

ACCESSORY ORGANS

MAJOR COMPONENTS

Salivary glands

Mouth (oral cavity)

Pharynx

Esophagus

Liver

Gallbladder

Pancreas

Stomach

Small intestine

Large intestine (colon)

Rectum

Anus

Strategies for Change

Dietary Guidelines

Based on nutritional research, the United States Department of Agriculture (USDA) has compiled the RDA (Recommended Daily Allowances) tables. The USDA has also developed the following guidelines for all Americans older than age 2 to help ensure lifelong optimal health and lower the risk of chronic diseases:

✔ *Eat a variety of foods.* Choosing among different types of foods every day helps ensure that you get the protein, vitamins, and minerals you need.

✔ *Maintain a healthy weight.* Excess pounds can increase your risk of high blood pressure, heart disease, stroke, certain cancers, and the most common kind of diabetes.

✔ *Choose a diet low in fat, saturated fat, and cholesterol.* Fat contains more than twice the calories of an equal amount of protein or carbohydrates and increases your risk of heart disease and certain types of cancer.

✔ *Choose a diet with plenty of vegetables, fruits, and grain products.* These foods provide vitamins, minerals, fiber, and complex carbohydrates.

✔ *Use sugars only in moderation.* Sugars, or simple carbohydrates, provide few nutrients for their calories and can contribute to tooth decay.

✔ *Use salt and sodium only in moderation.* Excessive sodium intake may increase your risk of high blood pressure. The Food and Drug Administration recommends that all adults restrict sodium to no more than 2400 milligrams a day.

✔ *If you drink alcoholic beverages, do so only in moderation.* Alcohol, which has a very low *nutrient density* (nutritional value compared to calories), can lead to dependence and other health problems.

The Food Guide Pyramid

The USDA's Food Guide Pyramid (see Figure 5-2), adopted in 1992, replaced the traditional Basic Four Food Groups—meats, milk products, fruits and vegetables, breads and cereals—with five categories. These categories are not considered nutritional equals. For the sake of good health, you need some food from all the groups every day, but in different amounts.

"The idea of the pyramid is to get people to eat more of the foods at its base (grains, fruits, and vegetables) and fewer of those toward the top (meat, milk products, sugars, and fats)," says Ann Shaw, Ph.D., a nutritionist with the federal Agriculture Research Service.[2] Foods in one group cannot substitute for those in another. Although the new guide doesn't ban any foods from plates or palates, the pyramid clearly advises less of some favorites, including meat.

The foods that should take center stage at mealtime are grain products. "They've been staples of the American diet for years," Shaw notes, "but we used to view them as fillers that we ate to satisfy our appetites and fill us up. Now we recognize their value as a source of nutrients, fiber, and energy." College students generally do not eat well-balanced diets. According to the National College Health Risk Behavior Survey, only 25% of undergraduate women and 28% of undergraduate men eat five or more servings of fruit or vegetables every day. Yet 84.9% of the women and 69.6% of the men have two or more servings of high-fat foods.[3] (See Campus Focus: "Nutrition on Campus.")

Breads, Cereals, Rice, and Pasta (6–11 servings a day)

These foods are the foundation of a healthy diet because they are a good source of complex **carbohydrates**. Both **simple** and **complex carbohydrates** (starches) have 4 calories per gram. Sugars provide little more than a quick spurt of energy, whereas complex carbohydrates are rich in vitamins, minerals, and other nutrients. Less than 25% of the daily calories in a typical American diet comes from complex carbohydrates; ideally, they should account for 50% to 60%.

A typical serving in this category might be one slice of bread and 1 ounce of ready-to-eat cereal (or one-half cup of cooked cereal, rice, or pasta). Although many people think of these foods as fattening, it's actually what you put on them, such as butter on a roll or cream sauce on pasta, that adds extra calories.

Here are suggestions for getting more grains in your diet:

● Add brown rice or barley to soups.

● Check the labels of rolls and bread and choose those with at least 2 to 3 grams of fiber per slice.

● Go for pasta power. Pasta has 210 calories per cooked cup and only 9 calories from fat. Like whole-grain breads, whole-grain pastas may provide more nutrients than those made with refined flour.

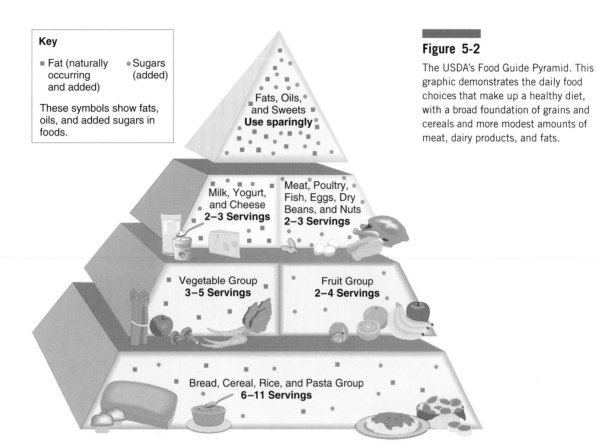

Figure 5-2

The USDA's Food Guide Pyramid. This graphic demonstrates the daily food choices that make up a healthy diet, with a broad foundation of grains and cereals and more modest amounts of meat, dairy products, and fats.

Key
- Fat (naturally occurring and added)
- Sugars (added)

These symbols show fats, oils, and added sugars in foods.

Fats, Oils, and Sweets
Use sparingly

Milk, Yogurt, and Cheese
2–3 Servings

Meat, Poultry, Fish, Eggs, Dry Beans, and Nuts
2–3 Servings

Vegetable Group
3–5 Servings

Fruit Group
2–4 Servings

Bread, Cereal, Rice, and Pasta Group
6–11 Servings

Vegetables
(3–5 servings a day)

Naturally low in fat and high in fiber, vegetables provide crucial vitamins (such as A and C) and minerals (such as iron and magnesium). As discussed later in this chapter and in Chapter 10, numerous studies linking diet to cancer have found "extraordinarily consistent scientific evidence" supporting the protective role of certain vegetables as well as fruits in preventing cancers of the lung, stomach, colon, bladder, pancreas, esophagus, mouth, larynx, cervix, ovary, endometrium, and breast. These benefits are so great that some have dubbed the switch to more produce as a "nutrition revolution."[4]

A serving in this category consists of one cup of raw leafy vegetables, one-half cup of other vegetables (either cooked or raw), three-quarters cup of vegetable juice, or one potato or ear of corn. Since different types of vegetables provide different nutrients, it's best to eat a variety. Dark green vegetables are especially good sources of vitamins and minerals; certain greens (such as collards, kale, turnip, and mustard) provide calcium and iron. Winter squash, carrots, and the plant family that includes broccoli, cabbage, kohlrabi, and cauliflower

(the **crucifers**) are high in fiber, rich in vitamins, and excellent sources of **indoles**, chemicals that help lower cancer risk.

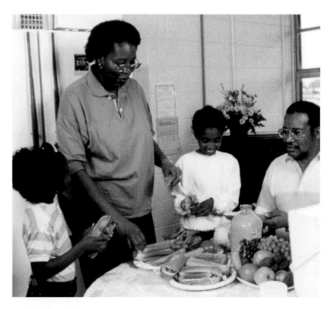

Including more vegetables in your diet doesn't mean eating like a rabbit—order the vegetable pizza instead of the pepperoni next time and add extra vegetables to your sandwiches and soups.

CAMPUS FOCUS: NUTRITION ON CAMPUS

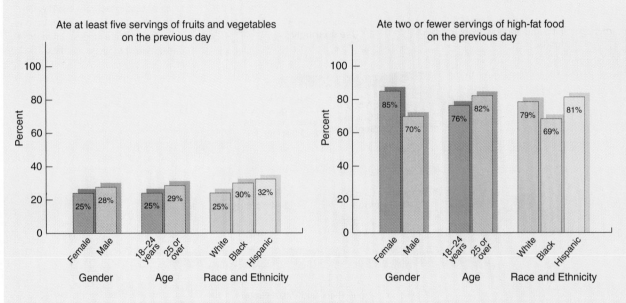

SOURCE: Douglas, Kathy, et al. "Results from the 1995 National College Health Risk Behavior Survey." *American Journal of College Health*, Vol. 46, September 1997.

Here are ways to increase your vegetable intake:

- Make or order sandwiches with extra tomatoes or other vegetable toppings.

- Add extra vegetables whenever you're preparing soups, sauces, and so on.

- If you can't find fresh vegetables, use frozen. They contain less salt than canned veggies.

- Use raw vegetables instead of chips for dipping.

Fruit (2–4 servings a day)

Like whole grains and vegetables, fruits are excellent sources of vitamins, minerals, and fiber. Along with vegetables, fruits may protect against cancer; those who eat little produce have a cancer rate twice that of people who eat the most fruits and vegetables.[5] A serving consists of a medium apple, banana, or orange; a half-cup of chopped, cooked, or canned fruit; or three-quarters of a cup of fruit juice.

Try the following suggestions to get more fruit into your daily diet:

- Carry a banana, apple, or package of dried fruit with you as a healthy snack.

- Eat fruit for dessert or a snack. Try poached pears, baked apples, or fresh berries.

- Start the day with a daily double: a glass of juice and a banana or other fruit on cereal.

- Add citrus fruits (such as slices of grapefruit, oranges, or apples) to green salads, rice, grains, and chicken, pork, or fish dishes.

- Squeeze fresh lemon or lime juice over seafood, fruit salads, or vegetable dishes.

Meat, Poultry, Fish, Dry Beans, Eggs, and Nuts (2–3 servings a day)

These foods are excellent sources of **protein**, which forms the basic framework for our muscles, bones, blood, hair, and fingernails and is essential for growth and repair. In addition, they supply phosphorus, iron, zinc, vitamin B-6, niacin, and other vitamins and minerals.

A serving in this category consists of 2 or 3 ounces of lean, cooked meat, fish, or poultry (roughly the size of an average hamburger or the amount of meat on half a medium chicken breast). An egg or one-half cup of cooked dry beans can substitute for 1 ounce of lean meat. Thus, one day's total protein intake might include an egg at breakfast, a serving of beans or 2 ounces of sliced chicken in a sandwich at lunch, and 3 ounces of fish for dinner.

To pick the best protein, try these recommendations:

- Choose the leanest meats, such as beef round or sirloin, pork tenderloin, or veal. Broil or roast instead of fry. Trim fat before cooking, which can lower the fat content by more than 10%. Marinate low-fat cuts to increase tenderness.

- Cook stews, boiled meat, or soup stock ahead of time, refrigerate, and remove the hardened fat before using. Drain fat from ground beef after cooking.

- Watch out for processed chicken and turkey products; for example, bolognas and salamis made from turkey can contain 45% to 90% fat.

- Select small chickens when you shop: They're leaner than large ones. Broiler-fryers are lowest in fat, followed by roasters. Remove skin before eating poultry.

- Choose fish as a leaner alternative to meat. It's high in protein and packed with vitamins and minerals. Fatty acids help lower the risk of cardiovascular disease.[6]

- Substitute bean-based dishes, such as chili or lentil stew, for meat entrees.

Milk, Yogurt, and Cheese (2–3 servings a day)

Most milk products are high in calcium, riboflavin, protein, and vitamins A and B-12. The Food Guide Pyramid recommends two servings of milk, yogurt, or cheese for most adults and three for women who are pregnant or breast-feeding. In addition, teenagers and young adults up to age 24 should also get three servings of milk products a day. Dairy products, such as milk and yogurt, are the best calcium sources, but be sure you choose products that are low-fat or preferably nonfat. A serving in this category consists of an 8-ounce cup of milk, one cup of plain yogurt, 1½ ounces of hard cheese, or 1 tablespoon of cheese spread. An 8-ounce glass of nonfat milk is a more nutritious choice than a tablespoon of a high-fat cheese spread.

To make sure you get more milk with less fat, try the following:

- Gradually switch from whole milk to 2%-fat (reduced fat) milk, then to 1%-fat (low-fat) milk, then to nonfat (skim) milk.

- Substitute fat-free sour cream or nonfat plain yogurt for sour cream.

- Use part-skim or low-fat cheeses whenever possible.

- Note that cottage cheese is lower in calcium than most cheeses. Thus, one cup of cottage cheese counts as only one-half serving of milk.

Fats, Oils, and Sweets

The Food Guide Pyramid places fats, oils, and sweets at the very top so that Americans will realize they should use them only in very small amounts. These foods supply calories but little or no vitamins or minerals.

Added sugars include sweeteners used in processing or at the table (such as jams, jellies, syrups, corn sweetener, molasses, fruit-juice concentrate, and the sugar in candy, cake, and cookies). These foods often are hidden in favorites—such as soft drinks (9 teaspoons of sugar per can), low-fat fruit yogurt (7 teaspoons per cup), fruit pie (6 teaspoons per serving), and catsup (a teaspoon in every tablespoon).

Try the following:

- Avoid temptation by not keeping a stash of cookies or candies.

- Put a small, child-sized spoon in the sugar bowl.

- When you crave a sweet, reach for nature's candy: fruit.

- If you want a daily sweet, have it as dessert, when you'll eat less of it, rather than as a snack.

- Drink fruit juices and water instead of sugar-laden soft drinks.

Water

The Food Guide Pyramid doesn't include water, but that doesn't mean it isn't important. Water makes up 85% of the blood, 70% of the muscles, and about 75% of the brain.[7] You lose about 64 to 80 ounces of water a day— the equivalent of eight to ten 8-ounce glasses—through urine, perspiration, bowel movements, and normal exhalation.[8] You lose water more rapidly if you're ill, live in a dry climate, are at a high altitude, drink a lot of coffee or alcohol (which increase urination), skip a meal, exercise, or travel on an airplane. Drink water before and during exercise to prevent dehydration. A general guideline is to drink one or two 8-ounce glasses of water 30 minutes to an hour before exercising and half to three-quarters of a glass of water every 10 to 20 minutes during a workout.

To keep up your water supply, try these tips:

- Don't substitute soft drinks, coffee, tea, or alcoholic beverages for water.

- Take regular water breaks to prevent mild dehydration. Keep a water bottle or pitcher nearby whenever possible.

- Respond quickly to thirst, which is a good but not foolproof indicator of dehydration. If you're ill, exercising, or at a high altitude, you need more fluid than usual, even if you don't feel thirsty.

- Check your urine. Dark yellow urine means your kidneys had to concentrate waste material into a smaller volume of water, while pale urine is a sign of good hydration.

The Payoffs of the Pyramid

The benefits of following the Food Guide Pyramid are many. By heeding its recommendations for eating a nutritious variety of foods, you'll be able to lower fat, increase fiber, get more vitamins and minerals, and possibly protect yourself from many illnesses.

Less Fat

Fats are a concentrated form of energy, providing 9 calories per gram—more than twice the amount in carbohydrates or proteins. A high-fat diet can lead to obesity and increase the risk of heart disease, certain cancers, and other health problems. (See Pulsepoints: "Top Ten Ways to Cut Fat.")

Forms of Fat

Fat can be saturated or unsaturated. **Saturated fats**, found mainly in meat, lard, butter, and "tropical" vegetable oils (such as coconut and palm), are most dangerous because they can increase the risk of heart disease and certain cancers, including those of the colon and breast. **Unsaturated fats**, which are usually liquid at room temperature, include polyunsaturates, such as those in oils derived from corn, soybeans, sunflowers, sesame, and cotton plants, and monounsaturates, such as those in olive and canola oils. Monounsaturated fats may be most healthful because they lower the levels of harmful forms of cholesterol. Polyunsaturates in liquid oils can do the same, although they may also reduce beneficial cholesterol forms.

Pulsepoints   Top Ten Ways to Cut Fat

1. Eat less meat. Rather than making meat the heart of a meal, think of it as a flavoring ingredient.

2. Forget frying. Instead, steam, boil, bake, or microwave vegetables or meats.

3. Switch to reduced-fat and nonfat dairy products. Rather than buying whole-fat dairy products, choose skim milk, fat-free sour cream, and low- or nonfat yogurts.

4. Season with herbs and spices. Avoid using fatty sauces, butter, or margarine. The abundance of herbs and spices in stores (or grown in a personal garden) makes them an attractive seasoning alternative.

5. Avoid high-fat fast foods. Hot dogs, fried foods, packaged snack foods, and pastries are most likely to be high in fat.

6. Say no to ice cream. As a tasty treat, try frozen ices and nonfat frozen yogurt instead.

7. Read labels carefully. Remember that "cholesterol-free" doesn't necessarily mean fat-free. Avoid products that contain highly saturated coconut oil, palm oil, or lard.

8. Check the numbers. When buying prepared foods, choose items that contain no more than 3 grams of fat per 100 calories.

9. Remove all visible fat. When you do serve meat, make sure to choose lean cuts and trim fat before and/or after cooking.

10. Think small. Remember that a dinner-size serving of meat should be about the size of a deck of cards or the palm of your hand. As you cut back on meat portions, serve larger amounts of fresh fruits and vegetables, grains, and beans.

Although Americans have long been advised to curtail dietary fat, particularly saturated fat, a 1997 report suggested that the type of fat—not the quantity eaten—may have a greater impact on heart health. Based on data from 80,000 nurses followed for 14 years, researchers concluded that most dangerous of all may be so-called **trans fats**, formed when liquid vegetable oils are processed to make hard or semisoft table spreads and cooking fats. Trans fats also are found in beef and dairy foods.

When you do use them, which fats should you choose? Olive oil, which is high in monounsaturated fats, is one of the best vegetable oils for salads and cooking. It has been used for thousands of years in countries around the Mediterranean, which have relatively low levels of heart disease. Canola oil is lowest in saturated fat and can be used for baking, stir-frying, and salad dressings.

In 1998, products made of Olean (also known by its generic name, olestra), the first calorie-free fat-replacement ingredient that can be used to fry foods, entered the national marketplace. Because the ingredients of Olean are processed in a special way, the body doesn't break them down, so Olean doesn't add fat or calories to foods. On the basis of more than 150 research studies, the FDA approved Olean for use in savory snacks, such as chips and crackers, and many medical organizations, including the American Dietetic Association, have supported its use as one way to reduce fat and calories in the diet. However, some participants in early tests have reported gastrointestinal side effects, and consumer advocacy groups, such as the Center for Science in the Public Interest, have warned that fat-replacement products may pose potential risks that could outweigh their benefits.[9]

The Cholesterol Connection

Dietary fats can increase blood levels of **cholesterol**, a lipid (fat) known mainly for its role in the development of heart disease. Foods high in saturated fat raise blood cholesterol levels more than any other foods, even those high in cholesterol.[10] Cutting back on fats, a strategy that has been proven healthful for adults, also is a safe and beneficial means of lowering high cholesterol levels in children over the age of 2.[11]

More Fiber

The increased servings of grains, fruits, and vegetables called for in the Food Guide Pyramid provide an added benefit: more of the indigestible leaves, stems, skins, seeds, and hulls of grains and plants containing dietary **fiber**. *Insoluble fibers*—cellulose, lignin, and some hemicellulose—increase bulk in feces, prevent constipation and diverticulosis (a painful inflammation of the bowel), and may lower the risk of colon cancer, heart disease, and stroke.[12] Whole grains also may help prevent chronic diseases, such as diabetes.[13] Good sources of insoluble fiber are wheat and corn bran (the outer layer), leafy greens, and the skins of fruits and root vegetables. *Soluble fibers*—pectin, gums, and some hemicellulose—lower blood cholesterol and may help control blood sugar levels.[14] Good sources of soluble fiber are oats, beans, barley, and the pulp of many fruits and vegetables, such as apples and citrus fruits. Foods rich in fiber also have higher levels of many other beneficial components, such as vitamins that may protect against cancer and heart disease.

Despite the benefits of fiber, few Americans eat enough. The National Cancer Institute recommends that a person consume 20 to 35 grams a day, but the average intake is about 11 to 13 grams. More servings of fruit and vegetables could make a big difference in fiber intake. One apple or half a grapefruit can add 2 grams of fiber to your diet.

If you have not been eating a high-fiber diet, increase grains, fruits, and vegetables gradually. A sudden increase in fiber intake can result in intestinal gas, bloating, cramps, and diarrhea—the consequences of fermentation of fiber and sugars in the colon. Try to spread out your fiber intake throughout the day and increase total consumption gradually to avoid these effects.

Knowing What You Eat

For years, many manufacturers advertised products as "nutritious," "healthy," or otherwise good for you, but offered little or no proof to back up such claims. Today, thanks to the Nutrition Labeling and Education Act, enacted in 1994, food manufacturers must provide information about fat, calories, and ingredients in large type on packaged food labels that must show how a food item fits into a daily diet of 2000 calories. The law also restricts nutritional claims for terms such as *healthy*, *low fat*, or *high fiber*.[15]

Figuring Out Food Labels

As Figure 5-3 shows, the "Nutrition Facts" on food labels present a wealth of information—if you know what to

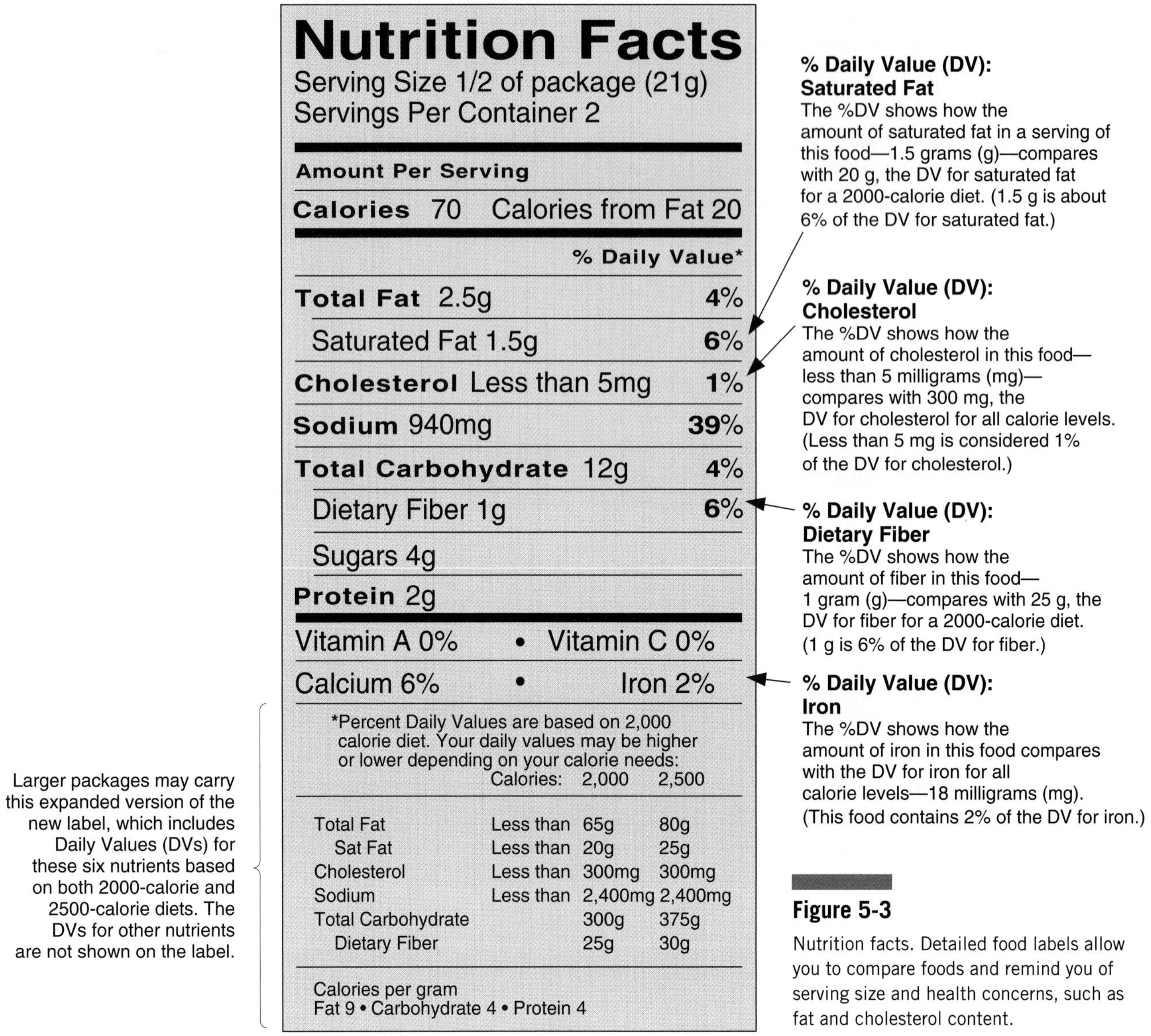

Nutrition Facts

Serving Size 1/2 of package (21g)
Servings Per Container 2

Amount Per Serving

Calories 70   Calories from Fat 20

% Daily Value*

Total Fat 2.5g	**4%**
Saturated Fat 1.5g	**6%**
Cholesterol Less than 5mg	**1%**
Sodium 940mg	**39%**
Total Carbohydrate 12g	**4%**
Dietary Fiber 1g	**6%**
Sugars 4g	
Protein 2g	

Vitamin A 0%	•	Vitamin C 0%	
Calcium 6%	•	Iron 2%	

*Percent Daily Values are based on 2,000 calorie diet. Your daily values may be higher or lower depending on your calorie needs:

		Calories:	2,000	2,500
Total Fat	Less than		65g	80g
Sat Fat	Less than		20g	25g
Cholesterol	Less than		300mg	300mg
Sodium	Less than		2,400mg	2,400mg
Total Carbohydrate			300g	375g
Dietary Fiber			25g	30g

Calories per gram
Fat 9 • Carbohydrate 4 • Protein 4

% Daily Value (DV):
Saturated Fat
The %DV shows how the amount of saturated fat in a serving of this food—1.5 grams (g)—compares with 20 g, the DV for saturated fat for a 2000-calorie diet. (1.5 g is about 6% of the DV for saturated fat.)

% Daily Value (DV):
Cholesterol
The %DV shows how the amount of cholesterol in this food— less than 5 milligrams (mg)— compares with 300 mg, the DV for cholesterol for all calorie levels. (Less than 5 mg is considered 1% of the DV for cholesterol.)

% Daily Value (DV):
Dietary Fiber
The %DV shows how the amount of fiber in this food— 1 gram (g)—compares with 25 g, the DV for fiber for a 2000-calorie diet. (1 g is 6% of the DV for fiber.)

% Daily Value (DV):
Iron
The %DV shows how the amount of iron in this food compares with the DV for iron for all calorie levels—18 milligrams (mg). (This food contains 2% of the DV for iron.)

Figure 5-3

Nutrition facts. Detailed food labels allow you to compare foods and remind you of serving size and health concerns, such as fat and cholesterol content.

Larger packages may carry this expanded version of the new label, which includes Daily Values (DVs) for these six nutrients based on both 2000-calorie and 2500-calorie diets. The DVs for other nutrients are not shown on the label.

look for. The label focuses on those nutrients most clearly associated with disease risk and health: total fat, saturated fat, cholesterol, sodium, total carbohydrate, dietary fiber, sugar, and protein.

- *Calories.* **Calories** are the measure of the amount of energy that can be derived from food. The label lists two numbers for calories: calories per serving and calories from fat per serving. This allows consumers to calculate how many calories they'll consume and to determine the percentage of fat in an item.

- *Serving size.* Rather than the tiny portions manufacturers sometimes used in the past to keep down the number of calories per serving, the new labels reflect more realistic portions.

- *Daily Values (DVs).* DVs refer to the total amount of a nutrient that the average adult should aim to get or not exceed on a daily basis. The DVs for cholesterol, sodium, vitamins, and minerals are the same for all adults. The DVs for total fat, saturated fat, carbohydrate, fiber, and protein are based on a 2000-calorie daily diet—the amount of food ingested by many American men and active women.

- *Percent Daily Values (%DV).* The goal for a full day's diet is to select foods that together add up to 100% of the DVs. The %DVs shows how a particular food's nutrient content fits into a 2000-calorie diet.

- *Calories per gram.* The bottom of the food label lists the number of calories per gram for fat, carbohydrates, and protein.

What Should You Look For?

Different people may zero in on different figures on the food label—for example, calories if they're watching their weight or specific ingredients if they have **food allergies**. Among the useful items to check are the following:

- *Calories from fat.* Get into the habit of calculating the percentage of fat calories in a food before buying or eating it.

- *Total fat.* Since the average person munches on fifteen to twenty food items a day, it's easy to overload on fat. Saturated fat is a figure worthy of special attention because of its reported link to several diseases (discussed later in this chapter).

- *Cholesterol.* Cholesterol is made by and contained in products of animal origin only. Many high-fat products, such as potato chips, contain 0% cholesterol because they're made from plants and are cooked in vegetable fats. However, the vegetable fats they contain can be processed and made into saturated fats that are more harmful to the heart than cholesterol itself.

- *Sugars.* There is no DV for sugars because health experts have yet to agree on a daily limit. The figure on the label includes naturally present sugars, such as lactose in milk and fructose in fruit, as well as those added to the food, such as table sugar, corn syrup, or dextrose.

- *Fiber.* A "high-fiber" food has 5 or more grams of fiber per serving. A "good" source of fiber provides at least 2.5 grams. "More or added" fiber means at least 2.5 grams more per serving than similar foods—10% more of the DV for fiber.

- *Calcium.* "High" equals 200 milligrams (mg) or more per serving. "Good" means at least 100 mg, while "more" indicates that the food contains at least 100 mg or more calcium—10% more of the DV—than the item usually would have.

- *Sodium.* Since many foods contain sodium, most of us routinely get more than we need. It's important to read labels carefully to avoid excess sodium, which can be a health threat.[16]

- *Vitamins.* A DV of 10% of any vitamin makes a food a "good" source; 20% qualifies it as "high" in a certain vitamin.

More Vitamins and Minerals

Vitamins and **minerals** are nutrients that are essential to regulating growth, maintaining tissue, and releasing energy from foods. Vitamins help put proteins, fats, and carbohydrates to use. Together with the enzymes in the body, they help produce the right chemical reactions at the right times. They're also involved in the manufacture of blood cells, as well as hormones and other compounds.

Some vitamins are produced within the body. Vitamin D, for example, is manufactured in the skin after exposure to sunlight and changed to an active form through processes in the liver and then the kidney. However, most vitamins must be ingested. Vitamins such as A, D, E, and K are *fat-soluble*—absorbed through the intestinal membranes and stored in the body. The B vitamins and vitamin C are *water-soluble*—absorbed directly into the blood and then used up or washed out of the body in urine and sweat. They must be replaced daily (see Table 5-1).

The elements carbon, oxygen, hydrogen, and nitrogen make up 96% of our body weight. The other 4% consists of minerals, which help build bones and teeth, aid in muscle function, and help our nervous systems transmit messages. We need daily about a tenth of a gram (100 mg) or more of each of the *major minerals*: sodium, potassium, chloride, calcium, phosphorus, and magnesium. We also need daily about a hundredth of a gram (10 mg) or less of each of the *trace minerals*: iron (more than that for premenopausal women), zinc, selenium, molybdenum, iodine, cobalt, copper, manganese, fluoride, and chromium (see Table 5-2).

Antioxidants: The Promise of Prevention

Antioxidants are substances that prevent the harmful effects caused by oxidation within the body. There has been great general and scientific interest in the antioxidant vitamins, particularly vitamin C, vitamin E, and beta carotene (a form of vitamin A). The proven health benefits of these vitamins are many. Vitamin C speeds healing, helps prevent infection, and prevents scurvy. Vitamin E helps prevent heart disease by stopping the oxidation of low-density lipoprotein (the harmful form of cholesterol), strengthens the immune system, and may help prevent Alzheimer's disease, cataracts, and some forms of cancer. Beta carotene aids eyesight and resistance to infection and keeps skin, hair, teeth, gums, and bones healthy.[17]

Table 5-1 Key Information About the Vitamins

Vitamin	Major Dietary Sources	Major Functions	Signs of Severe, Prolonged Deficiency	Signs of Extreme Excess
Fat-Soluble				
A	Fat-containing and fortified dairy products; liver; provitamin carotene in orange and deep green fruits and vegetables	Antioxidant; retinoic acid affects gene expression; needed for epithelial cells and all new cell synthesis; still under intense study	Night blindness; dry, scaling skin; increased susceptibility to infection	Damage to liver, bone; headache, irritability, vomiting, hair loss, blurred vision; some fetal defects; yellowed skin
D	Fortified and full-fat dairy products, egg yolk (diet often not as important as sunlight exposure)	Promotes absorption and use of calcium and phosphorus	Rickets (bone deformities) in children; osteomalacia (bone softening) in adults	Calcium deposition in tissues leading to cerebral, cardiovascular, and kidney damage
E	Vegetable oils and their products; nuts, seeds	Antioxidant to prevent cell membrane damage; still under intense study	Possible anemia and neurological effects	Generally nontoxic, but may worsen clotting defect in vitamin K deficiency
K	Green vegetables; tea; dairy products; produced internally by intestinal bacteria	Aid in formation of certain proteins, especially those for blood clotting	Defective blood coagulation, causing severe bleeding on injury	Liver damage and anemia from high doses of the synthetic form menadione
Water-Soluble				
Thiamin (B-1)	Pork, legumes, peanuts, enriched or whole-grain products	Coenzyme used in energy metabolism	Nerve changes; sometimes edema; heart failure; beriberi	Generally nontoxic, but repeated injections may cause shock reaction
Riboflavin (B-2)	Dairy products, meats, eggs, enriched grain products, green leafy vegetables	Coenzyme used in energy metabolism	Skin lesions	Generally nontoxic
Niacin	Nuts, meats; provitamin tryptophan in most proteins	Coenzyme used in energy metabolism	Pellagra (multiple vitamin deficiencies including niacin)	Flushing of face, neck, hands; potential liver damage
B-6	High-protein foods in general; bananas, potatoes, avocados	Coenzyme used in amino acid metabolism	Nervous, skin, and muscular disorders; anemia	Unstable gait, numb feet, poor coordination
Folic acid	Green vegetables, orange juice, nuts, legumes, grain products	Coenzyme used in DNA and RNA metabolism; single carbon utilization; needed for hemoglobin synthesis	Megaloblastic anemia; pernicious anemia when due to an inadequate intrinsic factor; nervous system damage	Thought to be nontoxic
Pantothenic acid	Animal products and whole grains; widely distributed in foods	Coenzyme used in energy metabolism	Fatigue, numbness, and tingling of hands and feet	Generally nontoxic; occasionally causes diarrhea
Biotin	Widely distributed in foods	Coenzyme used in energy metabolism	Scaly dermatitis	Thought to be nontoxic
C (ascorbic acid)	Fruits and vegetables, especially broccoli, cabbage, cantaloupe, cauliflower, citrus fruits, green pepper, kiwi fruit, strawberries	Functions in synthesis of collagen; is an antioxidant; aids in detoxification; improves iron absorption; still under intense study	Scurvy; petechiae (minute hemorrhages around hair follicles); weakness; delayed wound healing; impaired immune response	Gastrointestinal upsets, confounds certain lab tests

Source: Shils, M. E., and V. R. Young, eds. *Modern Nutrition in Health and Disease.* Philadelphia: Lea & Febiger, 1988.

Antioxidants also may prevent damage to our cells caused by *free radicals* (oxygen molecules formed by normal metabolic processes) as well as by smog, smoke, radiation, and cancer-promoting chemicals. These free radicals act like biological terrorists in the body, damaging or killing healthy cells so they cannot perform their usual functions. For example, free radicals may alter a cell's DNA (deoxyribonucleic acid), the basic genetic blueprint, in ways that could lead to uncontrolled cell growth—that is, to cancer. They also may play a role in the buildup of cholesterol in the arteries.[18]

Because there currently is no conclusive scientific evidence for the effectiveness of antioxidants or for the safety of taking large amounts of these substances over many years, the FDA does not recommend antioxidant supplements.

TABLE 5-2 KEY INFORMATION ABOUT MANY ESSENTIAL MINERALS

Mineral	Major Dietary Sources	Major Functions	Signs of Severe, Prolonged Deficiency	Signs of Extreme Excess
Major Minerals				
Calcium	Milk, cheese, dark green vegetables, legumes	Bone and tooth formation; blood	Stunted growth; perhaps less bone mass; clotting; nerve transmission	Depressed absorption of some other minerals; perhaps kidney damage
Magnesium	Whole grains, green leafy vegetables	Component of enzymes	Neurological disturbances	Neurological disturbances
Sodium	Salt, soy sauce, cured meats, pickles, canned soups, processed cheese	Body water balance; nerve function	Muscle cramps; reduced appetite	High blood pressure in genetically predisposed individuals
Potassium	Meats, milk, many fruits and vegetables, whole grains	Body water balance; nerve function	Muscular weakness; paralysis	Muscular weakness; cardiac arrest
Trace Minerals				
Iron	Meats, eggs, legumes, whole grains, green leafy vegetables	Components of hemoglobin, myoglobin, and enzymes	Iron deficiency anemia, weakness, impaired immune function	Acute: shock, death Chronic: liver damage; cardiac failure
Iodine	Marine fish and shellfish, dairy products, iodized salt, some breads	Component of thyroid hormones	Goiter (enlarged thyroid)	Iodide goiter
Fluoride	Drinking water, tea, seafood	Maintenance of tooth (and maybe bone) structure	Higher frequency of tooth decay	Acute: gastrointestinal distress Chronic: mottling of teeth; skeletal deformation
Zinc	Meats, seafood, whole grains	Component of enzymes	Growth failure; scaly dermatitis; reproductive failure; impaired immune function	Acute: nausea; vomiting; diarrhea Chronic: adversely affects copper metabolism, anemia; and immune function
Selenium	Seafood, meat, whole grains	Component of enzymes functions in close association with vitamin E	Muscle pain; maybe heart muscle deterioration	Nausea and vomiting; hair and nail loss

SOURCE: Shils, M. E. "Magnesium." In Shils, M. E., and V. R. Young, eds., *Modern Nutrition in Health and Disease.* Philadelphia: Lea & Febiger, 1988. Fairbanks, V. F., and E. Beutler. "Iron." In Shils and Young, eds., *Modern Nutrition.* Solomons, N. W. "Zinc and Copper." In Shils and Young, eds., *Modern Nutrition.* Underwood, E. J. *Trace Elements in Human and Animal Nutrition.* New York: Academic Press, 1977.

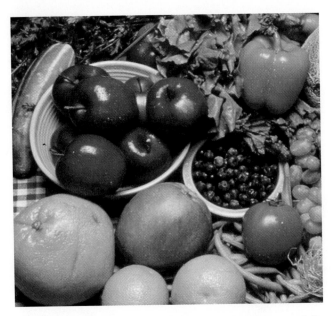

Antioxidant salad. Believe it or not, it's easy to get your daily antioxidant fix directly from food. Just eat an orange for breakfast and half a carrot for lunch and you'll have all the vitamin A (1000 retinal equivalents) and vitamin C (60 milligrams) you need for the day.

Do You Need Supplements?

An estimated 100 million Americans spend $6.5 billion a year on vitamins and minerals, according to the Council for Responsible Nutrition in Washington, D.C., a trade group for the vitamin supplement industry. So many people are taking supplements to prevent cancer, protect their hearts, lengthen their lives, or enhance their energy that some say "vitamania" is sweeping the country.[19]

Many health experts feel that the best way to make sure your body gets the vitamins and minerals it needs is to follow the Food Guide Pyramid and eat a wide variety of foods. If you rely on vitamin/mineral pills and fortified foods to make up for poor nutrition, you may shortchange yourself. However, supplements can benefit people whose diets do not provide adequate nutrients. For instance, supplements of the antioxidant selenium may help lower the risk of lung, colorectal, and prostate cancers in people living in areas with low soil selenium.[20] Selenium may also prevent these cancers in individuals with a history of skin cancer.[21,22]

Beginning in 1998, food manufacturers began adding folic acid, or folate, a B vitamin, to America's food. The primary reason is that insufficient levels of folic acid increase the risk of neural tube defects (abnormalities of the brain and spinal cord), such as spina bifi-da, in which a piece of the spinal cord protrudes from the spinal column.

Calcium, the most abundant mineral in the body, builds strong bone tissue throughout our lives and plays a vital role in heart and brain functioning. Adequate calcium is especially critical for pregnant or nursing women, who need it to meet the additional needs of their babies' bodies. Calcium may also help control high blood pressure and prevent colon cancer in adults.

Adequate calcium intake during the teens and twenties may be crucial to prevent osteoporosis, the bone-weakening disease that strikes one out of every four women over the age of 60. Dietary calcium can significantly increase the bone density of children, safeguarding against osteoporosis in later life. Research has shown that elderly men and women who consume adequate calcium can keep their bones strong and prevent fractures.[23] Although calcium-rich foods should provide the bulk of calcium intake, supplements may be needed to ensure adequate calcium intake.

Getting enough iron can be a big problem for women, whose iron stores are drained by menstruation, pregnancy, and nursing. Half of all women of childbearing age get less than the RDA of 15 mg, and 5% suffer from iron-deficiency anemia.

The symptoms of iron deficiency are sensitivity to cold, chronic fatigue, edginess, depression, sleeplessness, and susceptibility to colds and infections. Don't take supplements unless you've had a blood test that indicates you should. Excess iron can cause severe constipation and other complications.

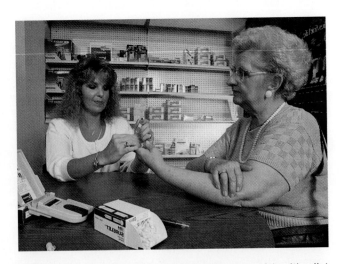

Women are more susceptible to anemia than men. A healthy diet that includes whole-grain cereals, broccoli, and foods rich in vitamin C is a good strategy for boosting iron stores.

Even though there's little proof that multivitamin supplements help, many people figure that taking them certainly can't hurt. As they see it, supplements serve as a nutritional insurance policy, something to fall back on in case they don't get everything they need from whole foods. For the most part, this is true. "If you have a good diet and you take a multivitamin supplement, there's probably no danger," says nutritionist Ann Shaw. "But if you take megadoses of a single vitamin or several different vitamins, you could run into problems."[24]

Large doses of vitamins can be especially dangerous for individuals with certain health conditions. Excessive intake of vitamin C or D may precipitate the formation of kidney stones in the urinary tract. Too much vitamin B-6 may inhibit milk production in breast-feeding mothers. In individuals suffering from epilepsy, folate may interfere with their drug therapy.

The Way We Eat

For centuries, Native Americans ate a diet of corn, beans, fish, game, wild greens, wild fruits, squash, and tomatoes. Over time the United States—a nation of immigrants—has imported a wide variety of ethnic cuisines. Many people think of hamburgers, steak, potatoes, cheesecake, and ice cream as "all-American" favorites. But in addition, most cities across the country feature the tastes of dozens of different cultural cuisines.

Dietary Diversity

Whatever your cultural heritage, you have probably sampled Chinese, Mexican, Indian, Italian, and Japanese foods. If you belong to any of these ethnic groups, you may eat these cuisines regularly. Each type of ethnic cooking has its own nutritional benefits and potential drawbacks (see Figure 5-4). In addition, different foods or eating rituals may have special religious or cultural significance.

Vegetarian Diets

Not all vegetarians avoid all meats. Some, who call themselves "lact-ovo-pesco-vegetarians," eat dairy products, eggs, chicken, and fish, but not red meat. **Lacto-vegetarians** eat dairy products as well as grains, fruits, and vegetables; **ovo-lacto-vegetarians** also eat eggs.

Figure 5-4

Diet and life expectancy. Nutritionists in various countries have different ideas about what constitutes a healthful diet. Putting science aside, here's a look at eating habits and longevity in several developed countries around the world.

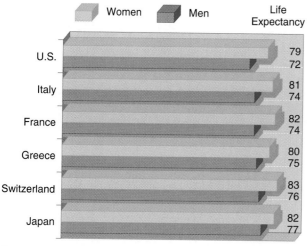

Country	Life Expectancy (Women / Men)
U.S.	79 / 72
Italy	81 / 74
France	82 / 74
Greece	80 / 75
Switzerland	83 / 76
Japan	82 / 77

Source: *1994 World Almanac.*

Country	Traditional Diet
U.S.	High in meat, fat, sugar, processed foods. Low in seafood, grains, fresh fruits and vegetables.
Italy	High in cheese, olive oil, meat, grains, wine. Low in processed foods.
France	High in butter, cheese, wine. Low in meat, processed foods.
Greece	High in olives, olive oil, yogurt, seafood, cheese, nuts. Low in meat, processed foods.
Switzerland	High in animal fat, cheese and meat. Low in seafood.
Japan	High in seafood, soy products, rice. Low in fat, cheese, meat.

Source: *American Health,* December 1994.

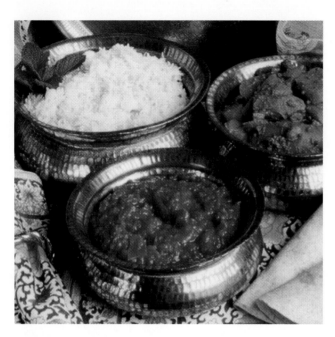
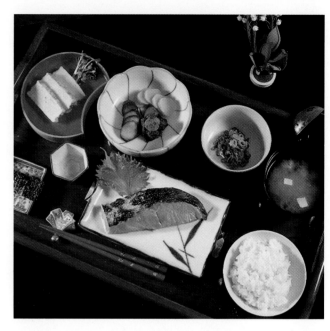

All-American diversity. The rice and beans of Mexico are healthy and high in protein, but too much cheese can cancel some of the benefits. The Japanese diet is high in seafood and rice and low in fats, cheese, and meat.

Pure vegetarians, called **vegans**, eat only plant foods; often they take vitamin B-12 supplements, because that vitamin is normally found only in animal products. If they select their food with care, vegetarians can get sufficient amounts of protein, vitamin B-12, iron, and calcium without supplements (see Figure 5-5).

The key to getting sufficient protein from a vegetarian diet is understanding the concept of **complementary proteins**. Meat, poultry, fish, eggs, and dairy products are **complete proteins** that provide the nine essential **amino acids**—substances containing carbon, hydrogen, oxygen, and nitrogen that the human body cannot produce itself. **Incomplete proteins**, such as legumes and nuts, may have relatively low levels of one or two essential amino acids, but fairly high levels of others. By combining complementary protein sources, you can make sure that your body makes the most of the nonanimal proteins you eat. Many cultures rely heavily on complementary foods for protein. In Middle Eastern cooking, sesame seeds and chick-peas are a popular combination; in Latin American dishes, beans and rice or beans and tortillas; in Chinese cuisine, soy and rice.

Vegetarian diets have proven health benefits. Studies show that vegetarians' cholesterol levels are low, and vegetarians are seldom overweight. As a result, they're less apt to be candidates for heart disease than those who consume large quantities of meat. Vegetarians also have lower incidences of breast, colon, and prostate cancer; high blood pressure; and osteoporosis.

Strategies for Prevention

A Guide to Fast Foods

✔ For breakfast, avoid croissants or muffins stuffed with eggs or meat; they pack as many as 700 calories. Better options include plain scrambled eggs (150–180 calories), pancakes without butter or syrup (400 calories), and English muffins (185 calories each).

✔ For lunch or dinner, if you want meat, go for plain hamburgers (no cheese), which average 275 to 350 calories. An even better choice is roast beef, which is lower in fat and calories.

✔ Be wary of fast-food fish. With frying oil trapped in the breading and creamy tartar sauce on top, fried-fish sandwiches supply more calories (425–500) and fat than regular hamburgers.

✔ Avoid fried chicken; the coatings tend to retain grease. If you want bite-sized chicken, select bites made of chicken breast, not processed chicken (which contains fatty, ground-up skin).

✔ Ask for unsalted items; they are available. (Many chains have also reduced the amount of sodium used in cooking.)

✔ If you sample the salad bar, steer clear of mayonnaise, bacon bits, oily vegetable salads, and rich dressings.

Figure 5-5

Vegetarian Food Guide Pyramid. This version of the Food Guide Pyramid has been modified for use by vegetarians. Compare it to the Food Guide Pyramid shown in Figure 5-2.

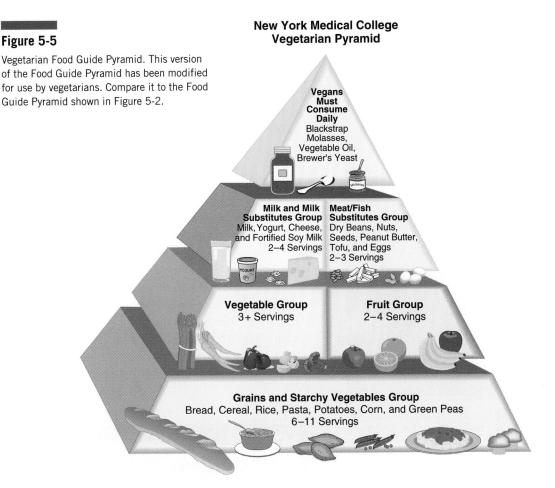

New York Medical College
Vegetarian Pyramid

Vegans Must Consume Daily
Blackstrap Molasses, Vegetable Oil, Brewer's Yeast

Milk and Milk Substitutes Group
Milk, Yogurt, Cheese, and Fortified Soy Milk
2–4 Servings

Meat/Fish Substitutes Group
Dry Beans, Nuts, Seeds, Peanut Butter, Tofu, and Eggs
2–3 Servings

Vegetable Group
3+ Servings

Fruit Group
2–4 Servings

Grains and Starchy Vegetables Group
Bread, Cereal, Rice, Pasta, Potatoes, Corn, and Green Peas
6–11 Servings

When combined with exercise and stress reduction, vegetarian diets have led to reductions in the buildup of harmful plaque within the blood vessels of the heart.

Fast Food: Nutrition on the Run

Not all fast foods are junk foods—that is, high in calories, sugar, salt, and fat, and low in nutrients. But while it's not all bad, fast food has definite disadvantages. A meal in a fast-food restaurant may cost twice as much as the same meal prepared at home and may provide half your daily calorie needs. The fat content of many items is extremely high. A Burger King Whopper with cheese contains 723 calories and 48 grams of fat, 18 grams from saturated fat. A McDonald's Sausage McMuffin with egg has 517 calories and 33 grams of fat, 13 grams from saturated fat. Many fast-food chains have switched from beef tallow or lard to unsaturated vegetable oils for frying, but the total fat content of the foods remains the same.

In response to criticism by health professionals and consumers in general, many fast-food outlets have also added lighter menu items, such as salads, grilled chicken sandwiches on whole-grain buns, and nonfat yogurt.

Some have reduced sodium in their products, removed additives from fish breading, and taken MSG out of sausages.

At regular restaurants or cafeterias, with a little extra attention, you can usually get a better nutritional value for the calories you consume. For example, you can request that your entree be baked or broiled without fat. You can also ask that fresh vegetables be steamed without salt or butter. When possible, ask for luncheon rather than dinner-sized portions. Or order appetizers and side dishes instead of an entree, for instance, tomato soup, a salad, and vegetables. Ask for your salad dressing on the side, request low-calorie dressing if available, or make your own dressing with lemon juice or vinegar.

Food Safety

Increasingly, Americans are concerned not just with whether the food they eat is nutritious, but whether it's safe. As the amount of processing our food goes through increases, we must consider the effects of new high-tech methods for growing and preparing food.

focused on low-dose irradiation to delay ripening and destroy insects. In 1997 the FDA approved the irradiation of red meat as a means of eliminating dangerous bacteria that could cause food poisoning. Irradiation had previously been approved for poultry, where it was used to kill disease-causing bacteria like salmonella, and fruits and vegetables, where it is used in low doses to kill fungi and molds.[25]

While many people worry about pesticides or additives in their food, a much bigger threat to the safety of our food supply is food-borne infections. Someone in the United States is stricken with food poisoning approximately every second of every day, says the Council for Agricultural Sciences and Technology. Every year as many as 35 million Americans suffer from food poisoning; some 9000 die as a result. In a study of food-borne illnesses, the General Accounting Office estimated that such illnesses cost the economy some $22 billion annually. The World Health Organization describes food as "the major source of exposure to disease-causing agents—biological and chemical—from which no one

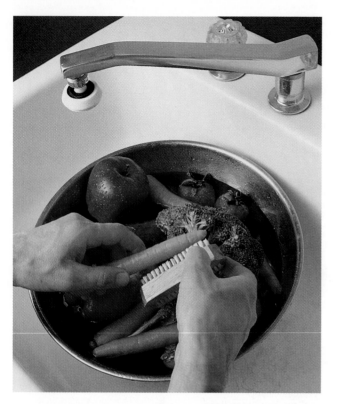

Clean food from a clean kitchen. Wash produce thoroughly in fresh water to remove dirt and any pesticide residue, scrubbing when necessary to clean off soil.

Fearful of potential risks in pesticides, many consumers are purchasing **organic** foods. The term *organic* refers to foods produced without the use of commercial chemicals at any stage. Some independent groups certify foods as organic if they have no detected residues of pesticides, even though pesticides may have been used in their cultivation. Foods that are truly organic are cleaner and have much lower levels of residues than standard commercial produce. There's no guarantee that the organic produce you buy at a grocery or health-food store is more nutritious than other produce. However, buying organic foods is one way to work toward a healthier environment.

Irradiation is the use of radiation, either from radioactive substances or from devices that produce X rays, on food. It doesn't make the food radioactive. Its primary benefit is to prolong the shelf life of food. Like the heat in canning, irradiation can kill all the microorganisms that might grow in a food, and the sterilized food can then be stored for years in sealed containers at room temperature without spoiling. Are irradiated foods safe to eat? The best available answer is a qualified yes, because we don't have complete data yet. Most of the research conducted so far has

Strategies for Prevention

Protecting Yourself from Food Poisoning

✔ Clean food thoroughly. Wash produce thoroughly. Wash utensils, plates, cutting boards, knives, blenders, and other cooking equipment with very hot water and soap after preparing raw meat, poultry, or fish to avoid contaminating other foods or the cooked meat.

✔ Don't eat raw eggs. Since raw eggs can be contaminated with salmonella, don't use them in salad dressings or other dishes. Avoid eggnog.

✔ Cook chicken thoroughly. About a third of all poultry sold contains harmful organisms. Thorough cooking eliminates any danger.

✔ Cook pork to an internal temperature of 170°F to kill parasites called trichina occasionally found in the muscles of pigs.

✔ Keep foods hotter than 140°F or colder than 40°F. The temperatures in between are a danger zone. If you must leave foods out—perhaps at a buffet or picnic—don't let them stay in the temperature danger zone for more than 2 hours. After that time, throw the food away.

Health Online

CyberDiet Nutritional Profile http://www.CyberDiet.com/index.html

This comprehensive nutrition site helps you develop an individualized nutritional profile, plan healthy meals, assess your current diet, and learn more about fast foods. There is also a huge database of foods with their nutritional values and healthy recipes you can print out and use.

Think about it ...

- Write down everything you eat in a day and then enter the items in the diet assessment program. How does your typical diet compare with your ideal nutritional profile? What areas are particularly poor—vitamins, minerals, fat, calories, sodium? In which areas is your diet strong?

- See if you can put together a menu that would meet all your nutritional requirements for 1 day. Does it sound appetizing? Try eating this way for 1 day and see how you feel.

- If you were to write a page for this site on "Healthy Eating Tips for College Students," what might you include?

---

in either the developing or developed countries is spared."[26]

Food-borne infections generally produce nausea, vomiting, and diarrhea from 12 hours to 5 days after infection. The symptoms and severity depend on the specific microorganism and the victim's overall health. Although the illnesses tend to be short term and not usually severe, they can be fatal to those whose immune systems are impaired or whose general health is poor.

Making This Chapter Work for You

A Food Guide for the 21st Century

- Nutrition—the science that explores the connections between our bodies and the food we eat—has shown that our daily diet affects our long-term health prospects more than any other factor within our control.

- Health officials recommend that Americans reduce fat intake, eat more grains, fruits, and vegetables, and consume only moderate amounts of salt, sugar, and alcohol.

- The USDA's Food Guide Pyramid reflects scientific recognition of the health benefits of complex carbohydrates (plant-based foods such as whole grains, vegetables, and fruits), which should form the core of our daily diet. Americans should eat fewer servings of animal products, such as dairy products, meats, poultry, and eggs. Added fats and sugars should be used sparingly.

- The benefits of following the Food Guide Pyramid include less dietary fat, increased fiber, and more vitamins and minerals.

- Saturated fats, found in meat and animal products, can increase the risk of heart disease and certain cancers, including those of the colon and breast. When converted to liquid form in vegetable oils, polyunsaturated fats form potentially harmful substances known as trans fatty acids. Monounsaturates, the most beneficial form of fat, are found in olive and canola oils. Dietary fats, especially saturated ones, can increase cholesterol levels.

- Fiber (found in whole grains, vegetables, and fruit) helps keep the intestines healthy and aids elimination, prevents diverticulosis, is low in calories, and may lessen the risks of certain illnesses, such as heart disease, colon cancer, and diabetes.

- The Nutrition Labeling and Education Act requires food manufacturers to provide substantial information about fat, calories, and ingredients. Food labels must state serving size, calories per serving, fat per serving, daily values (the total amount of a nutrient that the average adult should not exceed on a daily basis), and percentage of daily values (an indication of how a particular food's nutrition content fits into a 2000-calorie diet).

■ Vitamins and minerals may play an important role in preventing disease. Certain antioxidant vitamins (particularly vitamin C, vitamin E, and beta carotene, a form of vitamin A) may prevent damage to our cells caused by free radical oxygen molecules.

■ Most people eating a balanced diet don't need vitamin supplements. However, certain people may benefit from a supplement of folic acid, calcium, iron, or a multivitamin.

■ An increasing number of people are cutting down on meats or adopting a vegetarian diet, which may or may not include dairy products, fish, or poultry.

■ Food safety has become an increasingly important issue because of the possible dangers of food-borne illnesses, additives, antibiotics and hormones in meat, pesticides, and irradiation.

After reading this chapter, you may conclude that eating isn't simple anymore. You're right. Every time you grill bacon for breakfast, grab a quick cheeseburger for lunch, or heat up a burrito for dinner, you're making a choice that could have a long-term negative impact on your health.

While we must eat to live, eating can also bring a special joy and satisfaction to living. Here are some eating guidelines for physical and psychological well-being:

■ Eat with people you like.

■ Talk only of pleasant things while eating.

■ Eat slowly. Focus on the taste of each food you're eating.

■ When you eat, eat—don't write, work, or talk on the phone.

■ Eat because you're hungry, not to change how you feel.

■ After eating, take time to be quiet and rest.

Key Terms

The terms listed here are used within the chapter. Page numbers are included for each term. A definition of each term is given in the green Glossary pages at the end of this book.

amino acids *82*	**fiber** *75*	**organic** *84*
antioxidants *77*	**food allergies** *77*	**ovo-lacto-vegetarians** *81*
calories *76*	**incomplete proteins** *82*	**protein** *72*
carbohydrates *70*	**indoles** *71*	**saturated fats** *74*
cholesterol *75*	**irradiation** *84*	**simple carbohydrates** *70*
complementary proteins *82*	**lacto-vegetarians** *81*	**trans fats** *75*
complete proteins *82*	**minerals** *77*	**unsaturated fats** *74*
complex carbohydrates *70*	**nutrients** *69*	**vegans** *82*
crucifers *71*	**nutrition** *69*	**vitamins** *77*

Review Questions

1. List at least six guidelines for a healthy diet. Why are these important?

2. What nutrients are necessary to maintain a healthy body? Give examples of good sources of each.

3. What food groups make up the Food Guide Pyramid? How many servings of each should you eat each day? How many do you eat?

4. What types of people would benefit from vitamin supplements?

5. Do you think it's a good idea to eat organic foods? Why or why not?

Critical Thinking Questions

1. Scientists are using genetic engineering to develop foods, such as tomatoes that won't bruise easily, cows that will produce more milk, and corn that will grow larger ears. Some consumer advocates argue that these items shouldn't be put on the market because they haven't been studied carefully enough. What do you think of these foods?

2. Is it possible to meet nutritional requirements on a limited budget? Have you ever been in this situa-tion? What would you recommend to someone who wanted to eat healthfully on $30 a week?

3. Consider the number of times a week you eat fast food. How much money would you have saved if you had eaten home-prepared meals? What different foods from the bottom levels of the Food Guide Pyramid might you have eaten instead?

Connections to Personal Health Interactive

*To enhance your understanding of the material covered in this chapter, check out the following study aids on the **Personal Health Interactive CD-ROM**.*

- Personal Insights: How Nutritious Is Your Diet?
- **Online Research**: Nutrition

- Point of View: Dietician
- Glossary & Key Term Review

References

1. Center for Science in the Public Interest.
2. Shaw, Ann. Personal interview.
3. Douglas, Kathy, et al. "Results from the 1995 National College Health Risk Behavior Survey." *Journal of American College Health*, Vol. 46, September 1997.
4. "Nutrition Revolution." *University of California, Berkeley Wellness Letter*, Vol. 13, No. 12, September 1997.
5. "More Evidence for Antioxidants." *Harvard Women's Health Watch*, Vol. 2, No. 5, January 1995.
6. Uauy-Dagach, Ricardo, and Alfonso Valenzuela. "Marine Oils: The Health Benefits of n-3 Fatty Acids." *Nutrition Reviews*, Vol. 54, No. 11, November 1996. Nair, Sudheera, et al. "Prevention of Cardiac Arrhythmia by Dietary (n-3) Polyunsaturated Fatty Acids and Their Mechanisms of Action." *Journal of Nutrition*, Vol. 127, No. 3, March 1997.
7. Conkling, Winifred. "Water: How Much Do We Need?" *American Health*, May 1995.
8. Ibid.
9. "What the Experts Say About Olean." Procter & Gamble Press Information, February 1998.
10. Callaway, Wayne. "Reexamining Cholesterol and Sodium Recommendations." *Nutrition Today*, Vol. 29, No. 5, September–October 1994.
11. The Writing Group for the DISC Collaborative Research Group. "Efficacy and Safety of Lowering Dietary Intake of Fat and Cholesterol in Children with Elevated Low-Density Lipoprotein Cholesterol." *Journal of the American Medical Association*, Vol. 273, No. 18, May 10, 1995.

12. Elash, Anita. "Powerful Grains and Beans." *Maclean's*, Vol. 110, No. 43, October 27, 1997.
13. Hunter, Beatrice. "The Neglected Wholegrains." *Consumers' Research Magazine*, Vol. 80, No. 7, July 1997. Maki, Kevin, et al. "Fiber Intake and Risk of Developing Non-Insulin-Dependent Diabetes Mellitus." *Journal of the American Medical Association*, Vol. 277, No. 22, June 11, 1997. Salmeron, Jorge, et al. "Dietary Fiber, Glycemic Load, and Risk of Non-Insulin-Dependent Diabetes Mellitus in Women." *Journal of the American Medical Association*, Vol. 277, No. 6, February 12, 1997.
14. Mee, Karen, and David Gee. "Apple Fiber and Gum Arabic Lower Total and Low-Density Lipoprotein Cholesterol Levels in Men with Mild Hypercholesterolemia." *Journal of the American Dietetic Association*, Vol. 97, No. 4, April 1997.
15. Byrd-Bredbenner, Carol. "Designing a Consumer Friendly Nutrition Label." *Journal of Nutrition Education*, Vol. 26, No. 4, July–August 1994. Lytle, Victoria. "What's Behind the New Food Labels?" *NEA Today*, Vol. 13, No. 2, September 15, 1994. DeVries, Jonathon, and Amy Nelson. "Meeting Analytical Needs for Nutrition Labeling." *Food Technology*, Vol. 48, No. 7, July 1994. Mermelstein, Neil H. "Nutrition Labeling Regulatory Update." *Food Technology*, Vol. 48, No. 7, July 1994.
16. Kurtzweil, Paula. "Scouting for Sodium: and Other Nutrients Important to Blood Pressure." *FDA Consumer*, Vol. 28, No. 7, September 1994.

17. Butler, Robert. "Vitamin E Supplements." *Geriatrics*, Vol. 52, No. 7, July 1997.

18. Norvell, C. "Have You Had Your Antioxidants Today?" *Current Health,* Vol. 21, No. 8, April 1995.

19. Brody, Jane. "In Vitamin Mania, Millions Take a Gamble on Health." *New York Times*, October 26, 1997.

20. Fleet, James. "Dietary Selenium Repletion May Reduce Cancer Incidence in People at High Risk Who Live in Areas with Low Soil Selenium." *Nutrition Reviews*, Vol. 55, No. 7, July 1997.

21. Barone, Jeanine. "Foods:The Best Source for Nutrients." *The 1998 World Book Health & Medical Annual.* Chicago: World Book, 1998.

22. "Selenium May Prevent Some Cancers in Patients with History of Skin Cancer." *Geriatrics*, Vol. 52, No. 2, February 1997.

23. Prince, Richard. "Diet and the Prevention of Osteoporotic Fracture." *New England Journal of Medicine*, Vol. 227, No. 10, September 4, 1997.

24. Shaw, Ann. Personal interview.

25. Kolata, Gina. "F.D.A., Saying Process Is Safe, Approves Irradiating Red Meat." *New York Times*, December 3, 1997.

26. Gavzer, Bernard. "We Can Make Our Food Safer." *Parade*, October 19, 1997.

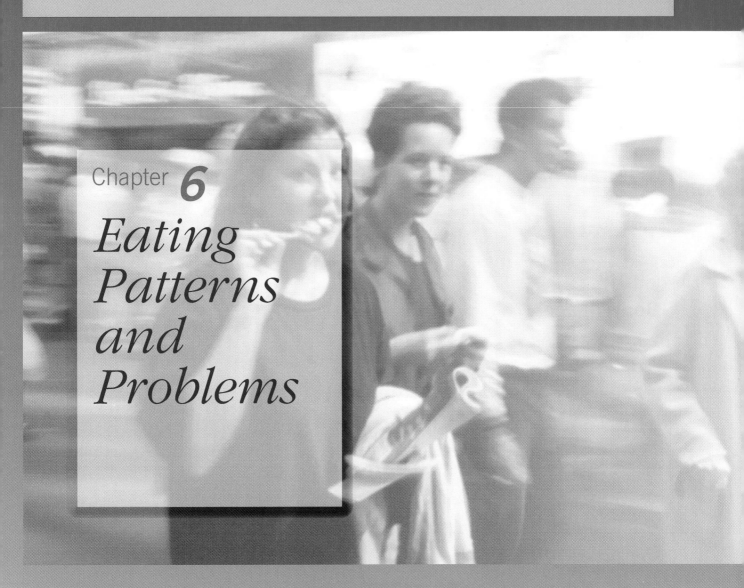

Chapter 6

Eating Patterns and Problems

After studying the material in this chapter, you should be able to:

- **Describe** three different methods for determining your ideal body weight.

- **Identify** several factors that influence food consumption.

- **Identify** and **describe** the symptoms and dangers associated with abnormal eating behaviors and eating disorders.

- **Define** obesity and **describe** its relationship to genetics, lifestyle, and major health problems.

- **Explain** how health problems are created by fad diets.

- **Design** a personal plan for sensible weight management.

This chapter explores our national preoccupation with slimness, examines unhealthy eating patterns and eating disorders, explains what obesity is and why excess pounds are dangerous, shows why fad diets don't work, and tells how to control weight safely, sensibly, and permanently.

Body Image

Throughout most of history, bigger was better. The great beauties of centuries past, as painted by such artistic masters as Rubens and Renoir, were soft and fleshy, with rounded bellies and dimpled thighs. Many developing countries still regard a full figure, rather than a thin one, as the ideal standard for health and beauty.

On the eve of the 21st century in the United States, men and women are paying more attention to their body image than ever before. "We've become a nation of appearance junkies and fitness zealots driven to think, talk, strategize, and worry about our bodies with the same fanatical devotion we applied to putting a man on the moon," says psychologist Judith Rodin, Ph.D.[1] Such self-absorption can affect self-esteem and confidence and lead to a preoccupation with weight and potentially dangerous forms of dieting.[2]

Even though studies show that men don't necessarily consider the slimmest women the most attractive, young women—especially white women—grow up thinking that thin is better.[3] African-American women often have more positive attitudes toward their bodies, feeling more satisfied with their weight and seeing themselves as more attractive.[4] However, there are no significant differences between African-American and white women *dieters* in terms of self-esteem and body dissatisfaction.[5]

A preoccupation with weight and appearance, in and of itself, can be harmful. "The quest for the perfect body is, like most wars, a costly one—emotionally and physically, to say nothing of financially," notes Rodin, who argues that "what your body really needs is moderate exercise, healthy foods, sensual pleasures, and relaxation. Give it those, and it will respond by treating you better." And in the process, you'll feel better about yourself.

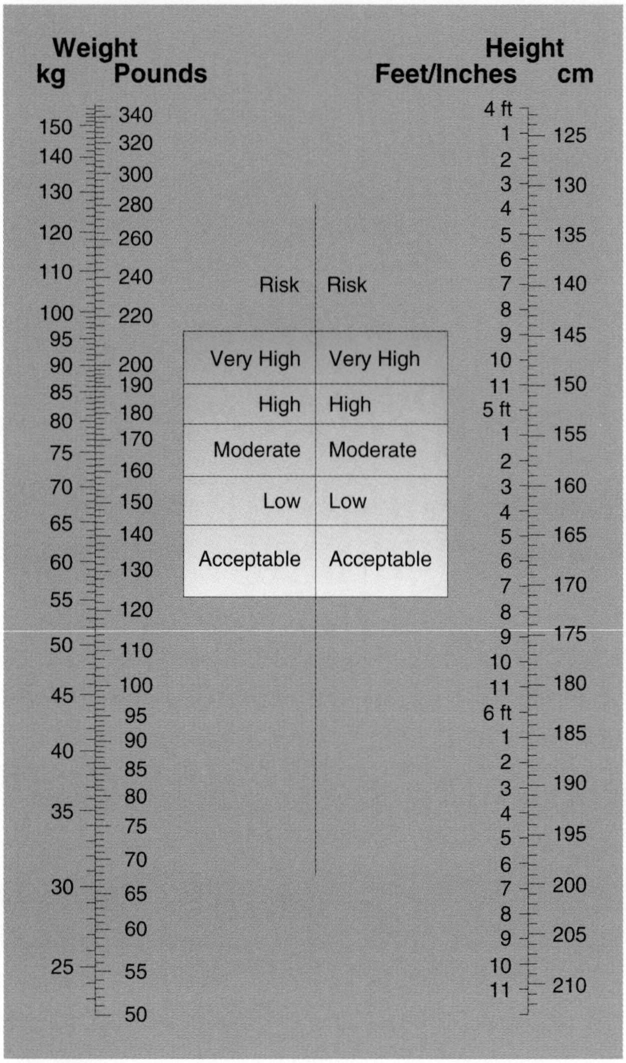

Figure 6-1

Calculating your Body-Mass Index (BMI) and risk. To find out if your current level of body fat increases your health risks, draw a straight line from your weight to your height. Your level of risk is determined by where you cross the center line. Beware, too, that at the bottom of the acceptable range, health risks begin to increase again.

Weight and Body Composition

Many factors determine what you weigh: heredity, eating behavior, food selection, amount of daily exercise. For any individual of a given height, there is no single best weight, but a range of healthy weights. The traditional weight tables prepared by the insurance industry relate weight and height to how long policyholders live, not to their health, vitality, or appearance.

Increasingly, medical experts are paying less attention to total weight and focusing on body composition—that is, on the relative amounts of lean body mass (bones, muscles, and organs) and fatty tissue. One of the best indicators of a healthy ratio of lean to fatty tissue is the **Body-Mass Index (BMI)**, a standard index assessing the ratio of a person's weight to height (Figure 6-1). The National Institutes of Health have defined a reading higher than 25 as an indicator that a person is overweight; a reading of 30 or above indicates obesity (Table 6-1). By this calculation, more than half of all Americans are overweight.

Another means of assessment is measuring body fat. The lowest health risks are associated with a body fat percentage of weight below 20 for men and 25 for women. Body fat may be assessed in different ways. **Skin calipers**, which pinch skin folds at the arms, waist, and back, are the most widely used method, although they may be less accurate than other techniques. Proper use of these instruments by trained personnel is critical in getting a precise reading. **Hydrostatic weighing**—weighing a person in water to distinguish buoyant fat from denser muscle—is far more precise. Other methods include whole-body

TABLE 6.1 THE BODY-MASS INDEX

Federal health authorities are using this index to determine who is overweight. Under new guidelines, a body mass of **25** or more is considered overweight. On this chart, your Body-Mass Index is at the intersection of your height and weight.

Body mass is generally calculated in kilograms and meters, but for those accustomed to pounds and feet, this formula works: 1. Multiply weight by 703. 2. Multiply height in inches by height in inches. 3. Divide the answer in Step 1 by the answer in Step 2 for your Body-Mass Index.

25 OVERWEIGHT LIMIT   OVERWEIGHT

HEIGHT / WEIGHT	100	105	110	115	120	125	130	135	140	145	150	155	160	165	170	175	180	185	190	195	200	205
5' 0"	20	21	21	22	23	24	25	26	27	28	29	30	31	32	33	34	35	36	37	38	39	40
5' 1"	19	20	21	22	23	24	25	26	26	27	28	29	30	31	32	33	34	35	36	37	38	39
5' 2"	18	19	20	21	22	23	24	25	26	27	27	28	29	30	31	32	33	34	35	36	37	37
5' 3"	18	19	19	20	21	22	23	24	25	26	27	27	28	29	30	31	32	33	34	35	35	36
5' 4"	17	18	19	20	21	21	22	23	24	25	26	27	27	28	29	30	31	32	33	33	34	35
5' 5"	17	17	18	19	20	21	22	22	23	24	25	26	27	27	28	29	30	31	32	32	33	34
5' 6"	16	17	18	19	19	20	21	22	23	23	24	25	26	27	27	28	29	30	31	31	32	33
5' 7"	16	16	17	18	19	20	20	21	22	23	23	24	25	26	27	27	28	29	30	31	31	32
5' 8"	15	16	17	17	18	19	20	21	21	22	23	24	24	25	26	27	27	28	29	30	30	31
5' 9"	15	16	16	17	18	18	19	20	21	21	22	23	24	24	25	26	27	27	28	29	30	30
5' 10"	14	15	16	17	17	18	19	19	20	21	22	22	23	24	24	25	26	27	27	28	29	29
5' 11"	14	15	15	16	17	17	18	19	20	20	21	22	22	23	24	24	25	26	26	27	28	29
6' 0"	14	14	15	16	16	17	18	18	19	20	20	21	22	22	23	24	24	25	26	26	27	28
6' 1"	13	14	15	15	16	16	17	18	18	19	20	20	21	22	22	23	24	24	25	26	26	27
6' 2"	13	13	14	15	15	16	17	17	18	19	19	20	21	21	22	22	23	24	24	25	26	26
6' 3"	12	13	14	14	15	16	16	17	17	18	19	19	20	21	21	22	22	23	24	24	25	26
6' 4"	12	13	13	14	15	15	16	16	17	18	18	19	19	20	21	21	22	23	23	24	24	25

SOURCES: *Shape Up America, National Institutes of Health*

counting, which measures the total amount of K-40, a naturally occurring form of potassium found primarily in lean tissue; imaging methods, such as computerized tomography (CT) and magnetic resonance imaging (MRI); ultrasonography, which uses high-frequency sound waves; and bioelectrical impedance assessment (BIA), which measures the resistance of the body to a flow of alternating electric current.

The distribution of weight and the location of fat storage also are important. Fat at the hips, which is more common in women and more difficult to lose than abdominal fat, is stored primarily for special purposes, such as extra energy needs during pregnancy and nursing. Abdominal fat seems more dangerous. The bigger the waist and belly, the higher the risk of various diseases, such as diabetes, heart disease, and stroke. Figure 6-2 illustrates how to calculate your waist-to-hip ratio.

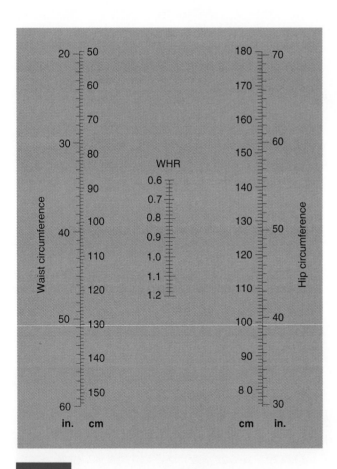

Figure 6-2

Determining waist-to-hip ratio (WHR). Use a straightedge to draw a line from your waist circumference (left) to your hip circumference (right). The point at which the line crosses the center column is your WHR. Recommended waist-to-hip ratios: less than 0.80 for women and less than 0.95 for men.

SOURCE: Data from Gray, G. A., and D. S. Gray. "Obesity: Part 1: Pathenogensis." *Western Journal of Medicine*, Vol. 149, 1988.

Strategies for Change

Rethinking Your Weight Goals

Regardless of what you weigh, chances are that in your mind's eye you're fatter than you really are—or fatter than you want to be. Stop looking at your bathroom scale or in your mirror and look inside. Answer these questions as honestly as you can:

✔ If you could choose your weight, what would it be? Why? At what weight do you have enough energy to make it through an average day, yet not feel hungry all the time?

✔ What's the weight range that's best for your height and body-frame size? How does this compare with what you consider your ideal weight? (See Table 6-2 for a formula to use in calculating your ideal weight.)

✔ What do you think is a realistic weight for you to strive for? Have you ever gotten to, and stayed at, this weight? If you had to choose between the weight that was best for your health and the one you thought most attractive, which would you choose? Why?

Calories: How Many Do You Need?

Calories are the measure of the amount of energy that can be derived from food. Science defines a **calorie** as the amount of energy required to raise the temperature of 1 gram of water by 1°C. In the laboratory, the caloric content of food is measured in 1000-calorie units called *kilocalories*. The calorie referred to in everyday usage is actually the equivalent of the laboratory kilocalorie.

An average adult woman—with a height of 5'4" and a weight of 138 pounds—generally needs 1900 to 2200 calories. An average man—with a height of 5'10" and a weight of 174 pounds—generally consumes 2300 to 2900 calories. How many calories you need depends on your gender, age, body-frame size, weight, percentage of body fat, and your **basal metabolic rate (BMR)**—the number of calories needed to sustain your body at rest.

Your activity level also affects your calorie requirements. Regardless of whether you consume fat, protein, or carbohydrates, if you take in more calories than required to maintain your size and don't work them off in some sort of physical activity, your body will convert the excess to fat (Table 6-3).

TABLE 6-2 CALCULATING YOUR IDEAL WEIGHT

Here are two widely used formulas for calculating your ideal weight, based on body-fat percentages of less than 20% for men and less than 26% for women. For men, the first formula is as follows:

$$\text{Height (in inches)} \times 4 - 128 = \text{Ideal Weight}$$

If you have a large frame, add 10% to the total. Thus, a 6' tall man with a large frame would make the following calculations:

$$72 \times 4 = 288$$
$$288 - 128 = 160$$
$$160 \times 0.10 = 16$$
$$160 + 16 = 176 \text{ pounds, Ideal Weight}$$

For women, the formula is slightly different:

$$\text{Height (in inches)} \times 3.5 - 108 = \text{Ideal Weight}$$

A 5' 4" woman with a medium frame would perform these calculations:

$$64 \times 3.5 = 224$$
$$224 - 108 = 116 \text{ pounds, Ideal Weight}$$

The second, even simpler formula for men is to allow 106 pounds for the first 5 feet of height and to add 6 pounds for each additional inch thereafter. Thus, for a 6' man, the calculations would be as follows:

$$106 + (12 \times 6) = 106 + 72 = 178 \text{ pounds, Ideal Weight}$$

The second formula for women is to allow 100 pounds for the first 5 feet of height and to add 5 pounds for each additional inch thereafter. For a 5' 4" woman, the calculations would be as follows.

$$100 + (4 \times 5) = 100 + 20 = 120 \text{ pounds, Ideal Weight}$$

Notice that the results from applying these two formulas don't match perfectly: This underscores the fact that there is a range of at least 5–10 pounds in the ideal weight for every height.

Hunger, Satiety, and Set Point

Why do you wake up starving or feel your stomach rumbling during a late afternoon lecture? The simple answer is **hunger**: the physiological drive to consume food. More than a dozen different signals may influence and control our desire for food.

Appetite—the psychological desire to eat—usually begins with the fear of the unpleasant sensation of hunger. We learn to avoid hunger by eating a certain amount of food at certain times of the day, just as dogs in the laboratory learn to avoid electric shocks by jumping at the sound of a warning bell.

We stop eating when we feel satisfied; this is called **satiety**, a feeling of fullness and relief from hunger. According to the **set-point theory**, each individual has an unconscious control system for regulating appetite and satiety to keep body fat at a predetermined level, or *set point*. If our fat stores fall too low, our appetite gnaws at us, so we eat more. Conversely, appetite subsides if we overeat.

From this perspective, diets are doomed to fail because they pit the dieter against tireless internal enemies: the set point and its enforcer, appetite. The only effective alternative is lowering, or resetting, the set point. And the safest, most effective way to do so is through physical activity, which dampens appetite in the short run and lowers the set point for the long term. Moderate activity not only works up an appetite but also helps work it off.

TABLE 6-3 HOW MANY CALORIES DO YOU NEED DAILY?

Desirable Weight (lb)	High Activity	Medium Activity	Low Activity
Women			
99	1700	1500	1300
110	1850	1650	1400
121	2000	1750	1550
128	2100	1900	1600
132	2150	1950	1650
143	2300	2050	1800
154	2400	2150	1850
165	2550	2300	1950
Men			
121	2400	2150	1850
132	2550	2300	1950
143	2700	2400	2050
154	2900	2600	2200
165	3100	2800	2400
176	3250	2950	2500
187	3300	3100	2600

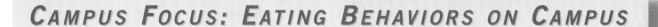

CAMPUS FOCUS: EATING BEHAVIORS ON CAMPUS

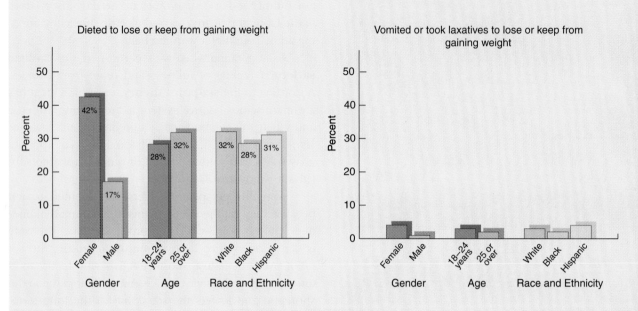

SOURCE: Douglas, Kathy, et al. "Results from the 1995 National College Health Risk Behavior Survey." *Journal of American College Health*, Vol. 46, September 1997.

Unhealthy Eating Behavior

Sooner or later many people *don't* eat the way they should. They may skip meals, thereby increasing the likelihood that they'll end up with more body fat, a higher weight, and a higher blood cholesterol level. Others live on "diet" foods, but consume so much of them that they gain weight anyway. Still others engage in more extreme forms of what health professionals call "disordered eating." They continuously go on and off diets, eat compulsively, or binge on high-fat treats. Such behaviors can be warning signs of potentially serious eating disorders that should not be ignored.[6]

College students—particularly women—are at risk for unhealthy eating behaviors. As "Campus Focus: Eating Behaviors on Campus" shows, about one in five undergraduates is overweight. Among women, 42.1% have dieted to lose or keep from gaining weight; 16.7% of the men have done the same. Seven percent of undergraduate women have taken diet pills; 4.2% have vomited or used laxatives for weight control.[7]

The prevalence of disordered eating symptoms and eating disorders has increased dramatically in the last 20

years. In some studies as many as 64% of college women have reported at least one unhealthy eating behavior. One reason may be the pressure some young women feel to attain what has been called the "Super Woman" ideal. As they try to excel in multiple roles, they diet, induce vomiting, or restrict food intake for the sake of meeting their idealized standards for appearance.[8] Sorority women, some researchers have found, may have an even greater fear of becoming fat. They tend to be more dissatisfied with their bodies and are more concerned with weight and dieting than college women in general.[9]

Extreme Dieting

"Extreme" dieters go beyond cutting back on calories or increasing physical activity and become preoccupied with what they eat and weigh. Although their weight never falls below 85% of normal, their weight loss is severe enough to cause uncomfortable physical consequences, such as weakness and sensitivity to cold. Technically, these dieters do not have *anorexia nervosa* (discussed later in the chapter), but they are at increased risk for it.

Extreme dieters may think they know a great deal about nutrition, yet many of their beliefs about food and weight are misconceptions or myths. For instance, they may eat only protein because they believe complex carbohydrates, including fruits and breads, are fattening. When they're anxious, angry, or bored, they focus on food and their fear of fatness. Dieting and exercise become ways of coping with any stress in their lives.

Sometimes nutritional education alone can help change this eating pattern. However, many avid dieters who deny that they have a problem with food may need counseling (which they usually agree to only at their family's insistence) to correct dangerous eating behavior and prevent further complications.

Compulsive Overeating

Individuals who eat compulsively cannot stop putting food in their mouths. They eat fast; they eat a lot; they eat even when they're full; and they may eat round the clock rather than at set meal times—often in private because of embarrassment over how much they consume.

Some mental health professionals describe compulsive eating as a food addiction that is much more likely to develop in women. According to Overeaters Anonymous (OA), an international support agency, many women who eat compulsively view food as a source of comfort against feelings of inner emptiness, low self-esteem, and fear of abandonment.

Strategies for Change

Recognizing Compulsive Overeating

The following behaviors may signal a potential problem:

✔ Turning to food when depressed or lonely, when feeling rejected, or as a reward.

✔ A history of failed diets and anxiety when dieting.

✔ Thinking about food throughout the day.

✔ Eating quickly and without pleasure.

✔ Frequent talking about food or refusing to talk about food.

✔ Fear of not being able to stop eating once you start. Continuing to eat even when you're no longer hungry.

Recovery from compulsive overeating can be challenging because people with this problem cannot give up entirely the "substance" they abuse. Like everyone else, they must eat. However, they can learn new eating habits and ways of dealing with underlying emotional problems. An OA survey found that most of its members joined to lose weight but later felt the most important effect was their improved emotional, mental, and physical health. As one woman put it, "I came for vanity but stayed for sanity."

Binge Eating

Binge eating—the rapid consumption of an abnormally large amount of food in a relatively short time—often occurs in compulsive eaters. Individuals with a binge-eating disorder typically eat a larger-than-ordinary amount of food during a relatively brief period, feel a lack of control over eating, and binge at least twice a week for at least a 6-month period. During most of these episodes, individuals experience at least three of the following:

- Eating much more rapidly than usual.

- Eating until they feel uncomfortably full.

- Eating large amounts of food when not feeling physically hungry.

- Eating large amounts of food throughout the day with no planned mealtimes.

- Eating alone because they are embarrassed by how much they eat and by their eating habits.

It is not clear whether dieting leads to binge eating, or vice versa.[10] Binge eaters may spend up to several hours eating and consume 2000 or more calories of food in a single binge—more than many people eat in a day. After such binges, they usually do not induce vomiting, use laxatives, or rely on other means (such as exercise) to control weight. They simply get fatter. As their weight climbs, they become depressed, anxious, or troubled by other psychological symptoms to a much greater extent than others of comparable weight.[11]

About 2% of Americans—some 5 million in all—may have binge-eating disorder.[12] It is most common among young women in college and, increasingly, in high school. Persons who binge eat may require professional help to change their behavior. Treatment includes education, behavioral approaches, cognitive therapy, and psychotherapy. As they recognize the reasons for their behavior and begin to confront the underlying issues, individuals usually are able to resume normal eating patterns.

Eating Disorders

Just a few decades ago there was no official psychiatric diagnosis for behaviors that are now collectively called **eating disorders**, the most common of which are anorexia nervosa and bulimia nervosa. Even though these problems involve food, researchers increasingly view them as "dieting disorders" that affect and are affected by a person's body image and that can threaten psychological and physical well-being.[13]

If someone you know has an eating disorder, let your friend know you're concerned and that you care. Don't criticize or make fun of his or her eating habits. Encourage your friend to talk about other problems and feelings and suggest that he or she talk to the school counselor or someone at the mental health center, the family doctor, or another trusted adult. Offer to go along if you think that will make a difference.

Anorexia Nervosa

Although *anorexia* means loss of appetite, most individuals with **anorexia nervosa** are, in fact, hungry all the time. For them, food is an enemy—a threat to their sense of self, identity, and autonomy. In the distorted mirror of their mind's eye, they see themselves as fat or flabby even at a normal or below-normal body weight. Some simply feel fat; others think that they are thin in some places and too fat in others, such as the abdomen, buttocks, or thighs.

In the *restricting* type of anorexia, individuals lose weight by avoiding any fatty foods and by dieting, fasting, and exercising.[14] Some start smoking as a way of controlling their weight.[15] In the *binge-eating/purging* type, they engage in binge eating, purging (through self-induced vomiting, laxatives, diuretics, or enemas), or both. Obsessed with an intense fear of fatness, they may weigh themselves several times a day, measure various parts of their body, check mirrors to see if they look fat, and try on different items of clothing to see if they feel tight.

The causes of anorexia nervosa are complex; genetic, biochemical, and developmental factors may play a role.[16] Its consequences are serious: Menstrual periods stop in women; testosterone levels decline in men. Adolescents with this disorder do not undergo normal sexual maturation, such as breast development, and may not reach their anticipated height. Even individuals who look and feel reasonably healthy may have

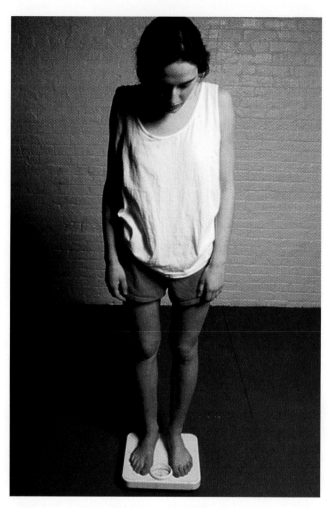

Anorexia nervosa is complex in its causes, and successful treatment usually involves medical, nutritional, and behavioral therapy.

Strategies for Change
● ●

Recognizing Anorexia Nervosa

The characteristics of anorexia nervosa include:

✔ A refusal to maintain normal body weight.

✔ An intense fear of gaining weight or becoming fat, even though underweight.

✔ A distorted body image, so that the person feels fat even when emaciated.

✔ In women, the absence of at least three menstrual cycles.

subtle or hidden abnormalities, including heart irregularities and arrhythmias that can increase their risk of sudden death. Women who do not menstruate for 6 months or more may develop osteoporosis and suffer irreversible weakening and thinning of their bones as a result.[17]

According to current practice guidelines, treatment of anorexia nervosa includes medical therapy (such as "refeeding" to overcome malnutrition) and behavioral, cognitive, psychodynamic, and family therapy (described in Chapter 3). Antidepressant medication sometimes can help, particularly when there is a personal or family history of depression. Most people who get help do return to normal weight, but it can take a long time for their eating behaviors to become normal and for them to deal with troubling body image issues.[18]

Bulimia Nervosa

Individuals with **bulimia nervosa** go on repeated eating binges and rapidly consume large amounts of food, usually sweets, stopping only because of severe abdominal pain or sleep or because they are interrupted. Those with *purging* bulimia induce vomiting or take large doses of laxatives to relieve guilt and control their weight. In *nonpurging* bulimia, individuals use other means, such as fasting or excessive exercise, to compensate for binges.[19]

Many factors, including psychological, developmental, and biochemical influences, can contribute to bulimia nervosa.[20] This disorder often begins after a rigid diet of several weeks to a year that may have altered brain chemistry in such a way as to disrupt the normal mechanisms for appetite and satiety. Because they're so distressed when they break their diet and binge, dieters may begin to purge. Once they realize that vomiting reduces the anxiety triggered by gorging, they no longer fear overeating and fall into a regular binge–purge habit.

Bulimia may continue for many years, with binges alternating with periods of normal eating. Often dentists are the first to detect bulimia because they notice damage to teeth and gums, including erosion of the enamel from the stomach acids in vomit. Repeated vomiting can lead to other complications as it robs the body of essential nutrients and fluids, causes dehydration and electrolyte imbalances, and impairs the ability of the heart and other muscles to function. Bulimia can trigger cardiac arrhythmias and, occasionally, sudden death.[21]

Strategies for Change

Recognizing Bulimia Nervosa

The characteristics of bulimia nervosa include:

✔ Repeated binge eating.

✔ A feeling of lack of control over eating behavior.

✔ Regular reliance on self-induced vomiting, laxatives, or diuretics.

✔ Strict dieting or fasting, or vigorous exercise, to prevent weight gain.

✔ A minimum average of two binging episodes a week for at least 3 months.

✔ A preoccupation with body shape and weight.

Most mental health professionals treat bulimia with a combination of nutritional counseling, psychodynamic, cognitive-behavioral therapy, individual or group psychotherapy, and medication. The drug most often prescribed is an antidepressant medication such as Prozac or fluoxetine, which increases levels of the neurotransmitter serotonin. About 70% of those who complete treatment programs reduce their binging and purging, although flareups are common in times of stress.

Obesity

Obesity is characterized by excess fat in the body and a body weight of 20% or more above the ideal weight for a person of that height and gender. *Mild obesity* refers to a body weight that is 20% to 40% above the ideal weight; *moderate obesity*, to a body weight that is 41% to 100% above the ideal weight; and *severe obesity*, to a body weight that is 100% or more above the ideal weight for a person of that height and gender.

Although more people in certain regions of the country are likely to be heavy, obesity affects all racial and ethnic groups. A third of white American women are obese, as are nearly 50% of African-American and Mexican-American women. In some Native American communities, up to 70% of all adults are dangerously overweight.[22]

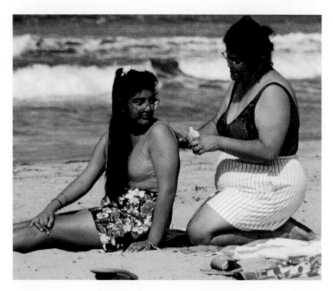

Obesity tends to run in families, so heredity may play a role in your weight. But environment and behavior also matter. If you eat high-calorie, high-fat foods, you're likely to become overweight.

What Causes Obesity?

Are some people fated to be fat? Scientists have identified a gene for a protein that signals the brain to halt food intake or to step up metabolic rate to make use of extra calories. If this gene is defective or malfunctions, it could contribute to weight problems. The discovery of a genetic predisposition to excess weight could explain, at least in part, why children with obese parents tend to be obese themselves, especially if both parents are obese.[23] A protein named leptin also may play a role. When laboratory mice are injected with high doses of leptin, they initially decrease their food intake, increase their metabolic rate, and become much thinner. Eventually, the body adapts to the high levels of leptin and becomes resistant to its effects.[24]

Yet genes are not the sole culprits. As scientists now realize, obesity is a complex and serious disorder with multiple causes.[25] These include:

- *Developmental factors.* Some obese people have a high number of fat cells, others have large fat cells, and the most severely obese have both more *and* larger fat cells. Whereas the size of fat cells can increase at any time in life, the number is set during childhood, possibly as the result of genetics or overfeeding at a young age.

- *Social determinants.* In affluent countries, people in lower socioeconomic classes tend to be more obese. For reasons unknown, those in the upper classes, who can afford as much food as they want, tend to be leaner. Education may be one factor; another is that a healthy, nonfattening diet with plenty of fresh fruits and vegetables is more expensive.

- *Physical activity.* Obesity tends to go with a sedentary lifestyle. In countries where many people tend to work at physically demanding jobs, obesity is rare. Physical activity prevents obesity by increasing caloric expenditure, decreasing food intake, and increasing metabolic rate.

- *Emotional influences.* Obese people are neither more nor less psychologically troubled than others. Psychological problems, such as irritability, depression, and anxiety, are more likely to be the result of obesity than the cause. However, emotions do play some role in weight problems. Just as some people reach for a drink or a drug when they're upset, others cope by overeating, binging, or purging.[26]

- *Lifestyle.* People who watch more than 3 hours of TV a day are twice as likely to be obese as those who watch less than an hour. Even those who log between 1 and 2 hours are fatter than those who watch just 1 hour.

The Dangers of Obesity

Obesity has long been singled out as a major health threat that increases the risk of many chronic diseases. Obese people have three times the normal incidence of high blood pressure and diabetes. Very heavy women have a threefold higher risk of heart attack and chronic chest pain than very lean women. Excess weight in women has been linked with an increased incidence of high blood pressure, ovarian cancer, and breast cancer. Obese men have an increased chance of heart disease and cancer of the colon, rectum, and prostate. If overweight individuals have surgery, they're more likely to develop complications. Even relatively small amounts of excess fat—as little as 5 pounds—can add to the dangers in those already at risk for hypertension and diabetes.

Moreover, in our calorie-conscious and thinness-obsessed society, obesity can be a heavy psychological burden and is often seen as a sign of failure, laziness, or inadequate willpower. As a result, overweight men and women often blame themselves for becoming heavy and feel guilty and depressed as a result. In fact, the psychological problems once considered the cause of obesity may be its consequence.[27]

Pulsepoints

Top Ten Ways to Lose Weight

1. Take charge of your weight. Successful dieters often simply decide that they no longer are going to be fat.

2. Make a commitment. Join a group, such as an on-campus support group.

3. Bite and write. As an exercise, for a week, record every morsel that goes into your mouth. Reread your diary to find out what, how much, when, and where you eat—and why.

4. Don't skip meals. People who eat three meals a day burn off 10% more calories than meal skippers.

5. Snack sensibly. Avoid high-fat snack foods. Reach for plain popcorn, rice cakes, vegetables, and fruit instead.

6. Eat at a moderate pace. Slow down and savor each bite. And avoid that second helping—the "little bit more" you don't really need.

7. Narrow your options. While you should eat an assortment of food, be wary of too many tempting tastes at one meal. We eat more when offered many different foods at once.

8. Graze, don't gorge. Spread calorie intake over the day rather than stuffing yourself at any one meal. Potential pay-

offs include better performance, greater stamina, and less likelihood of a weight gain.

9. Get a buddy. If you want to lose weight, don't go it alone. Dieters who double up with a friend or spouse lose more weight and are more likely to keep it off.

10. Move it and lose it. Don't lie down when you can sit; don't sit when you can stand; don't stand when you can walk; don't walk when you can run. The more active you are, the more calories you use up.

Overcoming Weight Problems

Each year an estimated 80 million Americans go on a diet, but no matter how much weight they lose, 95% gain it back within 5 years.[28] At any given time, more than 25% of the adults in this country are trying to lose weight, while millions of others are trying to keep off the weight they lost. Most dieters cut back on food, not because they want to *feel* better, but because they want to *look* better. Individuals who drastically reduce their food intake and make weight loss a major part of their lives may be jeopardizing their physical and psychological well-being.

The best approach to obesity depends on how overweight a person is. For extreme obesity, medical treatments, including surgery, may be necessary to overcome the danger to a person's health and life. People who are moderately or mildly obese can lose weight through different approaches, including behavioral modification (monitoring food intake, altering eating style, avoiding eating "triggers," and similar strategies), cognitive therapy (changing thoughts or beliefs that lead to overeating), and social support (participating in groups such as Overeaters Anonymous).[29] The keys to overcoming obesity are acknowledging biological limits, addressing individual differences, altering unrealistic expectations, and individualizing treatment. (See Pulsepoints: "Top Ten Ways to Lose Weight.") Although research is still at very

preliminary stages, there have been reports of various drugs that, at least in laboratory animals, have led to reductions in body fat.

Strategies for Change

Evaluating a Diet

If you hear about a new diet that promises to melt away fat, don't try it until you get answers to the following questions:

✔ Does it include a wide variety of nutritious foods?

✔ Does it provide at least 1200 calories a day?

✔ Is it designed to reduce your weight by one-half to two pounds per week?

✔ Does it emphasize moderate portions?

✔ Does it use foods that are easy to find and prepare?

✔ Can you follow it wherever you eat—at home, work, restaurants, or parties?

✔ Is its cost reasonable?

If the answer to any of these questions is no, don't try the diet; then ask yourself one more question: Is losing weight worth losing your well-being?

A Practical Guide to Weight Management

Even experienced dieters who've tried dozens of ways of losing weight often know little about the most effective ways to shed pounds and keep them off. In studies of successful dieters, those who were highly motivated, who monitored their food intake, increased their activity, set realistic goals, and received social support from others were most likely to lose weight. Another key to long-term success is tailoring any weight-loss program to an individual's gender, lifestyle, and cultural, racial, and ethnic values.[30]

A Customized Weight-Loss Plan

"If there's one thing we've learned in decades of research into weight management, it's that the one-diet-fits-all approach doesn't work," says clinical psychologist David Schlundt, Ph.D., of Vanderbilt University.[31] The key is recognizing the ways you tend to put on weight and developing strategies to overcome them. Here are some examples:

- Do you simply like food and consume lots of it? If so, keep a diary of everything you eat and tally up your daily total in calories and fat grams. The numbers may stun you. Look for where most of the calories come from—probably high-fat foods such as whole milk, chocolate, cookies, fried foods, potato chips, steaks—and cut down on how much and how often you eat them.

- Do you eat when you're bored, sad, frustrated, or worried? If so, you may be especially susceptible to "cues" that trigger eating. "People get in the habit of using food to soothe bad feelings or cope with boredom," says Schlundt. "Sometimes the real issue is a self-esteem or body-image problem." Dealing with these concerns is generally more helpful in the long run than dieting.

- Do you "graze," nibbling on snacks rather than eating regular meals? If so, limit yourself to low-calorie, low-fat foods, like carrots, celery, grapes, or air-popped popcorn. Take sips of water regularly to freshen your mouth. Even if you're only having a few crackers or carrots, put them on a plate and try to eat in the same place, preferably while seated. This helps you break the habit of putting food in your mouth without thinking.

Diet Traps to Avoid

Whatever your eating style, there are only two effective strategies for losing weight: eating less and exercising more. Unfortunately, most people search for easier alternatives that almost invariably turn into dietary dead ends. The following are among the most common traps to avoid.

Diet Foods

According to the Calorie Control Council, 90% of Americans choose some foods labeled "light."[32] But even though these foods keep growing in popularity, Americans' weights keep rising. There are several reasons: Many people think choosing a food that's lower in calories, fat-free, or "light" gives them a license to eat as much as they want. What they don't realize is that many foods that are low in fat are still high in sugar and calories. And too much of any food, even one with zero fat and relatively few calories per serving, can sabotage a diet and lead to weight gain.

What about the artificial sweeteners and fake fats that appear in many diet products? Nutritionists caution to use them in moderation and not to substitute them for basic foods, such as grains, fruits, and vegetables.

The Yo-Yo Syndrome

On-and-off-again dieting, especially by means of very-low-calorie diets (under 800 calories a day), can be self-defeating and dangerous. Some studies have shown that "weight cycling" may make it more difficult to lose weight or keep it off. Repeated cycles of rapid weight loss followed by weight gain may even change food preferences. Chronic crash dieters often come to prefer foods that combine sugar and fat, such as cake frosting.[33]

There is a way to avoid weight cycling and overcome its negative effects: exercise. Researchers at the University of Pennsylvania found that when overweight women who exercised went off a very-low-calorie diet, their metabolism did not stay slow but bounced back to the appropriate level for their new lower body weights.[34] The reason may be exercise's ability to preserve muscle tissue. The more muscle tissue you have, the higher your metabolic rate.

Very-Low-Calorie Diets

Any diet that promises to take pounds off fast can be dangerous. For reasons that scientists don't fully understand, rapid weight loss is linked with increased mortality. Most risky are very-low-calorie diets that provide fewer than 800 calories a day. Whenever people cut back drastically on calories, they immediately lose several pounds because of a loss of fluid. As soon as they return to a more normal way of eating, they regain this weight.

On a very-low-calorie diet, as much as 50% of the weight you lose may be muscle (so you'll actually look flabbier). Because your heart is a muscle, it may become so weak that it no longer can pump blood through your body. In addition, your blood pressure may plummet, causing dizziness, lightheadedness, and fatigue. You may develop nausea and abdominal pain. You may lose hair. If you're a woman, your menstrual cycle may become irregular, or you may stop menstruating altogether. As you lose more water, you also lose essential vitamins, and your metabolism slows down. Even reaction time slows, and crash dieters may not be able to respond as quickly as usual.[35]

Once you go off an extreme diet—as you inevitably must—your metabolism remains slow, even though you're no longer restricting your food intake. The human body appears to alter its energy use to compensate for weight loss. In a 1995 study, researchers found that individuals who'd lost 10% of their weight on a liquid-formula diet burned fewer calories than before their diet. These metabolic changes may make it harder for people to maintain a reduced body weight after dieting.[36]

Diet Pills and Products

In their search for a quick fix to weight problems, millions of people have tried often-risky remedies. In the 1920s, some women swallowed patented weight-loss capsules that turned out to be tapeworm eggs. In the 1960s and 1970s, addictive amphetamines were common diet aids. In the 1990s, new appetite suppressants known as fen-phen ("fen" referring to fenfluramine [Pondimin] or dexfenfluramine [Redux], appetite depressants, and the "phen" referring to phentermine, a type of amphetamine) became popular. An estimated 6 million Americans, most of them women, took fen-phen, which helped control cravings by boosting the brain chemical serotonin.[37] In September 1997, fen-phen was taken off the market after these agents were linked to heart valve problems.[38]

The search for the perfect diet drug continues—with plenty of economic incentives for drug makers. By some estimates, the potential market for weight-loss pills totals at least $5 billion. Other diet products, including diet sodas and low-fat foods, also are a very big business. Yet people who use these products aren't necessarily sure to slim down. In fact, people who consume such

---

Strategies for Prevention

Protecting Yourself from Diet Hucksters

The National Council Against Health Fraud cautions dieters to watch for warnings of dangerous or fraudulent programs, including:

✔ Promises of very rapid weight loss.

✔ Claims that the diet can eliminate "cellulite" (a term for dimply fatty tissue on the arms and legs).

✔ "Counselors" who are really salespersons pushing a product or program.

✔ No mention of any risks associated with the diet.

✔ Unproven gimmicks, such as body wraps, starch blockers, hormones, diuretics, or "unique" pills or potions.

✔ No maintenance program.

---

products often gain weight because they think that they can afford to add high-calorie treats to their diet.

Liquid Diets

Liquid diets, such as Optifast, Medifast, and other programs, supply 420 to 800 calories a day and include sufficient protein to preserve muscle tissue. For several months, dieters on these plans eat no solid food, consuming only the special liquid formula and water. These extreme diets, generally reserved for those at least 40% or more overweight, do result in rapid loss, but they can be hazardous. Only 10% to 20% of those who enroll in liquid-diet programs manage to stay within 10 pounds of their target weight a year and a half after entering the program.

Exercise: The Best Solution

You may think that exercise will make you want to eat more. Actually, it has the opposite effect. The combination of exercise and cutting back on calories may be the most effective way of taking weight off and keeping it off. As recent research has shown, exercise keeps your metabolic rate up while you're dieting—and afterward. Exercise, along with a healthy diet, can lead to weight losses of up to 10 pounds.[39]

Exercise has other benefits: It increases energy expenditure, it builds up muscle tissue, and it burns off

Strategies for Change

Working Off Weight

✔ *Get moving.* Take the stairs instead of the elevator. Get off the bus a few blocks from your home and walk the rest of the way.

✔ *Walk.* Most people find it hard to make excuses for not walking 15 minutes every day. Once you start, increase gradually so that you go farther and faster.

✔ *Exercise daily.* You're more likely to lose and keep weight off if you exercise regularly. Try to burn 1800 to 2000 calories a week through exercise—the equivalent of 18 to 20 miles of walking or jogging.

✔ *Get physical.* There are more ways to burn calories than traditional exercise activities: Dancing, hiking, gardening can all help you get in shape. Check your campus bulletin boards and newspapers for information on rock-climbing, kayaking, skiing, and other fun forms of working out.

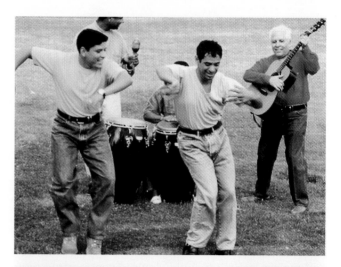

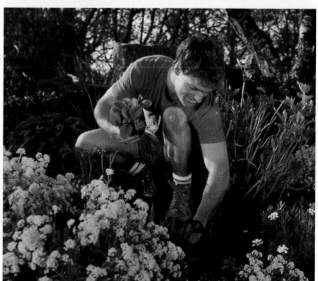

Exercise isn't just tennis or jogging. You can increase your daily exercise by such simple changes as taking the stairs instead of the escalator. Walking, gardening, hiking, and other not-so-strenuous activities can provide enjoyment as well as exercise.

fat stores.[40] Exercise also may reprogram metabolism so that individuals burn up more calories during and after a workout.

Once you start an exercise program, keep it up. Individuals who've started an exercise program during or after a weight-loss program are consistently more successful in keeping off most of the pounds they've shed.[41]

Making This Chapter Work for You

Weighing in for a Healthy Future

■ Weight has become a central preoccupation in many people's lives. However, an obsession with appearance can be dangerous to physical and psychological well-being. People who want to look or be thinner may develop unhealthy eating behaviors, such as extreme dieting and binging, that can undermine their health and diminish their self-esteem.

■ Many factors determine what a person should weigh: heredity, eating behavior, food selection, amount of daily exercise. For any individual of a given height, there is no single best weight, but a range of healthy weights. Standardized tables that give healthy ranges of Body-Mass Index (BMI), a standard index for assessing the ratio of a person's weight to height, are a good indicator of overweight and obesity.

■ Health experts generally advise keeping body fat below 20% of weight for men and 25% for women. The most common ways of measuring an individual's body fat include skin calipers (which pinch skin folds at the arms, waist, and back) and hydrostatic immersion testing (which weighs a person in water to distinguish buoyant fat from denser muscle).

■ A person's waist-hip ratio can indicate health risks. Abdominal fat seems more dangerous than fat stored on the hips, thighs, and buttocks. The bigger the waist and belly, the higher the risk of various diseases, such as diabetes, heart disease, and stroke.

■ The number of calories you need every day depends on your gender, age, size, and activity level. An "average" adult woman—with a height of 5'4" and a weight of 138 pounds—generally needs 1900 to 2200 calories. An average man—with a height of 5'10" and a weight of 174 pounds—generally needs 2300 to 2900 calories.

■ Hunger, the physiological drive to consume food, stimulates our appetite or desire for food. We stop eating when we achieve a state of satisfaction called satiety. According to the set-point theory, each individual has an unconscious control system for regulating appetite and satiety to keep body fat at a predetermined level, or set point.

■ Unhealthy eating behaviors, such as extreme or chronic dieting, compulsive overeating, and binge eating (the rapid consumption of an abnormally large amount of food in a relatively short time) can be early warning signals of more serious eating disorders.

■ The eating disorders anorexia nervosa and bulimia nervosa are most common among young women.

■ The causes of anorexia nervosa are complex; genetic, biochemical, and developmental factors may play a role. Its consequences include extreme weight loss, cessation of menstrual periods in women, decline in testosterone levels in men, heart irregularities, and arrhythmias that can increase the risk of sudden death. Because of their fear of fatness, many people with this disorder resist seeking help. A combination of medical therapy and psychotherapy can lead to recovery.

■ Individuals with bulimia nervosa go on repeated eating binges and rapidly consume large amounts of food, usually sweets. Those with purging-type bulimia induce vomiting or take large doses of laxatives to control their weight. Individuals with nonpurging bulimia use other means, such as fasting or excessive exercise, to compensate for binges. Complications include damaged tooth enamel, dehydration, electrolyte imbalance, cardiac arrhythmias, and even sudden death. Most mental health professionals treat bulimia with a combination of nutritional counseling, psychotherapy, and medication.

■ People gain weight whenever they take in more calories than they burn off. About a third of the adults in the United States are obese. Many different factors contribute to obesity, including heredity, environment, culture, and development. Mild obesity refers to a person being 20% to 40% above his or her ideal weight. An individual who is 41% to 100% above his or her ideal weight is moderately obese, and a per-

son who is more than 100% above his or her ideal weight is severely obese.

■ Obese people are at risk for developing high blood pressure, diabetes, heart disease, certain kinds of cancer, and other life-threatening conditions.

■ In studies of successful dieters, those who were highly motivated, who monitored their food intake, set realistic goals, and received social support from others were most likely to lose weight.

■ Many people fall into diet traps, such as an overreliance on low or reduced fat and other "light" foods, a pattern of off-and-on or yo-yo dieting, very-low-calorie diets, appetite suppressants, diet aids (such as gum, powders, or potions, and low- or no-calorie soft drinks and snacks), and liquid diets.

■ Exercise in combination with diet is the most effective means of losing excess pounds and keeping them off. Exercise increases energy expenditure, builds up muscle tissue, and burns off fat stores. Exercise also may reprogram your metabolism so that you burn up more calories during and after a workout.

If you are overweight, the insight and information in this chapter can help you set up an effective weight-loss program. But losing weight is only the first step. You also have to keep off the pounds you've shed. Here are some ways to do so:

■ **Become a slow eater.** Your brain needs 20 minutes to register that you're full. Eat at a moderate pace, chew each bite thoroughly, and pause regularly throughout your meal. Always wait before taking second helpings.

■ **Develop alternative pleasures.** Learn to indulge your other senses. Listen to music. Soak in a bubble bath. Take up hiking, gardening, yoga.

■ **Treat your taste buds.** If you're giving up or cutting down on rich foods, try highly spiced dishes, such as a hot Indian curry or a spicy Mexican entree, as a main course.

■ **Develop strategies for social occasions.** Always eat something that's filling and low in calories before a party. Decide in advance which items you'll eat and which you won't—pretzels and carrot sticks, but not chips, for instance.

■ **Set a danger zone.** Don't let your weight climb more than 3 or 4 pounds above your ideal weight. If you do, take action immediately rather than waiting until you gain an additional 5 or 10 pounds.

Health Online

Healthy Body Calculator   http://www.dietitian.com/ibw/ibw.html

The Healthy Body Calculator allows you to input your age, gender, height, activity level, and frame size. It then determines your healthy weight range. You can also enter your weight goal, information about your nutrient intake, and your waist-to-hip ratio for more detailed results.

Think about it ...

- According to the Healthy Body Calculator, are you within your healthy weight range? If not, are you willing to take steps to change your weight?

- What are three things you could do each day to become more physically active? And what three specific changes could you make to your diet to make it healthier?

- Do you have any older relatives or friends who are overweight? Have they suffered any physical problems that might be related to their weight?

Key Terms

The terms listed here are used within the chapter. Page numbers are included for each term. A definition of each term is given in the green Glossary pages at the end of this book.

anorexia nervosa *96*	**bulimia nervosa** *97*	**obesity** *97*
appetite *93*	**calorie** *92*	**satiety** *93*
basal metabolic rate (BMR) *92*	**eating disorders** *96*	**set-point theory** *93*
binge eating *95*	**hunger** *93*	**skin calipers** *91*
Body-Mass Index (BMI) *91*	**hydrostatic weighing** *91*	

Review Questions

1. What is a calorie? How many calories are needed to maintain a healthy body?
2. What is the set-point theory? Why does the set point make it difficult to diet? How can this problem be overcome?
3. What are the symptoms of anorexia? Of bulimia? How can each of these eating disorders be overcome?
4. How much overweight does a person have to be to be considered obese? What role do genetics, lifestyle, and overeating play in determining whether an individual becomes obese?
5. What is the best way to lose weight? What are some of the dangers associated with dieting?
6. What is your ideal weight? How does your actual weight compare? What changes, if any, do you need to make in your lifestyle to achieve and maintain your ideal weight?

Critical Thinking Questions

1. Ask your friends—particularly your women friends—how they feel about their bodies. Chances are they'll mention something they hate: their hair, their hips, their height, and most often of all, their weight. What do you think leads to such dissatisfaction? What can individuals do to feel better about the way they look?

2. Different cultures have different standards for body weight and attractiveness. Within our society, even men and women often seem to follow different standards. What influences have shaped your personal feelings about desired weight?

3. If you could choose skin calipers or hydrostatic immersion testing, which would you select to determine your body fat? Explain the reasons for your choice.

 ## Connections to Personal Health Interactive

To enhance your understanding of the material covered in this chapter, check out the following study aids on the **Personal Health Interactive CD-ROM**.

■ Personal Insights: Do You Like to Eat?
■ Diet Tips
■ **Online Research:** Weight Management

■ Personal Voices: Anorexia Nervosa
■ Glossary & Key Term Review

 ## References

1. Rodin, Judith. "Cultural and Psychosocial Determinants of Weight Concerns." *Annals of Internal Medicine*, October 1, 1993.

2. Rumpel, Catherine, and Tamara Harris. "The Influence of Weight on Adolescent Self-Esteem." *Journal of Psychosomatic Research*, Vol. 38, No. 6, August 1994. Tordjman, Sylvie, et al. "Preliminary Study of Eating Disorders Among French Female Adolescents and Young Adults." *International Journal of Eating Disorders*, Vol. 16, No. 3, November 1994. Stice, Eric, and Heather Shaw. "Adverse Effects of the Media Portrayed Thin Ideal on Women and Linkages to Bulimic Symptomatology." *Journal of Social and Clinical Psychology,* Vol. 13, No. 3, Fall 1994.

3. Alley, Thomas, and Katherine Scully. "The Impact of Actual and Perceived Changes in Body Weight on Women's Physical Attractiveness." *Basic & Applied Social Psychology*, Vol. 15, No. 4, December 1994. Levine, Michael, et al. "The Relation of Sociocultural Factors to Eating Attitudes and Behaviors Among Middle School Girls." *Journal of Early Adolescence*, Vol. 14, No. 4, November 1994.

4. Allison, David, et al. "Weight-Related Attitudes and Beliefs of Obese African-American Women." *Journal of Nutrition Education*, Vol. 27, No. 1, January–February 1995. Stevens, June, et al. "Attitudes Toward Body Size and Dieting." *American Journal of Public Health*, Vol. 84, No. 8, August 1994.

5. Caldwell, Marcia, et al. "Relationship of Weight, Body Dissatisfaction, and Self-Esteem in African American and White Female Dieters." *International Journal of Eating Disorders*, Vol. 22, No. 2, September 1997.

6. Hunter, Beatrice Trum. "Eating Disorders: Perilous Compulsions." *Consumers' Research Magazine*, Vol. 80, No. 9, September 1997.

7. Douglas, Kathy, et al. "Results from the 1995 National College Health Risk Behavior Survey." *Journal of American College Health*, Vol. 46, September 1997.

8. Hart, Kathleen, and Maureen Kenny. "Adherence to the Super Woman Ideal and Eating Disorder Symptoms Among College Women." *Sex Roles: A Journal of Research*, Vol. 36, No. 7–8, April 1997.

9. Schulken, Ellen, et al. "Sorority Women's Body Size Perceptions and Their Weight-Related Attitudes and Behaviors." *Journal of American College Health*, Vol. 46, September 1997.

10. Bulik, Cynthia, et al. "Initial Manifestations of Disordered Eating Behavior: Dieting Versus Binging." *International Journal of Eating Disorders*, Vol. 22, No. 2, September 1997.

11. Antony, Martin, et al. "Psychopathology Correlates of Binge Eating and Binge Eating Disorder." *Comprehensive Psychiatry*, Vol. 35, No. 5, September–October 1994. Nangle, Douglas, et al. "Binge Eating Disorder and the Proposed DSM-IV Criteria: Psychometric Analysis of the Questionnaire of Eating and Weight Patterns." *International Journal of Eating Disorders*, Vol. 16, No. 2, September 1994.

12. American Psychiatric Association. *Diagnostic and Statistical Manual of Mental Disorders*. 4th ed. Washington, DC: American Psychiatric Association, 1994.

13. Beumont, Pierre, et al. "Diagnoses of Eating or Dieting Disorders: What May We Learn from Past Mistakes?"

International Journal of Eating Disorders, Vol. 16, No. 4, December 1994. Fairburn, Christopher, and Sarah Beglin. "Assessment of Eating Disorders: Interview or Self-Report Questionnaire?" *International Journal of Eating Disorders*, Vol. 16, No. 4, December 1994.

14. Fernstrom, Madelyn, et al. "Twenty-Four-Hour Food Intake in Patients with Anorexia Nervosa and in Healthy Control Subjects." *Biological Psychiatry*, Vol. 36, No. 10, November 1994.

15. Ogden, Jane, and Pauline Fox. "Examination of the Use of Smoking for Weight Control in Restrained and Unrestrained Eaters." *International Journal of Eating Disorders*, Vol. 16, No. 2, September 1994.

16. Walters, Ellen, and Kenneth Kendler. "Anorexia Nervosa and Anorexic-Like Syndromes in a Population-Based Female Twin Sample." *American Journal of Psychiatry*, Vol. 152, No. 1, January 1995.

17. Hersen, Michel, and Samuel M. Turner. "Eating Disorders." In *Diagnostic Interviewing*. 2nd ed. New York: Plenum Press, 1994. Garner, David, and Lionel Rosen. "Eating Disorders." In *Handbook of Aggressive and Destructive Behavior in Psychiatric Patients*. New York: Plenum Press, 1994.

18. Hales, Dianne, and Robert E. Hales. *Caring for the Mind: The Comprehensive Guide to Mental Health*. New York: Bantam Books, 1995.

19. van der Ster Wallin, G., et al. "Binge Eating Versus Non-purged Eating in Bulimics: Is There a Carbohydrate Craving After All?" *Acta Psychiatrica Scandinavica*, Vol. 89, No. 6, June 1994.

20. Leal, Linda, et al. "The Relationship Between Gender, Symptoms of Bulimia, and Tolerance for Stress." *Addictive Behaviors*, Vol. 20, No. 1, January–February 1995. Boumann, Christine, et al. "Risk Factors for Bulimia Nervosa: A Controlled Study of Parental Psychiatric Illness and Divorce." *Addictive Behaviors*, Vol. 19, November–December 1994. Weiss, Lillie, et al. "Bulimia Nervosa: Definition, Diagnostic Criteria, and Associated Psychological Problems." In *Understanding Eating Disorders: Anorexia Nervosa, Bulimia Nervosa, and Obesity*. Philadelphia: Taylor & Francis, 1994.

21. Sansone, Randy, and Lori Sansone. "Bulimia Nervosa: Medical Complications." In *Understanding Eating Disorders: Anorexia Nervosa, Bulimia Nervosa, and Obesity*. Philadelphia: Taylor & Francis, 1994.

22. Centers for Disease Control and Prevention. Polednak, Anthony. "Weight/Height Ratio in Hispanic Adults Surveyed by Telephone." *Health Values*, Vol. 19, No. 2, March–April 1995.

23. Magid, Barry. "Is Biology Destiny After All?" *Journal of Psychotherapy Practice & Research*, Vol. 4, No. 1, Winter 1995.

24. Spector, Rosanne. "Researchers Discover New Target for Obesity Drugs." *Stanford University Medical News*, October 1, 1997.

25. Brownell, Kelly, and Thomas Wadden. "Etiology and Treatment of Obesity: Understanding a Serious, Prevalent, and Refractory Disorder." *Journal of Consulting & Clinical Psychology*, August 1992.

26. Zwaan, Martina de, et al. "Eating Related and General Psychopathology in Obese Females with Binge Eating Disorder." *International Journal of Eating Disorders*, Vol. 15, No 1, January 1994. Telch, Christy, and Stewart Agras. "Obesity, Binge Eating and Psychopathology: Are They Related?" *International Journal of Eating Disorders*, Vol. 15, No. 1, January 1994. Webber, Eleanor. "Psychological Characteristics of Binging and Nonbinging Obese Women." *Journal of Psychology*, Vol. 128, No. 3, May 1994.

27. Karlsson, Jan, et al. "Predictors and Effects of Long-Term Dieting on Mental Well-Being and Weight Loss in Obese Women." *Appetite*, Vol. 23, No. 1, August 1994. Ross, Catherine. "Overweight and Depression." *Journal of Health & Social Behavior*, Vol. 35, No. 1, March 1994.

28. Horowitz, Janice, and Lawrence Mondi. "Fat Times." *Time*, January 16, 1995.

29. Foster, Gary, and Philip Kendall. "The Realistic Treatment of Obesity: Changing the Scales of Success." *Clinical Psychology Review*, Vol. 14, No. 8, 1994. Sperry, Len. "Helping People Control Their Weight: Research and Practice." In *Addictions: Concepts and Strategies for Treatment*. Gaithersburg, MD: Aspen Publishers, 1994.

30. "Weight Loss Programs and Weight Maintenance." *American Family Physician*, Vol. 55, No. 7, November 15, 1997.

31. Schlundt, David. Personal interview.

32. Margolis, Dawn. "The Lowfat Trap." *American Health*, May 1995.

33. Brownell, K. D., and Judy Rodin. "Medical, Metabolic, and Psychological Effects of Weight Cycling." *Archives of Internal Medicine*, June 27, 1994.

34. Ibid.

35. "Cutting Calories Too Much Can Slow Reaction Time." *Tufts University Health & Nutrition Letter*, Vol. 14, No. 6, August 1997. Raloff, Janet. "Dieting Impairs Reaction Time." *Science News*, Vol. 151, No. 21, May 24, 1997.

36. Rudolph L., et al. "Changes in Energy Expenditure Resulting from Altered Body Weight." *New England Journal of Medicine*, Vol. 332, No. 10, March 9, 1995. Roust, L. R., et al. "Effects of Isoenergetic, Low-Fat Diets on Energy Metabolism in Lean and Obese Women." *American Journal of Clinical Nutrition*, October 1994. Sintsova, N. "Adaptation to Low-Calorie Diet in Obese Patients." *Human Physiology*, September–October 1993.

37. "The Painful Business of Losing Weight." *The Economist*, Vol. 344, No. 8032, August 30, 1997.

38. Kolata, Gina. "How Fen-Phen, a Diet 'Miracle,' Rose and Fell." *New York Times*, September 23, 1997. Cowley, Geoffrey, and Karen Springen. "After Fen-Phen." *Newsweek*, Vol. 130, No. 13, September 29, 1997.

39. Parr, Richard. "Exercising to Lose 10 to 20 Pounds." *Physician & Sportsmedicine*, Vol. 25, No. 4, April 1997.

40. Linkowish, Mary Desmond. "Winning at Losing: Some Optimism about Weight-loss Maintenance." *Patient Care*, Vol. 31, No. 17, October 30, 1997.

41. Katoh, Junichi, et al. "Effects of Exercise on Weight Reduction in Middle-Aged Obese Women." *Current Therapeutic Research*, Vol. 55, No. 9, September 1994.

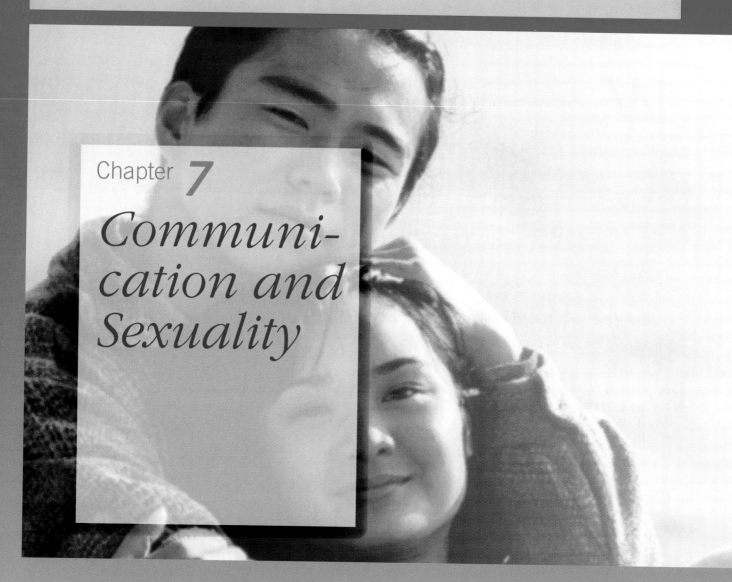

Chapter 7

Communi-cation and Sexuality

After studying the material in this chapter, you should be able to:

- **Compare** and **contrast** the behavioral expectations for friendship, dating, and mature love.

- **Describe** the typical progress of a relationship from dating to mature love.

- **Explain** how the institution of marriage has changed over the last 50 years and what factors predict marital success.

- **Describe** the male and female reproductive systems and the functions of the individual components of each system.

- **Describe** some issues unique to women's sexual health and men's sexual health.

- **Describe** some ways to make responsible decisions about your sexuality.

We are born social. From our first days of life, we reach out to others, struggle to express ourselves, and strive to forge connections. As adults, sexual intimacy can be one of our most rewarding kinds of relationship. But while sexual expresssion and experience can provide intense joy, they also involve sexual responsibility. This chapter is an introduction to your social and sexual self. It provides information and insight you can use in making decisions and choosing behaviors that are responsible for all concerned.

Personal Communication

Getting to know someone is one of life's greatest challenges and pleasures. When you find another person intriguing—as a friend, as a teacher, as a colleague, as a possible partner—you want to find out as much as you can about him or her and to share more and more information about yourself. Roommates may talk for endless hours. Friends may spend years getting to know each other. Partners in committed relationships may delight in learning new things about each other.

Communication stems from a desire to know and a decision to tell. Each of us chooses what information about ourselves we want to disclose and what we want to keep private. But in opening up to others, we increase our own self-knowledge and understanding.

Communicating Feelings

A great deal of daily communication focuses on facts: on the who, what, where, when, and how. Information is easy to convey and comprehend. Emotions are not. Some people have great difficulty saying "I appreciate you" or "I care about you," even though they are genuinely appreciative and caring. Others find it hard to know what to say in response and how to accept such expressions of affection.

Sometimes people convey strong emotions with a kiss or a hug, a pat or a punch, but such actions aren't precise enough to communicate exact thoughts. Stalking out of a room and slamming the door may be clear signs of anger, but they don't explain what caused the anger

---

Strategies for Change

How to Enhance Communication

✔ *Use "I" statements.* Describe what's going on with you. Say, "I worry about being liked" or "I get frustrated when I can't put my feelings into words." Avoid generalities such as, "You never think about my feelings" or "Nobody understands me."

✔ *Gently ask how the other person feels.* If your friend or partner describes thoughts rather than feelings, ask for more adjectives. Was he or she sad, excited, angry, hurt?

✔ *Become a very good listener.* When another person talks, don't interrupt, ask why, judge, or challenge. Nod your head. Use body language and facial expression to show you're eager to hear more.

✔ *Respect confidences.* Treat a friend's or partner's secrets with the discretion they deserve. Consider them a special gift entrusted to your care.

---

or suggest what to do about it. You must learn how to communicate all feelings clearly and appropriately if you hope to become truly close to another person.

As two people build a relationship, they must sharpen their communication skills so that they can discuss all the issues they may confront. They must learn how to communicate anger as well as affection, hurt as well as joy—and they must listen as carefully as they speak. If and when love grows, they will find themselves as concerned with the other as with the self.

Gender Differences in Communication

Every man and every woman is unique, but researchers who've carefully observed each gender have noticed differences in the way many—but not necessarily all—men and women use language. There are complex reasons why men and women may use words in different ways. Deborah Tannen, Ph.D., a professor of linguistics at Georgetown University and author of *You Just Don't Understand: Women and Men in Conversation,* theorizes that men and women communicate for different reasons. In many public situations, men speak to convey information, to challenge others, to achieve status in a group, or to put themselves in a "one-up" situation.

Figure 7-1

Relationships begin with signals. The more effective our signals—verbal as well as gestures and expressions—the more likely we are to build good relationships.

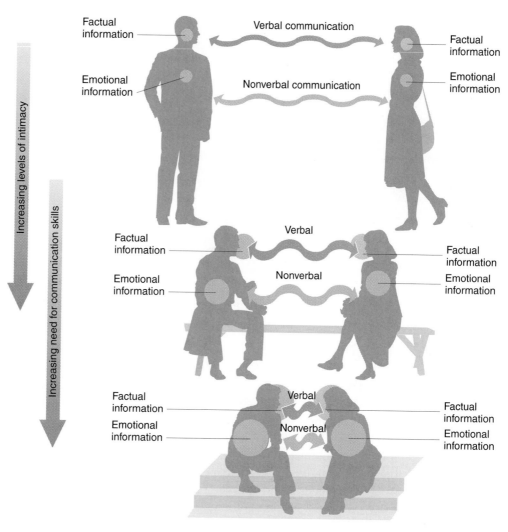

Increasing levels of intimacy

Increasing need for communication skills

Factual information

Verbal communication

Factual information

Emotional information

Nonverbal communication

Emotional information

Factual information

Verbal

Factual information

Emotional information

Nonverbal

Emotional information

Factual information

Verbal

Factual information

Emotional information

Nonverbal

Emotional information

Many women, on the other hand, feel more comfortable with private conversations among friends and family. They talk to achieve and nurture intimacy, to promote closeness and equality in a group, and to build better connections to others.[1]

The existence of gender differences in communication styles does not mean that one gender's preference is right, wrong, better, or worse than the other's. However, recognition of the fact that the sexes use language differently can help both men and women avoid jumping to erroneous conclusions and overcome potential obstacles to their mutual understanding and acceptance.

Nonverbal Communication

More than 90% of communication may be nonverbal. While we speak with our vocal cords, we communicate with our facial expressions, tone of voice, hands, shoulders, legs, torsos, posture. "Body language is a very elementary level of communication that people react to

without realizing why," observes Albert Mehrabian, Ph.D., a professor of psychology at the University of California, Los Angeles (UCLA) and author of *Silent Messages.* "It's the building block upon which more advanced verbal forms of communication rest."[2]

Culture has a great deal of influence on body language. In some cultures, for example, establishing eye contact is considered hostile or challenging; in others, it conveys friendliness. People's sense of personal space—the distance they feel most comfortable in keeping from others—also varies in different societies. Nonverbal messages also reveal something important about the individual. "Nonverbal messages come from deep inside of you, from your own sense of self-esteem," says Marilyn Maple, Ph.D., an educator at the University of Florida. "To improve your body language, you have to start from the inside and work out. If you're comfortable with yourself, it shows. People who have good self-esteem, who give themselves status and respect, who know who they are, have a relaxed way of talking and moving and always come across best."[3]

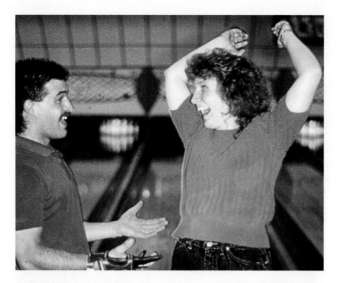

Body language. Cultural influences aside, people who have good self-esteem are comfortable with themselves and the world.

Forming Relationships

We first learn how to relate in our families, as children. Our relationships with parents and siblings change dramatically as we grow toward independence. Relationships between friends also change as they move or develop different interests; between lovers, as they come to know more about each other; between spouses, as they pass through life together; and between parents and children, as youngsters develop and mature.

Strategies for Change

Getting Your Signals Straight

✔ *Tune into your body talk.* Notice details about the way you speak, gesture, and move. If possible, watch yourself on videotape. Analyze the emotions you're feeling at the time and think of how they may be influencing your body language.

✔ *Learn to establish good eye contact, but don't glare or stare.* If you sense that someone feels uncomfortable with an intense eye grip, shift your focus so that your gaze hits somewhere between the eyes and the chin, rather than pupil-to-pupil.

✔ *Avoid putting up barriers.* If you fold your arms across your chest, you'll look defensive or uninterested in contact. Crossing your legs or ankles also can seem like a way of keeping your distance.

But throughout life, close relationships, tested and strengthened by time, allow us to explore the depths of our souls and the heights of our emotions.

I, Myself, and Me

The way we perceive ourselves as individuals affects all the ways we reach out and relate to others. If we feel unworthy of love, others may share that opinion. Self-esteem and self-love (discussed in Chapter 3) provide a positive foundation for our relationships with others. Self-love doesn't mean vanity or preoccupation with our own needs; rather, it is a genuine concern and respect for ourselves so that we remain true to our own feelings and beliefs. We can't know or love or accept others until we know and love and accept ourselves, however imperfect we may be.

If we're lacking in self-esteem, our relationships may suffer. According to research on college students by psychologists at the University of Texas, individuals with negative views of themselves seek out partners (friends, roommates, dates) who are critical and rejecting—and who confirm their low opinions of their own worth.[4]

Friendship

Friends can be a basic source of happiness, a connection to a larger world, a source of solace in times of trouble. Although we have different friends throughout life, often the friendships of adolescence and young adulthood are the closest we ever form. They ease the normal break from parents and the transition from childhood to independence.

Friendship transcends all boundaries of distance and differences and enhances feelings of warmth, trust, love, and affection between two people. It is a common denominator of human existence that cuts across major social categories: In every country, culture, and language, human beings make friends. Friendship is both a universal and a deeply satisfying experience.

Dating

A date is any occasion during which two people share their time. It can be a Friday night dance, a bicycle ride, dinner for two, or a walk in the park. Friends and lovers go on dates; so do complete strangers. Some men date other men; some women date other women. We don't expect to love, or even like, everyone we date. Yet the people you date reveal something about the sort of person you are.

Strategies for Change

Being a Good Friend

✔ *Be willing to open up.* The more you share, the deeper the bond between you and your friend will become.

✔ *Be sensitive to your friend's feelings.* Keep in mind that, like you, your friend has unique needs, desires, and dreams.

✔ *Express appreciation.* Be generous with your compliments. Let your friends know you recognize their kindnesses.

✔ *Know that friends will disappoint you from time to time.* They, too, are only human. Accept them as they are. Admitting their faults need not reduce your respect for them.

✔ *Talk about your friendship.* Evaluate the relationship periodically. If you have any gripes or frustrations, air them.

Dating can do more than help you meet people. By dating, you can learn how to make conversation, get to know more about others as well as yourself, and share feelings, opinions, and interests. In adolescence and young adulthood, dating also provides an opportunity for exploring your sexual identity. Some people date for months and never share more than a good-night kiss. Others may fall into bed together before they fall in love or even "like."

It's often difficult to sort out your emotional feelings about someone you're dating from your sexual desires. The first step to making responsible sexual decisions is respecting your sexual values and those of your partner. If you care about the other person—not just his or her body—and the relationship you're creating, sex will be an important, but not the all-important, factor while you're dating. (Sexual decision making and etiquette are discussed later in this chapter.)

Sexual Attraction

What draws two people to each other and keeps them together: chemistry or kismet, survival instincts or sexual longings? "Probably it's a host of different things," reports sociologist Edward Laumann, Ph.D., coauthor of *Sex in America*, a landmark survey of 3432 men and women conducted by the National Opinion Research Center at the University of Chicago.[5] "But what's remarkable is that most of us end up with partners much like ourselves—in age, race, ethnicity, socioeconomic class, education."

Why? "You've got to get close for sexual chemistry to occur," says Laumann. "Sparks may fly when you see someone across a crowded room, but you only see a preselected group of people—people enough like you to be in the same room in the first place. This makes sense because initiating a sexual relationship is very uncertain. We all have such trepidations about being too fat, too ugly, too undesirable. We try to lower the risk of rejection by looking for people more or less like us."

In the University of Chicago survey, most men and women chose sexual and marital partners of the same race, the same or similar religion and socioeconomic class, and within 5 years of their own age. More than 75% selected partners of similar education levels.[6] Physical attractiveness also plays a role in sexual attraction—at least for men, who consistently place more emphasis on looks than do women.[7]

Intimate and Committed Relationships

The term **intimacy**—the open, trusting sharing of close, confidential thoughts and feelings—comes from the Latin word for *within*. Intimacy doesn't happen at first sight or in a day or a week or in a number of weeks. Intimacy requires time and nurturing; it is a process of revealing rather than hiding, of wanting to know another and to be known by that other (see Figure 7-2 for the elements of love). Although intimacy doesn't require sex, an intimate relationship often includes a sexual relationship, heterosexual or homosexual.

Romantic Love

Falling in love is an intense, dizzying experience. A person not only enters our life but takes possession of it as well. We are intrigued, flattered, delighted—but is this love, or a love of loving? At the time you're experiencing it, you may not care. You're in such a state of giddy elation that it doesn't matter, at least for the moment, whether it stems from a strong sexual attraction, a fear of loneliness, loneliness itself, or a hunger for approval.

We like to think of this powerful force, this source of both danger and delight, as something that defies analysis. However, in recent years, as scientists have attempted to study love objectively, they have provided new perspectives on its nature.

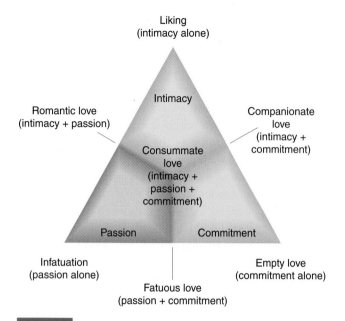

Figure 7-2

This love triangle illustrates the three components of love and the various kinds of love as reflected in different combinations of the three components. *Note:* Nonlove is the absence of all three components.

The heart is the organ we associate with love, but the brain may be where the action really is. According to research on neurotransmitters (messenger chemicals within the brain), love sets off a chemical chain reaction that causes our skin to flush, our palms to sweat, and our lungs to breathe more deeply and rapidly. The "love chemicals" within the brain—dopamine, norepineph-

rine, and phenylethylamine (PEA)—have effects similar to those of amphetamines, stimulant drugs that intensify physiological reactions.[8]

Infatuation may indeed be a natural high, but like other highs, this rush doesn't last—possibly because the body develops tolerance for love-induced chemicals, just as it does with amphetamines. However, as the initial lovers' high fades, other brain chemicals may come into play: the endorphins, morphinelike chemicals that can help produce feelings of well-being, security, and tranquillity. These feel-good molecules may increase in partners who develop a deep attachment.

Mature Love

Social scientists have distinguished between passionate love—characterized by intense feelings of elation, sexual desire, and ecstasy—and companionate love, which is characterized by friendly affection and deep attachment. Often relationships begin with passionate love and evolve into a more companionate love. Sometimes the opposite happens and two people who know each other well discover that their friendship has "caught fire" and the sparks have flamed an unexpected passion.

Mature love is a complex combination of sexual excitement, tenderness, commitment, and—most of all—an overriding passion that sets it apart from all other love relationships in one's life. This passion isn't simply a matter of orgasm, but also entails a crossing of the psychological boundaries between oneself and one's lover. You feel as if you're becoming one with your partner while simultaneously retaining a sense of yourself. (For other characteristics of mature, healthy love, see Pulsepoints: "Ten Characteristics of a Good Relationship" on p. 114.)

When Love Ends

Breaking up is indeed hard to do. Sometimes two people grow apart gradually, and both of them realize that they must go their separate ways. More often, one person falls out of love first. It hurts to be rejected; it also hurts to inflict pain on someone who once meant a great deal to you. In surveys, college students say it's more difficult to initiate a breakup than to be rejected. Those who decided to end a relationship reported greater feelings of guilt, uncertainty, discomfort, and awkwardness than those with whom they broke up.[9]

While the pain does ease over time, it can help both parties if they end their relationship in a way that shows kindness and respect. Your basic guideline should be to think of how you would like to be treated if someone

---

Strategies for Change

Is It Infatuation, "Like," or Love?

A romantic relationship shows definite promise if:

✔ You feel at ease with your new partner.

✔ You feel good about your new partner both when you're together and when you're not.

✔ Your partner is open with you about his or her life—past, present, and future.

✔ You can say no to each other without feeling guilty.

✔ You feel cared for, appreciated, and accepted as you are.

✔ Your partner really listens to what you have to say.

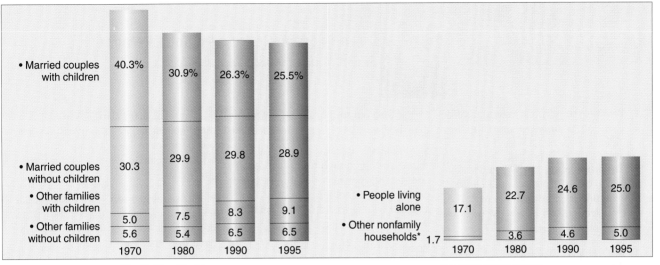

Figure 7-3

The changing American household. More Americans are living alone, and there are fewer married couples with children at home.

were breaking up with you. Would it hurt more to find out from someone else? Would it be more painful if the person you cared for lied to you or deceived you, rather than admitted the truth? Saying, "I don't feel the way I once did about you; I don't want to continue our relationship," is hard, but it's also honest and direct.

Strategies for Change

Dealing with Rejection

✔ Remind yourself of your own worth. You are no less attractive, intelligent, interesting, or lovable because someone ends a relationship with you.

✔ Accept the rejection as a statement of the other person's preference rather than trying to debate or defend yourself.

✔ Think of other people who value or have valued you, who accept and even see as appealing the same characteristics the rejecting person viewed as undesirable.

✔ Don't withdraw from others. Although you may not want to risk further rejection, it's worth the gamble to get involved again. The only individuals who've never been rejected are those who've never reached out to connect with another.

Living Together

Although couples have always shared homes in informal relationships without any official ties, "living together," or **cohabitation**, has become more common in the United States, increasing by 80% in the last two decades. There are about 7 unmarried couples for every 100 married ones. Often young people live together in a trial marriage, getting to know each other better to see whether they're compatible—although this does not necessarily lead to a more successful marriage. People who have been married and divorced may be content just sharing their lives with one another.

Unmarried couples aren't very different from married couples: They share, they talk, they quarrel. They're also gaining legal recognition; some U.S. cities have "domestic partnership" laws that grant a variety of spousal rights—such as insurance benefits and bereavement leave—to partners, heterosexual or homosexual, who live together. Couples counselors in some cities say that more than half of the partners they see aren't married. Men and women who live together are equally likely to split up or to marry.

Marriage

Contemporary marriage has been described as an institution that everyone on the outside wants to enter and everyone on the inside wants to leave. About 90% of

Pulsepoints

Ten Characteristics of a Good Relationship

1. Trust. Partners are able to confide in each other openly, knowing their confidences will be respected.

2. Togetherness. In a healthy relationship, two people create a sense of both intimacy and autonomy. They enjoy each other's company but also pursue solitary interests.

3. Expressiveness. Partners in healthy relationships say what they feel, need, and desire.

4. Staying power. Couples in committed relationships keep their bond strong through tough times by proving that they will be there for each other.

5. Security. Because a good relationship is strong enough to absorb conflict and anger, partners know they can express their feelings honestly. They also are willing to risk vulnerability for the sake of becoming closer.

6. Laughter. Humor keeps things in perspective—always crucial in any sort of ongoing relationship or enterprise.

7. Support. Partners in good relationships continually offer each other encouragement, comfort, and acceptance.

8. Physical affection. Sexual desire may fluctuate or diminish over the years, but partners in loving, long-term relationships usually retain some physical connection.

9. Personal growth. In the best relationships, partners are committed to bringing out the best in each other and have the other's best interests at heart.

10. Respect. Caring partners are aware of each other's boundaries, need for personal space, and vulnerabilities. They do not take each other or their relationship for granted.

Strategies for Prevention

When to Think Twice About Getting Married

Don't get married if:

✔ You or your partner is constantly asking the other such questions as, "Are you sure you love me?"

✔ You spend most of your time together disagreeing and quarreling.

✔ You're both under the age of 20.

✔ You're really looking in the relationship for a mother or father, not an equal.

✔ Your boyfriend or girlfriend has behaviors (such as non-stop talking), traits (such as bossiness), or problems (such as drinking too much) that really bother you and that you're hoping will change after you're married.

✔ Your partner wants you to stop seeing your friends, quit a job you enjoy, or change your life in some other way that diminishes your overall personal satisfaction.

all American adults marry—for as long as they both love, if not live. According to the Census Bureau, the marriage rate has dropped dramatically, with a lower percentage of couples tying the knot in the 1990s than in previous decades.[10] This trend may reflect a variety of new social forces, such as increases in cohabitation and divorce.

With more than half of all marriages ending in divorce, there's little doubt that modern marriages aren't made in heaven. Are some couples doomed to divorce even before they swap "I do's"? Could counseling before a marriage increase its odds of success? According to recent research findings, the answer to both questions is yes.[11]

Generally, men and women marry people from the geographical area they grew up in and from the same social background. Differences in religion and race can add to the pressures of marriage, but they also can enrich the relationship if they aren't viewed as obstacles. Generally speaking, in our culturally diverse society, interracial and crosscultural marriages are becoming more common and widely accepted. According to the Census Bureau, there are four times as many interracial couples today as there were in 1970, with as many as one marriage out of every fifty crossing racial lines.

Some of the things that appeal to us in a date become less important when we select a mate; others become key ingredients in the emotional cement holding two people together. According to psychologist Robert Sternberg of Yale University, the crucial ingredients for commitment are the following:

- Shared values.

- A willingness to change in response to each other.

- A willingness to tolerate flaws.

- A match in religious beliefs.

- The ability to communicate effectively.

The single best predictor of how satisfied one will be in a relationship, according to Sternberg, is not how one feels toward a lover, but the difference between how one would like the lover to feel and how the lover actually feels. Feeling that the partner you've chosen loves too little or too much is, as he puts it, "the best predictor of failure."[12]

Divorce

More than 1.2 million marriages end in divorce every year. The divorce rate soared in the 1960s and 1970s but peaked at a rate of 5.3 per 1000 in 1981. Since then it has slowly declined (see Figure 7-4). In 1996 there were about 1.17 million divorces and about 2.33 million marriages.[13] However, the U.S. divorce rate remains the highest in the world, even though divorce is becoming more common everywhere.

More than one in every five men and women who have ever been married have been divorced. Increasingly, therapists and family counselors are urging couples to try to work out their differences for their own and

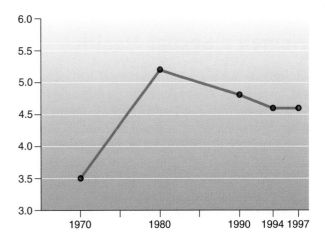

Figure 7-4

The divorce rate. The divorce rate—the number of divorces in a given year per 1000 persons in the population—has declined slightly in recent years.

Source: Bureau of the Census.

their children's sake. As many people have discovered, divorce hurts.

Even after their hopes for happiness with one spouse end, men and women still yearn to mesh two personalities, two life histories, and two persons' dreams into a marriage. Eighty percent of divorced men and women remarry, and the remarriage rate increases with the number of times an individual has been divorced. The remarriage rate after a second divorce is 90%; after a third divorce, it's even higher.

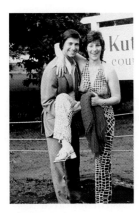
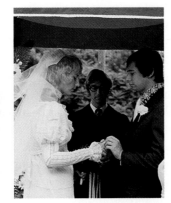
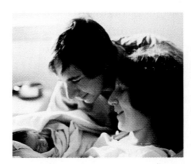
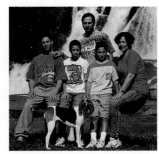

A relationship is just as alive as the individuals who create it. It grows if there is caring, it can blossom if there is emotional nourishment, and it endures if there is commitment.

Women's Sexual Health

Only recently has medical research devoted major scientific investigations to issues in women's health. In fact, until 1993, the National Institutes of Health routinely excluded women from experimental studies because of concerns about menstrual cycles and pregnancy. In clinical settings, women are more likely to have their symptoms dismissed as psychological and not to be referred to a specialist than are men with identical complaints. Some physicians are suggesting the creation of a new medical specialty (distinct from obstetrics and gynecology) devoted to women's health to provide more comprehensive care and overcome the current gender gap in health services.[14]

Female Sexual Anatomy

As illustrated in Figure 7-5a, the **mons pubis** is the rounded, fleshy area over the junction of the pubic bones. The folds of skin that form the outer lips of a woman's genital area are called the **labia majora**. They cover soft flaps of skin (inner lips) called the **labia minora**. The inner lips join at the top to form a hood over the **clitoris**, a small elongated erectile organ and the most sensitive spot in the entire female genital area. Below the clitoris is the **urethral opening**, the outer opening of the thin tube that carries urine from the bladder. Below that is a larger opening, the mouth of the **vagina**, the canal that leads to the primary internal organs of reproduction. The **perineum** is the area between the vagina and the anus (the opening to the rectum and large intestine).

At the back of the vagina is the **cervix**, the opening to the womb, or **uterus** (see Figure 7-5b). The uterine walls are lined by a layer of tissue called the **endometrium**. The **ovaries**, about the size and shape of almonds, are located on either side of the uterus and contain egg cells called **ova** (singular, **ovum**). Extending outward and back from the upper uterus are the **fallopian tubes**, the canals that transport ova from the ovaries to the uterus. When an egg is released from an ovary, the fingerlike ends of the adjacent fallopian tube "catch" the egg and direct it into the tube.

The Menstrual Cycle

As shown in Figure 7-6, the hypothalamus monitors hormone levels in the blood and sends messages to the pituitary gland to release follicle stimulating hormone (FSH) and luteinizing hormone (LH). In the ovary, these hormones stimulate the growth of a few of the immature eggs, or ova, stored in every woman's body. Usually, only one ovum matures completely during each monthly cycle. As it does, it increases its production of the female sex hormone estrogen, which in turn triggers the release of a larger surge of LH.

At midcycle, the increased LH hormone levels trigger **ovulation**, the release of the egg cell. Estrogen levels drop, and the remaining cells of the follicle then enlarge, change character, and form the **corpus luteum**, or yellow body. In the second half of the menstrual cycle, the corpus luteum secretes estrogen and larger amounts of progesterone. The endometrium (uterine lining) is stimulated by progesterone to thicken and become more engorged with blood in preparation for nourishing an implanted fertilized ovum.

If the ovum is not fertilized, the corpus luteum disintegrates. As the level of progesterone drops, **menstruation** occurs; the uterine lining is shed during the course of a menstrual period. If the egg is fertilized and pregnancy occurs, the cells that eventually develop into the placenta secrete *human chorionic gonadotropin (HCG),* a messenger hormone that signals the pituitary not to start a new cycle. The corpus luteum then steps up its production of progesterone. Many women experience physical or psychological changes, or both, during their monthly cycles. Usually the changes are minor, but more serious problems can occur.

Premenstrual Syndrome (PMS)

Women with **premenstrual syndrome (PMS)** experience bodily discomfort and emotional distress for up to 2 weeks, from ovulation until the onset of menstruation. Of these women 3% to 15% develop very severe symptoms. In some studies, as many as 40% to 45% of women have reported at least one premenstrual symptom.

The most common symptoms of PMS are mood changes, anxiety, irritability, difficulty concentrating, forgetfulness, impaired judgment, tearfulness, digestive symptoms (diarrhea, bloating, constipation), hot flashes, palpitations, dizziness, headache, fatigue, changes in appetite, cravings (usually for sweets or salt), water retention, breast tenderness, and insomnia. For a diagnosis to be made, women—using a self-rating symptom scale or calendar—must report troubling premenstrual symptoms in the period before menstruation in at least two successive menstrual cycles.[15]

Treatments for PMS depend on specific symptoms. Diuretics (drugs that speed up fluid elimination) can

Figure 7-5

The female sex organs and reproductive structure.

A. External structure

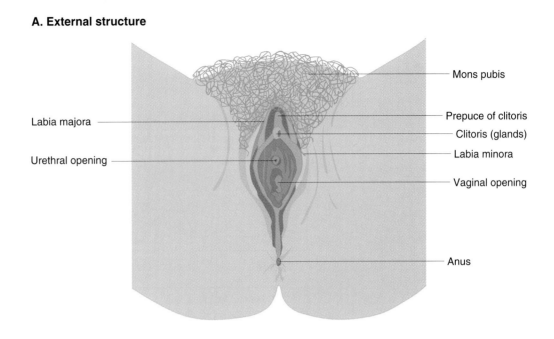

Labia majora

Urethral opening

Mons pubis

Prepuce of clitoris

Clitoris (glands)

Labia minora

Vaginal opening

Anus

B. Internal structure

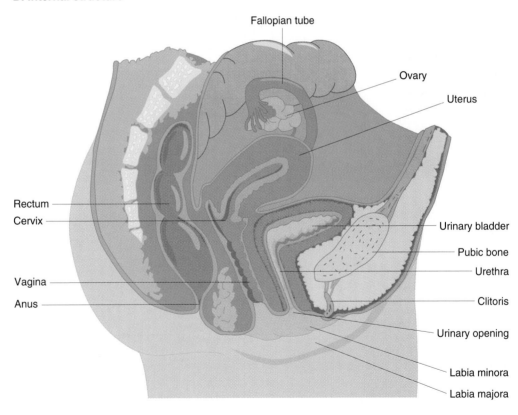

Fallopian tube

Ovary

Uterus

Rectum

Cervix

Vagina

Anus

Urinary bladder

Pubic bone

Urethra

Clitoris

Urinary opening

Labia minora

Labia majora

relieve water retention and bloating. Relaxation techniques have led to a 60% reduction in anxiety symptoms. Sleep deprivation, or the use of bright light to adjust a woman's circadian or daily rhythm, also has proven beneficial. Behavioral approaches, such as exercise or charting cycles, help by letting women know when they're vulnerable. Psychiatric drugs that boost the neurotransmitter serotonin, such as the antidepressants Prozac and Zoloft, also have provided significant relief for symptoms such as tension, depression, irritability, and mood swings.

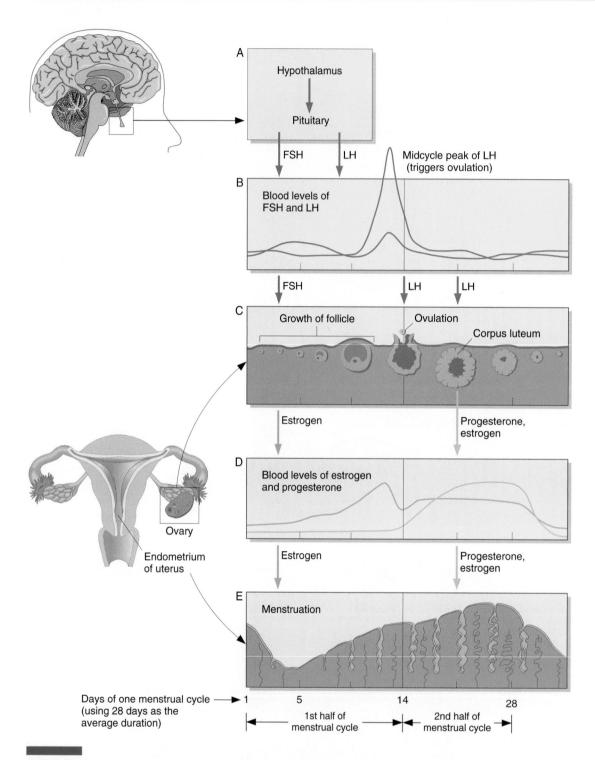

Figure 7-6

The menstrual cycle. Levels of the gonadotrophins (FSH and LH) rise and then fall to stimulate the cycle. These changes affect the levels of the hormones estrogen and progesterone, which in turn react with LH and FSH. As a result, the lining of the uterus prepares to receive a fertilized egg while the ovarian follicle matures and then ruptures, releasing the ovum (egg) into a fallopian tube. If a fertilized egg is deposited, pregnancy begins. But if the egg is not fertilized, progesterone production decreases and the uterine lining is shed (menstruation). At this point both estrogen and progesterone levels have dropped, so the pituitary responds by producing FSH, and the cycle begins again.

Men's Sexual Health

Because the male reproductive system is simpler in many ways than the female, it's often ignored—especially by healthy young men. However, just like women, men should make regular self-exams part of their routine.

Male Sexual Anatomy

The visible parts of the male sexual anatomy are the **penis** and **scrotum**, the pouch that contains the **testes** (see Figure 7-7a). The testes manufacture testosterone and **sperm**, the male reproductive cells. Immature sperm are stored in the **epididymis**, a collection of coiled tubes adjacent to each testis.

The penis contains three hollow cylinders loosely covered with skin. The two major cylinders, the *corpora cavernosa,* extend side by side through the length of the penis. The third cylinder, the *corpus spongiosum,* surrounds the **urethra**, the channel for both seminal fluid and urine (see Figure 7-7b).

When hanging down loosely, the average penis is about 3¾ inches long. During erection, its internal cylinders fill with so much blood that they become rigid, and the penis stretches to an average length of 6¼ inches. About 90% of all men have erect penises measuring between 5 and 7 inches in length. There is no relation, however, between penis size and female sexual satisfaction; a woman's vagina naturally adjusts during intercourse to the size of her partner's penis.

Inside the body are several structures involved in the production of seminal fluid, or **semen**, the liquid in which sperm cells are carried out of the body during ejaculation. The **vas deferens** are two tubes that carry sperm from the epididymis into the urethra. The **seminal vesicles**, which make some of the seminal fluid, join with the vas deferens to form the **ejaculatory ducts**. The **prostate gland** produces some of the seminal fluid, which it secretes into the urethra during ejaculation. The **Cowper's glands** are two pea-sized structures on either side of the urethra (just below where it emerges from the prostate gland) and connected to it via tiny ducts. When a man is sexually aroused, the Cowper's glands often secrete a fluid that appears as a droplet at the tip of the penis. This fluid is not semen, although it occasionally contains sperm.

Circumcision

In its natural state, the tip of the penis is covered by a fold of skin called the foreskin. About 60% of baby boys in the United States undergo **circumcision**, the surgical removal of the foreskin. However, increasingly more parents are opting for the natural look.

The most common medical benefit of circumcision is that it prevents the accumulation of oils and secretions under the foreskin, which could cause swelling or infection. However, careful washing of the genitals and good general hygiene can lower this risk. In an analysis of data on 1410 men, uncircumcised men were no more likely to contract sexually transmitted diseases than circumcised ones.[16]

The disadvantages of circumcision include risks associated with anesthesia and surgery, bleeding, and possible infection. Because of concern about pain, increasing numbers of physicians apply a topical painkiller or inject a local anesthetic agent into the penis to reduce or eliminate pain.[17]

Figure 7-7
The male sex organs and reproductive structure.

A. External structure

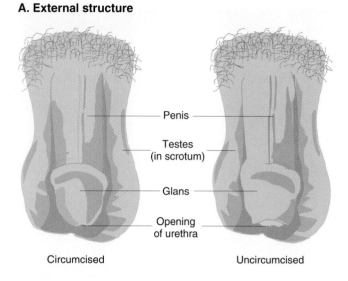

Penis

Testes
(in scrotum)

Glans

Opening
of urethra

Circumcised   Uncircumcised

B. Internal structure

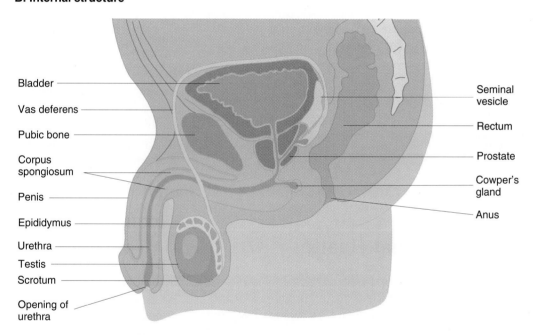

Bladder

Vas deferens

Pubic bone

Corpus
spongiosum

Penis

Epididymus

Urethra

Testis

Scrotum

Opening of
urethra

Seminal
vesicle

Rectum

Prostate

Cowper's
gland

Anus

Responsible Sexual Decision Making

"The new openness about sex and the greater threat of physical danger from sex suggest a need for increased responsibility, better communication, and more respect for individuals," state the student authors of *Sexual Etiquette 101*.[18] As they note, today's students are confronting many difficult issues as they make choices about their sexual lives. Sexual decision making always takes place within the context of an individual's values and perceptions of right and wrong behavior. Making sexually responsible decisions means considering all the possible consequences of sexual behavior for both yourself and your partner. It must always take into account, not just personal preferences and desires, but the very real risks of unwanted pregnancy, sexually transmitted diseases (STDs), and long-term medical consequences (such as impaired fertility). You also must consider the emotional consequences of a sexual relationship—not just for yourself but also for your partner.

Pulsepoints

Top Ten Rules of Sexual Etiquette

1. Be sure sexual activity is consensual. Coercion can take many forms: physical, emotional, and verbal. All cause psychological damage and undermine trust and respect.

2. No means no. At any point in a relationship, whether the couple is dating or married, either individual has the right to say no.

3. In sexual situations, always think ahead. For the sake of safety, think about potential dangers—parking in an isolated area, going into a bedroom with someone you hardly know, and the like—and options to protect yourself.

4. Be aware of your own and your partner's alcohol and drug intake. The use of such substances impairs judgment and reduces the ability to say no. While under their influence, you may engage in sexual behavior you'll later regret.

5. Be prepared. If there's any possibility that you may be engaging in sex, be sure you have the means to protect yourself against unwanted pregnancy and sexually transmitted diseases (STDs).

6. Communicate openly. If you or your partner cannot talk openly and honestly about your sexual histories and contraception, avoid having sex. For the sake of protecting your sexual health, you have to be willing to ask—and answer—questions that may seem embarrassing.

7. Share responsibility in a sexual relationship. Both partners should be involved in protecting themselves and each other from STDs and, if heterosexual, unwanted pregnancy.

8. Respect sexual privacy. Revealing sexual activities violates the trust between two partners. Bragging about a sexual conquest demeans everyone involved.

9. Do not sexually harass others. Pinches, pats, sexual comments or jokes, and suggestive gestures are offensive and disrespectful.

10. Be considerate. A public display of sexual affection can be extremely embarrassing to others. Roommates, in particular, should be sensitive and discreet in their sexual behavior.

SOURCE: Adapted from: Hatcher, Robert, et al. *Sexual Etiquette 101.* Atlanta, GA: Emory University School of Medicine.

The following sections may help ensure that the sexual decisions you make are responsible ones.

Informing Yourself

Most people grow up with a lot of myths and misconceptions about sex. Rather than relying on what peers say or what you've always thought was true, find out the facts. This textbook is a good place to start. The student health center and the library can provide additional materials on sexual identity, orientation, behavior, and health, as well as on options for reducing your risk of acquiring sexually transmitted diseases or becoming pregnant.

Talking About Sex

Many—if not most—people feel awkward or embarrassed discussing sex. Yet few topics are more important to bring up. Honest, open, caring communication is the key to a satisfying sexual relationship. Ideally, you should spend time talking about other personal subjects,

getting to know a potential sexual partner, and enjoying each other's company before sex becomes the major focus of what you say or do together.

Prior to any sexual activity that involves a risk of sexually transmitted infection or pregnancy, both partners should talk about their prior sexual histories (including number of partners and exposure to STDs) and other high-risk behavior, such as the use of injection drugs. They should also discuss the issue of birth control and which methods might be best to use. If you know someone well enough to consider having sex, you should be able to talk about such sensitive subjects. If a potential partner is unwilling to talk or hedges on crucial questions, you shouldn't engage in sex.

Styles of communicating vary among white Americans, African Americans, Hispanic Americans, and Asian Americans. While white and African Americans may openly discuss sex with partners, Hispanic American couples generally do not discuss their sexual relationship. Asian Americans also are less inclined to discuss sex and to value nonverbal, indirect, and intuitive communication over explicit verbal interaction.[19]

Deciding to Abstain

If practiced for the sake of avoiding pregnancy, **abstinence** is defined as refraining from intercourse. If practiced to prevent the transmission of STDs, it means no exchange of body fluids. Individuals who abstain from sexual activity, not just for a weekend or a summer vacation but as a lifestyle choice, are described as celibate.

Because engaging in sexual intercourse is never 100% risk-free, abstinence is the safest possible option, especially for young people. Realizing this, increasing numbers of adolescents and young adults are choosing to remain virgins until they enter a committed, permanent, monogamous relationship. Rather than saying "no" to sex, they are saying, "not yet."

"Having sex" refers to the motions two people go through to achieve sexual pleasure; "making love" is a profound sharing of emotion and experience. Which do you want? Here are some other questions to consider as you think about the significance of becoming sexually intimate with a partner:

- What role do I want relationships and sex to have in my life at this time?

- What are my values as they pertain to sexual relationships? Do I believe that intercourse should be reserved for a permanent partnership or committed relationship?

- Will a decision to engage in sex enhance my positive feelings about myself or my partner? Do I have questions about my sexual orientation or the kinds of people who attract me?

- Do I and my partner both want to have sex? Is my partner pressuring me in any way? Am I pressuring my partner? Am I making this decision for myself or my partner?

- Have my partner and I discussed our sexual histories and risk factors? Have I spoken honestly about any STDs I've had in the past? Am I sure that neither my partner nor I have a sexually transmitted infection?

- Have we taken precautions against unwanted pregnancy and STDs?

The Right to Say No

Whether couples are on a first date or have been married for years, each partner always has the right *not* to have sex. Unfortunately, no sometimes seems to mean different things to men and women. In a 1994 survey by University of Chicago researchers, 22.8% of the women said they had been forced to do something sexually that they did not want to, usually by their spouse or someone they knew well or loved. Yet only 2.8% of the men felt that they had ever forced a woman to perform a sexual act. Why the discrepancy? The researchers speculate that men don't perceive their behavior as coercive, even when women feel pressured into unwanted sexual activities.[20]

Heeding basic rules of sexual etiquette (see Pulsepoints: "Ten Top Rules of Sexual Etiquette" on p. 121) can help couples avoid such situations. At some campuses, such as Antioch College in Ohio, freshmen must attend workshops on sexual consent and adhere to a campus policy that requires "willing and verbal consent" for each sexual act.

Strategies for Change

How to Say No to Sex

✔ First of all, recognize your own values and feelings. If you believe that sex is something to be shared only by people who've already become close in other ways, be true to that belief.

✔ If you're at a loss for words, try these responses: "I like you a lot, but I'm not ready to have sex." "You're a great person, but sex isn't something I do to prove I like someone." "I'd like to wait until I'm married to have sex."

✔ If you're feeling pressured, let your date know that you're uncomfortable.

✔ If you're a woman, monitor your sexual signals. Men impute more sexual meaning to gestures (such as casual touching) that women perceive as friendly and innocent.[21]

✔ Communicate your feelings to your date sooner rather than later. It's far easier to say, "I don't want to go to your apartment," than to fight off unwelcome advances once you're there.

✔ Remember that if saying no to sex puts an end to a relationship, it wasn't much of a relationship in the first place.

CAMPUS FOCUS: COLLEGE STUDENTS AND SEXUALITY

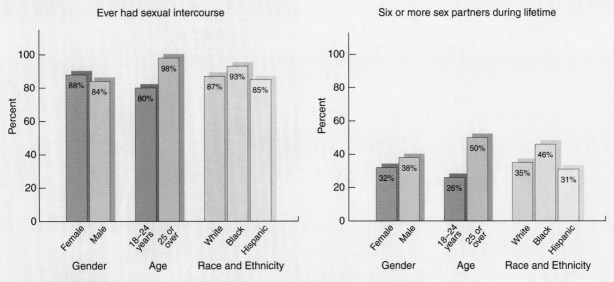

SOURCE: Douglas, Kathy, et al. "Results from the 1995 National College Health Risk Behavior Survey." *American Journal of College Health*, Vol. 46, September 1997.

Sex on Campus

As seen in Campus Focus: "College Students and Sexuality," most college students—87.8% of women and 84% of men—have had sexual intercourse. A much smaller but significant percentage—31.8% of women and 37.8% of men—had six or more sex partners during their lifetime.[22]

Yet most students, as indicated by a report on 272 students at a midwestern university, don't believe it's embarrassing to be a virgin. Of those who are sexually active, many college students worry about STDs, yet they don't always take precautions to reduce the risk of disease, often because they believe that HIV and other infections simply couldn't happen to them. But concern about STDs has had some impact on the sexual habits of college students. In a study of 132 women students, 41% said that they used condoms during intercourse, an increase over reported use in previous decades.[23] As the women became seriously involved with men, however, they tended to use less, rather than more, protection. This is a potentially dangerous practice, since just knowing someone better doesn't make sex safer. Today's students also seem just as willing as their counterparts of

two decades ago to engage in oral or anal sex and to have multiple partners.[24]

Sexual Orientation

Human beings are diverse in all ways, including sexual preferences and practices. Physiological, psychological, and social factors attract us to members of a certain sex; this attraction is our **sexual orientation**. Sigmund Freud argued that we all start off **bisexual**, or attracted to both sexes. But by the time they reach adulthood, most males prefer female sexual partners, and most females prefer male partners. **Heterosexual** is the term used for individuals whose primary orientation is toward members of the other sex. In virtually all cultures, some men and women are **homosexuals**, preferring partners of their own sex.

In our society, we tend to view heterosexuality and homosexuality as very different. In reality, these orientations are opposite ends of a spectrum of sexual preferences. Sex researcher Alfred Kinsey devised a seven-point continuum representing sexual orientation in American society. At one end of the continuum are those exclusively attracted to members of the opposite sex; at the other end are people exclusively attracted to members of the same sex. In between are varying degrees of homosexual and heterosexual orientation.

Bisexuality

Bisexuality—sexual attraction to both males and females—can develop at any point in one's life. In some cultures, bisexual activity is considered part of normal sexual experimentation. Among the Sabmia Highlanders in Papua New Guinea, for instance, boys perform oral sex on one another as part of the rites of passage into manhood.[25]

Some people identify themselves as bisexual even if they don't behave bisexually. Some are "serial" bisexuals—that is, they are sexually involved with same-sex partners for a while and then with partners of the other sex, or vice versa. An estimated 7 to 9 million men, about twice the number thought to be exclusively homosexual, could be described as bisexual during some extended period of their lives. The largest group are married, rarely have sexual relations with women other than their wives, and have secret sexual involvements with men.

Fear of HIV infection has sparked great concern about bisexuality, particularly among heterosexual women who worry about becoming involved with a bisexual man. About 20% to 30% of women with AIDS were infected by bisexual partners, and health officials fear that bisexual men who hide their homosexual affairs could transmit HIV to many more women (see Chapter 9).

Homosexuality

Homosexuality—social, emotional, and sexual attraction to members of the same sex—exists in almost all cultures. Men and women homosexuals are commonly referred to as *gay*; women homosexuals are also called *lesbians*.

Homosexuality threatens and upsets many people, perhaps because homosexuals are viewed as different, or perhaps because no one understands why some people are heterosexual and others homosexual. Homophobia has led to an increase in "gay bashing" (attacking homosexuals) in many communities, including college campuses. Some blame this on the emergence of AIDS as a societal danger. However, researchers have found that fear of AIDS has not created new hostility but has simply given bigots an excuse to act out their hatred.

For decades, behavioral and medical specialists have debated whether homosexuality is biologically or socially determined. Some say that sexual orientation is genetically determined. Others contend that prenatal hormones

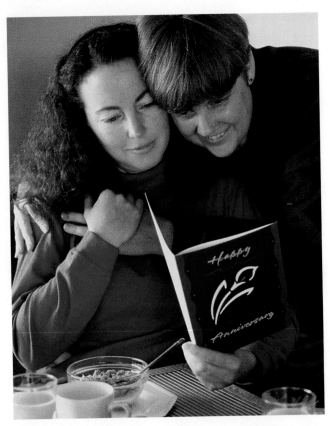

Happy together. Close-couple homosexual relationships are similar to stable heterosexual relationships.

influence sexual preference. Some psychotherapists have argued that mothers foster homosexuality by loving their sons too much and their daughters too little. Others have traced homosexuality to broken homes, seductive friends, and failure at "dating and mating."

Researchers have found structural differences in the brains of heterosexual and homosexual men that might indicate a biological basis for sexual orientation. In gay men, one segment of the hypothalamus, part of the forebrain, is typically about one-quarter to one-half the size of the same region in heterosexual men. Also, a cord of nerve fibers that allows the two halves of the brain to communicate with one another is larger in homosexual men than in either heterosexual men or in women. Such findings have raised many questions and controversies about the roots and nature of sexual orientation.[26]

Extensive studies of male and female homosexuals have shown that only a minority have problems coping with their homosexuality. The happiest and best adjusted tend to be those in close-couple relationships, the equivalent of stable heterosexual partnerships. An estimated 3 to 5 million gays and lesbians have conceived children in heterosexual relationships; others have become parents through adoption or artificial insemination. These men and women describe their families as

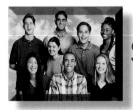

Spotlight on Diversity
Cultural Variations in Sexual Arousal

While the biological mechanisms underlying human sexual arousal and response are essentially universal, the particular sexual stimuli or behaviors that people find arousing are greatly influenced by cultural conditioning. For example, in Western societies, where the emphasis during sexual activity tends to be heavily weighted toward achieving orgasm, genitally focused activities are frequently defined as optimally arousing. In contrast, devotees to Eastern Tantric traditions (where spirituality is interwoven with sexuality) often achieve optimal pleasure by emphasizing the sensual and spiritual aspects of shared intimacy rather than orgasmic release.

Kissing on the mouth, a universal source of sexual arousal in Western society, may be rare or absent in many other parts of the world. Certain North American Eskimo people and inhabitants of the Trobriand Islands would rather rub noses than lips, and among the Thonga of South Africa, kissing is viewed as odious behavior. The Hindu people of India are also disinclined to kiss because they believe such contact symbolically contaminates the act of sexual intercourse. In their survey of 190 societies, Clellan Ford and Frank Beach found that mouth kissing was acknowledged in only 21 societies and practiced as a prelude or accompaniment to coitus in only 13.

Foreplay in general, whether it be oral sex, sensual touching, or passionate kissing, is subject to wide cultural variation. In some societies, most notably those with Eastern traditions, couples may strive to prolong intense states of sexual arousal for several hours. While varied patterns of foreplay are common in Western cultures, these activities often are of short duration as lovers move rapidly toward the "main event" of coitus. In still other societies, foreplay is either sharply curtailed or absent altogether. For example, the Lepcha farmers of the southeastern Himalayas limit foreplay to men briefly caressing their partners' breasts, and among the Irish inhabitants of Inis Beag, precoital sexual activity is limited to mouth kissing and rough fondling of the woman's lower body by her partner.

Source: Robert Crooks and Karla Bauer, *Our Sexuality*, 7th edition. Pacific Grove, CA: Brooks/Cole, 1999.

---

much like any other, and studies of lesbian mothers have found that their children are essentially no different from average in self-esteem, gender-related issues and roles, sexual orientation, and general development.

Different ethnic groups respond to homosexuality in different ways. To a greater extent than white homosexuals, gays and lesbians from minority groups tend to stay in the closet longer rather than risk alienation from their families and communities. Often they feel forced to choose between their gay and ethnic identities.

In general, the African-American community has stronger negative views of homosexuals than whites, possibly because of the influence of strong fundamentalist Christian beliefs. Hispanic culture, with its emphasis on machismo, also has a very negative view of male homosexuality. Asian cultures, which tend to view an individual as a representative of his or her family, tend to view open declarations of sexual orientation as shaming the family and challenging its reputation and future.[27]

Sexual Activity

Part of learning about your own sexuality is having a clear understanding of human sexual behaviors. Understanding frees us from fear and anxiety, so that we may accept ourselves and others as the natural sexual beings we all are.

Masturbation

Not everybody masturbates, but most people do. Kinsey estimated that seven out of ten women and nineteen out of twenty men masturbate (and admit they do). Their reason is simple: It feels good. **Masturbation** produces the same physical responses as sexual activity with a partner and can be an enjoyable form of sexual release.

Masturbation has been described as immature; unsocial; tiring; frustrating; and a cause of hairy palms, warts, blemishes, and blindness. None of these myths is true. Even Freud felt that masturbation was normal for children. Sex educators recommend masturbation to adolescents as a means of releasing tension and becoming familiar with their sexual organs. Throughout adulthood, masturbation often is the primary sexual activity of individuals not involved in a sexual relationship and can be particularly useful when illness, absence, divorce, or death deprives a person of a partner. In a University of Chicago survey, about 25% of men and 9% of women said they masturbate at least once a week.

Kissing and Touching

A kiss is a universal sign of affection. It can be just a kiss—a quick press of the lips—or it can lead to much more. Usually kissing is the first sexual activity that couples engage in, and even after years of sexual experimentation and sharing, it remains an enduring pleasure for partners.

Touching is a silent form of communication between friends and lovers. Although a touch to any part of the body can be thrilling, some areas, such as the breasts and genitals, are especially sensitive. Stimulating these **erogenous** regions can lead to orgasm in both men and women. Though such forms of stimulation often accompany intercourse, more couples are gaining an appreciation of these activities as primary sources of sexual fulfillment—and as safer alternatives to intercourse.

Intercourse

Vaginal **intercourse**, or coitus, refers to the penetration of the vagina by the penis (see Figure 7-8). This is the preferred form of sexual intimacy for most heterosexual couples, who may use a wide variety of positions. The most familiar position for intercourse in our society is the so-called missionary position, with the man on top, facing the woman. An alternative is the woman on top, either lying down or sitting upright. Many couples move into several different positions for intercourse during a single episode of lovemaking; others may have a personal favorite or may choose different positions at dif-

ferent times. (See Spotlight on Diversity: "Cultural Variations in Sexual Arousal" on p. 125.)

Vaginal intercourse, like other forms of sexual activity involving an exchange of bodily fluids, carries a risk of sexually transmitted diseases, including HIV infection. In many other parts of the world, in fact, heterosexual intercourse is the most common means of HIV transmission.

Oral-Genital Sex

The formal terms for oral sex are **cunnilingus**, which refers to oral stimulation of the woman's genitals, and **fellatio**, oral stimulation of the man's genitals. For many couples, oral-genital sex is a regular part of their lovemaking. For others, it's an occasional experiment. Oral sex with a partner carrying a sexually transmitted disease, such as herpes or HIV infection, can lead to infection, so a condom should be used (with cunnilingus, a condom cut in half to lay flat can be used).

Anal Stimulation and Intercourse

Because the anus has many nerve endings, it can produce intense erotic responses. Stimulation of the anus by the fingers or mouth can be a source of sexual arousal; anal intercourse involves penile penetration of the anus. An estimated 25% of adults have experienced anal intercourse at least once.[28] However, anal sex involves important health risks, such as damage to sensitive rectal tissues and the transmission of various intestinal infections, hepatitis, and STDs, including HIV.

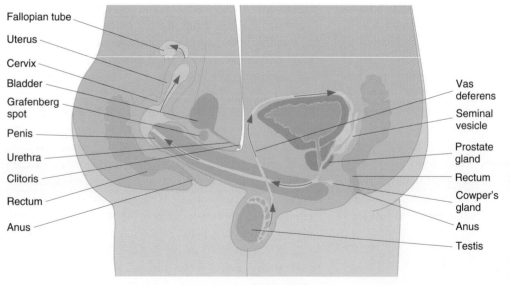

Fallopian tube
Uterus
Cervix
Bladder
Grafenberg spot
Penis
Urethra
Clitoris
Rectum
Anus

Vas deferens
Seminal vesicle
Prostate gland
Rectum
Cowper's gland
Anus
Testis

Figure 7-8

A cross-sectional view of sexual intercourse. Sperm are formed in each of the testes and stored in the epididymis. When a man ejaculates, sperm, in semen, travel up the vas deferens. (The prostate gland and seminal vesicles contribute components of the semen.) The semen is expelled from the penis through the urethra and deposited in the vagina, near the cervix. During sexual excitement and orgasm in a woman, the upper end of the vagina enlarges and the uterus elevates. After orgasm, these organs return to their normal states, and the cervix descends into the pool of semen.

Sexual Response

Sexuality involves every part of you: mind and body, muscles and skin, glands and genitals. The pioneers in finding out exactly how human beings respond to sex were William Masters and Virginia Johnson, who first studied more than 800 individuals in their laboratory in the 1950s. They discovered that sexual response is a well-ordered sequence of events, so predictable it could be divided into four phases: excitement, plateau, orgasm, and resolution (see Figure 7-9). In real life, individuals

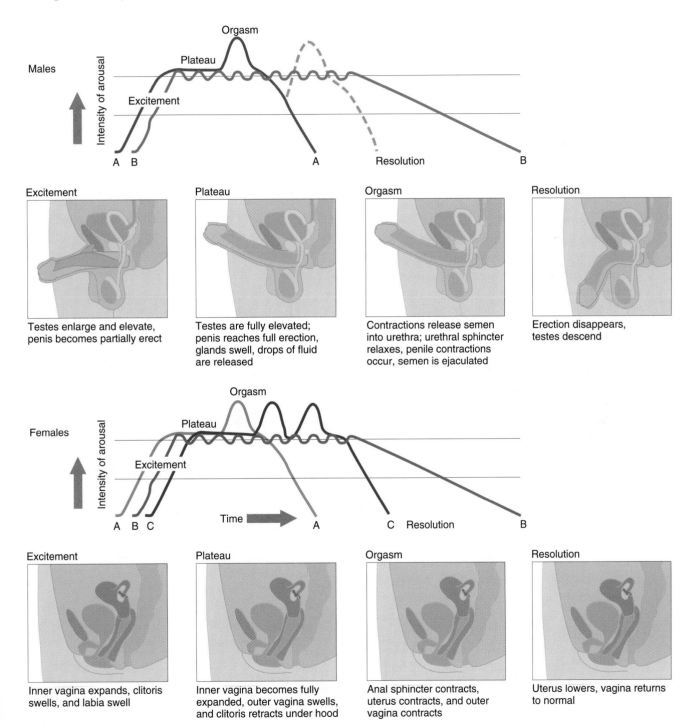

Figure 7-9

Human sexual response is a well-ordered sequence: excitement, plateau, orgasm, and resolution.

don't necessarily follow this well-ordered pattern. But the responses for both sexes are remarkably similar. And sexual response always follows the same sequence, whatever the means of stimulation.

- *Excitement*. Stimulation is the first step: a touch, a look, a fantasy. In men, sexual stimuli set off a rush of blood to the genitals, filling the blood vessels in the penis. Because these vessels are wrapped in a thick sheath of tissue, the penis becomes erect. The testes lift. Women respond to stimulation with vaginal lubrication within 10 to 20 seconds of exposure to sexual stimuli. The clitoris becomes larger, as do the vaginal lips (the labia), the nipples, and later the breasts. The vagina lengthens, and its inner two-thirds increase in size. The uterus lifts, further increasing the free space in the vagina.

- *Plateau*. During this stage, the changes begun in the excitement stage continue and intensify. The penis further increases in both length and diameter. The outer one-third of the vagina swells. During intercourse, the vaginal muscles grasp the penis to increase stimulation for both partners. The upper two-thirds of the vagina become wider as the uterus moves up; eventually its diameter is 2½ to 3 inches.

- *Orgasm*. Men and women have remarkably similar **orgasm** experiences. Both men and women typically have three to twelve pelvic muscle contractions approximately four-fifths of a second apart and lasting up to 60 seconds. Both undergo contractions and spasms of other muscles, as well as increases in breathing, pulse rates, and blood pressure. Both can sometimes have orgasms simply from kisses, stimulation of the breasts or other parts of the body, or fantasy alone.

  The process of **ejaculation** (the discharge of semen by a male) requires two separate events. First, the vas deferens, the seminal vesicles, the prostate, and the upper portion of the urethra contract. The man perceives these subtle contractions deep in his pelvis just before the point of no return, which therapists refer to as the point of "ejaculatory inevitability." Then, seconds later, muscle contractions force semen out of the penis via the urethra.

  Female orgasms follow several patterns. Some women experience a series of mini-orgasms—a response sometimes described as "skimming." Another pattern consists of rapid excitement and plateau stages, followed by a prolonged orgasm.

This is the most frequent response to stimulation by a vibrator.

Female orgasms are primarily triggered by stimulating the clitoris. When stimulation reaches an adequate level, the vagina responds by contracting. Although it sometimes seems that vaginal stimulation alone can set off an orgasm, the clitoris is usually involved—at least indirectly during full penile penetration.

Some researchers have identified what they call the *Grafenberg (or G) spot* (or area) just behind the front wall of the vagina, between the cervix and the back of the pubic bone (see Figure 7-8). When this region is stimulated, women report various sensations, including slight discomfort, a brief feeling that they need to urinate, and increasing pleasure. Continued stimulation may result in an orgasm of great intensity, accompanied by ejaculation of fluid from the urethra. However, other researchers have failed to confirm the existence and importance of the G spot, and sex therapists disagree about its significance for a woman's sexual satisfaction.

- *Resolution*. The sexual organs of men and women return to their normal nonexcited state during this final phase of sexual response. Heightened skin color quickly fades after orgasm, and the heart rate, blood pressure, and breathing rate soon return to

Strategies for Change

Improving a Sexual Relationship

✔ Use "I" statements, such as "I really enjoy making love, but I'm so tired right now that I won't be a responsive partner. Why don't we get the kids to bed early tomorrow so we can enjoy ourselves a little earlier?"

✔ When your partner is talking, do not dismiss what he or she is saying as crazy, irrational, or selfish.

✔ If your partner has temporarily lost interest in sex, express concern and ask what the two of you might do to make things better. Don't blame yourself.

✔ Speak up if something hurts during sex. Be specific.

✔ If you would like to try something different, say so. Practice saying the words first if they embarrass you. If your partner feels uncomfortable, don't force the issue, but do try talking it through.

normal. The clitoris also resumes its normal position and appearance very shortly thereafter, whereas the penis may remain somewhat erect for up to 30 minutes.

Sexual Concerns

Many sexual concerns stem from myths and misinformation. There is no truth, for instance, behind the misconception that men are always capable of erection, that sex always involves intercourse, that partners should experience simultaneous orgasms, or that people who truly love each other always have satisfying sex lives.

The concept of sexual normalcy differs greatly in different times, cultures, and racial and ethnic groups. In certain times and places, only sex between a husband and wife has been deemed normal. In other circumstances, "normal" has been applied to any sexual behavior—alone or with others—that does not harm others or produce great anxiety and guilt. The following are some of the most common contemporary sexual concerns.

Safer Sex

Having sex is never completely safe; the only 100% risk-free sexual choice is abstinence. If you choose to be sexually active, you can greatly reduce your risk by restricting sexual activity to the context of a mutually exclusive, monogamous relationship in which both partners know, on the basis of laboratory testing, that neither has an STD or HIV antibodies.

For centuries, sexually transmitted diseases, such as gonorrhea and syphilis, caused great suffering and many deaths. Modern medicine has developed effective treatments for these health threats, but other STDs, such as herpes and chlamydia, have become serious health problems. However, no STD in recent history has had as terrifying an impact as infection with HIV, which causes AIDS, a disease that has taken the lives of thousands of people in their prime.

Sex with a person who has never been exposed to HIV or to other STDs is safe (for you), regardless of what type of sexual activity you engage in. The only way of knowing for certain that a prospective partner doesn't have an STD or is not infected with HIV is through laboratory testing (see Chapter 9). Sex educators and health professionals strongly encourage couples to abstain from any sexual activity that puts them at risk for STDs until they both undergo medical examinations and testing for STDs. This process greatly reduces

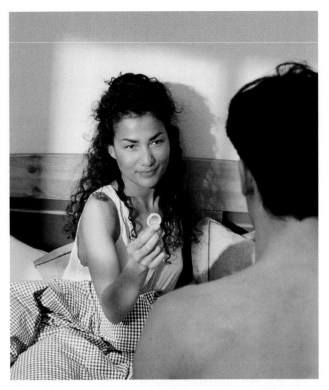

Don't forget. Be sexually responsible—for your own and your partner's sake. Using condoms is one way you can lower your risks of contracting STDs.

the danger of disease transmission and can also help foster a deep sense of mutual trust and commitment. Many campus and public health clinics provide exams or laboratory testing either free of charge or on a sliding scale determined by your income.

Sexual Difficulties

A sexual difficulty may occur anywhere in the sexual response sequence. The most frequent problem sex therapists and marriage counselors see is lack of sexual desire. Perfectly healthy couples, with no physical impairment, simply become bored with sex, even though they love each other. Often stress—perhaps caused by a recent move, a new baby, or a high-pressure job—is the real culprit.

A common sexual difficulty in men is erectile disorder, or **impotence**, the inability to achieve or maintain an erection. Psychological factors, such as anxiety about performance, may cause impotence. But in as many as 80% of cases, the problem has physical origins. There are many new treatments for impotence, including Viagra, a drug that relaxes smooth muscle cells. Viagra (sildenafil citrate) became the fastest selling new

Health Online

Online Sexual Disorders Screening

http://www.med.nyu.edu/Psych/screens/sdsf.html (women)
http://www.med.nyu.edu/Psych/screens/sdsm.html (men)

These pages from the New York University School of Medicine present separate questionnaires for men and women that screen for the possible presence of sexual disorders. There are also links to referrals for counseling and medical treatment and more information on sexual disorders.

Think about it ...

- Many of these symptoms are experienced by most people at one time or another. At what point do you think sexual problems become "disorders"?

- According to this screening test, do you have symptoms of a sexual disorder? If so, what do you think might be the causes of this problem?

---

drug in pharmaceutical history when it won FDA approval. However, its use has been linked to serious, even fatal, complications. Men and their partners may also be troubled by a different sort of problem, **premature ejaculation,** or an inability to delay ejaculation long enough to satisfy a responsive partner at least half the time. Men can learn to control their ejaculation by concentrating on their sexual response and by communicating with their partner about when to slow down or stop movements.

Some women experience **dyspareunia,** or pain during intercourse. An extreme form of painful intercourse is **vaginismus,** in which involuntary contractions of the muscles of the vagina close the vaginal opening. Relaxation techniques may help some women with vaginismus. Orgasmic dysfunction is a controversial sexual topic. Many women experience orgasm, but not during intercourse. Is intercourse without orgasm a sexual problem? The best answer is that it is a problem if a woman wants to experience orgasm during intercourse but doesn't. Counseling programs can teach women to masturbate and then to share with their partners what they have learned about their own sexual response.

Most forms of sexual difficulty are treatable. After any underlying physical problems are treated or ruled out, sex therapists work with couples on communication, reduction of performance anxiety, and exercises that enhance sexual intimacy. Contrary to common misconceptions, sex therapy does not involve conducting sexual activity in front of the therapist. The core of the program is the couple's "homework"—a series of exercises carried out in private that enhance their sensory awareness and improve nonverbal communication.

Making This Chapter Work for You
Relationships and Sexuality

- Sending clear messages through words, gestures, expressions, and behaviors is the essence of good communication. Effective communication helps create good relationships built on honesty, understanding, and mutual trust.

- Nonverbal communication refers to the unspoken messages people send with their gestures, expressions, and body movements.

- In today's society, friends often become an extended family, providing acceptance, warmth, and loyalty.

- Dating provides opportunities to get to know other people, to practice social skills, and to explore one's sexuality.

- Romantic love is characterized by intense passion. From a biochemical view, infatuation may trigger a rise in certain neurotransmitters that create a natural high that is very pleasurable, but not long-lasting.

- Mature love combines sexual excitement, tenderness, a commitment to bringing out the best in each other, mutual growth, a willingness to risk vulnerability, and the ability to enjoy time apart.

■ Most couples who choose to marry do so for love. The older and more similar two people are, the more likely they are to have a successful marriage.

■ Divorce rates have remained fairly stable, and more people are seeking help to make their marriages work.

■ Women and men have different sexual organs, hormones, and different health problems. Awareness of these differences can help individuals take better care of their own sexual health and be more sensitive to the needs of their partners.

■ A woman's menstrual cycle is a monthly process involving all her reproductive organs. Once a month, her ovary releases an egg cell, or ovum, that travels through a fallopian tube to the uterus. If the egg isn't fertilized, the uterine lining is shed during menstruation.

■ Making responsible sexual decisions—especially important in an age of sexual risks—requires accurate information, honest communication, consideration of all your options (including abstinence), and recognition of every person's right to say no.

■ Sexual orientation may be predominantly heterosexual, bisexual, or homosexual. Regardless of sexual orientation, healthy sexuality involves an understanding of your body, your partner's needs and desires, and responsible sexual behavior.

■ Sexual behaviors involve erotic fantasizing, masturbation, kissing and touching, intercourse, and oral sex.

■ Whatever the type of sexual stimulation, the body's response always follows the same sequence: excitement, plateau, orgasm, and resolution.

■ The safest sex practices are abstinence or sexual relations with only one partner who has never been exposed to HIV or other STDs.

■ Sexual concerns include safer sex, sexual anxiety, lack of sexual interest, sexual unresponsiveness, and sexual impairment.

▶ Key Terms

The terms listed here are used within the chapter. Page numbers are included for each term.
A definition of each term is given in the green Glossary pages at the end of this book.

Review Questions

1. What are the characteristics of a friendship? How does friendship develop and grow? Can you describe the different stages?
2. How does a relationship progress from dating to mature love? Define each stage and describe the steps involved.
3. Name the different parts of the male reproductive system and briefly explain the function of each part. Name the different parts of the female repro-

ductive system, and briefly explain the function of each part.
4. What is the human response cycle? List and briefly describe each step. Are there any differences in the sexual response cycles of males and females?
5. What are some preventive behaviors that can reduce an individual's chances of becoming HIV infected?

Critical Thinking Questions

1. What are your personal criteria for a successful relationship? Develop a brief list of factors you consider important and support your choices with examples or experiences from your own life.
2. Anita insists that her boyfriend, Bill, has never taken any sexual risks. But when she suggested that they get tested for STDs, he was furious and refused. Now Anita says she doesn't know what to believe. Is he telling the truth, or is he hiding something? She doesn't want to take any risks, but

she doesn't want to lose him either. What would you advise her to say or do?
3. Some people support the legalization of homosexual marriages. Some gay people feel that they will never be fully accepted in society unless they can legally marry. Other gay people oppose the idea as too imitative of straight couples. Some heterosexuals think that gay marriages would violate the sanctity of marriage. Do you think homosexual marriages should be legal? Why or why not?

Connections to Personal Health Interactive

*To enhance your understanding of the material covered in this chapter, check out the following study aids on the **Personal Health Interactive CD-ROM**.*

■ Personal Insights: Do People Understand You?
■ Glossary & Key Term Review

References

1. Tannen, Deborah. *You Just Don't Understand: Women and Men in Conversation*. New York: Ballantine, 1990.
2. Mehrabian, Albert. Personal interview.
3. Maple, Marilyn. Personal interview.
4. Swann, William, et al. "Socialization Patterns of Depressed and Non-Depressed College Students." *Journal of Abnormal Psychology*, Vol. 104, 1992.
5. Laumann, Edward. Personal interview.
6. Laumann, Edward, et al. *The Social Organization of Sexuality*. Chicago: University of Chicago Press, 1994.
7. Sprecher, Susan, et al. "Mate Selection Preferences." *Sex Roles*, June 1994. Feingold, Alan. "Sex Differences in the Effects of Similarity and Physical Attractiveness." *Basic & Applied Social Psychology*, September 1991; "Gender Differences in Effects of Physical Attractiveness on Romantic Attraction." *Journal of Personality & Social Psychology*, November 1990.
8. Ackerman, Diane. *A Natural History of Love*. New York: Vintage Books, 1995.
9. Baumeister, R., et al. "Unrequited Love: On Heartbreak, Anger, Guilt, Scriptlessness and Humiliation." *Journal of Personality & Social Psychology*, Vol. 64, 1993.
10. Bureau of the Census.
11. Gottman, John. *Why Marriages Succeed or Fail*. New York: Simon & Schuster, 1994.
12. Sternberg, Robert. Personal interview.
13. Statisical Summary. *Pediatrics*, December 1997.
14. Blumenthal, Susan. "Improving Women's Mental and Physical Health: Federal Initiative and Programs." *American Psychiatric Press Review of Psychiatry*, Vol. 14. Washington, DC: American Psychiatric Press, 1995. Pinn, Vivian. "Women's Health Research." *Journal of the American Medical Association*, October 14, 1992. Clancy, Carolyn, and Charlea Massion. "American Women's Health

Care." *Journal of the American Medical Association,* October 14, 1992.

15. "PMS: 66 Years of Research." *University of California, Berkeley Wellness Letter*, Vol. 14, No. 1, October 1997.

16. Crooks, Robert, and Karla Baur. *Our Sexuality.* 7th ed. Pacific Grove, CA: Brooks/Cole, 1999.

17. Wiswell, Thomas. "Circumcision Circumspection." *New England Journal of Medicine*, Vol. 336, No. 17, April 24, 1997.

18. Hatcher, Robert, et al. *Sexual Etiquette 101.* Atlanta, GA: Emory University School of Medicine.

19. Crooks and Baur, *Our Sexuality.*

20. Laumann, et al. *The Social Organization of Sexuality.*

21. Kowalski, Robin M. "Inferring Sexual Interest from Behavioral Cues: Effects of Gender and Sexually Relevant Attitudes." *Sex Roles: A Journal of Research*, Vol. 29, No. 2, July 1993.

22. Douglas, Kathy, et al. "Results from the 1995 National College Health Risk Behavior Survey." *Journal of American College Health*, Vol. 46, September 1997.

23. DeBuono, Barbara, et al. "Sexual Behavior of College Women in 1975, 1986 and 1989." *New England Journal of Medicine*, March 22, 1990.

24. Reinisch, June, et al. "High-Risk Sexual Behavior Among Heterosexual Undergraduates at a Midwestern University." *Family Planning Perspectives*, May–June 1992.

25. Crooks, and Baur. *Our Sexuality.*

26. Risch, Neil, et al. "Male Sexual Orientation and Genetic Evidence." *Science*, Vol. 262, December 24, 1993. LeVay, S. "A Difference in Hypothalamic Structure Between Heterosexual and Homosexual Men." *Science,* Vol. 253, 1991, pp. 1034–1037.

27. Crooks and Baur, *Our Sexuality.*

28. Seidman, Stuart, and Ronald Rieder. "Sexual Behavior Through the Life Cycle: An Empirical Approach." *American Psychiatric Press Review of Psychiatry*, Vol. 14. Washington, DC: American Psychiatric Press, 1995.

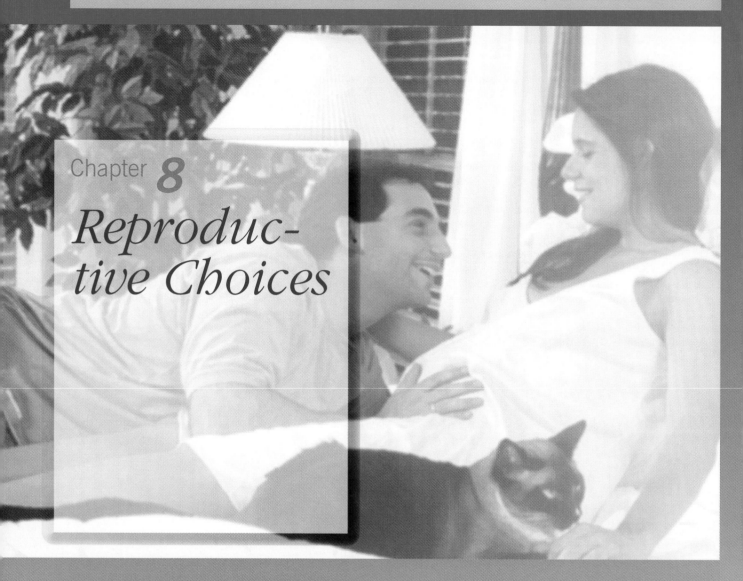

Chapter *8*

Reproduc-
tive Choices

After studying the material in this chapter, you should be able to:

- **Explain** the process of conception in humans.
- **List** the major options available for contraception and **explain** the advantages and risks of each.
- **Define** *abortion* and **list** the commonly used abortion methods.
- **Define** and **give examples** of *preconception care*.
- **Describe** the physiological effects of pregnancy on a woman, including the most frequent complications of pregnancy.
- Briefly **describe** the growth and development of a fetus from embryo to birth.
- **Describe** the three stages of labor and birth.
- **Explain** the options available to infertile couples wishing to have children.

*A*s human beings, we have a unique power: the ability to choose to conceive or not to conceive. No other species on earth can separate sexual activity and pleasure from reproduction. However, simply not wanting to get pregnant is never enough to prevent conception, nor is simply wanting to have a child ever enough to get pregnant. Both desires require individual decisions and actions.

Anyone who engages in vaginal intercourse must be willing to accept the consequences of that activity—the possibility of pregnancy and responsibility for the child who might be conceived—or take action to avoid those consequences. A heterosexual woman in Western countries spends 90% of her reproductive years trying to prevent pregnancy and

10% of these years trying to become or being pregnant.[1] This chapter provides information on conception, birth control, and the processes by which a new human life develops and enters the world.

Conception

The equation for making a baby is quite simple: One sperm plus one egg equals one fertilized egg, which can develop into an infant. But the processes that affect or permit **conception** are quite complicated. The creation of sperm, or **spermatogenesis**, starts in the male at puberty. The production of sperm is regulated by hormones. Sperm cells form in the seminiferous tubules of the testes and are passed into the epididymis, where they are stored until ejaculation (see Figure 8-1); a single male ejaculation may contain 500 million sperm. Each of the sperm released into the vagina during intercourse moves on its own, propelling itself toward its target, an ovum.

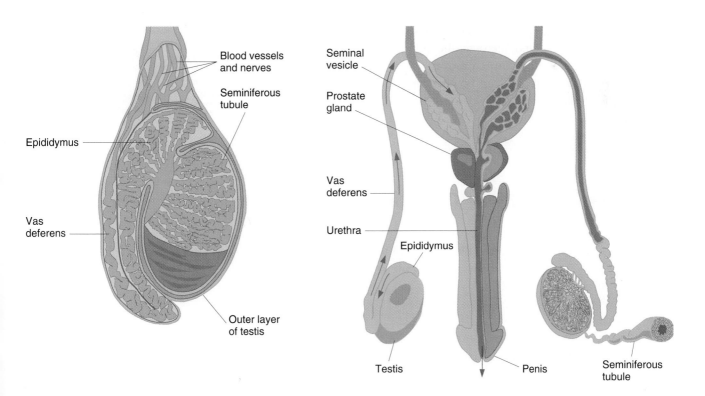

Figure 8-1

The testes. Spermatogenesis takes place in the testes. Sperm cells form in the seminiferous tubules and are stored in the coils of the epididymis. Eventually, the sperm drain into the vasa deferentia ready for ejaculation.

To reach its goal, the sperm must move through the acidic secretions of the vagina, enter the uterus, travel up the fallopian tube containing the ovum, then fuse with the nucleus of the egg **(fertilization)**. Just about every sperm produced by a man in his lifetime fails to accomplish its mission.

There are far fewer human egg cells than there are sperm cells. Each woman is born with her lifetime supply of ova, and between 300 and 500 eggs eventually mature and leave her ovaries during ovulation. Every month, one or the other of the woman's ovaries releases an ovum to the nearby fallopian tube. It travels through the fallopian tube until it reaches the uterus, a journey that takes 3 to 4 days. An unfertilized egg lives for about 24 to 36 hours, disintegrates, and during menstruation, is expelled along with the uterine lining.

Even if a sperm, which can survive in the female reproductive tract for 2 to 5 days, meets a ripe egg in a fallopian tube, its success is not assured. It must penetrate the layer of cells and a jellylike substance that surrounds each egg. Every sperm that touches the egg deposits an enzyme that dissolves part of this barrier. When a sperm bumps into a bare spot, it can penetrate the egg membrane and merge with the egg (see Figure 8-2). The fertilized egg travels down the fallopian tube, dividing to form a tiny clump of cells called a **zygote**. When it reaches the uterus, about a week after fertilization, it burrows into the endometrium, the lining of the uterus. This process is called **implantation**.

Conception can be prevented by **contraception**. Some contraceptive methods prevent ovulation or implantation, and others block the sperm from reaching the egg. Some methods are temporary; others permanently alter one's fertility.

The Basics of Birth Control

Today's sexually active couples have many choices in birth control (see Pulsepoints: "Ten Ways to Avoid Getting Pregnant"). According to the National Center for Health Statistics, the leading method of contraception in the United States is female sterilization, followed by oral contraceptives, the male condom, and male sterilization.[2]

Although many people are concerned about the risks associated with contraception, using birth control is safer and healthier than not using it. According to the Population Reference Bureau, the use of contraceptives, including oral contraceptives, saves millions of lives each year.[3] Some forms of contraception also reduce the risk of sexually transmitted diseases (STDs).

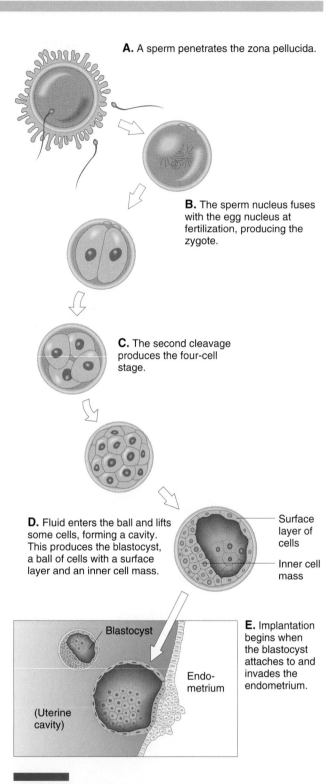

A. A sperm penetrates the zona pellucida.

B. The sperm nucleus fuses with the egg nucleus at fertilization, producing the zygote.

C. The second cleavage produces the four-cell stage.

D. Fluid enters the ball and lifts some cells, forming a cavity. This produces the blastocyst, a ball of cells with a surface layer and an inner cell mass.

Surface layer of cells

Inner cell mass

Blastocyst

Endo-metrium

(Uterine cavity)

E. Implantation begins when the blastocyst attaches to and invades the endometrium.

Figure 8-2

Fertilization. (A) The efforts of hundreds of sperm may allow one to penetrate the ovum's corona radiata, an outer layer of cells, and then the zona pellucida, a thick inner membrane. (B) The nuclei of the sperm and the egg cells approach. The nuclei merge, and the male and female chromosomes in the nuclei come together, forming a zygote. (C) The zygote divides into two cells, then four cells, and so on. (D) As fluid enters the ball, cells form a ball of cells called a blastocyst. (E) The blastocyst implants itself in the endometrium.

Pulsepoints

Ten Ways to Avoid Getting Pregnant

1. Abstain. The only 100% safe and effective way to avoid unwanted pregnancy is not to engage in heterosexual intercourse.

2. Limit sexual activity to "outercourse." You can engage in many sexual activities—kissing, hugging, touching, massage, oral-genital sex—without risking pregnancy.

3. Talk about birth control with any potential sex partner. If you are considering sexual intimacy with a person, you should feel comfortable enough to talk about contraception.

4. Know what doesn't work—and don't rely on it. There are lots of misconceptions about ways to avoid getting pregnant, such as having sex in a standing position or during menstruation. Only the methods described in this chapter are reliable forms of birth control.

5. Talk with a health-care professional. A great deal of information and advice is available—from written sources, from family planning counselors, from physicians on the Internet. Check it out.

6. Choose a contraceptive method that matches your personal habits and preferences. If you can't remember to take a pill every day, oral contraceptives aren't for you. If you're constantly forgetting where you put things, a diaphragm might not be a good choice.

7. Consider long-term implications. Since you may wish to have children in the future, find out about the reversibility of various methods and possible effects on future fertility.

8. Resist having sex without contraceptive protection "just this once." It only takes once—even the very first time—to get pregnant. Be wary of drugs and alcohol. They can impair your judgment and make you less conscientious about using birth control—or using it properly.

9. Use backup methods. If there's a possibility that a contraceptive method might not offer adequate protection (for instance, if it's been almost 3 months since your last injection of Depo-Provera), use an additional form of birth control.

10. Inform yourself about emergency contraception. Just in case a condom breaks or a diaphragm slips, find out about the availability of forms of after-intercourse contraception.

Choosing a Method

When it comes to deciding which form of birth control to use, there's no one "right" decision. However, good decisions are based on sound information. You should consult a physician or family-planning counselor if you have questions or want to know how certain methods might affect existing or familial medical conditions, such as high blood pressure or diabetes.

As Table 8-1 indicates, contraception doesn't always work. As you evaluate any contraceptive, always consider its **effectiveness** (the likelihood that it will indeed prevent pregnancy). Inevitably, theoretical effectiveness, based on statistical estimates, is greater than actual effectiveness. The **failure rate** for a contraceptive refers to the number of pregnancies that occur per year for every 100 women using a particular method of birth control.[4]

As many as 3 million unintentional pregnancies each year in the United States are the result of contraceptive failure, either from problems with the drug or device itself or from improper use. Half of the 1.5 million abortions performed in this country each year involve pregnancies that stem from failed birth control. Partners can lower the risk of unwanted pregnancy by using backup methods—that is, more than one form of contraception simultaneously. Emergency or postintercourse contraception (discussed later in this chapter) could prevent as many as 2.3 million unwanted pregnancies each year.[5]

Always discuss contraception with your partner. Men shouldn't automatically shift this responsibility to women simply because women are the ones who get pregnant. And women shouldn't assume that men don't want to be consulted or participate, nor should they hesitate to discuss sharing the costs with their partners. It takes two people to conceive a baby, and two people should be involved in deciding *not* to conceive a baby. In the process, they can also enhance their skills in communication, critical thinking, and negotiating.

TABLE 8-1 FACTORS TO CONSIDER WHEN CHOOSING A BIRTH CONTROL METHOD

Method	Failure Rate* If Used Correctly and Consistently	Typical Number* Who Become Pregnant Accidentally	Cost (in dollars per year for 100 occurrences of intercourse)
Abstinence	0	0	0
Estrogen-progestin pills	0.1	3	$130–$260 ($10–$20 per cycle)
Progestin-only pills	0.5	3	$130–$260 ($10–$20 per cycle)
Norplant	0.09	0.09	$130–$170 if kept 5 years
Depo-Provera	0.3	0.3	$140 ($35 per injection)
Condoms (male)	3	12	$50–$100 (50¢ to $1 each)
Condoms (female)	5	21	$250 ($2.50 each)
Diaphragm with spermicide	6	18	$155–$255 ($20 diaphragm, $50–$150 for fitting, $85 for spermicide)
Cervical cap			
Woman has become pregnant	26	36	Same as diaphragm
Woman never pregnant	9	18	
Spermicides	6	21	$85 (85¢ per application)
Progestasert T IUD	1.5	2	$160
Copper-T IUD	0.6	0.8	$160 1st year; less if kept more years
Tubal sterilization	0.4	0.4	$1,200–$2,500
Vasectomy	0.1	0.15	$250–$1,000
Fertility awareness: "rhythm" calendar, basal temperature, cervical mucus	1–9	20	0
Withdrawal	4	19	0
No method	85	85	0

* Number of women who become pregnant by the end of the first year of using a particular method.

SOURCE: Hatcher, et al., *Contraceptive Technology*. New York: Irvington, 1994.

Abstinence and "Outercourse"

The contraceptive methods discussed in this chapter are designed to prevent pregnancy as a consequence of vaginal intercourse. Couples who choose abstinence make a very different decision—to abstain from vaginal intercourse and other forms of sexual activity (any in which ejaculation occurs near the vaginal opening) that could result in conception. Abstinence is the only form of birth control that is 100% effective and risk-free. It is also an important, increasingly valued lifestyle choice.

Individuals who choose abstinence from vaginal intercourse often engage in activities sometimes called "outercourse," such as kissing, hugging, sensual touching, and mutual masturbation. Outercourse can prevent pregnancy, but couples must be careful to avoid any penis-vagina contact. If the man ejaculates near the vaginal opening, sperm can swim up into the vagina and fal-

TABLE 8-1 CONTINUED...

Advantages	Disadvantages
No medical side effects. Helps develop nonintercourse sexual intimacy	Risk of unplanned intercourse
Very effective; no interruption of sexual experience; reduced menstrual cramps and flow	Possible side effects; increased risk of pregnancy if forgotten
Very effective; no interruption of sexual experience; no estrogen-related side effects	Breakthrough bleeding
Very effective; no interruption of sexual experience; don't have to remember to take it; no estrogen-related side effects	Breakthrough bleeding; difficult removal
Very effective; no interruption of sexual experience; don't have to remember on daily basis; no estrogen-related side effects	Breakthrough bleeding side effects; clinic visit and injection every 3 months
Some protection from STDs; available without a prescription	Interruption of sexual experience; reduces sensation
Same as male condoms	Same as male condoms
No side effects; can be put in prior to sexual experience	Needs practice to use correctly
Same as diaphragm	Same as diaphragm
No prescription necessary; some protection from STDs	Interruption of sexual experience; skin irritation for some
Very effective; no interruption of sexual activity; don't have to remember to use	Side effects; increased menstrual flow and cramps; may be expelled
Highly effective; permanent	Not easy to reverse for fertility
Easier procedure than tubal sterilization	Not easy to reverse for fertility
Acceptable to Catholic Church; no medical side effects	Uncertainty of "safe times"; periods of abstinence from intercourse or use of other methods
No medical side effects	Interruption of intercourse
Acceptable only if pregnancy desired	

lopian tubes to fertilize an egg. Except for oral-genital and anal sex, outercourse also may lower the risk of contracting sexually transmitted diseases.

Hormone-Based Contraceptives

These reversible methods of birth control for women use forms of estrogen and progesterone to inhibit ovulation, alter the mucous lining of the cervix so that it blocks the passage of sperm, or prevent successful implantation of the fertilized egg in the uterus.

The Birth Control Pill

"The pill"—the popular term for **oral contraceptives**—is the method of birth control preferred by unmarried women and by those under age 30, including college students. Women 18 to 24 years old are most likely to choose oral contraceptives. In use for 30 years, the pill

CAMPUS FOCUS:
COLLEGE STUDENTS AND CONTRACEPTION

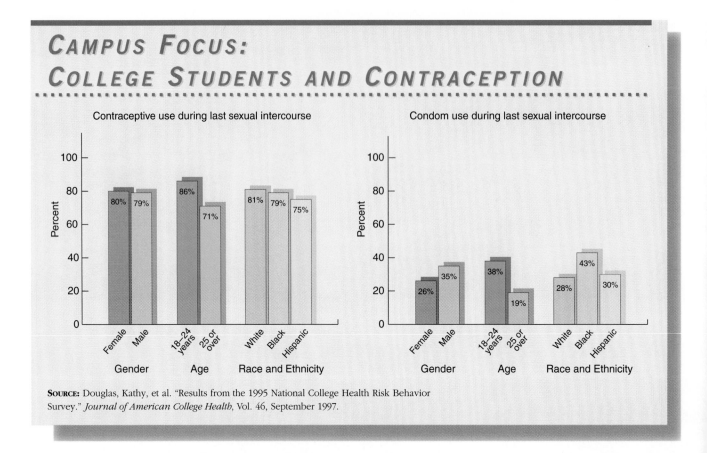

Contraceptive use during last sexual intercourse

Gender: Female 80%, Male 79%
Age: 18–24 years 86%, 25 or over 71%
Race and Ethnicity: White 81%, Black 79%, Hispanic 75%

Condom use during last sexual intercourse

Gender: Female 26%, Male 35%
Age: 18–24 years 38%, 25 or over 19%
Race and Ethnicity: White 28%, Black 43%, Hispanic 30%

SOURCE: Douglas, Kathy, et al. "Results from the 1995 National College Health Risk Behavior Survey." *Journal of American College Health*, Vol. 46, September 1997.

is one of the most researched, tested, and carefully followed medications in medical history.

Three types of oral contraceptives are currently widely used in the United States: the constant-dose combination pill, the multiphasic pill, and the progestin-only pill. The **constant-dose combination pill** releases two hormones, synthetic estrogen and progestin, which play important roles in controlling ovulation and the men-

strual cycle, at constant levels throughout the menstrual cycle. The **multiphasic pill** mimics normal hormonal fluctuations of the natural menstrual cycle by providing different levels of estrogen and progesterone at different times of the month. Multiphasic pills reduce total hormonal dose and side effects. The **progestin-only**, or **minipill**, contains a small amount of progestin and no estrogen. Unlike women who take constant-dose combination pills, those using minipills probably ovulate at least occasionally. The minipills make the mucus in the cervix so thick and tacky, however, that sperm can't enter the uterus. Minipills also may interfere with implantation by altering the uterine lining.

Advantages Birth control pills have several advantages: They are reversible, so a woman may easily stop using them. They do not interrupt sexual activity. Women on the pill have more regular periods, less cramping, and fewer tubal, or ectopic, pregnancies (discussed later in this chapter). The pill reduces the likelihood of benign breast lumps, ovarian cysts, and cancer of the lining of the uterus (endometrial cancer). In addition, the pill is one of the most effective forms of contraception. In actual use, the failure rate is 1% to 5% for estrogen/progesterone pills and 3% to 10% for minipills.

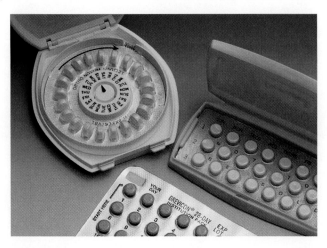

Oral contraceptives. The birth control pill.

Percentage of Women Using Contraception, by Method

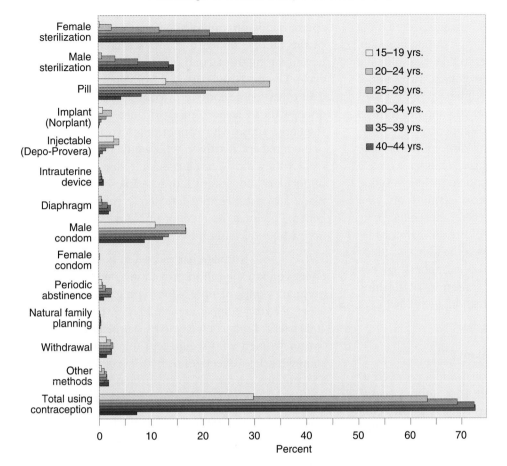

Figure 8-3

Percentage of women using contraception, by method.

SOURCE: Abma, J. C., et al. "Fertility Planning and Women's Health, new data from the 1995 National Survey of Family Growth." National Center For Health Statistics. *Vital Health Statistics*, Vol. 23, No. 19, 1997.

Disadvantages The pill does not protect against HIV infection and other sexually transmitted diseases, so condoms and spermicide should also be used. In addition, the hormones in oral contraceptives may cause various side effects, including spotting between periods, weight gain or loss, nausea and vomiting, breast tenderness, and decreased sex drive. Some women using the pill report emotional changes, such as mood swings and depression. Oral contraceptives can interact with other medications and diminish their effectiveness. There is a risk of cardiovascular problems associated with use of the pill, primarily for women over 35 who smoke and those with other health problems, such as high blood pressure. Women should inform any physician providing medical treatment that they are taking the pill.

Women generally worry more about the association of the newer pills with cancer than with cardiovascular disease. On the one hand, oral contraceptives may lower the risk of endometrial and ovarian cancer. On the other, some studies have found an increased risk of breast cancer, especially in women who take the pill when they're in their teens or early twenties.

Strategies for Prevention

Before You Take the Pill

Before starting on the pill, you should undergo a thorough physical examination that includes the following tests:

✔ Routine blood pressure test.

✔ Pelvic exam, including a Pap smear.

✔ Breast exam.

✔ Blood test.

✔ Urine sample.

You should also let your doctor know about any personal or family incidence of high blood pressure or heart disease, diabetes, liver dysfunction, hepatitis, unusual menstrual history, severe depression, sickle cell anemia, cancer of the breast, ovaries, or uterus, high cholesterol levels, or migraine headaches.

How to Use Oral Contraceptives The pill usually comes in 28-day packets: Twenty-one of the pills contain the hormones, and seven are "blanks," included so that the woman can take a pill every day, even during her menstrual period. If a woman forgets to take one pill, she should take it as soon as she remembers. However, if she forgets during the first week of her cycle or misses more than one pill, she should rely on another form of birth control until her next menstrual period.

Even if you experience no discomfort or side effects while on the pill, see a physician at least once a year for an examination, which should include a blood pressure test and a pelvic and breast exam. Notify your doctor at once if you develop severe abdominal pain, chest pain, coughing, shortness of breath, pain or tenderness in the calf or thigh, severe headaches, dizziness, faintness, muscle weakness or numbness, speech disturbance, blurred vision, a sensation of flashing lights, a breast lump, severe depression, or yellowing of your skin.

Contraceptive Implants (Norplant)

About 1% of women use hormonal implants, such as Norplant, which prevent pregnancy for up to 5 years.[6] Six thin silicone rubber capsules release a low, continuous dose of a synthetic form of progestin called levonorgestrel. Other implants are currently being developed.

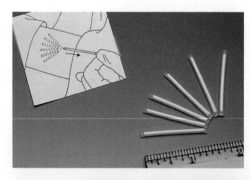

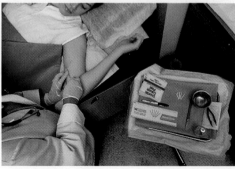

How Norplant works.

Norplant works primarily by suppressing ovulation, but it also thickens the cervical mucus (which inhibits sperm migration), inhibits the development and growth of the uterine lining, and limits secretion of progesterone during the second or luteal half of the menstrual cycle. The best candidates for Norplant are women who desire reversible long-term contraception, those who don't want to have to insert or ingest a contraceptive regularly, those who cannot take estrogen-containing oral contraceptives, those who would face high medical risks if they did become pregnant, and those who are undecided about sterilization. Adolescents using Norplant are considerably less likely than pill users to become pregnant unintentionally.[7] An estimated 1.8 million women have used Norplant worldwide.

Advantages Norplant has proven to be ten times more effective than the pill in preventing pregnancy, with a pregnancy rate of only 4 or 5 pregnancies per 1000 users per year, compared with 20 to 50 pregnancies per 1000 users of oral contraceptives. Norplant is most effective in women who weigh less than 110 pounds and somewhat less effective in those weighing more than 154 pounds. However, even in heavier women, Norplant is more effective than oral contraceptives.

Disadvantages Common side effects of Norplant include menstrual irregularities, spotting, and amenorrhea; these are most likely to occur in the first year of use. Other possible complications include ovarian cysts, headaches, acne, weight changes, breast discharge, and hair growth. Because Norplant doesn't include estrogen (as birth control pills do), there is no risk of clotting or high blood pressure. However, the FDA advises women with acute liver disease, unexplained vaginal bleeding, breast cancer, or blood clots in the lungs, legs, or eyes to avoid Norplant.

How to Use Norplant A qualified health-care professional, using a local anesthetic, implants the Norplant capsules with a needle under the skin of a woman's upper arms. The simple surgical procedure generally takes about 5 to 10 minutes. Once in place, the capsules can be felt and may be visible, particularly in slender women. Removal of the capsules again requires minor surgery, lasting 15 to 20 minutes, with a local anesthetic. Complications can occur during removal; the most common are bruising, slight bleeding, and pain at the removal site. After removal, fertility generally returns with the next menstrual cycle. According to various studies, most former users of Norplant began ovulating again within 7 weeks of implant removal, and most of those who wished to conceive did so within 1 year.

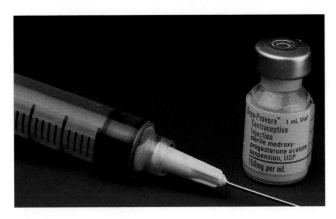

Depo-Provera, which is given by injection every 12 weeks.

Depo-Provera

One injection of Depo-Provera, a synthetic version of the natural hormone progesterone, provides 3 months of contraceptive protection. This long-acting hormonal contraceptive, approved for use in the United States in 1992, raises levels of progesterone, thereby simulating pregnancy.

Advantages   Because Depo-Provera contains only progestin, it can be used by women who cannot take oral contraceptives containing estrogen (such as those who've had breast cancer). Its main advantage is that women do not need to take a daily pill or use a barrier method during sexual activity. It also may have some protective action against endometrial and ovarian cancer.

Disadvantages   Depo-Provera provides no protection against HIV and other STDs. It causes menstrual irregularities in most users, a delayed return of fertility, excessive endometrial bleeding, and other side effects, including decreased libido, depression, headaches, dizziness, weight gain, frequent urination, and allergic reactions in a small percentage of users.

How to Use Depo-Provera   Women must receive an injection of Depo-Provera once every 12 weeks, ideally within 5 days of the beginning of menstruation.

Barrier Contraceptives

As their name implies, **barrier contraceptives** block the meeting of egg and sperm by means of a physical barrier (a condom, diaphragm, or a cervical cap) or a chemical one (vaginal spermicide in jellies, foams, creams, suppositories, or film). These forms of birth control have become increasingly popular because they can do more than prevent conception; they can also help reduce the risk of STDs.

The Male Condom

The male **condom** covers the erect penis and catches the ejaculate, thus preventing sperm from entering the woman's reproductive tract (see Figure 8-4). Most are made of thin surgical latex or sheep membrane; a new type is made of polyurethane, which is thinner, stronger, more heat-sensitive, and more comfortable than latex. Condoms with a spermicidal lubricant (nonoxynol-9) kill most sperm on contact and are thus more effective than other brands.

Although the theoretical effectiveness rate for condoms is 97%, the actual rate is only 80% to 85%. The condom can be torn during the manufacturing process or during its use; testing by the manufacturer may not be as strenuous as it could or should be. Careless removal can also decrease the effectiveness of condoms. However, the major reason that condoms have such a low actual effectiveness rate is that couples don't use them each and every time they have sex.

Advantages   Condoms made of latex or polyurethane, especially when used with spermicides containing nonoxynol-9, can help reduce the risk of certain STDs, including syphilis, gonorrhea, chlamydia, and herpes. They appear to lower a woman's risk of pelvic inflammatory disease (PID) and may protect against some parasites that cause urinary tract and genital infections. Public health officials view condoms as the best available defense against HIV infection.[8] They are available without a prescription or medical appointment, and their use does not cause harmful side effects. Some men appreciate the slight blunting of sensation they experience when using a condom because it helps prolong the duration of intercourse before ejaculation.

Disadvantages   Condoms are not 100% effective in preventing pregnancy or STDs, including infection with HIV or HPV (human papilloma virus). Condoms may have manufacturing defects, such as pinsize holes, or they may break or slip off during intercourse.[9] Some couples feel that putting on a condom interferes with sexual spontaneity; others incorporate it into their sex play. Some men dislike the reduced penile sensitivity or will not use them because they believe they interfere with sexual pleasure.

How to Use a Condom   Most physicians recommend prelubricated, spermicide-treated American-made latex or polyurethane condoms, not membrane condoms ("natural" or "sheepskin"). Before using a condom, check the expiration date and make sure it's soft and pliable. If it's yellow or sticky, throw it out. Don't check for leaks by blowing up a condom before using it; you may weaken or tear it.

The condom should be put on at the beginning of sexual activity, before genital contact occurs (Figure 8-4). There should be a little space at the tip of the condom to catch the semen. Wait until just before intercourse to apply spermicide. Any vaginal lubricant should be water-based. Petroleum based creams or jellies (such as Vaseline, baby oil, massage oil, vegetable oils, or oil-based hand lotions) can deteriorate the latex. After ejaculation, the condom should be held firmly against the penis so that it doesn't slip off or leak during withdrawal. Couples engaging in anal intercourse should use a water-based lubricant as well as a condom, but should never assume the condom will protect them from HIV infection or other STDs.

The Female Condom

The female condom, made of polyurethane, consists of two rings and a polyurethane sheath; it is inserted into the vagina with a tampon-like applicator. Once in place, the device loosely lines the walls of the vagina. Internally, a thickened rubber ring keeps it anchored near the cervix. Externally, another rubber ring, 2 inches in diameter, rests on the labia and resists slippage. The female condom should be used with a spermicide and water-based lubricant.

Advantages   The female condom gives women more control in reducing their risk of pregnancy and STDs. It does not require a prescription or medical appointment. One size fits all.

Disadvantages   The failure rate for the female condom is higher than for other contraceptives. The statistical failure rate is 12.2%, which means that 12 of every 100 women using the device could expect to get pregnant during a 1-year period. In clinical trials, the actual failure rate was even higher—20.6%. Since it does not have spermicide on it, the female condom does not provide as much risk reduction against STDs as do male condoms with spermicide.

How to Use the Female Condom   A woman removes the condom and applicator and inserts the condom slowly

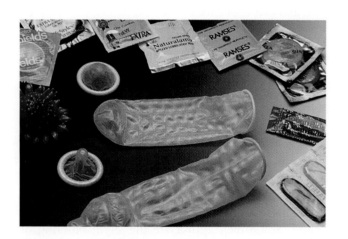

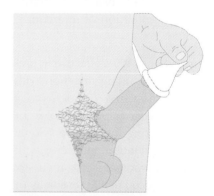

Pinch or twist the tip of the condom, leaving one-half inch at the tip to catch the semen.

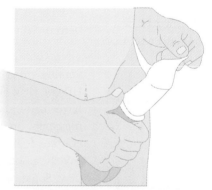

Holding the tip, unroll the condom over the penis.

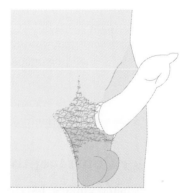

Unroll the condom until it reaches the pubic hairs.

Figure 8-4

The male condom. Condoms effectively reduce the risk of pregnancy as well as STDs. Using them consistently and correctly are important factors.

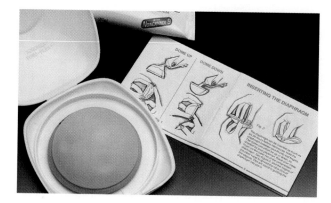

Figure 8-5

The diaphragm. When used correctly and consistently and with a spermicide, the diaphragm is effective in preventing pregnancy and STDs. It must be fitted by a health-care professional.

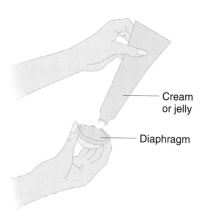

Cream or jelly

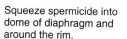

Diaphragm

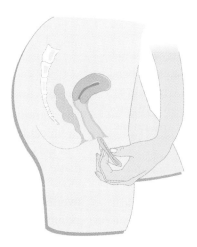

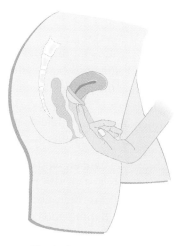

Squeeze spermicide into dome of diaphragm and around the rim.

Squeeze rim together; insert jelly-side up.

Check placement to make certain cervix is covered.

by gently pushing the applicator toward the small of the back. When properly inserted, the outer ring should rest on the folds of skin around the vaginal opening, and the inner ring (the closed end) should fit against the cervix.

The Diaphragm

The **diaphragm** is a bowl-like rubber cup with a flexible rim that is inserted into the vagina to cover the cervix and prevent the passage of sperm into the uterus during sexual intercourse (see Figure 8-5). When used with spermicide, the diaphragm is both a physical and a chemical barrier to sperm. The effectiveness of the diaphragm in preventing pregnancy depends on strong motivation (to use it faithfully) and a precise understanding of its use. If diaphragms with spermicide are used consistently and carefully, they can be 95% to 98% effective. Without a spermicide, the diaphragm is not effective.

Advantages Diaphragms have become increasingly popular, most likely because of concern about the side effects of hormonal contraceptives. Many women feel that using a diaphragm makes them more knowledgeable and comfortable about their bodies.

Disadvantages Some people find that the diaphragm is inconvenient and interferes with sexual spontaneity or that the spermicidal cream or jelly is messy, detracts from oral-genital sex, and may cause irritation. A poorly fitted diaphragm can cause discomfort during sex; some women report bladder discomfort, urethral irritation, or recurrent cystitis as a result of diaphragm use.

How to Use a Diaphragm Diaphragms are fitted and prescribed by a qualified health-care professional. The diaphragm's main function is to serve as a container for a spermicidal (sperm-killing) foam or jelly, which is available at pharmacies without a prescription. Do not use oil-based lubricants because they will deteriorate the latex. A diaphragm should remain in the vagina for at least 6 hours after intercourse to assure that all sperm are killed. If intercourse occurs again during this period, additional spermicidal cream or jelly must be inserted with an applicator tube.

The key to proper use of the diaphragm is having it available. A sexually active woman should keep it in the most accessible place—her purse, bedroom, bathroom. Before every use, a diaphragm should be checked for tiny leaks (hold up to the light or place water in the dome). A health-care provider should check its fit and condition every year when the woman has her annual Pap smear.

The Cervical Cap

Like the diaphragm, the **cervical cap**, combined with spermicide, serves as both a chemical and physical barrier blocking the path of sperm to the uterus. The rubber or plastic cap is smaller and thicker than a diaphragm and resembles a large thimble that fits snugly around the cervix. It is about as effective as a diaphragm.

Advantages Women who cannot use a diaphragm because of pelvic-structure problems or loss of vaginal muscle tone can often use the cap. Also, the cervical cap does not require additional applications of spermicide if intercourse occurs more than once within several hours.

Disadvantages Cervical caps are more difficult to insert and remove and may damage the cervix. Some women have difficulty getting a cervical cap that fits properly; others find it uncomfortable to wear.

How to Use a Cervical Cap

Like the diaphragm, the cervical cap is fitted by a qualified health-care professional. For use, the woman fills it one-third to two-thirds full with spermicide and inserts it by holding its edges together and sliding it into the vagina. The cup is then pressed onto the cervix. (Most women find it easiest to do so while squatting or in an upright sitting position.) The cap can be inserted up to 6 hours prior to intercourse and should not be removed for at least 6 hours afterward. It can be left in place up to 24 hours. Pulling on one side of the rim breaks the suction and allows easy removal. Oil-based lubricants should not be used with the cap because they can deteriorate the latex.

Vaginal Spermicides

The various forms of **vaginal spermicides** include chemical foams, creams, jellies, vaginal suppositories, and gels (see Figure 8-6). Some creams and jellies are made for use with a diaphragm; others can be used alone. Several vaginal suppositories claim high effectiveness, but no American studies have confirmed these claims. In general, failure rates for vaginal suppositories are as high as 10% to 25%.

Advantages Conscientious use of a spermicide together with another method of contraception, such as a condom, can provide safe and effective birth control and

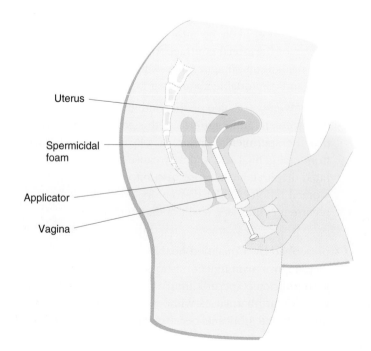

Uterus

Spermicidal foam

Applicator

Vagina

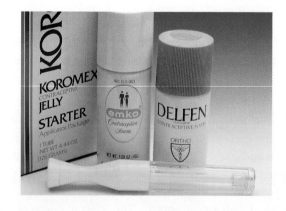

Figure 8-6

Vaginal spermicides. These various creams and jellies are available without a prescription and have minimal side effects. They are most effective in preventing pregnancy and STDs when used together with a condom.

reduce the risk of some vaginal infections, pelvic inflammatory disease, and STDs. The side effects of vaginal spermicides are minimal.

Disadvantages Even though spermicides can be applied in less than a minute, couples may feel that they interfere with sexual spontaneity. Some people are irritated by the chemicals in spermicides, but often a change of brand solves this problem. Others find foam spermicides messy or feel they interfere with oral-genital contact. Spermicidal suppositories that do not dissolve completely can feel gritty.

How to Use Vaginal Spermicides The various types of spermicide come with instructions that should be followed carefully for maximum protection. Contraceptive vaginal suppositories take about 20 minutes to dissolve and cover the vaginal walls. Foam, inserted with an applicator, goes into place much more rapidly. You must reapply spermicide before each additional intercourse. After sex, women should shower rather than bathe to prevent the spermicide from being rinsed out of the vagina and should not douche for at least 6 hours.

Vaginal Contraceptive Film (VCF)

Available from pharmacies without a prescription, the 2-inch-by-2-inch thin film known as the **vaginal contraceptive film (VCF)** is laced with spermicide. Once folded and inserted into the vagina, it dissolves into a stay-in-place gel. Its theoretical effectiveness is similar to that of other forms of spermicide; paired with a condom, it is almost 100% effective.

Advantages VCF film can be used by people allergic to foams and jellies. Unlike foams and jellies, it dissolves gradually and almost unnoticeably.

Disadvantages Some people feel that insertion, even though it takes only seconds, interrupts sexual spontaneity.

How to Use VCF A woman inserts the film by folding it and guiding it in with a finger so that it covers her cervix. VCF can be inserted from a minimum of 5 minutes to a maximum of 90 minutes before intercourse. It is effective for up to 2 hours and need not be removed. A new VCF must be inserted if intercourse occurs again after 2 hours.

The Intrauterine Device

The **intrauterine device (IUD)** is a small piece of molded plastic, with a nylon string attached, that is inserted into the uterus through the cervix. It prevents pregnancy by interfering with implantation. Once widely used, IUDs became less popular after most brands were removed from the market because of serious complications such as pelvic infection and infertility. However, the currently available IUDs have not been shown to increase the risk of such problems for women in mutually monogamous relationships.

Advantages The IUD is highly effective and easy to reverse. According to recent analyses, the Copper T is the cheapest and most cost-effective form of birth control. Current models cause fewer complications than the pill. The IUD does not interrupt sexual activity, and 98% of IUD users in one survey said they are happy with this method.[10]

Disadvantages The most serious disadvantage is the possibility of increased risk of PID, which can lead to scarring and infertility. Many gynecologists recommend other forms of birth control for childless women who someday may want to start a family. In addition, women with many sexual partners, who are at highest risk of PID, are not good candidates for this method. During insertion of an IUD, women may experience discomfort, cramping, bleeding, or pain, which may continue for a few days or longer. The hormonal IUD causes less excess bleeding and cramping than the Copper-T. An estimated 2% to 20% of users expel an IUD within a year of insertion.

How to Use an IUD A physician inserts an IUD during the woman's period, when the cervix is slightly softened and dilated. Antibiotics may be prescribed to lower any risk of infection. An IUD can be removed at any time during her cycle. A woman should check regularly, particularly after each menstrual period, for the nylon string attached to the IUD, because she may not otherwise notice if an IUD has been expelled.

Sterilization

The most popular method of birth control among married couples in the United States is **sterilization** (surgery to end a person's reproductive capability). Each year an estimated 1 million men and women in the United States undergo sterilization procedures.

Advantages Sterilization has no effect on sex drive in either men or women. Many couples report that their sexual activity increases after sterilization, because they're free from the fear of pregnancy or the need to deal with contraceptives.

Disadvantages Sterilization should be considered permanent and should be used only if both individuals are sure they want no more children. Although sterilization doesn't usually create psychological or sexual problems, it can worsen existing problems, particularly marital ones. Couples should discuss sterilization, together and with a physician, to understand fully the possible physical and emotional consequences. Although a link between vasectomy and an increased risk of prostate cancer was reported, the most recent research—including a study of almost 74,000 men in Denmark—did not find a correlation.[11]

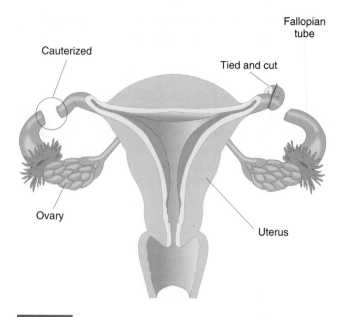

Figure 8-8
Female sterilization (tubal ligation).

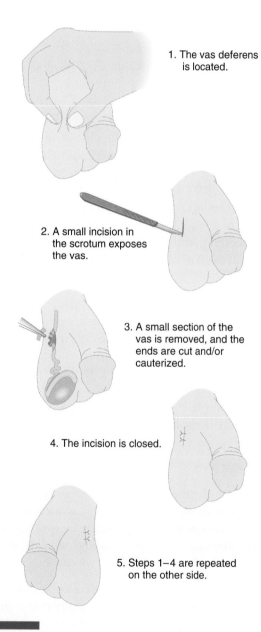

1. The vas deferens is located.

2. A small incision in the scrotum exposes the vas.

3. A small section of the vas is removed, and the ends are cut and/or cauterized.

4. The incision is closed.

5. Steps 1–4 are repeated on the other side.

Figure 8-7
Male sterilization, or vasectomy.

Male Sterilization An estimated 13% of married couples rely on male sterilization.[12] In men, the cutting of the *vas deferens,* the tube that carries sperm from one of the testes into the urethra for ejaculation, is called **vasectomy**. During the 15- or 20-minute office procedure, done under a local anesthetic, the doctor makes small incisions in the scrotum, lifts up each vas deferens, cuts them, and ties off the ends to block the flow of sperm (see Figure 8-7). Sperm continue to form, but they are broken down and absorbed by the body.

Female Sterilization Female sterilization procedures modify the fallopian tubes, which each month normally carry an egg from the ovaries to the uterus. These operations may soon surpass the pill as the first contraceptive choice among women. The two terms used to describe female sterilization are **tubal ligation** (the cutting or tying of the fallopian tubes) and **tubal occlusion** (the blocking of the tubes). The tubes may be cut or sealed with thread, a clamp, or a clip, or by cauterization (burning) to prevent the passage of eggs from the ovaries (see Figure 8-8). They can also be blocked with bands of silicone.

Methods Based on the Menstrual Cycle (Fertility Awareness Methods)

Awareness of a woman's cyclic fertility can help in both conception and contraception. The different methods of birth control based on a woman's menstrual cycle are sometimes referred to as natural family planning or fertility awareness methods. They include the cervical mucus method, the calendar method, and the basal-body-temperature method (all described below).

Advantages Birth control methods based on the menstrual cycle involve no expense, no side effects, and no need for prescriptions or fittings. On the days when the couple can have intercourse, there is nothing to insert, swallow, or check. In addition, abstinence during fertile periods complies with the teachings of the Roman Catholic Church.

Disadvantages During times of possible fertility (usually 8 or 9 days a month), couples must abstain from vaginal intercourse—which some may find difficult—or use some form of contraception. Conscientious planning and scheduling are essential. Women with irregular cycles may not be able to rely on the calendar method. Others may find the mucus or temperature methods difficult to use. They also provide no protection against STDs. For all these reasons, this approach to birth control is less reliable than many others. In theory, the overall effectiveness rate for the various fertility awareness methods is 80%. In practice, of every 100 women using one of these methods for a year, 24 become pregnant. However, using a combination of the basal-body-temperature method *and* the cervical mucus method may be 90% to 95% effective in preventing pregnancy.

Cervical Mucus Method This method, also called the **ovulation method**, is based on the observation of changes in the consistency of the mucus in the vagina. At peak estrogen levels, the mucus is smooth, stretchable, slippery (like raw egg white), and very clear. Mucus with these characteristics is usually observed within 24 hours of ovulation and lasts 1 to 2 days, signaling maximum fertility. The mucus becomes sticky and cloudy again 3 days thereafter, and the second safe period begins. Most women using this method have to refrain from unprotected intercourse for about 9 days of each 28-day menstrual cycle.

Calendar Method This approach, often called the **rhythm method**, involves counting the days after menstruation begins to calculate the estimated day of ovulation. Ideally, a woman first keeps a chart of her monthly cycles for about a year so she knows the average length of her cycle. The first day of menstruation is day one. She counts the number of days until the last day of her cycle, which is the day before menstrual flow begins. To determine the starting point of the period during which she should avoid unprotected intercourse, she subtracts

18 from the number of days in her shortest cycle. For instance, if her shortest cycle was 28 days, day 10 would be her first high-risk day. To calculate when she can again have unprotected intercourse, she subtracts 10 from the number of days in her longest cycle. If her longest cycle is 31 days, she could resume intercourse on day 21. Other forms of sexual activity can continue from day 10 to day 21. This method requires careful timing to avoid the possible meeting of a ripe egg and active sperm in the woman's fallopian tube.

Basal-Body-Temperature Method In this method the woman charts her **basal body temperature**, the body temperature upon waking in the morning, using a specially calibrated rectal thermometer, which is more precise than an oral one. The basal body temperature remains relatively constant from the beginning of the menstrual cycle to ovulation. After ovulation, however, basal body temperature rises by more than 0.5°F. The woman knows that her safe period has begun when her temperature has been elevated for 3 consecutive days. After 8 to 10 months, she should have a sense of her ovulatory pattern, in addition to knowing her daily readings.

Emergency, or After-Intercourse, Contraception

In cases where unprotected intercourse has occurred, a condom has broken or slipped off, or another form of contraception has failed, there are options for preventing implantation of a fertilized egg and possible pregnancy. **After-intercourse methods** of birth control include higher doses of standard oral contraceptives; the so-called *morning-after pill*, which prevents implantation of a fertilized egg; insertion of an IUD; *menstrual extraction*, in which the uterine lining is suctioned out; and *dilation and curettage (D and C)*, in which the uterine contents are scraped out. Many individuals are not aware that options for post-intercourse contraception exist. Yet some methods have been used in rape crisis centers for more than 20 years and are available from physicians, family planning clinics, and more than 80% of college health centers.[13]

Abortion

The purposeful termination of a pregnancy—**elective abortion**—should not be considered a form of contraception, but an alternative to giving birth to an unplanned child. Abortion is too risky, too expensive, and too complex a procedure to be viewed as anything other than an emergency backup if contraception fails.

More than 1.5 million abortions are performed in the United States every year; about 25% of all pregnancies in the United States end in abortion.[14] Three of every 100 American women between the ages of 15 and 44 have chosen to terminate a pregnancy. About half of all abortions are performed because of failed contraception; the others occur in the 9% of sexually active women who don't use birth control. In this country, 90% of abortions are performed within 12 weeks of fertilization; only 2 of every 1000 are performed more than 20 weeks after fertilization.[15]

Thinking Through the Options

A woman faced with an unwanted pregnancy—often alone, unwed, and desperate—can find it extremely difficult to decide what to do. The political debate over the right to life almost always is secondary to practical and emotional matters, such as the quality of her relationship to the baby's father, their capacity to provide for the child, the impact on any children she already has, and other important life issues.

In deciding whether or not to have an abortion, women report asking themselves many questions, including the following:[16]

- How do I feel about the man with whom I conceived this baby? Do I love him? Does he love me? Is this man committed to staying with me?

- What sort of relationship, if any, have we had or might we have in the future?

- If I continue the pregnancy and give birth, could I love the baby?

- Who can help me gain perspective on this problem?

- Have I thought about adoption? Do I think I could surrender custody of my baby? Would it make a difference if the adoption process were open and I could know the adoptive parents?

- If I keep my child, can I care for him or her properly? How would the birth of another baby affect my other children?

- Do I have marketable skills, an education, an adequate income? Would I be able to go to school or keep my job if I have a child? Who would help me?

- Would this child be born with serious abnormalities? Would it suffer or thrive?

- How does each option fit with what I believe is morally correct? Could I handle each of the options emotionally?

Answering these questions honestly and objectively may help women as they think through the realities of their situation.

Abortion Methods

A hormonal compound called RU-486 (mifepristone), which is not yet available in the United States, can end a pregnancy if taken within 9 weeks of a woman's last menstrual period. RU-486, which is 96% effective in inducing abortion, blocks progesterone, the hormone that prepares the uterine lining for pregnancy. Two days after taking this compound, a woman takes a prostaglandin to increase uterine contractions. The uterine lining is expelled along with the fertilized egg. Women have compared the discomfort of this experience to severe menstrual cramps. Common side effects include excessive bleeding, nausea, fatigue, abdominal pain, and dizziness. About 1 woman in 100 requires a blood transfusion following her use of RU-486.

Suction curettage, usually done from 7 to 13 weeks after the last menstrual period, involves the gradual dilation (opening) of the cervix, often by inserting one or more sticks of *laminaria* (a sterilized seaweed that absorbs moisture and expands, thus gradually stretching the cervix). Some women feel pressure or cramping with the laminaria in place. Occasionally, the laminaria itself starts to bring on a miscarriage.

At the time of abortion, the laminaria is removed, and dilators are used to enlarge the cervical opening further, if needed. The physician inserts a suction tip into the cervix, and the uterine contents are drawn out via a vacuum system (see Figure 8-9). A curette (a spoon-shaped surgical instrument used for scraping) is used to check for complete removal of the contents of the uterus. With suction curettage, the risks of complication are low. Major complications, such as perforation of the uterus, occur in fewer than 1 in 100 cases. About 90% of the abortions performed in this country are done by this technique.

For early-second-trimester abortions, physicians generally use a technique called **dilation and evacuation (D and E)**, in which they open the cervix and use medical instruments to remove the fetus from the uterus. D and E procedures are performed under local or general anesthesia.

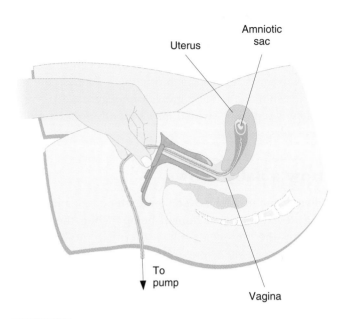

Uterus

Amniotic sac

To ▼ pump

Vagina

Figure 8-9

Suction curettage. The contents of the uterus are extracted through the cervix with a vacuum apparatus.

Psychological Responses After Abortion

The most common response of women who have just gotten an abortion is relief. While they may feel regret, sadness, or guilt following abortion, those with an unplanned pregnancy who obtain a legal abortion early in pregnancy typically report positive emotional effects. Moreover, emotional health and satisfaction typically continue to improve for 1 to 2 years following abortion. Researchers have found no evidence of so-called abortion trauma syndrome. The incidence of psychiatric illness and hospitalization is higher after childbirth than after abortion. Indeed, many women have reported that the decision to terminate a pregnancy was a "maturational point in their lives, one at which they experienced taking charge of their futures for the first time."[17]

The Politics of Abortion

Abortion is one of the most controversial political, religious, and ethical issues of our time. The issues of when life begins, a woman's right to choose, and an unborn child's right to survival are among the most divisive Americans have ever faced. Abortions were legal in the United States until the 1860s. For decades after that, women who decided to terminate unwanted pregnan-

cies did so by attempting to abort themselves or by obtaining illegal abortions—often performed by untrained individuals using unsanitary and unsafe procedures. In the late 1960s, some states began to change their laws to make abortions legal. In 1973, the U.S. Supreme Court, following a 1970 ruling on the case of *Roe v. Wade* by the New York Supreme Court, said that an abortion in the first trimester of pregnancy was a decision between a woman and her physician and was protected by privacy laws. The Court further ruled that abortion during the second trimester could be performed on the basis of health risks and that abortion during the final trimester could be performed only for the sake of the mother's health.

Since then, several laws have restricted the availability of legal abortions for low-income women. In 1989, the U.S. Supreme Court narrowed the interpretation of *Roe v. Wade* by upholding a law that sharply restricted publicly funded abortions and required doctors to test if a fetus could survive if they suspected a woman was more than 20 weeks pregnant. In 1992, in *Planned Parenthood v. Casey,* the Court upheld the right to legalized abortion but gave states the right to restrict abortion as long as they did not place an "undue burden" on a woman. This has limited the availability of abortion to young, rural, or low-income women.[18]

More than 25 years after *Roe v. Wade*, the debate over abortion continues to stir passionate emotion, with prolife supporters arguing that life begins at conception and that abortion is therefore immoral, and prochoice advocates countering that an individual woman should have the right to make decisions about her body and health. The

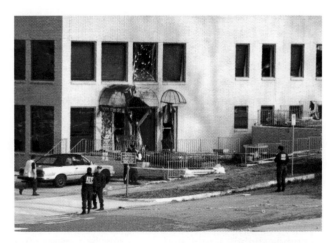

Opposition to legal abortions has often become violent. A security guard was killed and a nurse severely injured when a Birmingham, Alabama, abortion clinic was bombed in January 1998.

controversy over abortion has at times become violent: Physicians who performed abortions have been shot and killed; abortion clinics have been bombed, wounding and killing patients and staff members.

Pregnancy

After an upswing in the 1980s, the U.S. birth rate has declined, a trend that the Census Bureau expects to continue throughout the 1990s. The average age of mothers has risen, but about 70% of babies still are born to women in their twenties. Mothers are now averaging slightly fewer than two children each. Not every married couple is opting for parenthood. One-third of all married couples say that they plan *not* to have children; a generation ago, only one-fifth of all married couples were childless—and often not by choice. Childless couples are at least as likely—if not more likely—to be content with their marriages as couples with children.

Preconception Care: A Preventive Approach

The time *before* a child is conceived can be crucial in assuring that an infant is born healthy, full-size, and full-term. Women who smoke, drink alcohol, take drugs, eat poorly, are too thin or too heavy, suffer from unrecognized infections or illnesses, or are exposed to toxins at work or home may start pregnancy with one or more strikes against them and their unborn babies. The best chance for lowering the infant mortality rate and preventing birth defects is before pregnancy. **Preconception care**—the enhancement of a woman's health and well-being prior to conception to ensure a healthy pregnancy and baby—includes risk assessment (including evaluation of medical, genetic, and lifestyle risks), health promotion (such as teaching good nutrition guidelines), and interventions to reduce risk (such as treatment of infections and other diseases or assistance in quitting smoking or drug use).

How a Woman's Body Changes During Pregnancy

The 40 weeks of pregnancy transform a woman's body. At the beginning of pregnancy, the woman's uterus becomes slightly larger, and the cervix becomes softer and bluish due to increased blood flow. Progesterone and estrogen trigger changes in the milk glands and ducts in the breasts, which increase in size and feel somewhat tender. The pressure of the growing uterus against the bladder causes a more frequent need to urinate. As the pregnancy progresses, the woman's skin stretches as her body shape changes, her center of gravity changes as her abdomen protrudes, and her internal organs shift as the baby grows (see Figure 8-10). Pregnancy is typically divided into 3-month periods called trimesters.

How a Baby Grows

Silently and invisibly, over a 9-month period, a fertilized egg develops into a human being. When the zygote reaches the uterus, it's still smaller than the head of a pin. Once nestled into the spongy uterine lining, it becomes an **embryo**. The embryo takes on an elongated shape, rounded at one end. A sac called the **amnion** envelops it (see Figure 8-11). As water and other small molecules cross the amniotic membrane, the embryo floats freely in the absorbed fluid, cushioned from shocks and bumps. At 9 weeks the embryo is called a **fetus**.

A special organ, the **placenta**, forms. Attached to the embryo by the umbilical cord, it supplies the growing baby with fluid and nutrients from the maternal bloodstream and carries waste back to the mother's body for disposal (see Figure 8-12).

Emotional Aspects of Pregnancy

Almost all prospective parents worry about their ability to care for a helpless newborn. By talking openly about their feelings and fears, however, they can strengthen the bonds between them, so that they can work together as parents as well as partners. Psychological problems, such as depression, can occur during pregnancy. The availability of social support and other resources for coping with stress can make a great difference in the potential impact of emotional difficulties.[19]

The physiological changes of pregnancy can affect a woman's mood. In early pregnancy, she may feel weepy, irritable, or emotional. As the pregnancy continues, she may become calmer and more energetic. Men, too, feel a range of intense emotions about the prospect of having a child: pride, anxiety, hope, fears for their unseen child and for the woman they love. Although many men want to be as supportive as possible, they may think that they have to be strong and calm—and may therefore pull away from their wives. The more involved fathers become in preparing for birth, the closer they feel to their partners and babies afterward.

Figure 8-10

Physiological changes
of pregnancy.

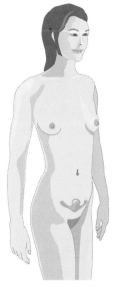

Before conception

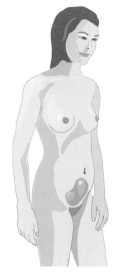

At 4 months

First Trimester

Increased urination because of hormonal changes and
the pressure of the enlarging uterus on the bladder.

Enlarged breasts as milk glands develop.

Darkening of the nipples and the area around them.

Nausea or vomiting, particularly in the morning.

Fatigue.

Increased vaginal secretions.

Pinching of the sciatic nerve, which runs from the buttocks
down through the back of the legs, as the pelvic bones
widen and begin to separate.

Irregular bowel movements.

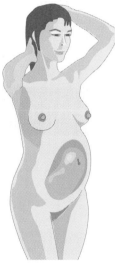

Second Trimester

Thickening of the waist as the uterus grows.

Weight gain.

Increase in total blood volume.

Slight increase in size and change in position of the heart.

Darkening of the pigment around the nipple and from
the navel to the pubic region.

Darkening of the face.

Increased salivation and perspiration.

Secretion of colostrum from the breasts.

Indigestion, constipation, and hemorrhoids.

Varicose veins.

At 7 months

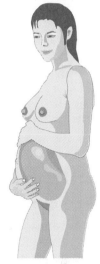

At 9 months

Third Trimester

Increased urination because of pressure from the uterus.

Tightening of the uterine muscles (called Braxton-Hicks
contractions).

Shortness of breath because of increased pressure
by the uterus on the lungs and diaphragm.

Heartburn and indigestion.

Trouble sleeping because of the baby's movements
or the need to urinate.

Descending ("dropping") of the baby's head into the
pelvis about 2 to 4 weeks before birth.

Navel pushed out.

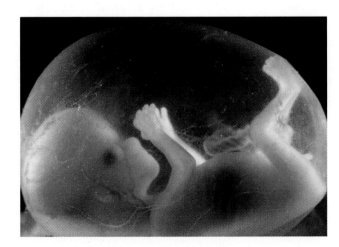

Figure 8-11

The amnion, or amniotic sac, surrounds and cushions the fetus.

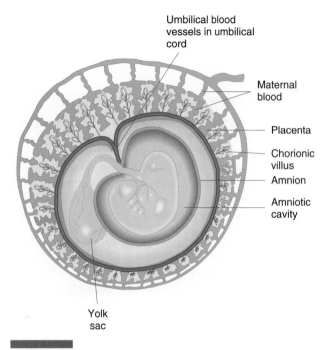

Umbilical blood
vessels in umbilical
cord

Maternal
blood

Placenta

Chorionic
villus

Amnion

Amniotic
cavity

Yolk
sac

Figure 8-12

The placenta. The placenta supplies the growing embryo with fluid
and nutrients from the maternal bloodstream and carries waste back
for disposal.

Prenatal Care: Taking Care of Yourself and Your Baby

A pregnant woman has to take good care of herself to provide good care for her unborn child. This means regular medical and dental checkups. A woman should have her first prenatal visit as soon as she discovers that she's pregnant. A study group of the American College of Obstetricians and Gynecologists (ACOG) has recommended seven or eight prenatal visits for women with low-risk pregnancies; women at higher risk require more frequent checkups.

Age

The risk of a poor pregnancy outcome increases with age. Women 30 or older face a 40% greater risk of late fetal death, compared with women ages 20 to 24. Women over 35 also face an increased risk of very low birth weight, preterm delivery, and small-for-gestational-age (SGA) infants. Preconception and prenatal care, including good nutrition and careful monitoring, increase the chances of a healthy baby for older mothers.

Nutrition

A well-balanced diet throughout pregnancy is critical for a mother and her fetus both before and at birth. If a

woman—regardless of her prepregnancy weight—gains too little weight, the risk to the growing fetus is high.[20]

No vitamin supplement can replace a well-balanced diet, but a multivitamin can help reduce or avoid deficiencies. According to the Centers for Disease Control and Prevention (CDC), women who take a simple daily multivitamin containing a B vitamin called folate (or folic acid) before conception can cut in half the risk that their children will suffer neural tube defects, which stem from faulty development of the spinal column.

Activity and Rest

Almost all pregnant women can benefit from exercise throughout pregnancy—as long as they don't push too hard or too far. Regular exercise (three times a week) is better, safer, and more effective than occasional workouts. While women who were athletic prior to pregnancy generally can continue their physical activity, they should be aware of warning signs such as faintness,

Strategies for Prevention

A Mother-to-Be's Guide to a Healthy Pregnancy

✔ ACOG recommends consuming about 300 more calories a day than before pregnancy and concentrating on eating the right foods, not on watching your weight. *Never* diet during pregnancy. Don't restrict salt intake either, unless specifically directed by your doctor.

✔ Drink six to eight glasses of liquids each day, including water, fruit and vegetable juices, and milk.

✔ Don't exercise strenuously for more than 15 minutes, ACOG advises. Avoid vigorous exercise in hot, humid weather. Never let your body temperature rise above 100°F or your heart rate climb above 140 beats per minute.

✔ Stretch and flex carefully because the joints and connective tissue soften and loosen during pregnancy. After the fourth month of pregnancy, don't do any exercises while lying on your back, as this could impair blood flow to the placenta.

✔ Walk, swim, and jog in moderation; and play tennis only if you played before pregnancy. Ski only if you're experienced, and stick to low altitudes and safe slopes. Do not water-ski, surf, or ride a horse.

dizziness, pain, or vaginal bleeding that could indicate a potential problem.[21]

Rest is as important as exercise; the pregnant woman who's not used to taking naps may have to make time in her schedule for rest periods. If insomnia or the frequent need to urinate during the night becomes a problem, she may have to rely on catnaps during the day. She should *not* take sleeping pills.

Substance Use

Smoking endangers two lives: the mother's and the fetus's. The sooner a mother-to-be stops smoking, the better the chances that the fetus will develop normally. Smoking increases the risk of miscarriage, stillbirth, low birth weight, heart defects, and premature birth; it also impairs growth.[22]

Approximately 16% of pregnant women report drinking in the month before conception.[23] According to the CDC, more than 8000 alcohol-damaged babies are born every year. One out of every 750 newborns has a cluster of physical and mental defects called **fetal alcohol syndrome (FAS)**: low birth weight, smaller-than-normal head circumference, smaller and shorter size, irritability as newborns, and permanent mental impairment as a result of their mothers' alcohol consumption. The milder forms of these problems, particularly impaired intellectual ability and school performance, are called fetal alcohol effects (FAE).

At least one out of every ten newborns is exposed to illegal drugs before birth. The consequences of drug use during pregnancy include severe damage to the child's brain and nervous system and birth defects. Marijuana smokers have smaller, sicker babies and a higher risk of stillbirths, according to some research. Drug use also may lead to "neurochemical" birth defects by disrupting normal development of the brain. Cocaine use increases the risk of premature birth, stillbirths, and malformations.

Complications of Pregnancy

Most pregnancies are free of complications. However, in about 10% to 15% of all pregnancies, there is an increased risk of some problem that might affect the mother and fetus. In an **ectopic pregnancy**, the fertilized egg remains in the fallopian tube instead of traveling to the uterus. Ectopic pregnancies have increased dramatically in recent years, and their major cause is STD infection. The misplaced egg develops normally until the cramped amniotic sac bursts, damaging the fallopian tube.

About 10% to 20% of pregnancies end in **miscarriage**, or spontaneous abortion, before the 20th week of gestation. Major genetic disorders may be responsible for 33% to 50% of pregnancy losses. Few medical events are more emotionally devastating than a pregnancy loss. Women and their partners often feel the loss acutely and should be allowed to grieve as they would for a lost child.

Approximately 10% of babies are born too soon, before the 37th week of pregnancy. According to a 1995 study, prematurity is the main underlying cause of stillbirth and infant deaths within the first few weeks after birth. The signs of premature labor include a dull, low backache, a feeling of pressure on the lower abdomen, and cramping.

Childbirth

A generation ago, delivering a baby was something a doctor did in a hospital. Today parents can choose from an almost bewildering array of birthing options. The first decision parents-to-be face is choosing a birth attendant, who can be a physician or a nurse-midwife. Certified nurse-midwives in the United States deliver more than 90,000 babies a year, mostly in hospitals and birth centers. Their approach is based on the belief that the typical pregnant woman can deliver her baby naturally without technological intervention. Lay midwives have a similar orientation but less formal training; only a handful of states permit lay midwives to deliver babies.

When interviewing physicians or midwives, look for the following:

- Experience in handling various complications.

- Extensive prenatal care.

- A commitment to be at the mother's side for the entire labor to spot complications quickly and provide assistance.

- A compatible philosophy toward childbirth and medical interventions.

Preparing for Childbirth

The most widespread method of childbirth preparation is **psychoprophylaxis**, or the **Lamaze method**. Fernand Lamaze, a French doctor, instructed women to respond to labor contractions with learned, controlled breathing techniques. As the intensity of each contraction increases, the laboring woman concentrates on increasing her breathing rate in a prescribed way. Her partner coaches her during each contraction and helps her cope with discomfort.

Women who have had childbirth preparation training tend to have fewer complications and require fewer medications. However, painkillers or anesthesia are always an option if labor is longer or more painful than expected. The lower body can be numbed with an **epidural block**, which involves injecting an anesthetic into the membrane around the spinal cord, or a **spinal block**, in which the injection goes directly into the spinal canal. General anesthesia is usually used only for emergency caesarean births.

Labor and Birth

There are three stages of **labor**. The first starts with *effacement* (thinning) and *dilation* (opening up) of the cervix. Effacement is measured in percentages, and dilation in centimeters (cm) or finger-widths. Around this time, the amniotic sac of fluids usually breaks, a sign that the woman should call her doctor or midwife.

The first contractions of the early, or *latent,* phase of labor are usually not uncomfortable; they last 15 to 30 seconds, occur every 15 to 30 minutes, and gradually increase in intensity and frequency. The most difficult contractions come after the cervix is dilated to about 8 cm, as the woman feels greater pressure from the fetus. The first stage ends when the cervix is completely dilated to a diameter of 10 cm (or five finger-widths) and the baby is ready to come down the birth canal (see Figure 8-13). For women having their first baby, this first stage of labor averages 12 to 13 hours. Women having another child often experience shorter first-stage labor.

When the cervix is completely dilated, the second stage of labor occurs, during which the baby moves into the vagina, or birth canal, and out of the mother's body. As this stage begins, women who have gone through childbirth preparation training often feel a sense of relief from the acute pain of the transition phase and at the prospect of giving birth.

This second stage can take up to an hour or more. Strong contractions may last 60 to 90 seconds and occur every 2 to 3 minutes. As the baby's head descends, the mother feels an urge to push. By bearing down, she helps the baby complete its passage to the outside.

As the baby's head appears, or *crowns,* the doctor may perform an *episiotomy*—an incision from the lower end of the vagina toward the anus to enlarge the vaginal opening. The purpose of the episiotomy is to prevent

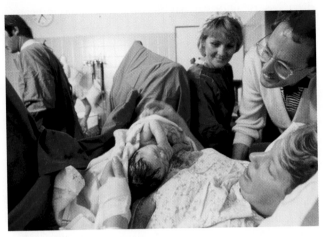

Family time. Fathers are routinely present at the birth of their children and often act as breathing coaches after both parents train in Lamaze techniques.

the baby's head from causing an irregular tear in the vagina, but routine episiotomies have been criticized as unnecessary. Women may be able to avoid this procedure by trying different birthing positions or having an attendant massage the perineal tissue.

Usually the baby's head emerges first, then its shoulders, then its body. With each contraction, a new part is born. However, the baby can be in a more difficult position, facing up rather than down, or with the feet or buttocks first (a **breech birth**), and a caesarean birth may then be necessary.

In the third stage of labor, the uterus contracts firmly after the birth of the baby, and usually within 5 minutes, the placenta separates from the uterine wall. The woman may bear down to help expel the placenta, or the doctor may exert gentle external pressure. If an episiotomy has been performed, the doctor sews up the incision. To help the uterus contract and return to its normal size, it may be massaged manually, or the baby may be put to the mother's breast to stimulate contraction of the uterus.

Caesarean Birth

In a **caesarean delivery** (also referred to as a caesarean section), the doctor lifts the baby out of the woman's body through an incision made in the lower abdomen and uterus. The most common reason for caesarean birth is "failure to progress," a vague term indicating that labor has gone on too long and may put the baby or mother at risk. Other reasons include the baby's position (if feet or buttocks are first) and signs that the fetus is in danger. Thirty years ago, only 5% of babies born in

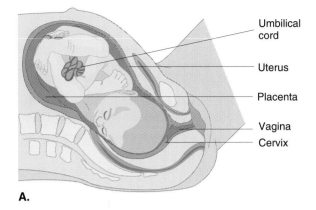

Umbilical cord
Uterus
Placenta
Vagina
Cervix

A.

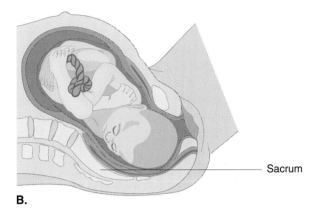

Sacrum

B.

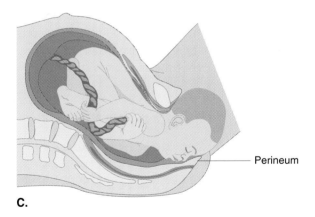

Perineum

C.

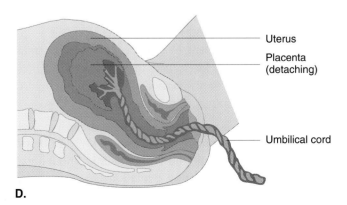

Uterus
Placenta (detaching)
Umbilical cord

D.

Figure 8-13

Birth. (A) The cervix is partially dilated, and the baby's head has entered the birth canal. (B) The cervix is nearly completely dilated. The baby's head rotates so that it can move through the birth canal. (C) The baby's head extends as it reaches the vaginal opening, and the head and the rest of the body pass through the birth canal. (D) After the baby is born, the placenta detaches from the uterus and is expelled from the woman's body.

America were delivered by caesarean birth; the current rate is 22.6%—substantially higher than in most other industrialized countries.

Following Birth

Hospital stays for new mothers have gotten shorter. The average length of stay is now only 2.6 days for a vaginal delivery and 4.1 days after a caesarean birth. A primary reason has been pressure to reduce medical costs. Obstetricians have voiced concern that the rush to release new mothers may jeopardize their well-being and the health of their babies, who are more likely to require emergency care for problems such as jaundice. The American College of Obstetricians and Gynecologists and the American Academy of Pediatrics recommend that women remain in the hospital 2 days after a vaginal delivery and 4 days after a caesarean birth.

For the new mother, the high of delivery may be followed by a low known as **postpartum depression**. This time of fatigue, anxiety, and fluctuating moods is so common that it is listed in obstetrics texts as a normal consequence of delivery. For most women, it is a temporary feeling. For others, the depression, combined with fatigue and the new demands of the newborn, can persist and deepen. If postpartum depression lasts more than 3 or 4 weeks, the woman should seek help from a qualified psychotherapist.

It takes a while for the mother's body to return to normal after having given birth. The woman usually loses about 11 pounds at delivery and an additional 4 to 5 pounds in the following weeks. Usually 4 to 8 weeks are required for the woman's reproductive organs, especially the uterus, to return to normal. Breast-feeding hastens this process, and exercises help restore the abdomen's size, shape, and tone. For 3 to 6 weeks after birth, there is a vaginal discharge called **lochia**, a mixture of blood from the site in the uterus where the placenta was attached and tissue from the uterine lining. If the mother doesn't breast-feed her infant, menstruation typically resumes about 4 to 10 weeks after giving birth.

Breast-Feeding Versus Bottle-Feeding

A generation ago, most middle- and upper-class women bottle-fed their babies. Today, an increasing number of mothers and medical professionals feel that breast milk is best. Breast-fed babies have fewer illnesses and a much lower hospitalization rate. Their mortality rate is also lower. Breast milk seems not only to prevent disease, but also to help bring infection under control. When breast-fed babies do get sick, they recover more quickly.

Despite the benefits of breast-feeding, there are valid reasons to choose bottle-feeding. According to the American Council on Science and Health, at least 20% of women are unable to breast-feed after their first deliveries, and 50% of new mothers encounter significant difficulties nursing. Sometimes the woman's breasts become inflamed, or she must take medications that would endanger her infant; sometimes the infant is unable to suckle vigorously enough to get an adequate milk supply. Another problem is that in certain areas of the country, the levels of pesticides and other chemical contaminants in mother's milk can be high.

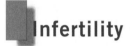

Infertility

The World Health Organization defines **infertility** as the failure to conceive after 1 year of unprotected intercourse. About 85% of couples will conceive during 1 year, rising to almost 90% by 2 years. The main causes of infertility are ovulation problems, tubal damage, or sperm dysfunction. Less common causes are endometriosis, cervical factors, or coital difficulties. Even after intensive investigation, 10% to 20% of couples have "unexplained infertility" in which no cause can be demonstrated.[24] Of the couples who marry this year, one in twelve won't be able to conceive a child, and 10% of couples already married won't be able to have additional children. About 6.1 million women reported impaired fertility in 1995, compared with 4.9 million in 1988. Infertility is a problem of the couple, not of the individual man or woman. In 40% of cases, infertility is caused by female problems; in 40% by male problems; in 10% by a combination of male and female problems; and in 10% by unexplained causes. A thorough diagnostic workup can reveal a cause for infertility in 90% of cases. Almost two-thirds of the couples who seek medical help for infertility eventually succeed in having a child.[25]

Medical treatment can identify the cause of infertility in about 90% of affected couples. The odds of successful pregnancy range from 30% to 70%, depending on the specific cause of infertility. One result of successful infertility treatments has been a boom in twins, triplets, and quadruplets. Some obstetricians have urged less aggressive treatment for infertility to avoid such high-risk multiple births.

Since the 1960s, **artificial insemination**—the introduction of viable sperm into the vagina by artificial means—has led to an estimated 250,000 births in the United States, primarily in couples in which the husband was infertile. However, some states do not recognize such children as legitimate; others do, but only if the woman's husband consented to the insemination.

Among the most promising techniques that can help couples overcome fertility problems is *in vitro fertilization,* which involves removing the ova, often with a long needle, from a woman's ovary just before normal ovulation would occur. The woman's egg and her mate's sperm are placed in a special fertilization medium (a substance that encourages fertilization) for a specific period of time and are then transferred to another medium to continue developing. If the fertilized egg cell shows signs of development, within several days it is returned to the woman's uterus by means of a hollow tube placed through the vagina and cervix. The egg cell implants itself in the lining of the uterus, and the pregnancy continues as normal. The success rate varies from center to center but is generally less than 20%, and the costs are high. In a 1994 study, in vitro fertilization costs per successful delivery ranged from $66,667 for the first cycle of IVF to $114,286 by the sixth attempt.[26]

Making This Chapter Work for You
Responsible Reproductive Choices

■ Simply not wanting to conceive is never enough to prevent conception. Before you become sexually active, you have to decide about birth control. The fact that women bear children does not mean that men aren't equally responsible for birth control.

■ A sexually active couple that doesn't use contraception has an 80% chance of conceiving a child within a year. If you decide to take that gamble, the stakes are your future, your partner's future, and the future of the child you may conceive.

■ To prevent conception, you can make the survival of sperm in the vagina more difficult or you can block the sperm's path into the vagina, uterus, and fallopian tubes. By preventing ovulation, you can make sure that the sperm doesn't find a ready, ripe egg; or

Health Online

Successful Contraception   http://www.arhp.org/success/index.html

Sponsored by the Association of Reproductive Health Professionals, this site includes an interactive program to help you choose the best birth control method. It takes into consideration your health history, lifestyle factors, and personal preferences. There is also information on assessing your birth control choices and details on each method.

Think about it ...

- Does this program recommend any birth control methods that you haven't considered before? What would be the advantages and disadvantages of these methods compared to the one you are currently using?

- What are your most important considerations in choosing a method of birth control? Cost, effectiveness, accessibility, convenience, or other factors?

- If you are not currently sexually active, have you thought about what method of contraception you might use if you do start having sex?

---

you can prevent the fertilized egg from implanting itself in the uterine wall.

- Abstinence and sexual activities that do not involve vaginal intercourse ("outercourse") are completely safe and 100% effective, as long as couples are committed to this practice and make sure that sperm are never ejaculated near the vaginal opening.

- Hormonally based birth control methods include oral contraceptives (the pill); hormone implants (Norplant), which inhibit ovulation and alter the cervical mucus so that sperm are prevented from entering the uterus; and Depo-Provera, an injectable hormone that provides 3 months of contraceptive protection.

- The barrier contraceptives provide a physical or chemical barrier that prevents sperm from reaching an egg. They include the condom, diaphragm, cervical cap, and spermicidal foam, jelly, suppositories, and film. Use of condoms with spermicides containing nonoxynol-9 can also reduce the risk of pregnancy and some sexually transmitted diseases.

- Intrauterine devices (IUDs), made with a hormonal compound or copper, prevent implantation of a fertilized egg. They are highly effective and long-acting but are recommended only for women in monogamous relationships.

- Couples using natural family planning or fertility awareness methods refrain from unprotected vaginal intercourse during the days just preceding and just following ovulation. They may use cervical mucus, a monthly calendar, or body temperature changes to determine a woman's period of greatest fertility.

- The most popular and effective, but permanent, birth control method among married couples is sterilization: vasectomy in a man and tubal ligation or occlusion in a woman.

- After-intercourse methods of birth control include higher doses of oral contraceptives; the so-called morning-after pill, which prevents implantation of a fertilized egg; insertion of an IUD; and menstrual extraction, in which the uterine lining is suctioned out.

- One of the most controversial and divisive issues today is legalized induced abortion, the termination of pregnancy by the removal of the uterine contents. A hormonal compound, RU-486, often called the abortion pill, available only at research centers, can terminate a pregnancy in its first weeks. Commonly used abortion methods in the United States are suction curettage, dilation and evacuation (D and E), prostaglandin injection, and hysterotomy.

■ Good prenatal care includes good nutrition; adequate rest and exercise; and avoiding risks, such as smoking, alcohol, caffeine, harmful drugs, and exposure to radiation.

■ Labor and delivery consists of three stages. During the first stage, the cervix thins and dilates to a diameter of 10 centimeters. In the next stage, the baby passes through the birth canal. The placenta is expelled during the third stage. A caesarean, or surgical, birth may be necessary to overcome certain risks. After birth, the woman's body begins to return to its prepregnant state. The woman may choose to breast-feed, which can help protect the newborn from various illnesses, or bottle-feed her baby.

■ Infertile couples may decide to attempt to have a child by such medical procedures as in vitro fertilization or other assisted forms of birth technology.

Choices about sexual behavior invariably lead to choices about reproduction. Sexual responsibility means recognizing that fact and acting with full awareness of the consequences of sexual activity. You must think not just of yourself, but also of your partner, because your decisions and actions may affect both of you, now and in the future. You must also consider the baby you might conceive if you don't use contraception. If you should decide to have a child, your responsibilities extend to the new life you helped to create.

Key Terms

The terms listed here are used within the chapter. Page numbers are included for each term. A definition of each term is given in the green Glossary pages at the end of this book.

Review Questions

1. What is conception? What is preconception care? Who should practice it? How? When does it occur?
2. What are some common methods of contraception? List an advantage and disadvantage for each method.

3. What is abortion? List and describe the various methods of abortion.
4. What happens to a woman when she becomes pregnant? Describe the physiological changes that occur during pregnancy.

Critical Thinking Questions

1. After reading about the various methods of contraception, which do you feel would be most effective for you? What factors enter into your decision (convenience, risks, effectiveness, etc.)?
2. In Wyoming, a pregnant woman went to the police station to report that her husband had beaten her. Instead of charges being brought against him, she was arrested for intoxication and charged with abusing her fetus by drinking. Across the country, other women who use hard drugs or alcohol while pregnant or whose newborns test positive for drugs have been arrested and put on trial for abusing their unborn children. Prosecutors argue that

they are defending the innocent victims of substance abuse. Some health officials, on the other hand, argue that addicted women need help, not punishment. What do you think? Why?
3. When Bobby McCaughey gave birth to septuplets in 1997, some people felt that the power of fertility drugs had gone too far. If you or your partner took fertility drugs and then became pregnant with seven fetuses, would you carry them all to term? What if you knew that the chances of all surviving were very slim and that eliminating some of them would improve the odds for the others? What ethical issues do cases like these raise?

Connections to Personal Health Interactive

*To enhance your understanding of the material covered in this chapter, check out the following study aids on the **Personal Health Interactive CD-ROM** .*

- Personal Insights: Do You Want to Be a Parent?
- Personal Insights: How Sexual Are You?
- Survey of Sexual Knowledge
- **Online Research:** Reproductive Choices
- Study Page: The Breast

- Study Page: Female Sexual Anatomy
- Study Page: Male Sexual Anatomy
- Study Page: Intercourse
- Glossary and Key Term Review

References

1. Mahoney, from Robert Brooks and Karla Baur, *Our Sexuality.* 7th ed. Pacific Grove, CA: Brooks/Cole, 1999.
2. Lancashire, Jeff. "New Report Documents Trends in Childbearing, Reproductive Health." National Center for Health Statistics, June 5, 1997.
3. "Family Planning Saves Millions of Women and Children's Lives." *WIN News*, Vol. 23, No. 2, Spring 1997.
4. Walling, Anne. "Overview of the Failure Rate of Contraceptive Methods." *American Family Physician*, Vol. 55, No. 1, January 1997.
5. Hanson, Vivien. "How to Provide Postcoital Contraception." *Patient Care*, April 15, 1997.
6. Lancashire. "New Report Documents Trends in Childbearing, Reproductive Health."

7. Berenson, Abbey, and Constance Wiemann. "Use of Levonorgestrel Implants Versus Oral Contraceptives in Adolescents: A Case-Controlled Study." *American Journal of Obstetrics & Gynecology*, Vol. 171, No. 4, April 1995.
8. Pinkerton, Steven, and Paul Abrahamson. "Condoms and the Prevention of AIDS." *American Scientist*, Vol. 85, No. 4, July–August 1997.
9. Lindberg, Laura Duberstein, et al. "Young Men's Experience with Condom Breakage." *Family Planning Perspectives*, Vol. 29, No. 3, May–June 1997.
10. Hatcher, Robert, et al. *Contraceptive Technology.* New York: Irvington, 1994.
11. Giovannucci, E., et al. "A Long-Term Study of Mortality in Men Who Have Undergone Vasectomy." New *England Journal of Medicine,* May 21, 1992.

12. Lancashire. "New Report Documents Trends in Childbearing, Reproductive Health."

13. Grimes, David. "Emergency Contraception—Expanding Opportunities for Primary Prevention." *New England Journal of Medicine*, Vol. 337, No. 15, October 9, 1997.

14. Gober, Patricia. "The Role of Access in Explaining State Abortion Rates." *Social Science & Medicine*, Vol. 44, No. 7, April 1997.

15. Hatcher et al. *Contraceptive Technology.*

16. Maloy, Katie, and Maggie Patterson. *Birth or Abortion? Private Struggles in a Political World.* New York: Plenum Press, 1992.

17. Stotland, Nada. "The Myth of the Abortion Trauma Syndrome." *Journal of the American Medical Association,* October 21, 1992.

18. Gober. "The Role of Access."

19. Seguin, Louise, et al. "Chronic Stressors, Social Support and Depression During Pregnancy." *Obstetrics & Gynecology*, Vol. 85, No. 4, April 1995.

20. Copper, Rachel, et al. "The Relationship of Maternal Attitude Toward Weight Gain During Pregnancy and Low Birth Weight." *Obstetrics & Gynecology*, Vol. 85, No. 4, April 1995.

21. Artal, Raul, and Philip Buckenmeyer. "Exercise During Pregnancy and Postpartum." *Contemporary Ob/Gyn*, May 1995. Stressguth, Ann, et al. "Prenatal Alcohol and Offspring Development: The First Fourteen Years." *Drug & Alcohol Dependence*, Vol. 36, No. 2, October 1994.

22. "Medical-Care Expenditures Attributable to Cigarette Smoking During Pregnancy—United States, 1995." *Journal of the American Medical Association*, Vol. 278, No. 23, December 17, 1997.

23. "Drinking in Pregnancy." *Morbidity & Mortality Weekly Report*, U.S. Centers for Disease Control, April 1997.

24. "Infertility: Its Investigation and Treatment." *WIN News*, Vol. 23, No. 2, Spring 1997.

25. "Infertility Statistics." *Focus on Fertility*, Vol. 1, No. 2, Spring 1995.

26. Neuman, P.J., et al. "The Cost of a Successful Delivery with In-Vitro Fertilization." *New England Journal of Medicine*, Vol. 331, 1994.

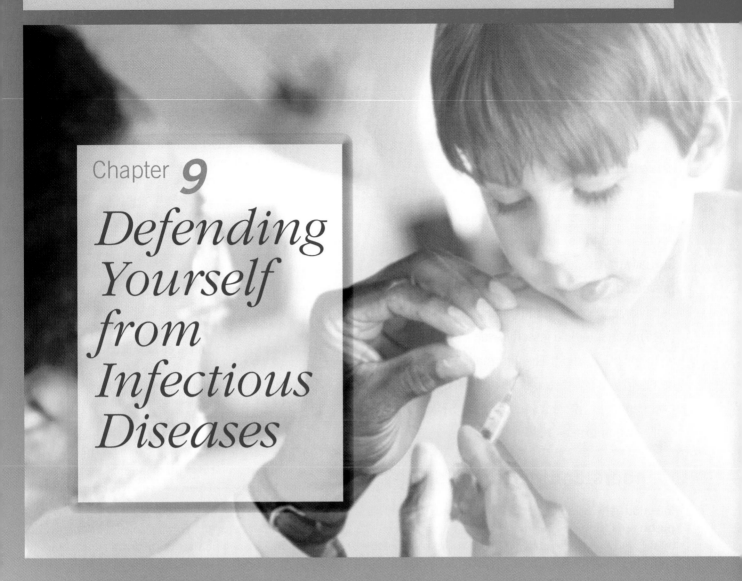

Chapter 9

Defending Yourself from Infectious Diseases

- **Explain** how the different agents of infection spread disease.
- **Describe** how your body protects itself from infectious disease.
- **List** and **describe** some common infectious diseases.
- **List** the sexually transmitted diseases and the symptoms and treatment for each.
- **Define** HIV infection, and **describe** its symptoms.
- **List** the methods of HIV transmission.
- **Explain** some practical methods for preventing HIV infection and other sexually transmitted diseases.

Although modern science has won many victories against the agents of infection, infectious illnesses have reemerged in recent years as a serious health threat.

Some of today's most common and dangerous infectious illnesses spread primarily through sexual contact, and their incidence has skyrocketed. Sexually transmitted diseases (STDs) cannot be prevented in the laboratory. Only you, by your behavior, can prevent and control them.

This chapter is a lesson in self-defense against all forms of infection. The information it provides can help you boost your defenses, recognize and avoid enemies, protect yourself from STDs, and realize when to seek help.

Understanding Infection

Infection is a complex process, triggered by various **pathogens** (disease-causing organisms) and countered by the body's own defenders. Physicians explain infection in terms of a **host** (either a person or a population) that contacts one or more agents in an environment. A **vector**—a biological or physical vehicle that carries the agent to the host— provides the means of transmission.

Agents of Infection

The types of microbes that can cause infection are viruses, bacteria, fungi, protozoa, and helminths (parasitic worms).

- *Viruses*. The tiniest pathogens—**viruses**—are also the toughest; they consist of a bit of nucleic acid (DNA or RNA, but never both) within a protein coat. Unable to reproduce on its own, a virus takes over a body cell's reproductive machinery and instructs it to produce new viral particles, which are then released to enter other cells.

- *Bacteria*. Simple one-celled organisms, **bacteria** are the most plentiful microorganisms as well as the most pathogenic. Most kinds of bacteria don't cause disease; some, like the *Escherichia coli* that aid in digestion, play important roles within our bodies.

Bacteria harm the body by releasing enzymes that digest body cells or toxins that produce the specific effects of such diseases as diphtheria or toxic shock. In self-defense the body produces specific proteins (called *antibodies*) that attack and inactivate the invaders. Tuberculosis, tetanus, gonorrhea, scarlet fever, and diphtheria are examples of bacterial diseases. Because bacteria are sufficiently different from the cells that make up our bodies, antibiotics can kill them without harming our cells.

- *Fungi*. Single-celled or multicelled organisms, **fungi** consist of threadlike fibers and reproductive spores. These plants, lacking chlorophyll, must obtain their food from organic material, which may include human tissue.

- *Protozoa*. These single-celled, microscopic animals release enzymes and toxins that destroy cells or interfere with their function. Diseases caused by **protozoa** are not a major health problem in this country, primarily because of public health measures. Around the world, however, some 2.24 billion people (more than 40% of the world's population) are at risk for acquiring one protozoa-caused disease—malaria—every year. Up to 3 million die of this disease annually.[1]

- *Helminths (Parasitic Worms)*. Small parasitic worms that attack specific tissues or organs and compete with the host for nutrients are called **helminths**. One major worldwide health problem is *shistosomiasis,* a disease caused by a parasitic worm, the fluke, that burrows through the skin and enters the circulatory system. Infection with another helminth, the tapeworm, may be contracted from eating undercooked beef, pork, or fish containing larval forms of the tapeworm. Helminthic diseases are treated with appropriate medications.

Transmission of Infectious Diseases

The major vectors, or means of transmission, for infectious disease are animals/insects, person-to-person, food, water, and air. Disease may be transmitted by house pets, livestock, or wild animals. Insects also spread a variety of diseases. The people you're closest to can transmit pathogens by coughing, sneezing, kissing, or sharing food or dishes with you. To avoid infection, stay out of range of anyone who's coughing, sniffling, or sneezing. Carefully wash your dishes, utensils, and hands, and abstain from sex or make self-protective decisions about sexual partners.

Every year foodborne illnesses strike millions of Americans, sometimes with fatal consequences. Bacteria account for two-thirds of foodborne infections, and thousands of suspected cases of infection with *Escherichia coli* bacteria in undercooked or inadequately washed food have been reported. Waterborne diseases, such as typhoid fever and cholera, are still widespread in less developed areas of the world.

The Process of Infection

If someone infected with the flu sits next to you on a bus and coughs or sneezes, tiny viral particles may travel into your nose and mouth. Immediately the virus finds or creates an opening in the wall of a cell, and the process of infection begins. During the **incubation period**, the time between invasion and the first symptom, you're unaware of the pathogen multiplying inside you. In some diseases, incubation may go on for months, even years; for most, it lasts several days or weeks.

The early stage of the battle between your body and the invaders is called the *prodromal* period. As infected cells die, they release chemicals that help block the invasion. Other chemicals, such as *histamines*, cause blood vessels to dilate, thus allowing more blood to reach the battleground. During all of this, you feel mild, generalized symptoms, such as headache, irritability, and discomfort. You're also highly contagious. At the height of the battle—the typical illness period—you cough, sneeze, sniffle, ache, feel feverish, and lose your appetite.

Recovery begins when the body's forces gain the advantage. With time, the body destroys the last of the invaders and heals itself. However, the body is not able to develop long-lasting immunity to certain viruses, such as colds, flu, or HIV.

How Your Body Protects Itself

Various parts of your body safeguard you against infectious diseases and provide **immunity**, or protection, from these health threats. Your skin, when unbroken, keeps out most potential invaders. Your tears, sweat, skin oils, saliva, and mucus contain chemicals that can kill bacteria. Cilia, the tiny hairs lining your respiratory passages, move mucus, which traps inhaled bacteria, viruses, dust, and foreign matter, to the back of the throat, where it is swallowed; the digestive system then destroys the invaders.

When these protective mechanisms can't keep you infection-free, your body's immune system, which is on constant alert for foreign substances that might threaten the body, swings into action. The immune system includes structures of the lymphatic system, which includes the spleen, thymus gland, lymph nodes, and vessels called lymphatics that help filter impurities from the body (see Figure 9-1). More than a dozen different types of white blood cells are concentrated in the organs of the lymphatic system or, by way of the blood and lymph vessels, patrol the entire body. The two basic types of immune mechanisms are humoral and cell-mediated.

Humoral immunity refers to the protection provided by antibodies, proteins derived from white blood cells called B lymphocytes or B cells. Humoral immunity is most effective during bacterial or viral infections. An *antigen* is any substance that enters the body and triggers production of an antibody. Once the body produces antibodies against a specific antigen—the mumps virus, for instance—you're protected against that antigen for life. If you're again exposed to mumps, the antibodies previously produced prevent another episode of the disease.

The various types of T cells are responsible for cellular, or **cell-mediated**, immunity. These lymphocytes are manufactured in the bone marrow and carried to the thymus for maturation. Cell-mediated immunity mainly protects against parasites, fungi, cancer cells, and foreign tissue. Thousands of different T cells work together to ward off disease. Some T cells activate other immune cells; others help in antibody-mediated responses; and still others suppress lymphocyte activity while others carry out different functions.

Immune Response

Attacked by pathogens, the body musters its forces and fights. Sometimes the invasion is handled like a minor border skirmish; other times a full-scale battle is waged throughout the body. Together, the immune cells work like an internal police force. When an antigen enters the body, the T cells aided by *macrophages* (large scavenger cells with insatiable appetites for foreign cells, diseased and run-down red blood cells, and other biological debris) engage in combat with the invader. Meanwhile, the B cells churn out antibodies, which rush to the scene and join in the fray. Also busy at surveillance are natural killer cells that, like the elite forces of a SWAT team, seek out and destroy viruses and cancer cells.

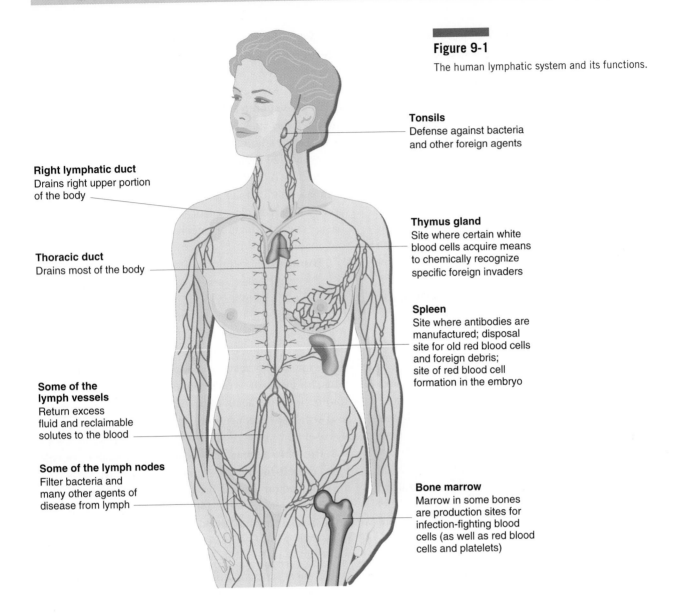

Figure 9-1
The human lymphatic system and its functions.

Tonsils
Defense against bacteria
and other foreign agents

Right lymphatic duct
Drains right upper portion
of the body

Thoracic duct
Drains most of the body

Thymus gland
Site where certain white
blood cells acquire means
to chemically recognize
specific foreign invaders

Spleen
Site where antibodies are
manufactured; disposal
site for old red blood cells
and foreign debris;
site of red blood cell
formation in the embryo

**Some of the
lymph vessels**
Return excess
fluid and reclaimable
solutes to the blood

Some of the lymph nodes
Filter bacteria and
many other agents of
disease from lymph

Bone marrow
Marrow in some bones
are production sites for
infection-fighting blood
cells (as well as red blood
cells and platelets)

The **lymph nodes**, or glands, are small tissue masses in which some protective cells are stored. If pathogens invade your body, many of them are carried to the lymph nodes, where they are then destroyed. This is why the lymph nodes often feel swollen when you have a cold or the flu.

If the microbes establish a foothold, the blood supply to the area increases, bringing oxygen and nutrients to the fighting cells. Tissue fluids, as well as antibacterial and antitoxic proteins, accumulate. You may develop redness, swelling, local warmth, and pain—the signs of **inflammation**. As more tissue is destroyed, a cavity, or **abscess**, forms and fills with fluid, battling cells, and dead white blood cells (pus). If the invaders aren't killed or inactivated, the pathogens are able to spread into the bloodstream and cause what is known as **systemic dis-**

ease. The toxins released by the pathogens cause fever, and the infection becomes more dangerous.

Immunity and Stress

Whenever we confront a crisis, large or small, our bodies produce powerful hormones that provide extra energy. However, this stress response dampens immunity, reducing the number of some key immune cells and the responsiveness of others.

As research into the field of psychoneuroimmunology (discussed in Chapter 3) has shown, psychological factors can affect immunity. When people are grieving for a loved one or lose their jobs, for instance, their immune systems show measurable impairment. People living with daily stress (caring for a parent with

Strategies for Prevention

Natural Ways to Bolster Immunity

✔ *Eat a balanced diet* to be sure you get essential vitamins and minerals. Severe deficiencies in vitamins B-6, B-12, and folic acid impair immunity. Keep up your iron and zinc intake. Iron influences the number and vigor of certain immune cells, whereas zinc is crucial for cell repair. Too little vitamin C may also increase susceptibility to infectious diseases.

✔ *Avoid fatty foods.* A low-fat diet can increase the activity of immune cells that hunt down and knock out cells infected with viruses.

✔ *Get enough sleep.* Without adequate rest, your immune system cannot maintain and renew itself.

✔ *Exercise regularly.* Aerobic exercise stimulates the production of an immune-system booster called interleukin-2.

✔ *Don't smoke.* Smoking decreases the levels of some immune cells.

✔ *Control your alcohol intake.* Heavy drinking interferes with normal immune responses and lowers the number of defender cells.

Alzheimer's disease, for example) or with episodic stress (such as final examinations in college) also have weakened immune responses. On the other hand, social contacts, through friendships, intimate relationships, or marriage, may bolster immunity.[2]

Immune Disorders

Sometimes our immune system overreacts to certain substances or mistakes the body's own tissues for enemies or doesn't react adequately. The result is an immune disorder. The most common are **allergies**, which essentially represent a hypersensitivity to a substance in one's environment or diet.

One of the most costly of chronic conditions, allergies run up annual tabs of $1.8 to $2 billion in doctor visits, diagnostic tests, prescriptions, and decreased productivity. Every year they account for more than 10 million workdays missed; every day they keep 10,000 children out of school.

Autoimmune disorders result when the immune system fails to recognize body tissue as self and attacks it. Many of these severely disabling diseases, such as myasthenia gravis, rheumatoid arthritis, and systemic lupus erythematosus, primarily strike women in their childbearing years. These diseases, which often worsen with time, may be treated with drugs that suppress the immune system.

Immunization: The Key to Prevention

One of the great success stories of American medicine has been the development of vaccines that provide protection against many infectious diseases. Unfortunately, many Americans, including large numbers of children in urban centers, haven't been properly immunized. As a result, some diseases that had been considered under control, such as measles, mumps, and whooping cough (pertussis), have been occurring more often. At particular risk are children in poorer sections of large American cities, who often aren't immunized against measles and other so-called childhood diseases because of the cost.[3]

As shown in Figure 9-2, the American Academy of Pediatrics recommends that all children be immunized against measles, mumps, German measles (rubella), diphtheria, tetanus, chickenpox, and hepatitis B. Although some vaccines confer lifelong protection, others do not. The protection provided by diphtheria and tetanus vaccinations, for example, diminishes over time, so booster vaccinations are required every 10 years. Health officials also recommend measles booster shots for students entering college and suggest that people born after 1956 be revaccinated for polio, measles, and other infectious diseases before visiting developing countries.

If you're uncertain about your past immunizations, check with family members or your doctor. If you can't find answers, a blood test can show whether you carry antibodies to specific illnesses.

If you're pregnant or planning to get pregnant within the next 3 months, do not get a measles, mumps, rubella, or oral polio vaccination. If you're allergic to neomycin, consult your doctor before getting a measles, mumps, rubella, or intramuscular polio vaccination. Those with egg allergies should check with a doctor before getting a measles, mumps, or flu vaccination. Also, never get a vaccination when you have a high fever.

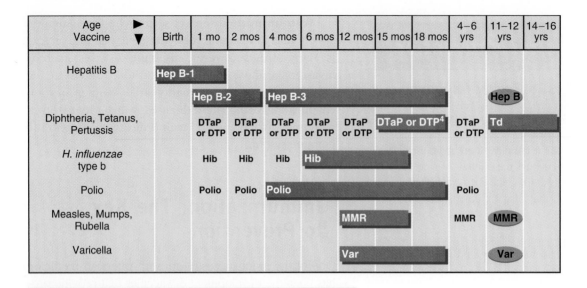

Age Vaccine ▶ ▼	Birth	1 mo	2 mos	4 mos	6 mos	12 mos	15 mos	18 mos	4–6 yrs	11–12 yrs	14–16 yrs
Hepatitis B	Hep B-1	Hep B-1	Hep B-2	Hep B-3	Hep B-3	Hep B-3				Hep B	
Diphtheria, Tetanus, Pertussis		DTaP or DTP	DTaP or DTP	DTaP or DTP	DTaP or DTP	DTaP or DTP	DTaP or DTP[4]		DTaP or DTP	Td	Td
H. influenzae type b		Hib	Hib	Hib	Hib	Hib					
Polio		Polio	Polio	Polio	Polio	Polio			Polio		
Measles, Mumps, Rubella						MMR	MMR		MMR	MMR	
Varicella						Var	Var			Var	

Figure 9-2 Recommended Childhood Immunization Schedule

Vaccines are listed under the routinely recommended ages. Bars indicate range of acceptable ages for immunization. Catch-up immunization should be done during any visit when feasible. Shaded ovals indicate vaccines to be assessed and given if necessary during the early adolescent visit.

Infectious Diseases

An estimated 500 microorganisms cause disease; no effective treatment exists for about 200 of these illnesses.[4] Although infections can be unavoidable at times, the more you know about their causes, the more you can do to protect yourself.

Who's at Highest Risk?

Like human bullies, the viruses responsible for the most common infectious illnesses tend to pick on those least capable of fighting back. Among the most vulnerable are the following groups:

- *Children and their families.* Youngsters get up to a dozen colds annually; adults average two a year. When a flu epidemic hits a community, about 40% of school-age boys and girls get sick, compared with only 5% to 10% of adults. But their parents get up to six times as many colds as other adults.[5]

- *The elderly.* Statistically, fewer older men and women are likely to catch a cold or flu, yet when they do, they face greater danger than the rest of the population. People over 65 who get the flu have a one in ten chance of being hospitalized for pneu-

monia or other respiratory problems and a one in fifty chance of dying from the disease.[6]

- *The chronically ill.* Lifelong diseases, such as diabetes, kidney disease, or sickle cell anemia, decrease an individual's ability to fend off infections. Individuals taking medications that suppress the immune system, such as steroids, are more vulnerable to infections, as are those with medical conditions that impair immunity, such as infection with HIV, the virus that causes AIDS.

- *Smokers and those with respiratory problems.* Smokers are a high-risk group for respiratory infections and serious complications, such as pneumonia. Chronic breathing disorders, such as asthma and emphysema, also greatly increase the risk of respiratory infections.

- *Those who live or work in close contact with someone sick.* Health-care workers who treat high-risk patients, nursing home residents, and others living in close quarters—such as students in dormitories—face greater odds of catching others' colds and flus.

- *Residents or workers in poorly ventilated buildings.* The technology of the 20th century has helped spread certain airborne illnesses, such as tuberculosis, via recirculated air. Indoor air quality may be closely linked with disease transmission in winter, when people spend a great deal of time in tightly sealed rooms.

The Common Cold

There are more than 200 distinct cold viruses, or rhinoviruses. Although in a single season you may develop a temporary immunity to one or two, you may then be hit by a third. Colds can strike in any season, but different cold viruses are more common at different times of year. Rhinoviruses cause most spring, summer, and early fall colds, and tend to cause more symptoms above the neck (stuffy nose, headache, runny eyes). Adenoviruses, parainfluenza viruses, corona viruses, influenza viruses, and others that strike in the winter are more likely to get into the bronchi and trachea (the breathing passages) and cause more fever and bronchitis. Cold viruses spread by coughs, sneezes, and touch. Cold sufferers who sneeze and then touch a doorknob or countertop leave a trail of highly contagious viruses behind them.[7]

Strategies for Prevention

Taking Care of Your Cold

✔ Drink plenty of liquids (except alcohol) to liquefy mucus, replace lost fluids, and prevent complications such as ear infections and bronchitis.

✔ If you have a sore throat, gargle with warm salty water. While sprays or lozenges can relieve the pain of a sore throat, none cures the inflammation causing the discomfort.

✔ If you have a cough, a cold-mist humidifier or steam vaporizer will liquefy secretions and help more than expectorants (drugs that bring up the mucus in your chest). If you do use an expectorant, make sure it contains guaifenesin, the only ingredient the FDA has found effective. The primary benefit of cough suppressants is that they allow a person with a dry, hacking cough to sleep through the night.

✔ Symptoms requiring medical attention include: fever lasting more than 4 or 5 days or rising over 104°F; yellow-green or rust-colored discharge from the nose or throat; significant pain in the throat, sinuses, eyes, or chest; or a cough that persists.

Strategies for Prevention

Protecting Yourself from Colds and Flus

✔ Wash your hands frequently with hot water and soap. In a public restroom, use a paper towel to turn off the faucet after you wash your hands and avoid touching the doorknob. Wash objects used by someone contagious with a cold.

✔ Take good care of yourself: Make sure you're getting adequate sleep. Eat a balanced diet. Exercise regularly. Don't share food or drinks.

✔ Spend as little time as possible in crowds, especially in closed places, such as elevators and airplanes. When out, keep your distance from sneezers and coughers. Don't touch your eyes, mouth, and nose after being with someone who has cold symptoms.

✔ Use tissues rather than cloth handkerchiefs, which may harbor viruses for hours or days.

✔ Try to avoid irritating air pollutants. Don't smoke, which destroys protective cells in the airways and worsens any cough. Limit your intake of alcohol, which depresses white blood cells and increases the risk of bacterial pneumonia in flu sufferers.

When cold symptoms develop, what should you do? According to the latest word from health experts, less treatment may be more effective. Aspirin and acetaminophen (Tylenol) may suppress the antibodies the body produces to fight cold viruses and may actually increase some symptoms, such as nasal stuffiness. If you want an alternative to relieve achiness, try ibuprofen (brand names include Motrin, Advil, and Nuprin), which doesn't seem to affect immune responses. Moreover, children, teenagers, and young adults should never take aspirin for a cold or flu, because of the danger of Reye's syndrome, a potentially deadly disorder that can cause convulsions, coma, swelling of the brain, and kidney damage.

Not too long ago millions of Americans gulped vitamin C to ward off colds, but large-scale research studies found no proof to back up this practice. Now many cold sufferers are thinking zinc, but the research remains inconclusive. In one study at the Cleveland Clinic Foundation, 100 adults who'd had cold symptoms for less than 24 hours sucked either on zinc gluconate lozenges or placebos every 2 hours during the day. The zinc users felt better in a median of 4.4 days, compared with 7.6 days for the others, and reported less coughing, hoarseness, nasal congestion, sore throat, and headache.[8]

Although pharmacy shelves are brimming with an estimated 800 different cold remedies, most contain the same basic ingredients. Physicians advise against multisymptom remedies, which usually provide medication (and side effects) for symptoms you don't have as well as those you do. Choose medications tailored to relieve specific symptoms, says Jack Gwaltney, M.D., head of the Division of Epidemiology and Virology at the University of Virginia and one of the nation's premier cold experts. His personal recommendation for a head cold is a 12-hour antihistamine and a nonsteroidal antiinflammatory drug (such as ibuprofen), taken from first symptom for 2 or 3 days.[9]

For a cough, the ingredient to look for in any suppressant is dextromethrophan, which turns down the brain's cough reflex. In expectorants, the only medicine the FDA has deemed effective is guaifenesin, which helps liquefy secretions so you can bring up mucus from the chest. Unless you're coughing up green or foul yellow mucus—signs of a "secondary" bacterial infection—antibiotics won't help. They have no effect against viruses and may make your body more resistant to such medications when you develop a bacterial infection in the future.

Your own immune system can do something modern science cannot: cure a cold. All that it needs is time, rest, and plenty of fluids. Warmth also is important, because the aptly named "cold" viruses replicate at lower temperatures. Hot soups and drinks (particularly those with a touch of something pungent, like lemon or ginger) both raise body temperature and help clear the nose. Even more important is getting off your feet. Taking it easy reduces demands on the body, which helps speed recovery.

Influenza

Although similar to a cold, **influenza**—or the flu—causes more severe symptoms that last longer (see Table 9-1). Some 25 to 50 million Americans come down with the flu every year. According to Centers for Disease Control (CDC) estimates, influenza and pneu-

TABLE 9-1 IS IT A COLD OR THE FLU?

	Cold	Flu
Symptoms		
Fever	Rare	Characteristic, high (102°F–104°F); lasts 3–4 days
Headache	Rare	Prominent
General aches, pains	Slight	Usual; often severe
Fatigue, weakness	Quite mild	Can last up to 2–3 weeks
Prostration (extreme exhaustion)	Never	Early and prominent
Stuffy nose	Common	Sometimes
Sneezing	Usual	Sometimes
Sore throat	Common	Sometimes
Chest discomfort, cough	Mild to moderate; hacking cough	Common; can become severe
Complications	Sinus congestion or earache	Bronchitis, pneumonia; can be life-threatening
Prevention	None	Annual vaccination; amantadine (an antiviral drug)
Treatment	Only temporary relief of symptoms	Amantadine within 24–48 hours after onset of symptoms

SOURCE: National Institutes of Health.

monia have accounted for 10,000 to 45,000 deaths in the last 20 years.

Flu viruses, transmitted by coughs, sneezes, laughs, and even normal conversation, are extraordinarily contagious, particularly in the first 3 days of the disease. The usual incubation period is 2 days, but symptoms can hit hard and fast. Two varieties of viruses—influenza A and influenza B—cause most flus. In recent years, the deadliest flu epidemics have been caused by various forms of influenza A viruses.

A vaccine against the flu is available, but it is not foolproof. "Because the flu virus is constantly changing, you need a new shot every year," explains Edwin Kilbourne, M.D., of New York Medical College, who has decided the components of each year's flu shots for 22 years. "And because it takes the body time to manufacture antibodies to the new viruses, you should get a vaccination at least 10 to 14 days before an outbreak hits your area."[10]

Other Infectious Diseases

- *Mononucleosis*. You can get **mononucleosis** through kissing or any other form of close contact. "Mono" is a viral disease that's most common among people 15 to 24 years old; its symptoms include a sore throat, headache, fever, nausea, and prolonged weakness. The spleen is swollen, and the lymph nodes are enlarged. You may also develop jaundice or a skin rash similar to German measles.

- *Chronic fatigue syndrome (CFS)*. More than 3 million Americans have the array of symptoms known as **chronic fatigue syndrome (CFS)**.[11] According to the CDC, symptoms include chills or low-grade fever, sore throat, tender lymph nodes, muscle pain and weakness, extreme fatigue that doesn't improve with rest, headaches, joint pain (without swelling), neurological problems (confusion, memory loss, visual disturbances), and sleep disorders. Symptoms may begin suddenly and persist for six months to several years. Depression and anxiety attacks generally develop after 10 months of illness.

  Once dismissed as the yuppie flu, CFS has long baffled scientists. Some researchers contend that a single agent, perhaps a retrovirus, triggers the collapse of the immune system. Others think that repeated, undetected infections by bacteria, viruses, fungi, and parasites may lead to a gradual decline. Another theory blames symptoms on chronic low blood pressure.

- *Hepatitis*. All forms of **hepatitis** target the liver, the body's largest internal organ. Symptoms include headaches, fever, fatigue, stiff or aching joints, nausea, vomiting, and diarrhea. The liver becomes enlarged and tender to the touch; sometimes the yellowish tinge of jaundice develops. Treatment consists of rest, a high-protein diet, and the avoidance of alcohol and drugs that may stress the liver until the disease runs its course. Alpha interferon, a protein that boosts immunity and prevents viruses from replicating, may be used for some forms.

  Hepatitis A, a less serious form, is generally transmitted by poor sanitation, primarily fecal contamination of food or water, and is less common in industrialized nations than in developing countries. Hepatitis B, a potentially fatal disease transmitted through the blood and other bodily fluids, infects an estimated 350,000 people around the world each year. Once spread mainly by contaminated tattoo needles, needles shared by drug addicts, or transfusions of contaminated blood, hepatitis B is now transmitted mostly through sexual contact. It can cause chronic liver infection, cirrhosis, and liver cancer. Hepatitis C, spread in the same way as hepatitis B, is the most common serious complication of blood transfusions. However, more effective screening tests have greatly reduced the risk of getting blood contaminated by hepatitis C virus.

- *Pneumonia*. An inflammation of the lungs, **pneumonia** fills the fine, spongy networks of the lungs' tiny air chambers with fluid. It can be caused by bacteria, viruses (including flu), or foreign material in the lungs (such as smoke). The symptoms of classic bacterial pneumonia are fever, shortness of breath, and general weakness. Along with influenza, pneumonia is the fifth-leading killer of Americans and the most common infectious cause of death.

- *Tuberculosis*. A bacterial infection of the lungs that was once the nation's leading killer, **tuberculosis (TB)** claims the lives of more people than any acute infectious disease other than pneumonia. In the United States, TB cases, after declining for decades, increased from the mid-1980s to the early 1990s. If you think you may have been exposed to TB or if you develop suspicious symptoms (loss of appetite and weight, low-grade fever, fatigue, chills, night sweats, coughing), see your doctor for a TB test.

- *Toxic shock syndrome*. **Toxic shock syndrome (TSS)** is a potentially deadly disease associated with

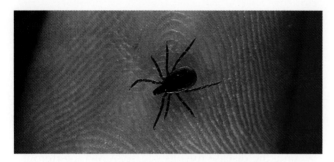

Ticks are responsible for the spread of Lyme disease. If you spot a tick, remove it as soon as possible with tweezers or small forceps. Put it in a plastic bag or sealed bottle and save it. If you develop a rash or other symptoms, take it with you to the doctor.

the use of tampons, particularly high-absorbency types. It is caused by *Staphylococcus aureus* and *Streptococcus pyogenes* bacteria that release toxins (poisonous waste products) into the bloodstream. Symptoms include a high fever; a rash that leads to peeling of the skin on the fingers, toes, palms, and soles; dizziness; dangerously low blood pressure; and abnormalities in several organ systems (the digestive tract and the kidneys) and in the muscles and blood.

- *Lyme disease.* **Lyme disease**, a bacterial infection, is spread by ticks carrying a kind of bacterium, the spirochete *Borrelia burgdorferi*. An infected person may have various symptoms, including joint inflammation, heart arrhythmias, blinding headaches, and memory lapses. The disease can also cause miscarriages and birth defects. Lyme disease is by far the most commonly reported vector-borne infectious disease in the United States.[12]

The Threat of Emerging and Resistant Infectious Diseases

As defined by the National Institute of Allergy and Infectious Diseases (NIAID), emerging infections are those that have been recently recognized, are increasing in humans, or threaten to spread to new areas in the near future. The most widespread is HIV, which is believed to have emerged from Central Africa fewer than 20 years ago. Other emerging viruses, such as Hantavirus, Ebola, dengue, Lassa, and Marburg, have been responsible for deadly outbreaks around the globe. The most well-known may be Ebola, a particularly virulent virus that is transmitted by direct contact with blood or bodily fluids. In several outbreaks in Africa, this filovirus has resisted all medication and killed up to 90% of its victims.[13]

Another threat comes from mutated, or changed, forms of familiar microbes (such as those that cause tuberculosis) that have become resistant to standard medications. Why, despite enormous scientific progress, do emerging and resistant microbes remain such a formidable foe? "Viruses and bacteria have the capacity to reinvent themselves rapidly," says John La Montagne, Ph.D, of NIAID. "Because they have few genes compared to people, one mutation can change an organism's ability to infect, spread, or cause disease."[14] There are other reasons why deadly infections are becoming a greater threat. As civilization spreads into previously undeveloped areas, such as the rainforests of Central Africa, and goods and animals are imported from distant lands, more human beings are encountering microbes that were once confined to very remote regions.

Reproductive and Urinary Tract Infections

Reproductive and urinary tract infections are very common. Many are not spread exclusively by sexual contact, and so they are not classified as sexually transmitted diseases (STDs), discussed later in this chapter.

The most common vaginal infections are **trichomoniasis**, and **candidiasis**. Protozoa (*Trichomonas vaginalis*) that live in the vagina can multiply rapidly, causing itching, burning, and discharge—all symptoms of trichomoniasis. Male carriers usually have no symptoms, although some may develop urethritis or an inflammation of the prostate and seminal vesicles.

Populations of a yeast called *Candida albicans*—normal inhabitants of the mouth, digestive tract, and vagina—are usually held in check. Under certain conditions, however (such as poor nutrition, stress, or antibiotic use), the microbes multiply, causing burning, itching, and a whitish discharge. Common sites for candidiasis, which is also called moniliasis, are the vagina, vulva, penis, and mouth. Vaginal medications, such as GyneLotrimin and Monistat, available as over-the-counter (OTC) drugs for women with recurrent infections, provide effective treatment. Male sexual partners may be advised to wear condoms during outbreaks of candidiasis. Women should keep the genital area dry and wear cotton underwear.

A urinary tract infection (UTI) can be present in any of the three parts of the urinary tract: the urethra, bladder, or kidney. Conditions that can set the stage for UTIs include irritation and swelling of the urethra or bladder as a result of pregnancy, bike riding, irritants (such as

Strategies for Prevention

How to Prevent UTIs

✔ Be conscientious about general cleanliness. Since a major cause of UTIs is the bacteria normally found in stools, be sure to wipe from front to back after bowel movements.

✔ Drink five to six glasses of water a day.

✔ Don't wait when you feel the urge to urinate.

✔ Don't use chemical irritants, such as perfumed hygiene sprays or bubble bath.

✔ If you use a diaphragm, have the fit checked regularly, especially after giving birth.

✔ If UTIs seem to follow sex, ask about prophylactic medication. Urinate immediately after intercourse.

✔ If you have a relapse after treatment or have recurrent infections, ask your partner to get a checkup too.

bubble bath, douches, or a diaphragm), urinary stones, enlargement in men of the prostate gland, vaginitis, and stress. Early diagnosis is critical, because infection can spread to the kidneys and, if unchecked, result in kidney failure. Symptoms include frequent burning, painful urination, chills, fever, fatigue, and blood in the urine.

Sexually Transmitted Diseases (STDs)

Venereal diseases (from the Latin *venus*, meaning "love" or "lust") are more accurately called **sexually transmitted diseases (STDs)**. Around the world, more than 250 million cases of STDs are diagnosed each year (more than a million are of HIV).[15] Almost 700,000 people are infected every day with one of the over twenty STDs tracked by world health officials. STDs are much more widespread (or "prevalent") in developing nations because of lack of adequate health standards, prevention practices, and access to treatment.

More Americans are infected with STDs now than at any other time in history. They are among the top ten most frequently reported diseases in the United States, and their annual economic cost is $17 billion.[16]

The major cause of preventable sterility in America, STDs have tripled the rate of ectopic (tubal) pregnancies, which can be fatal if not detected early. STD complications, including miscarriage, premature delivery, and uterine infections after delivery, affect more than 100,000 women annually. Moreover, infection with an STD greatly increases the risk of HIV transmission (discussed later in this chapter). The incidence of STDs is highest in young adults and homosexual men. Others affected by STDs include unborn and newborn children who can "catch" potentially life-threatening infections in the womb or during birth.

Although each STD is a distinct disease, all STD pathogens like dark, warm, moist body surfaces, particularly the mucous membranes that line the reproductive organs; they hate light, cold, and dryness. It is possible to catch or have more than one STD at a time. Curing one doesn't necessarily cure another, and treatments don't prevent another bout with the same STD (see Table 9-2).

Many STDs, including early HIV infection and gonorrhea in women, may not cause any symptoms. As a result, infected individuals can continue their usual sexual activity without realizing that they're jeopardizing others' well-being.

STDs, Adolescents, and Young Adults

STDs strike both sexes, all classes, and all ages. However, the young are at greatest risk. According to the CDC, 86% of all STDs in the United States occur among 15- to 29-year-olds; as many as half of all young people may develop an STD by age 30.[17]

The college years are a prime time for contracting sexually transmitted diseases. According to the American College Health Association, chlamydia and human papilloma virus (HPV) have reached epidemic levels at many schools—although many of those infected aren't even aware of it. Among college women who tested positive for chlamydia in a screening study, 79% had no symptoms.[18]

An estimated 1 to 2 per 100 college students are HIV-positive. While students are at lower risk of HIV infection than other groups, such as gay men or injecting drug users, they engage in many behaviors, such as alcohol and drug use and unsafe sexual practices, that place them at increased risk. Even though the current rates of HIV infection are relatively low, health officials feel that the potential exists for rapid spread of HIV on college campuses. Although studies show that many college students are well-informed about

TABLE 9-2 COMMON SEXUALLY TRANSMITTED DISEASES (STDs): MODE OF TRANSMISSION, SYMPTOMS, AND TREATMENT

STD	Transmission	Symptoms	Treatment
Chlamydial infection	The *Chlamydia trachomatis* bacterium is transmitted primarily through sexual contact. It may also be spread by fingers from one body site to another.	In women, PID (pelvic inflammatory disease) caused by *Chlamydia* may include disrupted menstrual periods, pelvic pain, elevated temperature, nausea, vomiting, headache, infertility, and ectopic pregnancy. In men, chlamydial infection of the urethra may cause a discharge and burning during urination. *Chlamydia*-caused epididymitis may produce a sense of heaviness in the affected testicle(s), inflammation of the scrotal skin, and painful swelling at the bottom of the testicle.	Doxycycline, azithromycin, or ofloxacin
Gonorrhea ("clap")	The *Neisseria gonorrhoeae* bacterium ("gonococcus") is spread through genital, oral–genital, or genital–anal contact.	The most common symptoms in men are a cloudy discharge from the penis and burning sensations during urination. If the disease is untreated, complications may include inflammation of scrotal skin and swelling at base of the testicle. In women, some green or yellowish discharge is produced but commonly remains undetected. Later, PID (pelvic inflammatory disease) may develop.	Dual therapy of a single dose of ceftriaxone, cefixime, ciprofloxacin, or ofloxacin plus doxycycline for 7 days
Non-gonococcal urethritis (NGU)	Primary causes are believed to be the bacteria *Chlamydia trachomatis* and *Ureaplasma urealyticum*, most commonly transmitted through coitus. Some NGU may result from allergic reactions or from *Trichomonas* infection.	Inflammation of the urethral tube. A man has a discharge from the penis and irritation during urination. A woman may have a mild discharge of pus from the vagina but often shows no symptoms.	Doxycycline or erythromycin
Syphilis	The *Treponema pallidum* bacterium ("spirochete") is transmitted from open lesions during genital, oral–genital, or genital–anal contact.	*Primary stage:* A painless chancre appears at the site where the spirochetes entered the body. *Secondary stage:* The chancre disappears and a generalized skin rash develops. *Latent stage:* There may be no visible symptoms. *Tertiary stage:* Heart failure, blindness, mental disturbance, and many other symptoms occur. Death may result.	Benzathine penicillin G, doxycycline, tetracycline, or erythromycin
Chancroid	The *Haemophilus ducreyi* bacterium is usually transmitted by sexual interaction.	Small bumps (papules) in genital regions eventually rupture and form painful, soft, craterlike ulcers that emit a foul-smelling discharge.	Single doses of either ceftriaxone or azithromycin or 7 days of erythromycin
Herpes	The genital herpes virus (HSV-2) seems to be transmitted primarily by vaginal, anal, or oral–genital intercourse. The oral herpes virus (HSV-1) is transmitted primarily by kissing.	Small, painful red bumps (papules) appear in the genital region (genital herpes) or mouth (oral herpes). The papules become painful blisters that eventually rupture to form wet, open sores.	No known cure; a variety of treatments may reduce symptoms; oral or intravenous acyclovir (Zovirax) promotes healing and suppresses recurrent outbreaks.

TABLE 9-2 CONTINUED...

STD	Transmission	Symptoms	Treatment
Genital warts (condylomata acuminata)	The virus is spread primarily through vaginal, anal, or oral-genital sexual interaction.	Hard and yellow-gray on dry skin areas; soft, pinkish-red, and cauliflowerlike on moist areas.	Freezing, application of topical agents like trichloroacetic acid or podofilox, cauterization, surgical removal, or vaporization by carbon dioxide laser
Viral hepatitis	The hepatitis B virus may be transmitted by blood, semen, vaginal secretions, and saliva. Manual, oral, or penile stimulation of the anus are strongly associated with the spread of this virus. Hepatitis A seems to be primarily spread via the fecal–oral route. Oral–anal sexual contact is a common mode for sexual transmission of hepatitis A.	Vary from nonexistent to mild, flulike symptoms to an incapacitating illness characterized by high fever, vomiting, and severe abdominal pain.	No specific therapy; treatment generally consists of bed rest and adequate fluid intake.
Bacterial vaginosis	The most common causative agent, the *Gardnerella vaginalis* bacterium, is sometimes transmitted through coitus.	In women, a fishy- or musty-smelling, thin discharge, like flour paste in consistency and usually gray. Most men are asymptomatic.	Metronidazole (Flagyl) by mouth or intravaginal applications of topical metronidazole gel or clindamycin cream
Candidiasis (yeast infection)	The *Candida albicans* fungus may accelerate growth when the chemical balance of the vagina is disturbed; it may also be transmitted through sexual interaction.	White, "cheesy" discharge; irritation of vaginal and vulval tissues.	Vaginal suppositories or topical cream, such as clotrimazole and miconazole, or oral fluconazole
Trichomoniasis	The protozoan parasite *Trichomonas vaginalis* is usually passed through genital sexual contact.	White or yellow vaginal discharge with an unpleasant odor; vulva is sore and irritated.	Metronidazole (Flagyl) for both women and men
Pubic lice ("crabs")	*Phthirus pubis*, the pubic louse, is spread easily through body contact or through shared clothing or bedding.	Persistent itching. Lice are visible and may often be located in pubic hair or other body hair.	Preparations such as A-200 pyrinate or Kwell (gamma benzene hexachloride)
Scabies	*Sarcoptes scabiei* is highly contagious and may be transmitted by close physical contact, sexual and nonsexual.	Small bumps and a red rash that itch intensely, especially at night.	5% permethrin lotion or cream
Acquired immuno-deficiency syndrome (AIDS)	Blood and semen are the major vehicles for transmitting HIV, which attacks the immune system. It appears to be passed primarily through sexual contact or needle sharing among injecting drug users.	Vary with the type of cancer or opportunistic infections that afflict an infected person. Common symptoms include fevers, night sweats, weight loss, chronic fatigue, swollen lymph nodes, diarrhea and/or bloody stools, atypical bruising or bleeding, skin rashes, headache, chronic cough, and a whitish coating on the tongue or throat.	Commence treatment early after seroconversion with a combination of three antiviral drugs ("triple drug therapy") plus other specific treatment(s), if necessary, of opportunistic infections and tumors.

Source: Crooks, Robert, and Baur, Karla. *Our Sexuality*, 7th ed. Pacific Grove, CA: Brooks Cole, 1999.

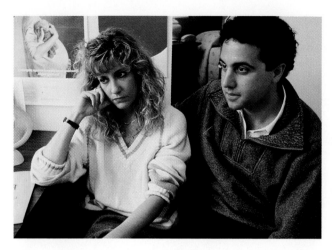

Talking openly about STDs and being tested with your partner protect your health and can foster a sense of trust and commitment.

Strategies for Prevention

Telling a Partner That You Have an STD

✔ *Talk before sex.* If you have a chronic STD, such as herpes, discuss it before you have sex. Emphasize that herpes is preventable and that you are committed to using proper precautions.

✔ *Be honest.* If you know or suspect you might have an STD, tell anyone with whom you have had sex exactly what it is.

✔ *Don't accuse.* If you suspect that your partner gave you an STD, you may well be angry. However, there is little to be gained by blaming. Inform your partner of your condition and suggest that he or she seek medical attention.

✔ *Try to be calm and clear.* If you respond with guilt, fear, or disgust, your partner is more likely to react in the same emotional way.

✔ *Be sensitive.* Rather than becoming defensive if your partner is angry or resentful, show that you're willing to listen and that you genuinely care.

✔ *Do not engage in sexual activities.* Wait until you both get a thorough medical evaluation, appropriate treatment, and reassurance that you are no longer contagious.

STDs, this knowledge often does not translate into behavioral change. Even students targeted as "opinion leaders"— individuals who serve as sources of information for a wide range of individuals and shape the opinions of many—are no better informed and no more likely to practice safer sex.[19]

Prevention and Protection

Abstinence is the only guarantee of sexual safety—and one that more and more young people are choosing. As discussed in Chapter 7, the choice of an abstinent (or celibate) lifestyle offers many advantages, both in the present and the future. By choosing not to be sexually active with a partner, individuals can safeguard their physical health, their fertility, and their future.

For men and women who are sexually active, a mutually faithful sexual relationship with just one healthy partner is the safest option. For those not in such relationships, safer sex practices are essential for reducing risks. (See Pulsepoints: "Ten Ways to Prevent Sexually Transmitted Diseases.") Some experts believe that condom use may be a more effective tactic than any drug or vaccine in preventing STDs.[20]

Chlamydia

The most widespread sexually transmitted bacterium in the United States is *Chlamydia trachomatis*, which causes 3 to 5 million **chlamydial infections** each year.[21] These infections are more common in younger than in older women, in African-American than in white women, and in unmarried than in married pregnant women. They also occur more often in both men and women with gonorrhea.

Those at greatest risk of chlamydial infection are individuals 25 years old or younger who engage in sex with more than one new partner within a 2-month period and women who use birth control pills or other nonbarrier contraceptive methods. Many physicians recommend testing for any woman who has more than one sexual partner in a year; for anyone who seeks medical treatment for an STD; for those seeking health care at adolescent or family planning clinics where chlamydia is seen often; and for young individuals, particularly in urban settings, with multiple sexual partners.

In men, *Chlamydia trachomatis* causes an estimated half of all cases of epididymitis (infection of the tube that leads out of the testicle) and nongonococcal urethritis (NGU) (inflammation of the urethra not caused by gonorrhea). About 30% of men with NGU develop no or few symptoms. Others experience symptoms similar to those of gonorrhea, including discharge from the penis and mild burning during urination.

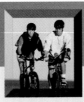

Pulsepoints

Ten Ways to Prevent Sexually Transmitted Diseases (STDs)

1. Abstain from sexual intercourse. You don't have to abstain from all sexual activity. Fantasizing, masturbating, touching, hugging, and petting are all safe and pleasurable.

2. Don't rush into a sexual relationship. Get to know a potential partner well over a period of several months or more. Share your sexual histories and build an honest, mutually caring, and trusting relationship.

3. Get checked out. The only accurate way to assess the risks of STDs is a thorough medical examination, including laboratory testing.

4. Maintain a mutually faithful sexual relationship with just one unin- fected partner. An exclusive sexual relationship with a person who has never been exposed to any STD is safe, regardless of what type of sexual activity you engage in.

5. Always use condoms and spermicides. Although their use reduces your risk, keep in mind that doing so does not guarantee protection.

6. Don't have sex with multiple partners. The risk of STDs increases along with the number of sexual partners. Also avoid sexual contact with individuals who've had multiple or anonymous sexual partners.

7. Inspect your partner's genitals before sex. Although some STDs produce no visible signs, it is possible to see herpes blisters, chancres, rashes, genital warts, and the like.

8. Wash your own—and your partner's—genitals before and after sex. Although it's not clear how effective soap and water are, washing—especially of the penis—is generally believed to have some benefits.

9. Don't have sexual contact with individuals who use injection drugs. Regardless of the type of drug—anabolic steroids, cocaine, heroin, and so on—users are at higher risk for several STDs, including hepatitis and HIV infection.

10. Keep a clear head. Don't make decisions about sexual activity while under the influence of alcohol or drugs that could affect your judgment.

According to CDC guidelines, the treatment of choice for uncomplicated chlamydia infections is a 7-day regimen of doxycycline or a single, 1-gram dose of azithromycin. Because chlamydia often occurs along with gonorrhea, some health practitioners prescribe 7 days of ofloxacin, a drug effective against both chlamydial and gonorrheal infections. The use of condoms with spermicide can reduce, but not eliminate, the risk of chlamydial infection. Sexual partners should be examined and treated if necessary.

Pelvic Inflammatory Disease (PID)

Infection of a woman's fallopian tubes or uterus, called **pelvic inflammatory disease (PID)**, is not actually an STD, but rather a complication of STDs. About one in every seven women of reproductive age has PID; by the year 2000, half of all adult women may have had it. Each year, about 1 million new cases are reported.

Ten to twenty percent of initial episodes of PID lead to scarring and obstruction of the fallopian tubes severe enough to cause infertility. Other long-term complications are ectopic pregnancy and chronic pelvic pain. The risk of these complications rises with subsequent PID episodes, bacterial vaginosis, and use of IUDs.

Smoking also may increase the likelihood of PID. Two bacteria—gonococcus (the culprit in gonorrhea) and chlamydia—are responsible for one-third to one-half of all cases of PID. Other organisms are responsible for the remaining cases.

Most cases of PID occur among women under age 25 who are sexually active. Gonococcus-caused cases tend to affect poor women; those caused by chlamydia range across all income levels. One-third to one-half of all cases are transmitted sexually, and others have been traced to some IUDs that are no longer on the market. Several studies have shown that women with PID are more likely to have used douches than those without the disease.[22]

PID is a silent disease that, in half of all cases, often produces no noticeable symptoms as it progresses and causes scarring of the fallopian tubes. Experts are encouraging women with mild symptoms, such as abdominal pain or tenderness, to seek medical evaluation and physicians to test these patients for infections.[23] Women may learn that they have PID only after discovering that they cannot conceive or after they develop an ectopic pregnancy. PID causes an estimated 15% to 30% of all cases of infertility every year and about half of all cases of ectopic pregnancy.

Gonorrhea

Gonorrhea (sometimes called the "clap" in street language) is one of the most common STDs in the United States and is increasing in occurrence. By some estimates, there may be approximately 1 million new cases every year. The incidence is highest among teenagers and young adults. Sexual contact, including oral-genital sex, is the primary means of transmission.

Most men who have gonorrhea know it. Thick, yellow-white pus oozes from the penis, and urination causes a burning sensation. These symptoms usually develop 2 to 9 days after the sexual contact that infected them. Men have a good reason to seek help: It hurts too much not to. Women also may experience discharge and burning on urination. However, as many as eight of ten infected women have no symptoms.[24]

If left untreated, gonorrhea spreads through the urinary-genital tract. In women, the inflammation travels from the vagina and cervix, through the uterus, to the fallopian tubes and ovaries. The pain and fever are similar to those caused by stomach upset, so a woman may dismiss the symptoms. Eventually these symptoms diminish, even though the disease spreads to the entire pelvis. Pus may ooze from the fallopian tubes or ovaries into the peritoneum (the lining of the abdominal cavity), sometimes causing serious inflammation. However, this, too, can subside in a few weeks. Gonorrhea, the leading cause of sterility in women, can cause PID. In pregnant women, gonorrhea becomes a threat to the newborn. It can infect the infant's external genitals and cause a serious form of conjunctivitis, an inflammation of the eye that may lead to blindness. As a preventive

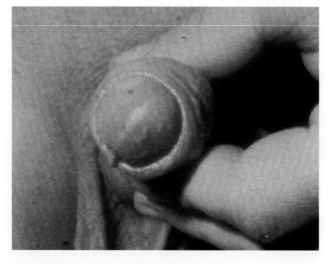

A cloudy discharge is symptomatic of gonorrhea.

step, newborns may have penicillin dropped into their eyes at birth.

In men, untreated gonorrhea can spread to the prostate gland, testicles, bladder, and kidneys. Among the serious complications are urinary obstruction and sterility caused by blockage of the vas deferens (the excretory duct of the testis). In both sexes, gonorrhea can develop into a serious, even fatal, bloodborne infection that can cause arthritis in the joints, attack the heart muscle and lining, cause meningitis, and attack the skin and other organs.

Nongonococcal Urethritis (NGU)

Nongonococcal urethritis (NGU) refers to any inflammation of the urethra that is not caused by gonorrhea. NGU is the most common STD in men, accounting for 4–6 million visits to a physician every year.[25]

In the United States, NGU is more common in men than gonoccocal urethritis. Male symptoms are similar to those of gonorrhea, including discharge from the penis (usually less than with gonorrhea) and mild burning during urination. Women frequently develop no symptoms or very mild itching, burning during urination, or discharge. Symptoms usually disappear after 2 or 3 weeks, but the infection may persist and cause cervicitis or PID in women and, in men, may spread to the prostate, epididymis, or both.

Syphilis

A corkscrew-shaped bacterium called *Treponema pallidum* causes **syphilis**. This frail germ dies in seconds if dried or chilled, but grows quickly in the warm, moist tissues of the body, particularly in the mucous membranes of the genital tract. Entering the body through any tiny break in the skin, the germ burrows its way into the bloodstream. Sexual contact, including oral sex or intercourse, is a primary means of transmission. Genital ulcers caused by syphilis may increase the risk of HIV infection, while individuals with HIV may be more likely to develop syphilis.

There are clearly identifiable stages of syphilis:

- *Primary syphilis.* The first sign of syphilis is a lesion, or chancre (pronounced "shanker"), an open lump or crater the size of a dime or smaller, teeming with bacteria. The incubation period before its appearance ranges from 10 to 90 days; 3 to 4 weeks are average. The chancre appears exactly where the bacteria entered the body: in the mouth, throat, vagina, rectum, or penis. Any contact with the chancre is likely to result in infection.

- *Secondary syphilis.* Anywhere from 1 to 12 months after the chancre's appearance, secondary-stage symptoms may appear. Some people have no symptoms. Others develop a skin rash or a small flat rash in moist regions on the skin; whitish patches on the mucous membranes of the mouth or throat; temporary baldness; low-grade fever; headache; swollen glands; or large, moist sores around the mouth and genitals. These are loaded with bacteria; contact with them, through kissing or intercourse, may transmit the infection. Symptoms may last for several days or several months. Even without treatment, they eventually disappear as the syphilis microbes go into hiding.

- *Latent syphilis.* Although there are no signs or symptoms, no sores or rashes at this stage, the bacteria are invading various organs inside the body, including the heart and brain. For 2 to 4 years, there may be recurring infectious and highly contagious lesions of the skin or mucous membranes. However, syphilis loses its infectiousness as it progresses: After the first 2 years, a person rarely transmits syphilis through intercourse.

- *Tertiary syphilis.* Ten to twenty years after the beginning of the latent stage, the most serious symptoms of syphilis emerge, generally in the organs in which the bacteria settled during latency. Syphilis that has progressed to this stage has become increasingly rare. Victims of tertiary syphilis may die of a ruptured aorta or of other heart damage, or may have progressive brain or spinal cord damage, eventually leading to blindness, insanity, or paralysis. About a third of those who are not treated during the first three stages of syphilis enter the tertiary stage later in life.

Health experts are urging screening for syphilis for everyone who seeks treatment for an STD, especially adolescents; for everyone using illegal drugs; and for the partners of these two groups. They also recommend that anyone diagnosed with syphilis be screened for other STDs and be counseled about voluntary testing for HIV. Early diagnosis of syphilis can lead to a complete cure.

Herpes

Herpes (from the Greek word that means "to creep") collectively describes some of the most common viral infections in humans. Characteristically, **herpes simplex** causes blisters on the skin or mucous membranes. It exists in several varieties. Herpes simplex virus 1 (HSV-1) generally causes cold sores and fever blisters around the mouth. Herpes simplex virus 2 (HSV-2) may cause blisters on the penis, inside the vagina, on the cervix, in the pubic area, on the buttocks, or on the thighs. With the increase of oral-genital sex, some doctors report finding HSV-2 lesions in the mouth and throat.

The incidence of herpes infection has soared. Since the late 1970s, the proportion of Americans with HSV-2 has increased by almost one-third. One in five women and one in seven men over age 12—some 45 million people—carry this virus. Two out of three people with the virus do not know they are infected and potentially contagious. Recent research with a new, more sensitive test reveals that individuals without any obvious symptoms shed the virus "subclinically" whether or not they have lesions.

HSV transmission occurs through close contact with mucous membranes or abraded skin. Condoms help prevent infection but aren't foolproof. When herpes sores are present, the infected person is highly contagious and should avoid bringing the lesions into contact with someone else's body through touching, sexual interaction, or kissing. However, HSV also can be transmitted when there are no signs or symptoms of the disease.

The virus that causes herpes never entirely goes away; it retreats to nerves near the lower spinal cord, where it remains for the life of the infected person. Herpes sores can return without warning weeks, months, or even years after their first occurrence, often during menstruation, times of stress, or with sudden changes in body temperature. Of those who experience HSV recurrence, 10% to 35% do so frequently—that is, about six or more

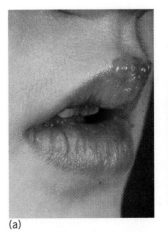 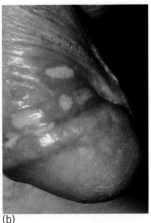

(a)   (b)

Herpes. (a) Herpes simplex virus 1, or HSV-1, as a mouth sore. (b) Herpes simplex virus 2, or HSV-2, usually causes genital sores.

times a year. In most people, attacks diminish in frequency and severity over time. Herpes, like other STDs, can trigger feelings of shame, guilt, and depression.

Acyclovir (Zovirax), a prescription drug, has proven effective in treating and controlling herpes. Available as an ointment, in capsules, and in injection form, it relieves the symptoms but doesn't kill the virus. Various other treatments—compresses made with cold water, skim milk, or warm salt water, ice packs, or a mild anesthetic cream—can relieve discomfort. Herpes sufferers should avoid heat, hot baths, or nylon underwear.

Human Papilloma Virus Infection (Genital Warts)

Infection with **human papilloma virus (HPV)**, a pathogen that can cause genital warts, is the most common viral STD. By some estimates, 20 million or more women in the United States are infected with HPV, as are three out of four of their male sexual partners.

HPV is transmitted primarily through vaginal, anal, or oral-genital sex. More than half of HPV-infected individuals do not develop any symptoms. Genital warts may appear from 3 weeks to 18 months after contact, with an average period of about 3 months after contact with an infected individual. These are treated by freezing, cauterization, chemicals, or surgical removal. Recurrences are common, for the virus remains in the body.

HPV infection may invade the urethra and cause urinary obstruction and bleeding. It greatly increases a woman's risk of developing a precancerous condition called cervical intraepithelial neoplasia, which can lead to cervical cancer. There also is a strong association between HPV infections and cancer of the vagina, vulva, urethra, penis, and anus.[26] Adolescent girls infected with HPV appear to be particularly vulnerable to developing cervical cancer. It is not known if HPV itself causes cancer or acts in conjunction with cofactors (such as other infections, smoking, or suppressed immunity). HPV transmission may be the reason women are five to eleven times as likely to get cervical cancer if their steady sexual partner has had twenty or more previous partners.

HPV-infected men, who may not develop any symptoms, can spread the infection to their partners. People with visible genital warts also may have asymptomatic or subclinical HPV infections that are extremely difficult to treat. No form of therapy has been shown to eradicate HPV completely, nor has any single treatment been uniformly effective in removing warts or preventing their recurrence.

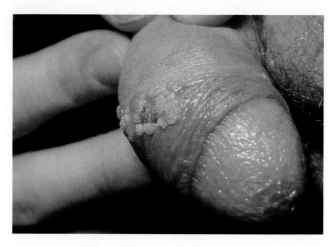

Human papilloma virus, which causes genital warts, is the most common viral STD.

Chancroid

A **chancroid** is a soft, painful sore or localized infection caused by the bacterium *Haemophilus ducrevi* and is usually acquired through sexual contact. Half of the cases heal by themselves. In other cases, the infection may spread to the lymph glands near the chancroid, where large amounts of pus can accumulate and destroy much of the local tissue. The incidence of this STD, widely prevalent in Africa and tropical and semitropical

Strategies for Change

What to Do If You Have an STD

✔ If you suspect that you have an STD, don't feel too embarrassed to get help through a physician's office or a clinic. Treatment relieves discomfort, prevents complications, and halts the spread of the disease.

✔ Following diagnosis, take oral medication (which may be given instead of or in addition to shots) exactly as prescribed.

✔ Try to figure out from whom you got the STD. Be sure to inform that person, who may not be aware of the problem.

✔ If you have an STD, never deceive a prospective partner about it. Tell the truth—simply and clearly. Be sure your partner understands exactly what you have and what the risks are.

regions, is rapidly increasing in the United States, with outbreaks in several states, including Louisiana, Texas, and New York. Chancroids, which may increase susceptibility to HIV infection, are believed to be a major factor in the heterosexual spread of HIV. This infection is treated with antibiotics and can be prevented by keeping the genitals clean and washing them with soap and water in case of possible exposure.

Pubic Lice and Scabies

These infections are sometimes, but not always, transmitted sexually. Pubic lice (or "crabs") are usually found in the pubic hairs, although they may migrate to any hairy areas of the body. Lice lay eggs called nits that attach to the base of the hair shaft. Irritation from the lice may produce intense itching. Scratching to relieve the itching can produce sores. Scabies is caused by a mite that burrows under the skin and lays eggs that hatch and undergo many changes in the course of their life cycle, producing great discomfort, including intense itching.

Lice and scabies are treated with applications of Kwell or A-200 pyrinate shampoo (which kills the adult lice but not always the nits) to all the areas of the body where there are concentrations of body hair (genitals, armpits, scalp). You must repeat treatment in 7 days to kill any newly developed adults. Wash or dry-clean clothing and bedding.

HIV/AIDS

Thirty years ago, no one knew what the **human immunodeficiency virus (HIV)** was. No one had ever heard of **acquired immunodeficiency syndrome**

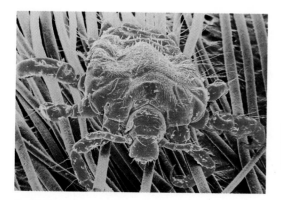

A pubic louse, or "crab."

Actual size

(AIDS). Today HIV/AIDS has been recognized as the most serious epidemic of our time. In the United States, the number of AIDS cases has been declining since 1995, with a 5% drop from 1995 to 1996 and a 12% decrease from 1996 to 1997. However, HIV infection and AIDS remain a grave health threat. Between 35,000 and 40,000 people are newly infected with HIV every year. According to the Centers for Disease Control and Prevention (CDC), an estimated 400,000 to 600,000 Americans are HIV-positive.[27]

Globally, HIV, once seen as an epidemic affecting primarily gay men and injecting drug users, has taken on a very different form. Today, heterosexuals in developing countries have the highest rates of infection and mortality.

The Spread of HIV

HIV came to the United States in the late 1970s. Several factors—including frequent sexual activity with multiple anonymous partners and high-risk sexual practices, such as anal intercourse—may have caused its quick spread through gay communities in the 1980s. As more became known about HIV transmission, many homosexual men adopted safer ways of sexual expression, reduced their number of sexual partners, or entered into monogamous relationships. As a result, the spread of HIV among gay men—especially older men in metropolitan areas—slowed. However, the incidence of AIDS in young gay men and homosexual men in rural or suburban areas increased steadily in the early 1990s.[28]

In the 1980s, HIV also spread among injecting drug users, who, by sharing contaminated needles, injected the virus directly into their bloodstream. Injection drug use has been the number-one source of HIV infection in heterosexual men and women in this country. Sex with an infected injecting drug user is also a major cause of HIV infection. Almost one-third of reported cases of AIDS have been directly or indirectly related to injection drug use. CDC-sponsored studies indicate that needle exchange programs that provide drug users with sterile needles could significantly reduce HIV transmission.[29]

HIV also spread through blood transfusions, blood products, and organ transplants from HIV-positive individuals during the period between 1978 and 1985, before testing to identify contaminated blood became routine. Today's blood and organ supply is much safer, primarily because of more sophisticated testing of donated blood, blood products used for hemophiliacs, and donated organs, tissues, and sperm.

Increasingly, HIV is being transmitted via heterosexual contact. More than 10% of known AIDS cases have occurred among heterosexuals. Although both men and women are at risk if they engage in unprotected sex, women are far more likely to contract HIV from an infected male partner than men are from an infected female partner.

HIV is transmitted to infants by HIV-positive mothers in three possible ways: before birth via circulation; during labor and birth; or after birth through infected breast milk. Every year about 7000 HIV-infected women give birth. Treatment of both mothers and newborns with zidovudine (AZT) can reduce the risk of HIV transmission from mother to child from one in four to less than one in ten—a 67.5% reduction.[30]

Accidental contact with HIV-contaminated blood or bodily fluids has led to some cases of HIV infection and AIDS. According to the CDC, HIV is transmitted among health-care workers in about 1 per 250 instances of their accidental injection with needles containing HIV-positive blood.

Reducing the Risk of HIV Transmission

HIV/AIDS can be so frightening that some people have exaggerated its dangers, whereas others understate them.

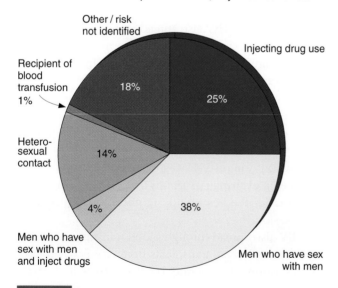

Adult and adolescent exposure to AIDS, July 1996–June 1997

Figure 9-3

Percent of adult and adolescent exposure to AIDS, from July 1996–June 1997

SOURCE: Centers for Disease Control, 1998.

The fact is that although no one is immune to HIV, you can reduce the risk if you abstain from sexual activity, remain in a monogamous relationship with an uninfected partner, and do not inject drugs. If you're not in a long-term monogamous relationship with a partner you're sure is safe and you're not willing to abstain from sex, there are things you can do to lower your risk of HIV infection.

Here's what you should know about HIV transmission (see Figure 9-4):

- Casual contact does *not* spread HIV infection. Compared to other viruses, HIV is extremely difficult to get.

- You cannot tell visually whether a potential sexual partner has HIV. A blood test is needed to detect the antibodies that the body produces to fight HIV, thus indicating infection.

- HIV can be spread in semen and vaginal fluids during a single instance of anal, vaginal, or oral sexual contact between heterosexuals, bisexuals, or homosexuals. The risk increases with the number of sexual encounters with an infected partner.

- Teenage girls may be particularly vulnerable to HIV infection because the immature cervix is easily infected.

- Anal intercourse is an extremely high-risk behavior because HIV may enter the bloodstream through tiny breaks in the lining of the rectum. HIV transmission is much more likely to occur during unprotected anal intercourse than vaginal intercourse.[31]

- Other behaviors that increase the risk of HIV infection include having multiple sex partners, engaging in sex without condoms or virus-killing spermicides, sexual contact with persons known to be at high risk (such as, prostitutes or injecting drug users), and sharing injection equipment for drugs.

- Individuals are at greater risk if they have an active sexual infection. Sexually transmitted diseases, such as herpes, gonorrhea, and syphilis, facilitate transmission of HIV during vaginal or rectal intercourse.

- No cases of HIV transmission by deep kissing have been reported, but it could happen. Social (dry) kissing is safe.

- Oral sex can lead to HIV transmission. The virus in any semen that enters the mouth could make its way into the bloodstream through tiny nicks or sores in the mouth.

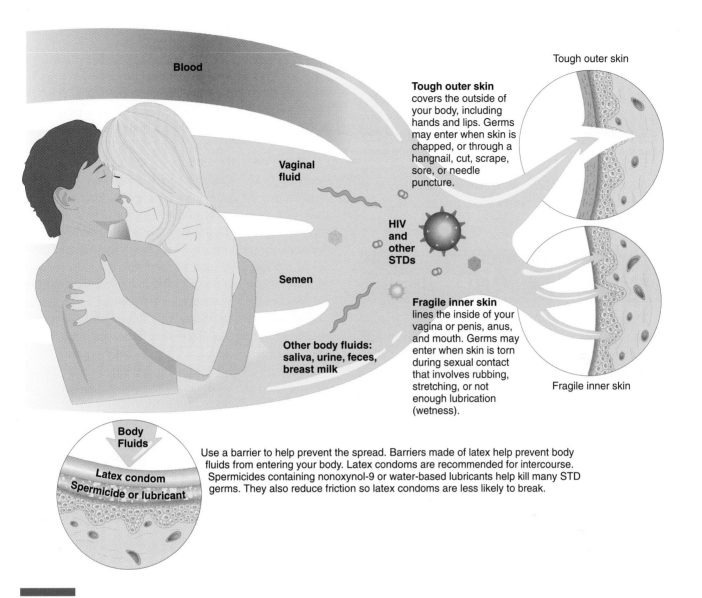

Figure 9-4

How HIV infection and other STDs are spread. Most STDs are spread by viruses, such as HIV, or bacteria carried in certain body fluids.

- HIV infection is not widespread among lesbians, although there have been documented cases of possible female-to-female HIV transmission. In each instance, one partner had had sex with a bisexual man or male injecting drug user or had injected drugs herself.[32]

HIV Infection

HIV infection refers to a spectrum of health problems that results from immunologic abnormalities caused by the virus when it enters the bloodstream. In theory, the body may be able to resist infection by HIV. In reality, in almost all cases, HIV destroys the cell-mediated immune system, particularly the CD4+ T-lymphocytes (also called T4 helper cells). The result is greatly increased susceptibility to various cancers and opportunistic infections (infections that take hold because of the reduced effectiveness of the immune system).

Shortly after becoming infected with HIV, individuals may experience a few days of flulike symptoms, which most ignore or attribute to other viruses. Some people develop a more severe mononucleosis-type syndrome. After this stage, individuals may not develop any signs or symptoms of disease for a period ranging from weeks to more than 12 years.

HIV infection can itself be a serious illness and is associated with a variety of HIV-related diseases, including different cancers and dangerous infections. HIV-infected individuals may develop persistent generalized lymphadenopathy, enlargement of the lymph nodes at two or more different sites in the body. This condition typically persists for more than 3 months without any other illness to explain its occurrence. Diminished mental function may appear before other symptoms. Tests conducted on infected, but apparently healthy, men have revealed impaired coordination, problems in thinking, or abnormal brain scans.

Strategies for Prevention

Lowering Your Risk of Exposure to HIV

✔ Abstain from sexual contact with anyone who is infected with HIV, whether or not he or she has symptoms, or with anyone who is at high risk of HIV infection because of his or her behavior.

✔ Avoid sexual contact with anyone who has had sex with people at risk of HIV infection. Avoid multiple or anonymous sex partners. Avoid sex with anyone who has had multiple or anonymous sex partners or with anyone who has had a sex partner infected with HIV.

✔ Use a condom during every sexual act, including oral sex, from start to finish. Also use a spermicide that provides extra protection against STDs.

✔ Don't have sexual contact with individuals who use injection drugs.

✔ Avoid receptive anal intercourse, as well as the insertion of fingers or objects into your anus, because these acts could tear your rectal tissues, allowing direct access to your bloodstream. Avoid contact with your partner's blood, semen, urine, and feces.

✔ Don't use amyl nitrite (poppers), a sexual stimulant that may be associated with the development of a cancer characteristic of AIDS.

✔ Don't have sex with prostitutes.

✔ Don't share needles (or other injection drug equipment), razor blades, or toothbrushes.

✔ In addition to their partner's use of a condom, women should use a diaphragm with a spermicide for extra protection.

Testing for HIV

The most widely used HIV antibody tests do not detect the virus itself but antibodies that the body forms in response to exposure to HIV. A negative result indicates no exposure to HIV. But since it can take 3 to 6 months for the body to produce the telltale antibodies, a negative result may not be accurate, depending on the timing of the test.

When perfectly performed, HIV tests can detect antibodies in 99.6% of infected people and can correctly give negative results in uninfected people at least 99% of the time. However, actual percentages of false reading are higher than the 99% implies. Most testing centers repeat the test if the initial results are positive. Experienced counselors can refer men and women with two positive readings to physicians who specialize in HIV-related problems.

Home HIV testing kits are available at health centers and pharmacies. By means of a finger prick, users produce a few drops of blood that they apply to a special card and mail to a laboratory. Usually within 7 days, thay can call a toll-free number, identify themselves by a number, and get results anonymously. According to preliminary reports from one manufacturer of HIV tests, 99% of those who use the home tests are HIV-negative. For those who do get positive results, it is important to undergo more precise laboratory testing and to take advantage of counseling services.

AIDS

Until recently, a diagnosis of AIDS was made only when an HIV-positive person developed one of more than twenty-three severe, debilitating illnesses, such as pneumonia or cancer. Since 1993, the definition of AIDS has been expanded to include anyone with HIV whose immune system is severely impaired, as indicated by a CD4 count of fewer than 200 cells per cubic millimeter of blood, compared to normal CD4 cell counts in healthy people not infected with HIV of 800 to 1200 per cubic millimeter of blood. In addition, the expanded definition includes those persons with HIV infection who experience recurrent pneumonia, invasive cervical cancer, or pulmonary tuberculosis.

People with AIDS also may experience persistent fever, diarrhea that persists for more than 1 month, or involuntary weight loss of more than 10% of normal body weight. Generalized lymphadenopathy may persist. Neurological disease—including dementia (confusion and impaired thinking) and other problems with thinking, speaking, movement, or sensation—may occur. Secondary infectious diseases that may develop in people with AIDS include *Pneumocystis carinii* pneumonia, tuberculosis, or oral candidiasis (thrush). Secondary cancers associated with HIV infection include Kaposi's sarcoma and cancer of the cervix.

The number of AIDS deaths in the United States has been declining. According to the Centers for Disease Control and Prevention, the number of deaths caused by AIDS declined by 47% in 1997, compared with 1996. AIDS no longer is one of the top ten killers of Americans.[33]

Treatments

The improvements in severe illness and death are due primarily to new forms of therapy, particularly protease inhibitor drugs, which have been remarkably effective in boosting levels of protective T cells and reducing "viral load"—the amount of HIV virus in the bloodstream.

This drug regimen is expensive and can run more than $10,000 to $12,000 a year. Only 20% of Americans who carry the HIV virus have insurance that pays this cost.[34] While this "cocktail therapy," as some call it, has had a dramatic effect, the benefits seem to decline in about half of those treated. After being knocked into temporary submission, levels of the HIV virus rise, even though patients often continue to feel well.[35]

The Personal Impact of HIV

In recent years, the announcements that celebrities such as basketball star Earvin (Magic) Johnson, Jr., are HIV positive have made many Americans far more aware of these problems. Because of greater awareness and medical advances, infection with HIV is viewed less as a death sentence than as a life sentence, and more individuals are living with AIDS.

In addition to medical dangers, many Americans infected with HIV, including children, have had to deal with physical or verbal abuse because of their disease. Individuals with HIV/AIDS have become more outspoken in defending their rights, in part because of a federal law, the Americans with Disabilities Act, which prohibits discrimination against all people with illnesses or disabilities. The courts have upheld the right of children with HIV infection to public education and the right of HIV-positive employees to remain on the job. However, in some cases, conflicts between personal rights and public health goals remain.

Strategies for Change

When a Friend Has HIV or AIDS

HIV has become so widespread among people in the prime of life that almost everyone knows someone either at risk or infected with the virus. While you may feel helpless or inadequate when a friend becomes seriously ill, you can offer comfort:

✔ Touch your friend. A simple squeeze of the hand or a hug can let him or her know that you care.

✔ Respond to your friend's emotions. Weep with your friend when he or she weeps. Laugh when your friend laughs. It's healthy to share these intimate experiences.

✔ Check in with your friend's partner or roommate and offer to take over any caregiving that is needed to provide him or her with a break.

✔ It's okay to ask about the illness, but be sensitive to whether your friend wants to discuss it. You can find out by asking, "Would you like to talk about how you're feeling?" But don't pressure your friend if the response is no.

Making This Chapter Work for You
Guarding Against Infectious Diseases

■ Infectious illnesses remain a serious health threat. Disease-causing organisms called pathogens, carried by various vectors, can infect a host (either a person or a population) in various ways.

■ The types of microbes that can cause infection are viruses, which invade a body cell and take over its reproductive processes; bacteria, one-celled organisms that release disease-causing toxins; fungi, microscopic plants that feed on human tissue; protozoa, one-celled organisms that release substances that destroy or damage cells; and helminths, parasitic worms that invade body tissue.

■ During the incubation period, a pathogen is multiplying; in the prodromal period, symptoms appear; during active infection, symptoms are most intense; during recovery, symptoms subside.

■ The body's natural defenses against pathogens include the skin; antibacterial substances in tears, sweat, saliva, and mucus; and the immune system, which includes many different types of defenders.

■ Immune system disorders include allergies, auto-immune disorders, and acquired immunodeficiency syndrome (AIDS).

■ Immunizations are the best method of prevention against infectious diseases. College-age men and women may be especially vulnerable to measles and may require revaccination.

■ Infectious diseases caused by viruses include the common cold, influenza, viral pneumonia, mononucleosis, and hepatitis. Bacterial infections include bacterial pneumonia, tuberculosis, toxic shock syndrome, and Lyme disease.

■ Emerging infections are those recently recognized, increasing in humans, or threatening to spread to new areas in the near future. They include HIV, Hantavirus, Ebola, dengue, Lassa, and Marburg, which have been responsible for deadly outbreaks around the globe.

■ Reproductive and urinary tract infections are very common and include trichomoniasis, candidiasis, and bacterial vaginosis, as well as infections of the urethra, bladder, or kidney.

■ The incidence of sexually transmitted diseases (STDs) is increasing. Because many STDs do not cause any symptoms in their initial stages, infected individuals may continue their usual sexual activity without realizing that they're jeopardizing others' well-being.

■ While STDs strike both sexes, all classes, and all ages, young Americans are at greatest risk. According to the CDC, as many as half of all young people may develop an STD by age 30.

■ The most widespread sexually transmitted bacterium in the United States is *Chlamydia trachomatis*, which causes 3 to 5 million infections each year, most in individuals 25 years old or younger.

■ Infection of a woman's fallopian tubes or uterus, called pelvic inflammatory disease (PID), is the second most serious STD affecting women (after HIV infection).

■ One of the most common and dangerous STDs in the United States is gonorrhea, which is caused by the gonococcus bacterium and is diagnosed with a blood test or a culture. The incidence is highest among teenagers and young adults.

■ Nongonoccal urethritis (NGU) refers to any inflammation of the urethra that is not caused by gonorrhea.

■ Syphilis, caused by a bacterium, is easily treated in its stages but can progress and, over time, invade various organs inside the body, including the heart and brain.

■ Herpes simplex virus causes painful blisters during flareups and never entirely leaves the body. Human papilloma virus (HPV) and chancroid infections are other STDs that are spreading rapidly.

■ Human immunodeficiency virus (HIV) is a retrovirus that attacks the body's immune system and causes various problems, ranging from symptomatic infection to generalized swelling of the lymph glands. It is spread through anal, vaginal, and oral sexual contact; contaminated needles of drug abusers; blood transfusions, blood products, and organ transplants from HIV-positive individuals; from HIV-positive mothers to their babies before, during, or after birth; and accidental contact with HIV-contaminated blood or bodily fluids.

■ Acquired immunodeficiency syndrome (AIDS) is diagnosed when HIV severely impairs a person's immune system, as indicated by a CD4 count of fewer than 200 cells per cubic millimeter of blood. People with AIDS also may experience persistent fever, diarrhea, involuntary weight loss, neurological disease, and secondary infectious diseases and cancers.

Infectious diseases threaten everyone's health, but—as with many other illnesses—you can do a great deal to reduce your odds of becoming a victim. Prevention is always the wisest course. Cleanliness is an important first step. The liberal use of soap and hot water kills many pathogens. Colds and flus are, in the long run, inevitable; but preventive measures, such as avoiding obvious carriers, can help reduce your risk.

Sexually transmitted diseases are a particularly personal responsibility. You owe it to yourself, to those you love, and to the children you might conceive to be aware of the signs, symptoms, and stages of STDs and to avoid exposure and take the protective steps described in Pulsepoints: "Ten Ways to Prevent Sexually Transmitted Diseases." You can do more than anyone else to prevent sexual infections. If you fear that you've been exposed, don't wait for serious symptoms to develop. Self-treatment doesn't work for STDs; you need a doctor's help.

Health Online

Cells Alive! http://www.cellsalive.com/

This site features interactive animations and other illustrations plus clear written descriptions to help explain how pathogens and the immune system work in the human body. Topics include HIV infection, making antibodies, penicillin, parasites, and streptococcus.

Think about it ...

- How does the HIV virus go about damaging the immune system? Where might researchers developing drugs to treat people with HIV try to interrupt this process?

- What are some recurring themes in the descriptions of infections and immunity? What could you do to make your immune system stronger?

- Do animated illustrations like these help you understand the process of infection better than still printed illustrations like those in this text?

 ## Key Terms

The terms listed here are used within the chapter. Page numbers are included for each term.
A definition of each term is given in the green Glossary pages at the end of this book.

abcess *166*

acquired immunodeficiency
   syndrome (AIDS) *181*

allergies *167*

autoimmune *167*

bacteria *164*

candidiasis *172*

cell-mediated *165*

chanchroid *180*

chlamydial infections *176*

chronic fatigue syndrome
   (CFS) *171*

fungi *164*

gonorrhea *178*

helminths *164*

hepatitis *171*

herpes simplex *179*

host *164*

human immunodeficiency virus
   (HIV) *181*

human papilloma virus
   (HPV) *180*

humoral *165*

immunity *165*

incubation period *165*

inflammation *166*

influenza *170*

Lyme disease *172*

lymph nodes *166*

mononucleosis *171*

nongonococcal urethritis
   (NGU) *178*

pathogens *164*

pelvic inflammatory disease
   (PID) *177*

pneumonia *171*

protozoa *164*

sexually transmitted diseases
   (STDs) *173*

syphilis *178*

systemic disease *166*

toxic shock syndrome
   (TSS) *171*

trichomoniasis *172*

tuberculosis (TB) *171*

vector *164*

viruses *164*

Review Questions

1. How does an agent of infection spread disease? Explain the process of transmission and infection using a common agent of infection as an example.
2. What is an infectious disease? Name some of the common ones and effective methods of prevention.
3. What are HIV infection and AIDS? How is HIV transmitted? Who is most at risk for contracting HIV?
4. How does a person contract a sexually transmitted disease? List and describe some different kinds of STDs, their symptoms, and treatment.
5. How can a person avoid HIV and other sexually transmitted diseases? What are the best methods of preventing STDs?

Critical Thinking Questions

1. What are several practices that you know of or use to avoid contracting infectious diseases? Briefly explain the convenience, advantages, and disadvantages of each practice.
2. The U.S. military and some employers routinely screen personnel for HIV. Some hospitals test patients and note their HIV status on their charts. Some insurance companies test for HIV before selling a policy. Do you believe that an individual has the right to refuse to be tested for HIV? Should a physician be able to order an HIV test without a patient's consent? Can a surgeon refuse to operate on an HIV-infected patient or one who refuses HIV testing? Do patients have the right to know if their doctors, dentists, or nurses are HIV-positive?
3. A man who developed herpes sued his former girlfriend. A woman who became sterile as a result of pelvic inflammatory disease (PID) took her ex-husband to court. A woman who contracted HIV infection from her dentist, who had died of AIDS, filed suit against his estate. Do you think that anyone who knowingly transmits a sexually transmitted disease should be held legally responsible? Do you think such an act should be a criminal offense?

Connections to Personal Health Interactive

To enhance your understanding of the material covered in this chapter, check out the following study aids on the ***Personal Health Interactive CD-ROM***.

■ Personal Insights: Do You Prevent Disease?
■ **Online Research:** Infectious Disease
■ Glossary & Key Term Review

References

1. Miller, Louis. "Malaria." *NIAID Tips Sheet for Science Writers*, February 21, 1995. Angier, Natalie. "Malaria's Genetic Game of Cloak and Dagger." *New York Times*, August 22, 1995.
2. Miles, Robert. Personal interview.
3. American Academy of Pediatrics. "Implementation of the Immunization Policy." *Pediatrics*, August 1995. Bowman, Marjorie, and Thomas Schwenk. "Family Medicine." *Journal of the American Medical Association*, Vol. 273, No. 21, June 7, 1995.
4. Centers for Disease Control and Prevention.
5. Sniadack, David. Medical epidemiologist, National Center for Infectious Diseases, Centers for Disease Control and Prevention, Atlanta. Personal interview.
6. Centers for Disease Control and Prevention.
7. Gwaltney, Jack M., Jr., and Scott B. Halstead. "Contagiousness of the Common Cold." *Journal of the American Medical Association*, Vol. 278, No. 3, July 16, 1997.
8. "Zinc Lozenges Reduce the Duration of Common Cold Symptoms." *Nutrition Reviews*, Vol. 55, No. 3, March 1997.
9. Gwaltney, Jack. Personal interview.
10. Kilbourne, Edwin. Personal interview.
11. Wessely, Simon, et al. "The Prevalence and Morbidity of Chronic Fatigue and Chronic Fatigue Syndrome." *American Journal of Public Health*, Vol. 87, No. 9, September 1997.
12. Fix, Alan, et al. "Tick Bite and Lyme Disease in an Endemic Setting." *Journal of the American Medical Association*, Vol. 279, No. 3, January 21, 1998.

13. Strausbaugh, Larry. "Emerging Infectious Diseases: A Challenge to All." *Journal of the American Medical Association*, Vol. 278, No. 5, August 6, 1997.

14. "Malicious Microbes Warrant Basic Biomedical Research." *NIAID News*, February 20, 1995.

15. Quinn, T. "Recent Advances in Diagnosis of Sexually Transmitted Disease." *NIAID News*, Vol. 21, 1994.

16. "Sexually Transmitted Diseases in the United States." *SIECUS Report*, Vol. 25, No. 3, February–March 1997.

17. Braverman, P., and Strasburger, V. "Adolescent Sexual Activity." *Clinical Pediatrics*, Vol. 32, 1994.

18. DePunzio, C., et al. "Epidemiology and Therapy of Chlamydia Trachomatis Genital Infection in Women." *Journal of Chemotherapy*, June 1992.

19. Schneider, Dona, et al. "Evaluating HIV/AIDS Education in the University Setting." *Journal of American College Health*, July 1994. O'Leary, A., et al. "Predictors of Safer Sex on the College Campus: A Social Cognitive Theory Analysis." *Journal of American College Health*, May 1992. Jaccard, James, et al. "Student Opinion Leaders and HIV/AIDS Knowledge and Risk Behavior." *Journal of American College Health*, March 1995.

20. Pinkerton, Steven, and Paul Abramsom. "Condoms and the Prevention of AIDS." *American Scientist*, Vol. 85, No. 4, July–August 1997.

21. Biro, F., et al. "A Comparison of Diagnostic Methods in Adolescent Girls With and Without Symptoms of Chlamydia Urogenital Infection." *Pediatrics*, Vol. 93, 1994. "*Chlamydia trachomatis* Antibody Testing Is More Accurate Than Hysterosalpingography in Predicting Tubal Factor Infertility." *Fertility and Sterility*, Vol. 61, 1994.

22. Zhang, Jun, et al. "Vaginal Douching and Adverse Health Effects." *American Journal of Public Health*, Vol. 87, No. 7, July 1997.

23. MacKay, Trent, et al. "PID: Suspect More, Treat More, Hospitalize Less." *Patient Care*, Vol. 31, No. 12, July 15, 1997.

24. Newland, Jamesetta. "Gonorrhea in Women." *American Journal of Nursing*, Vol. 97, No. 8, August 1997.

25. Schmid, George, and Phil Fontanarosa. "Evolving Strategies for Management of the Nongonococcal Urethritis Syndrome." *Journal of the American Medical Association*, Vol. 274, No. 7, August 16, 1995.

26. Braverman and Strasburger. "Adolescent Sexual Activity."

27. Centers for Disease Control and Prevention, February 1998.

28. Saag, Michael. "HIV Pathogenesis: The Evolving Understanding of HIV Disease." *HIV/AIDS Reporter*, Vol. 1, April 1995.

29. Marwick, Charles. "Released Report Says Needle Exchanges Work." *Journal of the American Medical Association*, Vol. 273, No. 13, April 5, 1995.

30. Wilbanks, George. "Protecting the Unborn Against AIDS." *ACOG Women's Health*, July 24, 1995.

31. Billy, J., et al. "The Sexual Behavor of Men in the United States." *Family Planning Perspectives*, 1993.

32. Seidman, S., and R. Rieder. "A Review of Sexual Behavior in the United States." *American Journal of Psychiatry*, Vol. 151, 1994.

33. Centers for Disease Control.

34. Lacayo, Richard. "Hope with an Asterisk." *Time*, Vol. 148, No. 29, December 30, 1996.

35. "Setbacks for Many on Drugs for AIDS." *New York Times*, September 30, 1997.

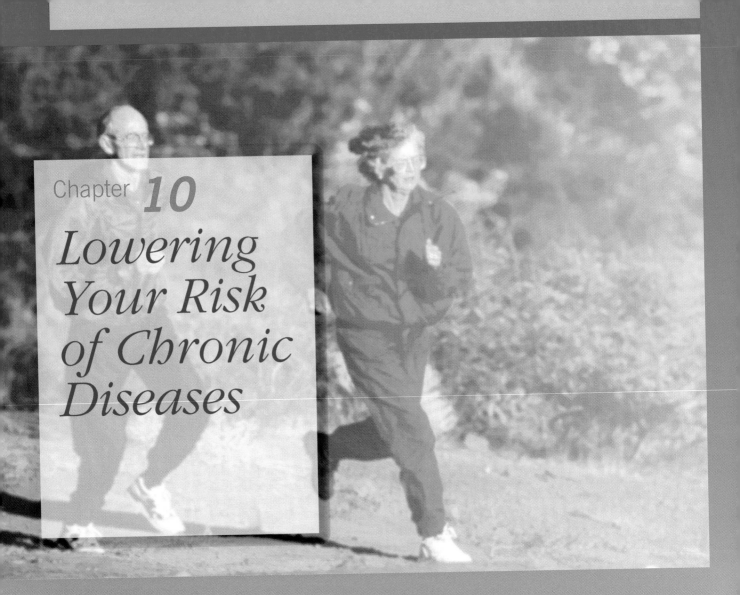

Chapter *10*

Lowering Your Risk of Chronic Diseases

- **Describe** how the heart functions.
- **List** and **explain** the controllable and uncontrollable risk factors for cardiovascular disease.
- **Define** the different kinds of heart disease and **explain** their cause, prevention, and treatment.
- **Define** cancer and **list** the seven warning signs.
- **List** the risk factors for cancer and **describe** practical behaviors to reduce the risk.
- **List** the major forms of cancer and **explain** their risk factors and prevention.
- **Describe** other major noninfectious illnesses.

Whether or not you will get a serious disease at some time in your life may seem to be a matter of odds. Genetic tendencies, environmental factors, and luck do affect your chances of having to face many health threats. However, you also have a lot of control over many of the major risk factors for chronic diseases like heart disease and cancer. The time to start preventing these diseases is now. This chapter provides the information you need about these diseases, their risk factors, and what you can do to minimize your chances of facing heart disease, cancer, or another serious chronic disease.

How Your Heart Works

The heart is a hollow muscular organ with four chambers that serve as two pumps (see Figure 10-1). It is about the size of a clenched fist. Each pump consists of a pair of chambers formed of muscles. The upper two—

each called an **atrium**—receive blood, which then flows through valves into the lower two chambers, the **ventricles**, which contract to pump blood out into the arteries through a second set of valves. A thick wall divides the right side of the heart from the left side; but even though the two sides are separated, they contract at almost the same time. Contraction of the ventricles is called **systole**; the period of relaxation between contractions is called **diastole**. The heart valves, located at the entrance and exit of the ventricular chambers, have flaps that open and close to allow blood to flow through the chambers of the heart.

Blood circulates through the body by means of the pumping action of the heart. The right ventricle (on your own right side) pumps blood, via the *pulmonary arteries*, to the lungs, where it picks up oxygen (a gas essential to the body's cells) and gives off carbon dioxide (a waste product of metabolism). The blood returns from the lungs via the *pulmonary veins* to the left side of the heart, which pumps it, via the **aorta**, to the arteries in the rest of the body.

The arteries divide into smaller and smaller branches, and finally into **capillaries**, the smallest blood vessels of all (only slightly larger in diameter than a single red blood cell). The blood within the capillaries supplies oxygen and nutrients to the cells of the tissues and takes up various waste products. Blood returns to the heart

Figure 10-1

The healthy heart. The heart muscle is nourished by blood from the coronary arteries, which arise from the aorta. The pericardium is the outer covering of the heart.

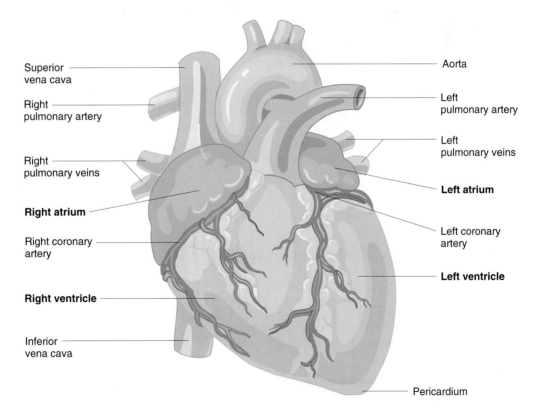

Superior vena cava

Right pulmonary artery

Right pulmonary veins

Right atrium

Right coronary artery

Right ventricle

Inferior vena cava

Aorta

Left pulmonary artery

Left pulmonary veins

Left atrium

Left coronary artery

Left ventricle

Pericardium

via the veins: The blood from the upper body (except the lungs) drains into the heart through the *superior vena cava*, while blood from lower body returns via the *inferior vena cava.*

The workings of this remarkable pump affect your entire body. If the flow of blood to or through the heart or to the rest of the body is reduced, or if a disturbance occurs in the small bundle of highly specialized cells in the heart that generate electrical impulses to control heartbeats, the result may at first be too subtle to notice. However, without diagnosis and treatment, these changes could develop into a life-threatening problem.

Preventing Heart Problems

According to a survey of 1503 college students, young adults are aware of the risk factors for heart disease, including high blood pressure, elevated cholesterol, smoking, and lack of exercise. However, only a third of

---

Strategies for Prevention

What You Can Do to Avoid Heart Disease

✔ *Eat a low-fat diet.* Get no more than 30% of your daily calories from fat in any form and no more than 10% from saturated fat. (See Chapter 5 for a discussion of types of fat.)

✔ *Limit your cholesterol intake to 300 milligrams a day.* (See Chapter 5.)

✔ *Exercise.* Regular aerobic exercise—walking, cycling, swimming, or jogging—is best.

✔ *Watch your weight.* Extra pounds can mean extra risk for high blood pressure and other forms of cardiovascular disease.

✔ *Don't smoke.* Smokers have twice the risk of heart attack and two to four times the risk of sudden cardiac death that nonsmokers have.

✔ *Limit your intake of alcohol.* Alcohol can increase blood pressure and directly affect the heart; drink no more than 3 ounces, or the equivalent of two alcoholic drinks, a day.

✔ *Hold the salt.* Along with losing weight, significantly cutting down on your intake of sodium can reduce blood pressure (see Chapter 5).

---

those surveyed exercised or had their cholesterol levels checked regularly. As with other health-related behaviors, there is a gap between what students know about the risks of heart disease and what they do to protect themselves.[1]

At any age, lifestyle changes can make a difference. Physical activity is particularly beneficial. Regular exercise reduces the risk of heart attack, helps maintain a desirable body weight, lowers blood pressure, and improves metabolism. If rigorous and frequent enough, it also may increase longevity.[2] Dietary changes (such as limiting total fat and cholesterol intake) also help prevent heart disease. Foods rich in cell-protecting **antioxidants**, as well as folic acid and supplements of vitamin E, have been linked with a lower risk of heart disease.[3]

Risk Factors for Cardiovascular Disease

Several major risk factors contribute to disorders of the heart and blood vessels. The greater the number or severity of these risk factors, the greater your overall risk.

Risks You Can Control

The choices individuals make and the habits they follow can have a significant impact on whether or not their hearts remain healthy. The following are potential risks that you can avoid for the sake of your heart's health.

Physical Inactivity

According to the Centers for Disease Control and Prevention (CDC), the leading culprit in deaths from heart attack is sedentary living. People who are not even somewhat physically active face a much greater risk of fatal heart attack than those who engage in some form of exercise or activity. Individuals who work out rigorously and regularly have the healthiest hearts and the lowest risks of heart disease.

Cigarette Smoking

Each year smoking causes more than 250,000 deaths from cardiovascular disease—far more than it causes from cancer and lung disease. Smokers who have heart attacks are more likely to die from them than are nonsmokers. Smoking is the major risk factor for *peripheral vascular disease,* in which the blood vessels that carry blood to the leg and arm muscles get hardened and clogged. Both active and passive smoking accelerate the process by which arteries become clogged and increase the risk of heart attacks and strokes.[4] Passive smoking also reduces beneficial blood fats and increases harmful ones in children.[5]

Cigarette smoking may damage the heart in several ways:

- The nicotine may repeatedly overstimulate the heart.

- Carbon monoxide may take the place of some of the oxygen in the blood, which reduces the oxygen supply to the heart muscle.

- The tars and other smoke residues may damage the lining of the coronary arteries, making it easier for cholesterol to build up and narrow the passageways.

- Smoking also increases blood clotting, leading to a higher incidence of clotting in the coronary arteries and subsequent heart attack. Clotting in the peripheral arteries is also increased, which can cause leg pain with walking and, ultimately, stroke.

- New research indicates that ex-smokers may have irreversible damage to their arteries.[6]

High Blood Pressure (Hypertension)

Blood pressure is a result of the contractions of the heart muscle, which pumps blood through your body, and the resistance of the walls of the vessels through which the blood flows. Each time your heart beats, your blood pressure goes up and down within a certain range. It's highest when the heart contracts; this is called *systolic blood pressure*. It's lowest between contractions; this is called *diastolic blood pressure*. A blood pressure reading consists of the systolic measurement "over" the diastolic measurement, recorded in millimeters of mercury (mmHg) by a sphygmomanometer.

High blood pressure, or **hypertension**, occurs when the artery walls become constricted so that the force exerted as the blood flows through them is greater than it should be. Physicians see blood pressure as a continuum: The higher the reading, the greater the risk of stroke and heart disease. However, you can control high blood pressure through diet, exercise, and medication (if necessary).

Blood Fats

Cholesterol is a fatty substance found in certain foods and also manufactured by the body. The measurement of cholesterol in the blood is one of the most reliable indicators of the formation of plaque, the sludgelike substance that builds up on the inner walls of arteries. You can lower blood cholesterol levels by cutting back on high-fat foods and exercising more, thereby reducing the risk of a heart attack. According to the National Heart, Lung, and Blood Institute (NHLBI), for every 1% drop in blood cholesterol, studies show a 2% decrease in the likelihood of a heart attack.

Triglycerides

These fats, which flow through the blood after meals, have been linked to increased risk of coronary artery disease, especially in women. **Triglyceride** levels tend to be highest in those whose diets are high in calories, sugar, alcohol, and refined starches. High levels of these fats may increase the risk of obesity, but cutting back on these foods can reduce high triglyceride levels.

Lipoproteins

Lipoproteins are compounds in the blood that are made up of proteins and fat. The different types are classified by their size or density. The heaviest are *high-density lipoproteins*, or HDLs, which have the highest portion of protein. These "good guys," as some cardiologists refer to them, pick up excess cholesterol in the blood and carry it back to the liver for removal from the body. *Low-density lipoproteins*, or LDLs, carry more cholesterol than HDLs and deposit it on the walls of arteries—they're the bad guys.

Diabetes Mellitus

Diabetes mellitus, a disorder of the endocrine system, increases the likelihood of hypertension and atherosclerosis, thereby increasing the risk of heart attack and stroke. A physician can detect diabetes and prescribe a diet, exercise program, and if necessary, medication to keep it in check. Even before developing diabetes, individuals at high risk for this disease—those who are overweight, have a family history of the disease, have mildly elevated blood pressure and blood sugar levels, and above-ideal levels of harmful blood fats—may already be at increased risk of heart disease.

Weight

According to the National Heart, Lung, and Blood Institute, losing weight at any age can help reduce the risk of heart problems. For women, obesity is as great a cause of excess death and disability from heart disease as smoking and heavy drinking. Even mild to moderately obese women are more likely to suffer chest pain or a heart attack than thinner women.[7]

Psychological Factors

The way we respond to everyday sources of stress can affect our hearts as well as our overall health. While we may not be able to control the sources of stress, we can change how we habitually respond to it. The significance of Type-A behavior has been debated for more than 30 years. Initial studies showed a clearly increased risk of coronary artery disease; more recent ones have not. Of all Type-A traits, anger and hostility have been most closely linked to heart disease. These negative emotions may send adrenaline and other stress hormones into the bloodstream, where they cause fat to be dumped into the blood, driving up cholesterol levels. Recent studies indicate that depression may increase the risk of heart disease as well.

Risks You Can't Control

Heredity

Anyone whose parents, siblings, or other close relatives suffered heart attacks before age 50 is at increased risk of developing heart disease. Certain risk factors, such as abnormally high blood levels of lipids, can be passed down from generation to generation. Although you can't rewrite your family history, individuals with an inherited vulnerability to cardiovascular disease can lower the danger by changing the risk factors within their control. Your heart's health depends to a great extent on your behavior, including the decisions you make about the foods you eat or the decision not to smoke.

Race and Ethnicity

African Americans are twice as likely to develop high blood pressure as are whites. African Americans also suffer strokes at an earlier age and of greater severity. Poverty may be an unrecognized risk factor for members of this minority group, who are less likely to receive medical treatments or undergo corrective surgery. Family history, lifestyle, diet, and stress may also play a role, starting early in life. However, researchers have found no single explanation for why African-American youngsters, like their parents, tend to have higher blood pressure than white children.[8]

Age

Almost four of five people who die of heart attacks are over age 65. Heart disease accounts for more than 40% of deaths among people between 65 and 74 and almost 60% at age 85 and above. However, the risk factors that are likely to cause heart disease later in life, including high blood pressure and cholesterol levels, may begin to develop in childhood. Nevertheless, although cardiovascular function declines with age, heart disease is not an inevitable consequence of aging. Many 80- and 90-year-olds have strong, healthy hearts.[9]

Gender

Men have a higher incidence of cardiovascular problems than women, particularly before age 40. Coronary artery disease tends to develop about a decade later in women than in men, possibly because younger women have high blood levels of heart-healthy HDLs. The female sex hormone estrogen may also have a protective effect by increasing HDL levels and decreasing harmful LDL levels. After menopause or surgical removal of the ovaries, women's estrogen levels drop and their LDL levels tend to go up. Postmenopausal hormone replacement therapy (HRT) can protect women against heart disease by keeping their HDL levels up and their LDL levels down. However, the question of which women should take estrogen remains controversial.[10]

The Cholesterol Connection

Cholesterol levels have dropped steadily among Americans since 1980; this change alone may account for an 8% to 17% decline in the incidence of heart disease.[11] For the sake of a healthy heart, all adults should know what their cholesterol level is, whether it's too high, and if it is, what they can do to lower it.

What's Normal?

According to the NHLBI:

- Total cholesterol should be below 200 mg/dL of blood for men and below 210 mg/dL for women.

- A total cholesterol reading of 201–239 mg/dL is considered borderline and presents a moderate to high risk for heart disease. Americans with cholesterol levels below 240 mg/dL account for more than 60% of the cases of coronary heart disease in this country.

- Total cholesterol levels of 240 or more mg/dL are dangerously high.

- LDL levels should be less than 130 mg/dL. A level of 160 mg/dL or more is high.

- HDL levels should be at least 35 mg/dL.

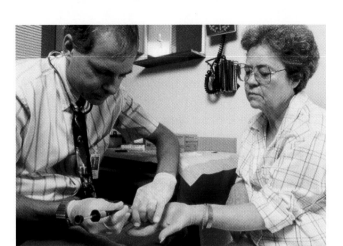

Getting a cholesterol test is a quick, simple, and relatively painless procedure.

Persons in the moderate- to high-risk categories (as many as half of all adults, according to some estimates) should undergo a test of the concentrations of the different types of lipoproteins (HDLs and LDLs), the protein-fat complexes that carry cholesterol in the blood.

Lowering Cholesterol Levels

There are various ways to reduce cholesterol levels—and the risk of heart disease. The best way to begin is by reducing cholesterol and fat in your diet. Your goal should be to limit all fats to no more than 30% of the calories you consume every day and saturated fats to no more than 10%. Controlling your weight and increasing physical activity also can help.

If cholesterol levels are dangerously high and exercise and diet therapy fail, medications to lower cholesterol can be highly effective. Researchers at the University of California's Lawrence Berkeley Laboratory found that, over several years, the combination of a low-fat diet and cholesterol-lowering drugs can reduce and even reverse clogging of the arteries.[12] The American College of Cardiology has reported that at least two cholesterol-lowering drugs, simvastatin and provastatin, can halt or delay the progression of heart disease and prolong life.[13] However, preventive treatment of individuals who have high cholesterol readings but no evidence of coronary artery disease with cholesterol-lowering drugs remains controversial.[14]

The Silent Killers

The two most common forms of cardiovascular disease in this country are high blood pressure (hypertension) and coronary artery disease, the gradual narrowing of the blood vessels of the heart. Often these two problems go together.

Pulsepoints

Ten Keys to a Healthy Heart

1. Don't smoke. There's no bigger favor you can do your heart—and lungs!

2. Watch your weight. Even relatively modest gains can have a big effect on your risk of heart disease.

3. Cut down on saturated fats and cholesterol. This could help prevent high blood cholesterol levels, obesity, and heart disease.

4. Get moving. Engage in regular physical activity. A little is better than none; more is even better.

5. Lower your stress levels. If too much stress is a problem in your life, try the relaxation techniques described in Chapter 2.

6. Know your family history. Inheriting a predispositon to high blood pressure or heart disease means that your heart needs extra preventive care.

7. Get your blood pressure checked regularly. Knowing your numbers can alert you to a potential problem long before you develop any symptoms.

8. Tame your temper. Hostility can be hazardous to the heart. Look for other ways of releasing anger and frustration.

9. Find out your cholesterol levels. You can't know if your heart is in danger unless you know if your cholesterol is too high. Get a blood test at your next physical and discuss the results with your physician.

10. Take appropriate medications. Those with high cholesterol or high blood pressure should seek their physicians' advice.

High Blood Pressure

Hypertension forces the heart to pump harder than is healthy. Because the heart must force blood into arteries that are offering increased resistance to blood flow, the left side of the heart often becomes enlarged (see Figure 10-2). The term *essential hypertension* indicates that the cause is unknown, as is usually the case. Occasionally, abnormalities of the kidneys or the blood vessels feeding them, or certain substances in the bloodstream, are identified as the culprits. Whatever its cause, hypertension is dangerous because excessive pressure can wear out arteries, leading to serious cardiovascular diseases, vision problems, and kidney disease.

More than 40 million Americans have high blood pressure that requires monitoring or treatment. While most are under age 65, hypertension has become increasingly common among people in their twenties and thirties. Physicians urge all adults to have their blood pressure checked at least once a year.

Normal blood pressure in most young adults is 120/80 mmHg (120 systolic pressure, 80 diastolic pressure) under relaxed conditions. Borderline hypertension is 140/90 to 160/95; definite hypertension is 160/95 and above. The lower, or diastolic, number has increasingly been used in categorizing high blood pressure, with 90 to 104 indicating mild hypertension; 105 to 114, moderate; and 115 and over, severe. A high diastolic reading indicates an increased risk of heart disease, even if the systolic pressure is normal (see Table 10-1). According to a 1995 report, people whose systolic blood pressure is slightly above normal also face increased health risks of heart disease and stroke, compared with those whose blood pressure is under 140.[15]

Lifestyle changes can help prevent high blood pressure. The can also serve as a nondrug (or nonpharmacologic) treatment for hypertension. (See Pulsepoints: "Ten Keys to a Healthy Heart.") However, there is no single ideal prescription for reducing high blood pressure in all patients. The most current recommendations are:

- Achieve and maintain appropriate body weight.

- Limit alcohol to 1 ounce a day.

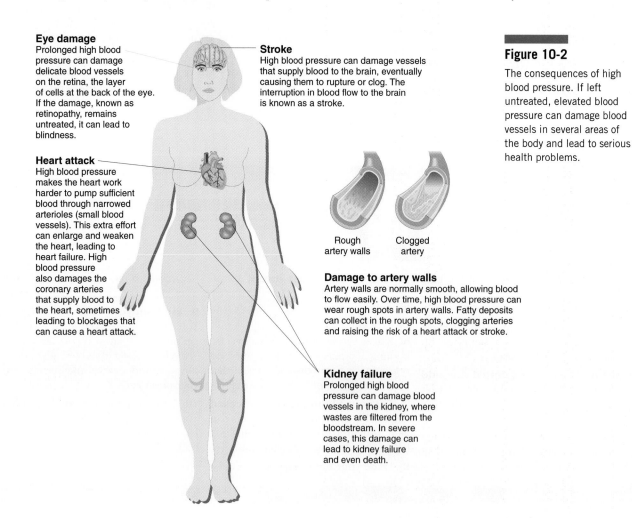

Eye damage
Prolonged high blood pressure can damage delicate blood vessels on the retina, the layer of cells at the back of the eye. If the damage, known as retinopathy, remains untreated, it can lead to blindness.

Stroke
High blood pressure can damage vessels that supply blood to the brain, eventually causing them to rupture or clog. The interruption in blood flow to the brain is known as a stroke.

Heart attack
High blood pressure makes the heart work harder to pump sufficient blood through narrowed arterioles (small blood vessels). This extra effort can enlarge and weaken the heart, leading to heart failure. High blood pressure also damages the coronary arteries that supply blood to the heart, sometimes leading to blockages that can cause a heart attack.

Rough artery walls   Clogged artery

Damage to artery walls
Artery walls are normally smooth, allowing blood to flow easily. Over time, high blood pressure can wear rough spots in artery walls. Fatty deposits can collect in the rough spots, clogging arteries and raising the risk of a heart attack or stroke.

Kidney failure
Prolonged high blood pressure can damage blood vessels in the kidney, where wastes are filtered from the bloodstream. In severe cases, this damage can lead to kidney failure and even death.

Figure 10-2

The consequences of high blood pressure. If left untreated, elevated blood pressure can damage blood vessels in several areas of the body and lead to serious health problems.

TABLE 10-1 CLASSIFICATION OF HIGH BLOOD PRESSURE

Category	Systolic Reading	Diastolic Reading	Followup Recommended
Normal	Less than 130	Less than 85	Check again in 2 years.
High normal	130–139	85–89	Check in 1 year. Many physicians recommend lifestyle modifications at this stage.
Hypertension			
Stage 1	140–159	90–99	Modify lifestyle. Begin drug treatment if lifestyle modifications are not effective within 6 months.
Stage 2	160–179	100–109	Begin drug treatment and modify lifestyle.
Stage 3	180–209	110–119	Begin drug treatment and modify lifestyle.
Stage 4	More than 210	More than 120	Immediate medical evaluation and treatment with drugs. Modify lifestyle.

SOURCE: Joint National Committee on Detection, Evaluation, Treatment of High Blood Pressure.

- Get some exercise daily.
- Keep sodium intake below 2.4 grams a day.
- Consume adequate dietary amounts of calcium and potassium.
- Don't smoke.
- Cut down on saturated fats, cholesterol, and "trans-fats."

If exercise, dietary changes, and restriction of salt intake fail to bring down blood pressure, some health experts argue that even those with mild hypertension should take drugs to prevent damage to the heart and blood vessels.

Coronary Artery Disease

The general term for any impairment of blood flow through the blood vessels, often referred to as "hardening of the arteries," is **arteriosclerosis**. The most common form is **atherosclerosis**, a disease of the lining of the arteries in which plaque—deposits of fat, fibrin (a clotting material), cholesterol, other cell parts, and calcium—narrows the artery channels.

Clogging the Arteries

Atherosclerosis, which may begin in childhood, worsens with the continued buildup of plaque on the arterial lining (see Figure 10-3). The arteries lose their ability to expand and contract. Blood moves with increasing difficulty through the narrowed channels,

making it easier for a clot (thrombus) to form, perhaps blocking the channel and depriving vital organs of blood. When such a blockage is in a coronary artery, the result is coronary thrombosis, one form of heart attack. When the clot occurs in the brain, the result is cerebral thrombosis, one form of stroke.

Unclogging the Arteries

For years, heart specialists said that clogged arteries couldn't be unclogged. However, recent research has shown that it is possible to reverse the buildup of plaque inside the arteries by means of cholesterol-lowering drugs and a low-fat diet. A strict program of

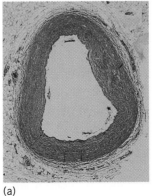 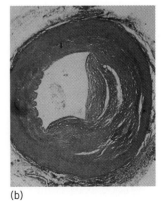

(a) (b)

Figure 10-3

(a) A healthy coronary artery. (b) An artery partially blocked by the buildup of atherosclerotic plaque.

dietary and lifestyle change without any medication, developed by Dean Ornish, M.D., of the University of California, San Francisco, also has proven effective in reversing coronary artery disease. Dr. Ornish's approach includes a very low-fat, vegetarian diet, moderate exercise, stress counseling, and daily relaxation techniques.[16]

Crises of the Heart

For many people, the first sign of heart disease is pain, ranging from mild to excruciating. They may be experiencing angina pectoris, spasms of the coronary artery, or myocardial infarction (heart attack). According to the American Heart Association (AHA), as many as 1.5 million men and women have heart attacks each year; almost 5 million Americans alive today have had a heart attack, chest pain, or both.

Angina Pectoris

A temporary drop in the supply of oxygen to the heart tissue causes feelings of pain or discomfort in the chest known as **angina pectoris**. Some people suffer angina only when the demands on their hearts increase, such as during exercise or when under stress. Many people have angina for years and yet never suffer a heart attack; in some, the angina even disappears. However, angina should be considered a warning of danger if it becomes more severe or more frequent, occurs with less activity or exertion, begins to waken a person from a sound sleep at night, persists for more than 10 to 15 minutes, or causes unusual perspiration.

Angina is most commonly treated with beta blockers, calcium channel blockers, or nitrates.

Coronary Artery Spasms

Sometimes the arteries tighten suddenly or go into a spasm, cutting off or reducing blood flow. Spasms can produce heart attacks, as well as angina, and can be fatal. Several factors that may trigger spasms in the heart include:

- *Clumping of platelets*. When *platelets* (a type of blood cell) clump together, they produce a substance called thromboxane A-2, which causes the narrowing of a blood vessel.

- *Smoking*. When some angina victims stop smoking, their chest pain declines or disappears.

Strategies for Prevention

What to Do If a Heart Attack Strikes

✔ If you develop chest discomfort that lasts for 2 minutes or more, call the local emergency rescue service immediately.

✔ If you're with someone who's exhibiting the classic signs of heart attack, and if they last for 2 minutes or more, act at once. Expect the person to deny the possibility of anything as serious as a heart attack, but insist on taking prompt action.

✔ Call for help. Bystanders should call the emergency medical system (available by dialing 911 in many places) immediately. The odds of survival are greatest if emergency teams get to a heart attack victim quickly and administer advanced cardiac life support. Individuals trained in **cardiopulmonary resuscitation (CPR)**, a combination of mouth-to-mouth breathing and chest compression for victims of cardiac arrest, should use this technique only after calling or having someone else call for emergency help.[17]

- *Stress*. No one knows exactly how stress may lead to spasms, but many heart specialists believe that it's a culprit.

- *Increased calcium flow*. Calcium regularly flows into smooth muscle cells; too much calcium, however, may lead to a spasm. (This calcium flow is not regulated by the amount of calcium in your diet.)

Myocardial Infarction (Heart Attack)

The medical name for a heart attack, or coronary, is **myocardial infarction (MI)**. The *myocardium* is the cardiac muscle layer of the wall of the heart. It receives its blood supply, and thus its oxygen and other nutrients, from the coronary arteries. If an artery is blocked by a clot or plaque, or by a spasm, the myocardial cells do not get sufficient oxygen, and the portion of the myocardium deprived of its blood supply begins to die (see Figure 10-4). Although such an attack may seem sudden, usually it has been building up for years, particularly if the person has ignored risk factors and early warning signs.

Individuals should seek immediate medical care if they experience the following symptoms:

Figure 10-4

The making of a heart attack. (a) The bulk of the heart is composed mainly of the myocardium, the muscle layer that contracts. (b) A clot in one of the arteries that feeds into the myocardium can cut off the blood supply to part of the myocardium, causing cells in that area to die. This is called a myocardial infarction, or heart attack.

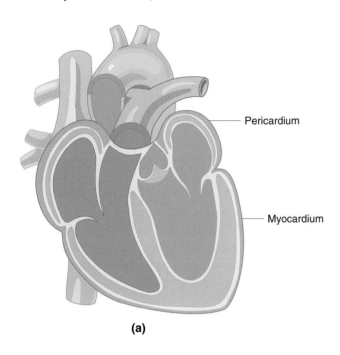

(a)

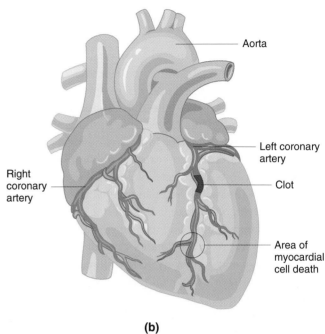

(b)

- A heavy, squeezing pain or discomfort in the center of the chest, which may last for several minutes.

- A pain that may radiate to the shoulder, arm, neck, back, or jaw.

- Anxiety.

- Sweating.

- Nausea and vomiting.

- Shortness of breath.

- Dizziness or fainting.

The 2 hours immediately following the onset of such symptoms are the most crucial period. About 40% of those who suffer an MI die within this time. According to the American Heart Association, most patients wait 3 hours after the initial symptoms begin before seeking help. By that time, half of the affected heart muscle may already be lost.

State-of the-art treatments for heart attacks include clot-dissolving drugs, early administration of medications to thin the blood, intravenous nitroglycerin and in some cases, a beta blocker (which blocks many of the effects of adrenaline in the body, particularly its stimulating impact on the heart).

Other Heart Problems

Sometimes the heart seems to skip a beat or experience premature (or early) heartbeats. In many cases, these irregularities are no cause for alarm, but they can be dangerous in an MI victim. Caffeine, long suspected of triggering irregular heartbeats, doesn't seem to be a culprit.

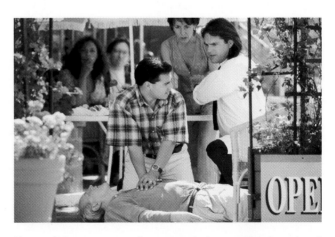

If you witness someone who appears to be experiencing a heart attack, the best thing you can do is call for emergency help immediately. Only after medical emergency personnel are called should you begin any CPR efforts.

Patients with very slow or irregular heartbeats who don't respond to drugs may need an implanted electrical pacemaker that stimulates contractions of the heart at a normal rate. Such pacemakers, compact battery-powered systems, deliver a series of small electrical impulses to the heart muscle.

When the heart's pumping power is well below normal capacity, fluid begins to collect in the lungs, hands, and feet. The heart is then said to be in failure. As blood fluids accumulate in the lungs, pulmonary congestion occurs, causing shortness of breath. In other parts of the body, fluid seeps through the thin capillary walls and causes swelling (edema), especially in the ankles and legs. **Congestive heart failure** usually results from myocardial infarction, but can also be the result of rheumatic fever, birth defects, hypertension, or atherosclerosis. It is treated by reducing the workload on the heart, modifying salt intake, administering drugs that rid the body of excess fluid, and using medications (such as digitalis) to improve the heart's pumping efficiency.

Approximately 8 of every 1000 children born in the United States have congenital heart disease. The most common defects are holes in the ventricular septum, the wall dividing the lower chambers of the heart. Holes may also occur in the atrial septum, the wall between the upper chambers. Sometimes the arteries delivering blood to the body and lungs are transposed and thus attached to the wrong ventricles. Such babies have a bluish color because their blood isn't carrying sufficient oxygen; they can die if this defect isn't corrected.

Heart Savers

A generation ago physicians had no way of detecting problems before the symptoms of heart disease began and could offer little more than bed rest as a therapy after they struck. The last decade, however, has brought tremendous progress in the diagnosis and treatment of heart problems. Today men and women with heart problems can learn of possible dangers much earlier than in the past and undergo treatments that may add years to their lives (see Figure 10-5).

Figure 10-5

WAYS TO REDUCE YOUR HEART ATTACK RISK

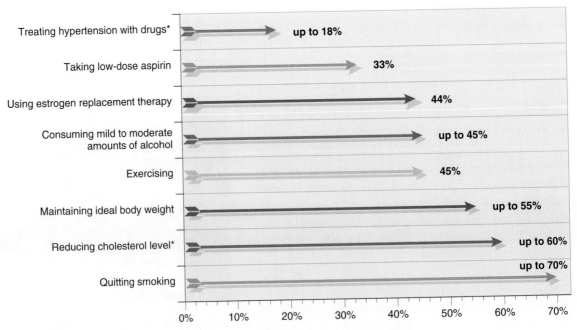

Treating hypertension with drugs*	up to 18%
Taking low-dose aspirin	33%
Using estrogen replacement therapy	44%
Consuming mild to moderate amounts of alcohol	up to 45%
Exercising	45%
Maintaining ideal body weight	up to 55%
Reducing cholesterol level*	up to 60%
Quitting smoking	up to 70%

0%   10%   20%   30%   40%   50%   60%   70%

*Because studies of these lifestyle changes have mostly involved men, the benefits are less clear for women.

SOURCE: *American Health*, March 1993, p. 14.

Diagnostic Tests

The **electrocardiogram (ECG, EKG)**, a recording of the electrical activity of the heart, is the traditional method of evaluating the heart's health. An exercise ECG—or *stress test*—is one method of finding out whether an area of the heart begins to run out of blood during the stress of an athletic workout. The subject walks or jogs on a treadmill while the ECG monitors the heart's response.

Thallium scintigraphy uses radioactive isotopes that are injected into the bloodstream. A special imaging device called a *scintillation*, or gamma camera, picks up the rays emitted by the isotopes; a computer translates these signals into images of the heart as it pumps.

In **coronary angiography**, the most complete and accurate diagnostic test for heart problems, a thin tube is threaded through the blood vessels of the heart, a radiopaque dye is injected, and X rays are taken to detect any blockage of the arteries. Angiography is extremely precise, but it's also costly and risky: About 1 of every 1500 patients dies as a result of the test.

Treatments

Most people with heart disease can be treated successfully with medications. Other alternatives are bypass surgery, balloon angioplasty, heart transplants, and external and implanted mechanical devices.

Medications

The main types of drugs used to treat high blood pressure and heart disease include diuretics; beta blockers; calcium channel blockers; and angiotensin converting enzyme (ACE) inhibitors, which block a hormone known as angiotensin that strongly influences blood pressure. Side effects range from lethargy and fatigue to an increased risk of chest pain and heart attack if certain drugs are discontinued abruptly. The newer, more expensive agents—calcium channel blockers and ACE inhibitors—have become more popular, even though they have not proved more effective than older medications such as diuretics and beta blockers. Unlike the older drugs, the new ones are less likely to cause side effects such as impotence, insomnia, lethargy, and depression. The newer drugs can be taken in lower doses with negligible side effects.

Surgical Procedures and Mechanical Aids

A **coronary bypass** is a procedure in which an artery from the patient's leg or chest wall is grafted onto a coronary artery to detour blood around the blocked area. Each year hundreds of thousands of coronary bypasses are performed in the United States; about 1% to 5% of these patients die as a result of surgical complications. But surgery is not a cure for the atherosclerotic process that caused the blockage; indeed, in as many as 80% of bypass patients, the grafts themselves develop blockages within 10 years.

Percutaneous transluminal coronary angioplasty (PTCA), also called balloon **angioplasty**, is now the most often perfomed heart operation. Less costly and less risky than bypass surgery, PTCA opens blood vessels in the heart that are narrowed but not completely blocked. PTCA involves a precise, time-consuming technique called *cardiac catheterization*—the threading of a narrow tube or catheter through an artery to the heart. An X ray taken with a special dye injected into the arteries reveals the location and extent of a blockage. By inflating a tiny balloon at the tip of the catheter, physicians can break up the clog and widen the narrowed artery. When they deflate the balloon, circulation is restored. Balloon angioplasties are not without risks, however, and balloon-opened arteries can clog up again.

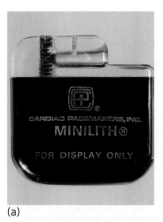 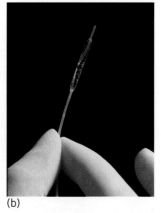

(a) (b)

Medical technology has more options now for treating heart disorders. (a) The pacemaker can be surgically implanted in the chest to deliver electrical impulses that normalize a weak or irregular heartbeat. (b) A catheter with a tiny balloon is used in balloon angioplasty to widen a clogged artery.

■ Stroke: From No Hope to New Hope

When the blood supply to a portion of the brain is blocked, a cerebrovascular accident, or **stroke**, occurs. About 500,000 people suffer strokes each year,

Strategies for Prevention

How to Prevent a Stroke

✔ Quit smoking. Smokers have twice the risk of stroke that nonsmokers have. When they quit, their risk drops 50% in 2 years. Within 5 years after quitting, their risk is nearly the same as nonsmokers.

✔ Keep blood pressure under control. Treating hypertension with medication can lead to a 40% reduction in fatal and nonfatal strokes.

✔ Eat a low-fat, low-cholesterol diet, which reduces your risk of fatty buildup in blood vessels.

✔ Avoid obesity, which burdens the blood vessels as well as the heart.

✔ Exercise. Moderate amounts of exercise improve circulation and may help dissolve deposits in the blood vessels that can lead to stroke.

and strokes rank third, after heart disease and cancer, as a cause of death in this country. After decades of steady decline, the number of strokes per year has begun to rise. The main reasons seem to be that more Americans are living longer, advanced medical care is allowing more people to survive heart disease, and doctors are better able to diagnose and detect strokes. Yet 80% of strokes are preventable, and key risk factors can be modified through either lifestyle changes or drugs.[18]

Risk factors for strokes, like those for heart disease, include some that can't be changed (such as gender and race) and some that can be controlled:

● *Gender.* Men have a greater risk of stroke than women do.

● *Race.* African Americans have a much greater risk of stroke than whites do. Hispanics also are more likely to develop hemorrhagic strokes than whites.[19]

● *Age.* A person's risk of stroke more than doubles every decade after age 55.

● *Hypertension.* Detection and treatment of high blood pressure are the best means of stroke prevention.

● *High red blood cell count.* A moderate to marked increase in the number of a person's red blood cells increases the risk of stroke.

● *Heart disease.* Heart problems can interfere with the flow of blood to the brain; clots that form in the heart can travel to the brain, where they may clog an artery.

● *Blood fats.* Although the standard advice from cardiologists is to lower harmful LDL levels, what may be more important for stroke risk is a drop in the levels of protective HDL.

● *Diabetes mellitus.* Diabetics have a higher incidence of stroke than nondiabetics.

Understanding Cancer

The declining rate of cancer deaths does not stem from research breakthroughs or development of a "magic bullet" to cure cancer. Most of the gains that have been made are the result of changes in lifestyle—most important, a reduction in smoking. Among white males, who have reduced smoking more than other groups in recent years, lung cancer death rates have dropped by more than 6%. Among white women, who have increased smoking, death rates from lung cancer have risen 6%.

Early detection also is helping to save lives. Thanks to refinements in diagnostic tests for breast cancer, for instance, tumors as small as 2 centimeters can now be detected; just a few years ago, only 3-centimeter tumors could be spotted on mammograms. This may be one reason why mortality rates from breast cancer also have dropped in the 1990s.[20]

The National Cancer Institute (NCI) estimates that approximately 7.4 million Americans alive today have a history of cancer. About 1,382,400 new cancers of various types (excepting basal and squamous-cell skin cancers) will be diagnosed this year. In the course of a lifetime, men in the United States have a one in two lifetime risk of developing cancer; for women, the risk is one in three.[21]

The uncontrolled growth and spread of abnormal cells cause cancer. Normal cells follow the code of instructions embedded in DNA (the body's genetic material); cancer cells do not. Think of the DNA within the nucleus of a cell as a computer program that controls the cell's functioning, including its ability to grow and reproduce itself. If this program or its operation is altered, the cell goes out of control. The nucleus no longer regulates growth. The abnormal cell divides to create other abnormal cells, which again divide, eventually forming **neoplasms** (new formations), or tumors.

Tumors can be either *benign* (slightly abnormal, not considered life-threatening) or *malignant* (cancerous). The only way to determine whether a tumor is benign is by microscopic examination of its cells. Cancer cells have larger nuclei than the cells in benign tumors. They vary more in shape and size and they divide more often.

Without treatment, cancer cells continue to grow, crowding out and replacing healthy cells. This process is called **infiltration**, or invasion. They may also **metastasize**, or spread to other parts of the body via the bloodstream or lymphatic system. For many cancers, as many as 60% of patients may have metastases (which may be too small to be felt or seen without a microscope) at the time of diagnosis.

Although all cancers have similar characteristics, each is distinct. Some cancers are relatively simple to

cure, whereas others are more threatening and mysterious. The earlier any cancer is found, the easier it is to treat and the better the patient's chances of survival. Cancers are classified according to the type of cell and the organ in which they originate, such as the following:

- *Carcinoma,* the most common kind, which starts in the epithelium, the layers of cells that cover the body's surface or line internal organs and glands.

- *Sarcomas,* which form in the supporting, or connective, tissues of the body: bones, muscles, blood vessels.

- *Leukemias,* which begin in the blood-forming tissues (bone marrow, lymph nodes, and the spleen).

- *Lymphomas,* which arise in the cells of the lymph system, the network that filters out impurities.

Leading Sites of New Cancer Cases and Deaths — U.S. 1998 Estimates

Figure 10-6

Some cancers appear to be on the rise, possibly because of environmental factors—and possibly because we now have the tests and the general awareness to be able to detect more cancers.

	Cancer Cases by Site and Sex*	Cancer Deaths by Site and Sex
Prostate	184,500	39,200
Lung	91,400	93,100
Colon and Rectum	64,200	27,900
Bladder	39,500	8,400
Lymphoma	34,800	13,700
Oral	20,600	5,300
Melanoma of the Skin	33,800	19,300
Kidney	17,600	7,100
Leukemia	16,100	12,000
Pancreas	14,100	14,000
Stomach	14,300	8,100
Larynx	9,000	3,400
Esophagus	9,300	9,100
Liver	9,300	7,900
Brain	9,800	7,300
All Sites	627,900	294,200

	Cancer Cases by Site and Sex*	Cancer Deaths by Site and Sex
Breast	178,700	43,500
Lung	80,100	67,000
Colon and Rectum	67,000	28,400
Uterus	13,700	4,900
Ovary	25,400	14,500
Bladder	14,900	4,100
Lymphoma	27,700	12,600
Oral	9,700	2,700
Melanoma of the Skin	19,300	3,400
Kidney	12,300	4,500
Leukemia	12,600	9,600
Pancreas	14,900	14,900
Liver	4,600	5,100
Brain	7,600	6,000
Stomach	8,300	5,600
Multiple Myeloma	6,600	5,500
All Sites	600,700	270,600

* Excluding basal and squamous-cell skin cancer and carcinoma in situ.

SOURCE: American Cancer Society, *Cancer Facts and Figures*, 1998.

Strategies for Prevention

The Seven Warning Signs of Cancer

If you note any of the following seven warning signs, immediately schedule an appointment with your doctor:

✔ **C**hange in bowel or bladder habits.

✔ **A** sore that doesn't heal.

✔ **U**nusual bleeding or discharge.

✔ **T**hickening or lump in the breast, testis, or elsewhere.

✔ **I**ndigestion or difficulty swallowing.

✔ **O**bvious change in a wart or mole.

✔ **N**agging cough or hoarseness.

After years of rising steadily, cancer incidence rates have begun to decline. In 1998 the National Cancer Institute and the American Cancer Society announced the first sustained decline in cancer mortality since national recordkeeping began in the 1930s. Since 1990 there have been declines in the incidence of cancers of the lung, prostate, colon-rectum, urinary bladder, and leukemia. Death rates for the four major cancers—lung, breast, prostate, colon-rectum—also decreased significantly.

Cancer Risk Factors That You Cannot Control

No one is immune from cancer, but many factors can influence an individual's risk.

Heredity

Heredity may account for about 10% of all cancers, and an estimated 13 to 14 million Americans may be at risk. Yet most people—and many physicians who haven't kept up with the dramatic breakthroughs in cancer genetics in recent years—don't realize that a person's genetic legacy can be a significant risk factor.[22]

In hereditary cancers, such as retinoblastoma (an eye cancer that strikes young children) or certain colon cancers, a specific cancer-causing gene is passed down from generation to generation. The odds of any child with one affected parent inheriting this gene and developing the cancer are fifty-fifty. In familial cancers, close relatives develop the same types of cancer, but no one knows exactly how the disease is transmitted. In the future, genetic tests may be able to identify individuals who are born with an increased susceptibility. Tracing cancers through a family tree is one simple way of checking your own risk.

Race and Culture

Cancer rates vary greatly among different ethnic and racial groups and in different cultures. In the United States, the cancer rate among African Americans is higher than that among whites, and a higher proportion of African Americans who get cancer die from the disease. The American Cancer Society (ACS) estimates that at least half of the differences in survival rates between African Americans and whites is due to poor access to medical care and late diagnosis of cancer among people who are economically disadvantaged.

An ACS study found that fewer public information materials are available in Spanish and that Latinos are less aware of symptoms and signs of cancer than are whites or African Americans. In addition, Latinos express greater fear of cancer and view it as a death sentence that they can do little, if anything, to change. This "fatalismo" may explain why, in three studies of women with cancer, the Latinos delayed seeking care for cancer-related symptoms or didn't go to the doctor until their symptoms were more advanced. Vietnamese-American women, whose cervical cancer rate is three times higher than it is for Caucasian Americans, also are less likely to undergo regular checkups and Pap smears.[23]

Viruses

Researchers have long known that viruses can cause tumors in animals, but only recently have they shown a connection between several different viruses and cancer in humans. Viruses have been implicated in certain leukemias (cancers of the blood system) and lymphomas (cancers of the lymphatic system), cancers of the nose and pharynx, liver cancer, and cervical cancer. Human immunodeficiency virus (HIV) can lead to certain lymphomas and leukemias and to a type of cancer called Kaposi's sarcoma. Human papilloma virus (HPV) has been linked to an increased risk of cervical cancer and cancer of the penis.[24]

Environmental Risks

Many chemicals used in industry today are carcinogens, and employees as well as people living near a factory that creates smoke, dust, or gases are at risk. Among the known dangers are nickel, chromate, asbestos, and vinyl chloride.

Three to five percent of all cancers might be caused by radiation, including medical, occupational, and environmental exposures. Large doses clearly cause cancer; the effects of lower doses are not as clear. Among those at greater risk are workers at and residents near nuclear facilities, pregnant women and their fetuses, and children exposed to nuclear fallout.

Cancer Risk Factors That You Can Control

Environmental factors may cause between 80% and 90% of cancers and, at least in theory, can be prevented by avoiding cancer-causing substances (such as tobacco and sunlight) or using substances that protect against cancer-causing factors (such as antioxidants and vitamin D).[25] How do you start protecting yourself? Simple changes in lifestyle—not smoking, protecting yourself from the sun, exercising regularly—are essential (see Pulsepoints: "Ten Ways to Protect Yourself from Cancer" for practical guidelines).

Cancer-Smart Nutrition

In a review of 156 studies linking diet to cancer, researchers found "extraordinarily consistent scientific evidence" that fruits and vegetables protect against a variety of cancers, including tumors of the breast, cervix, ovary, endometrium, lung, stomach, colon, bladder, pancreas, esophagus, mouth and larynx.[26] Which fruits and veggies are best? Researchers have identified beneficial antioxidants in many fresh fruits and vegetables, as well as specific cancer-blocking compounds in broccoli and other *crucifers*, such as brussels sprouts, cauliflower, and cabbage, and other potentially protective phytochemicals in carrots, greens (spinach, chicory, kale), tomatoes, and citrus fruits (see Chapter 5 on nutrition). However, your best bet is eating as many different types of fruits and vegetables as possible—for a total of five to nine servings a day.[27]

Another way to lower your cancer risk is to reduce the fat in your diet. There is solid evidence that cutting back on fat can lower the risks of colon, ovarian, and pancreatic cancer.[28] Pay attention to food processing

Pulsepoints

Ten Ways to Protect Yourself from Cancer

1. Don't smoke. Cigarette smoke is the number-one carcinogen in this country, responsible for one in every three cancers.

2. Stay out of the sun. Wearing sunscreen (with a Sun Protection Factor of at least 15) is better than not using any, but protective clothing is better—and staying in the shade is best.

3. Limit your intake of alcohol. Heavy drinkers are more likely to develop oral cancer and cancers of the larynx, throat, esophagus, liver, and breast.

4. Watch your weight. Obesity increases the risks of several cancers, including endometrial cancer and, particularly among postmenopausal women, breast cancer.

5. Get moving. Exercise—the heart strengthener and stamina builder—also can reduce the risk of colon can-

cer. Women who exercised early in life are less likely to develop breast cancer as adults.

6. Be sexually cautious. Cervical cancer has been linked with intercourse at an early age, multiple sex partners, and infection with the human papilloma virus (HPV), the virus that causes genital warts. The incidence of prostate cancer in men increases with multiple sexual partners and a history of frequent sexually transmitted diseases.

7. Check yourself out. Scan your skin for suspicious moles every month. If you're a woman, examine your breasts. If you're a man, check your testicles. Follow ACS recommendations for other cancer checkups.

8. Protect yourself from possible environmental carcinogens. Many chemicals used in industry can increase

the risk to employees and people living near a factory that creates smoke, dust, or gases. Follow safety precautions at work and check with local environmental protection officials about possible hazards in your community.

9. Watch what you eat. Cut down on fat; eat more fruits, vegetables, and whole grains. High-fat foods have been linked to several cancers, including breast, prostate, colon. Fruits, vegetables, and grains are rich in potentially protective antioxidants.

10. Inform yourself. Know the warning signs of cancer (see page 204), and see a physician if you develop any of them. Find out about any history of cancer in your family. Even though heredity accounts for a relatively small percentage of cancer cases, the more you know about potential risks, the more you can do to protect yours.

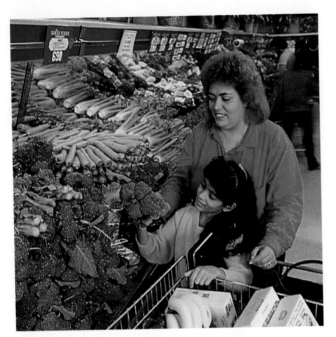

Eating cruciferous vegetables, including broccoli, brussels sprouts, and cabbage, can help reduce your cancer risk.

and preparation as well. Whenever possible, select foods close to their natural state, grown locally and without pesticides. Avoid cured, pickled, or smoked meats. When cooking, try not to fry or barbecue often;

Strategies for Prevention

Eating to Reduce Your Cancer Risk

✔ Eat at least five servings of fruits and vegetables a day: at least one rich in vitamin A (e.g., cantaloupe, carrots, spinach, or sweet potatoes), at least one high in vitamin C (e.g., grapefruit, oranges, cauliflower, or green peppers), at least one high-fiber selection (e.g., winter squash, corn, figs, or apples).

✔ Have cabbage family (cruciferous) vegetables several times a week.

✔ Don't fry or barbecue often. Safer cooking methods are baking, boiling, steaming, microwaving, poaching, and roasting.

✔ Choose foods without added chemicals or pesticides. Whenever possible, select foods that are close to their natural state, grown locally, and freshly picked.

these cooking methods can produce mutagens that induce cancer in animals.

Cigarette Smoke and Environmental Tobacco Smoke

Cigarette smoking is the single most devastating and preventable cause of cancer deaths in the United States. People who smoke two or more packs of cigarettes a day are fifteen to twenty-five times more likely to die of cancer than are nonsmokers. Cigarettes cause most cases of lung cancer and increase the risk of cancer of the mouth, pharynx, larynx, esophagus, pancreas, and bladder. Pipes, cigars, and smokeless tobacco also increase the danger of cancers of the mouth and throat.

Environmental tobacco smoke can increase the risk of cancer even among those who've never smoked. For example, researchers have found that exposure to others' tobacco smoke for as little as 3 hours a day can increase the risk of developing cancer threefold.[29]

Possible Carcinogens

Although it may not be possible to avoid all possible **carcinogens** (cancer-causing chemicals), you can take steps to minimize your danger. Many chemicals used in industry, including nickel, chromate, asbestos, and vinyl chloride, are carcinogens, and employees as well as people living near a factory that creates smoke, dust, or gases are at risk. If your job involves their use, follow safety precautions at work. If you are concerned about possible hazards in your community, check with local environmental protection officials.

Chemoprevention

In recent years scientists have focused on what has long seemed revolutionary: **chemoprevention**, the use of natural or laboratory-made substances to reduce the risk of developing cancer. Many of these substances resemble or are isolated from compounds found in foods. They are believed to work by halting or reversing the process by which a cell becomes cancerous.

To identify possible chemopreventive agents, scientists analyze data from studies of selected groups of people—for example, those with a lower than average rate of cancer—to determine whether they eat large amounts of certain types of foods. They then isolate compounds from these foods and test them in animals or in human cancer cells grown in the laboratory to see whether the compounds might halt or reverse the process of cancer development. If a substance shows promise, researchers may then evaluate it in clinical trials.

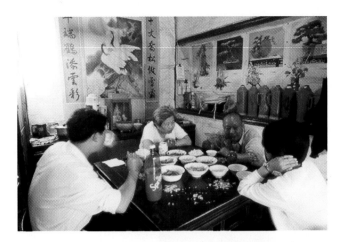

Chemoprevention is a growing area of study. Researchers seek to understand how dietary supplements lowered cancer risk in China but may have slightly increased certain cancer risks in Finland.

What to Do If You're High Risk

The only way of knowing if you are at risk for hereditary cancers is by learning your family history. Ask parents, aunts, uncles, and cousins whether close relatives developed cancer, which types, and at what age. If you discover several cases, talk with your physician, who may recommend genetic counseling, which is available at university medical centers throughout the country, or DNA tests to reveal whether family members have inherited specific genes that greatly increase their likelihood of developing cancer. (These tests are not recommended for the general population.) Table 10-2 presents a list of screening guidelines for high-risk individuals.

Types of Cancer

Cancer refers to a group of more than 100 diseases characterized by abnormal cell growth. The most common are discussed in the following sections.

Skin Cancer

Sunlight is the primary culprit in the 600,000 new cases of skin cancer that develop every year. Most damage is caused by exposure to the B range of ultraviolet light (UVB); the longer wavelength of light known as UVA also may be damaging to the skin. Tanning salons or sunlamps also increase the risk of skin cancer because they produce ultraviolet radiation. A half-hour dose of radiation from a sunlamp can be equivalent to the amount you'd get from an entire day in the sun (see Figure 10-7).

The most common skin cancers are basal-cell (involving the base of the epidermis, the top level of the skin) and squamous-cell (involving cells in the epider-

Strategies for Prevention

Scanning Your Skin

Here's how to screen yourself for possible changes that may indicate skin cancer:

✔ Once a month, stand in front of a full-length mirror to examine your front and back, and your left and right sides with your arms raised. Check the backs of your legs, the tops and soles of your feet, and the surfaces between your toes. Use a hand mirror to check the back of your neck, behind your ears, and your scalp.

✔ Watch for changes in the size, color, number, and thickness of moles. Suspicious moles are likely to be asymmetrical (one half doesn't match the other), with ragged, notched, or blurred edges. Also look for any signs of darkly pigmented growth, oozing, scaliness, bleeding, or a change in sensation, itchiness, tenderness, or pain.

✔ Don't put too much faith in sunscreens. Wearing sunscreen (with a Sun Protection Factor, or SPF, of at least 15) is good, but protective clothing is better—and staying in the shade is best.[30]

✔ Check your shadow. One simple guideline for reducing the risk of skin cancer risk is avoiding the sun anytime your shadow is shorter than you are. According to NCI, this shadow method—based on the principle that the closer the sun comes to being directly overhead, the stronger its ultraviolet rays—works for any location and at any time of year.

✔ Check for photosensitivity. If you are taking any drugs, ask your doctor or pharmacist to see if the medication could make you more sensitive to sun damage. Be especially cautious about sun exposure if you have been using a synthetic preparation derived from vitamin A (Retin A) as an acne or antiwrinkle treatment; it can increase your susceptibility.

mis). Smoking and exposure to certain hydrocarbons in asphalt, coal tar, and pitch may increase the risk of squamous-cell skin cancer. Both types can usually be treated with surgery. However, individuals who develop such cancers are at higher risk for developing subsequent tumors of the same type.

The incidence of the deadliest type, malignant melanoma, is rising by 4% to 5% per year. The overall risk of getting melanoma for Americans is about 1 in 120, but the risk increases for individuals with any of the following characteristics:

- Blond or red hair.

- Marked freckling of the upper back.

- Rough red bumps on the skin called actinic keratoses.

- A family history of melanoma.

- Three or more blistering sunburns in the teenage years.

- Three or more years at an outdoor summer job as a teenager.

Any one or two of these factors increases a person's risk of melanoma three or four times. A combination of three or more factors increases the risk twenty to twenty-five times. Other risk factors include occupational exposure to carcinogens and inherited skin disorders, such as xeroderma pigmentosum and familial atypical multiple-mole melanoma.

TABLE 10-2   WHAT TO LOOK FOR

Cancer	On your own	At the doctor's Test	What the test reveals
Breast	Lumps, swelling, or other changes found in manual self-exam	Mammogram yearly for women over 40; clinical manual exam	Lumps, swelling, or other abnormalities
Cervical	Unusual vaginal bleeding or discharge	Pap smear yearly	Precancerous or cancerous cells
Colorectal	Blood in the stool, change in bowel habits such as persistent and unexplainable diarrhea or constipation	Starting at age 50, digital rectal exam every 5 years	Lumps or lesions or other rectal abnormalities
		Fecal occult blood test yearly	Blood in the stool
		Sigmoidoscopy every 5 years	Unusual growths or lesions
Oral	Persistent sores or other lesions in the mouth or on the lips	Visual exam by a doctor or dentist yearly	Oral lesions
Prostate	Change in urinary habits, such as difficulty urinating (The cause is usually benign prostate enlargement, but the symptoms could indicate prostate cancer.)	Starting by age 50, digital rectal exam	Swelling of the prostate gland, lumps, or other abnormalities
		Prostate-specific antigen (PSA) test	Elevated levels of prostate-specific antigen (a protein produced by prostate cells), which may indicate prostate cancer
Skin	Changes or irregularities in the size of moles; unusual growths	Visual exam by a doctor every year for those over 40; every 3 years for ages 20–40.	Changes or irregularities in moles; precancerous lesions

SOURCE: *American Health,* September 1995.

Figure 10-7

Three types of skin cancer. Squamous-cell cancer; malignant melanoma, the deadliest form of skin cancer; and basal-cell cancer.

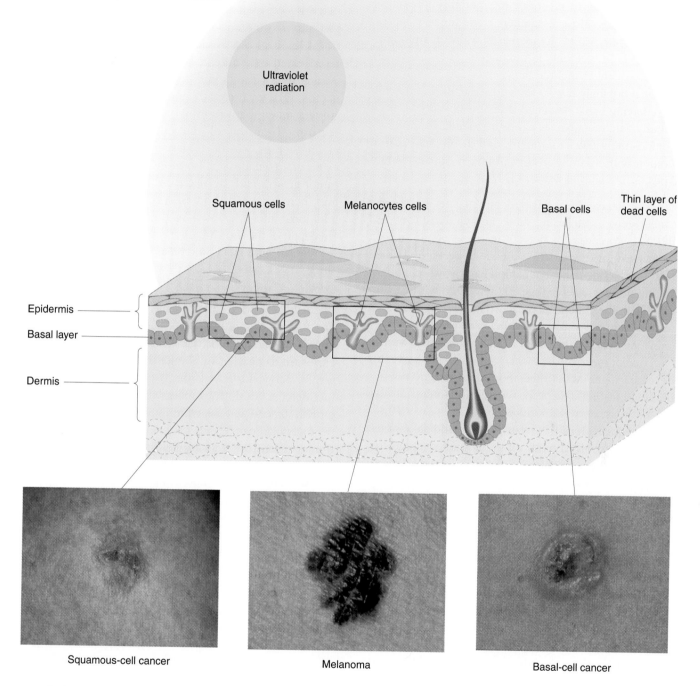

Ultraviolet radiation

Squamous cells

Melanocytes cells

Basal cells

Thin layer of dead cells

Epidermis

Basal layer

Dermis

Squamous-cell cancer

Melanoma

Basal-cell cancer

If detected early, melanoma is highly curable. However, once a tumor is thicker than an eighth of an inch—about the thickness of a dime—it probably has metastasized. Treatment may consist of surgery, radiation, electrodesiccation (tissue destruction by heat), cryosurgery (tissue destruction by cold), or a combination of these therapies. Individuals who've had melanoma may be at high risk for developing this cancer again.[31]

Breast Cancer

The disease American women fear most, according to a survey commissioned by the National Council on the Aging, is breast cancer. Yet, the number-one killer of

American women is heart disease, which claims the lives of one in every two women in the United States. By comparison, breast cancer accounts for 4% of annual deaths.[32] Although the incidence of breast cancer has remained steady in recent years, mortality rates have been declining. Most researchers credit the statistics on improved survival to the increased use of mammography and improvements in treatments. The risk factors for breast cancer include being over age 50, having a personal or family history of the disease, having no children, having had a first child after age 30, early onset of puberty, late menopause, exposure to radiation, obesity (for postmenopausal women), and in premenopausal women with a family history of breast cancer, certain types of benign breast disease.

Causes   Researchers have identified specific "breast cancer genes," including those known as BRCA1 and BRCA2. Women with defects in these genes have a greater risk of cancer than others. On average, women with at least one genetic mutation have a 56% chance of getting breast cancer by age 70 (compared with 13% for women in the general population) and a 16% chance of ovarian cancer (compared with 1.6%). However, genes aren't the only determinant of cancer risk, and a woman with one or more breast cancer genes will not inevitably develop cancer. At this time, most physicians do not recommend testing except for women in families at high risk of breast or ovarian cancer.[33]

The question of risk related to diet and alcohol use remains unresolved, with different studies suggesting different degrees of risk. There also is continuing controversy over the role of postmenopausal hormone replacement therapy (HRT) and an increased risk of breast cancer. Some studies have found an increased risk as high as 30% to 70%, whereas others have found no increased risk of breast cancer.[34]

Detection   To detect lumps or changes that could signal breast cancer, all women should perform monthly breast self-exams 7 to 10 days after their periods (see Figure 10-8) and have a professional breast exam yearly if over 40 and every 3 years if between ages 20 and 40.

The best tool for early detection is the diagnostic X-ray exam called **mammography**. Overall, screening mammograms could reduce breast cancer deaths by 25%. Mammograms can detect a tumor 2 to 3 years before it can be detected by manual exam. Although annual mammograms have long been routinely recommended for women over 50, there's been considerable controversy over screening recommendations for women in their forties. Ultimately, in March 1997, the ACS and

National Cancer Society recommended that all women begin routine mammographic screening by age 40.[35]

Treatment   If a mammogram detects a lump or suspicious area, a tissue biopsy is performed to confirm the diagnosis of cancer. Depending on the size and site of the tumor, surgeons may recommend **lumpectomy** (local removal of a tumor and surrounding tissue) or more extensive surgery, such as a **quadrantectomy** (which removes a larger area of the breast and lymph glands). These "breast-conserving" procedures lead to survival rates that are equal to those following **mastectomy** (removal of the entire breast). Followup chemotherapy with a drug such as tamoxifen blocks estrogens (female sex hormones) that can stimulate tumor growth and can decrease the risk of recurrences and increase survival times.[36] The use of adjuvant, or additional, therapies, such as the monoclonal antibody Herceptin or the drug Taxol, has extended survival times for women with metastatic breast cancer.

Cervical Cancer

The risk factors for cervical cancer include early age of first intercourse, multiple sex partners, genital herpes, human papilloma virus (HPV) infection, and significant exposure to passive smoking. The standard screening test for cervical cancer is the Pap smear. Each year this test detects about 1.2 million cases of abnormal cell growth. Since Pap tests were introduced, the death rate from cervical cancer has decreased by 70%. However, they can fail to detect cancerous cells in as many as 20%–40% of the women tested.

Warning signs for cervical cancer include irregular bleeding or unusual vaginal discharge. In precancerous stages, cervical cells may be destroyed by laser surgery or freezing in a doctor's office. More advanced cancer may require more extensive surgery, sometimes in combination with chemotherapy or radiation.[37]

Ovarian Cancer

Ovarian cancer is the leading cause of death from gynecological cancers, with 24,000 new cases diagnosed and 13,600 deaths each year. Risk factors include a family history of ovarian cancer; personal history of breast cancer; obesity; infertility (because the abnormality that interferes with conception may also play a role in cancer development); and low levels of transferase, an enzyme involved in the metabolism of dairy foods. Often women develop no obvious symptoms until the advanced stages, although they may experience painless swelling of the abdomen, irregular bleeding, lower

Looking

Stand in front of a mirror with your upper body unclothed. Look for changes in the shape and size of the breast, and for dimpling of the skin or "pulling in" of the nipples. Any changes in the breast may be made more noticeable by a change in position of the body or arms. Look for any of the above signs or for changes in shape from one breast to the other.

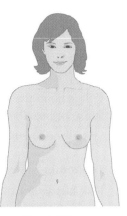 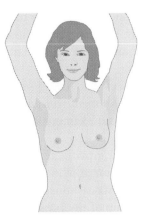 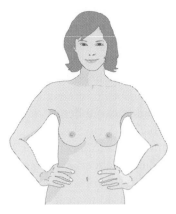

1. Stand with your arms down.

2. Raise your arms overhead.

3. Place your hands on your hips and tighten your chest and arm muscles by pressing firmly.

Feeling

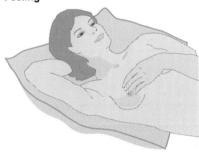 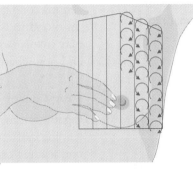 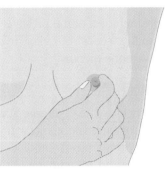

1. Lie flat on your back. Place a pillow or towel under one shoulder and raise that arm over your head. With the opposite hand, you'll feel with the pads, not the fingertips, of the three middle fingers for lumps or any change in the texture of the breast or skin.

2. The area you'll examine is from your collarbone to your bra line and from your breastbone to the center of your armpit. Imagine the area divided into vertical strips. Using small circular motions (the size of a dime), move your fingers up and down the strips. Apply light, medium, and deep pressure to examine each spot. Repeat this same process for your other breast.

3. Gently squeeze the nipple of each breast between your thumb and index finger. Any discharge, clear or bloody, should be reported to your doctor immediately.

Figure 10-8

Breast self-exam. The best time to examine your breasts is after your menstrual periods, every month.

abdominal pain, digestive and urinary abnormalities, fatigue, backache, bloating, and weight gain.

Colon and Rectal Cancer

Colon and rectal cancer claims about 60,000 lives a year. Most cases occur after age 50 and slightly more often among women than men. Risk factors include a personal or family history of colon and rectal cancer, polyps (growths) in the colon or rectum, and ulcerative colitis. Early signs of colorectal cancer are bleeding from the rectum, blood in the stool, or a change in bowel habits.

Treatment may involve surgery, radiation therapy, or chemotherapy. Regular exercise can lower the risk of colon and rectal cancer in both men and women. Hormone replacement after menopause may significantly reduce women's risk of colon cancer.[38]

Prostate Cancer

Prostate cancer is the most frequently diagnosed non-skin cancer among American men, with an estimated 200,000 new cases each year.[39] African-American men have the highest rate of prostate cancer in the world; their death rate from this cancer is twice that of white men.[40]

The risk of prostate cancer increases with age, family history, exposure to the heavy metal cadmium, high number of sexual partners, and history of frequent sexually transmitted diseases. (Researchers have found no evidence that vasectomies might increase prostate cancer risk, as had once been thought.) Saturated fats, those in animal products like butter and meat, do greatly increase the risk of prostate cancer.

Men whose brothers or fathers had the disease should begin screening at age 40. All men over age 50 should also undergo an annual rectal examination, in which a doctor inserts a gloved finger into the rectum and feels the prostate for abnormal growths that may indicate cancer. A chemoprevention trial is looking at the possible preventive benefits of Proscar (finasteride), a drug used to treat benign swelling of the prostate, a common problem in aging men.

Early warning signs of prostate cancer are frequent or difficult urination, blood in the urine, painful ejaculation, or constant lower back pain. Treatments include surgical removal of the prostate, conventional radiation, implanting "seeds" of radioactive iodine in the prostate, and hormone therapy.

Testicular Cancer

This cancer is not common, accounting for only 3% of cancers of the male genitals and urinary tract. What is more, it occurs mostly among young men between the ages of 18 and 35, who are not normally at risk of cancer. At highest risk are men with an undescended testicle (a condition that is almost always corrected in childhood to prevent this danger). To detect possibly

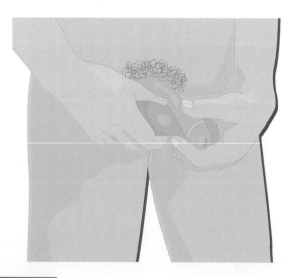

Figure 10-9

Testicular self-exam. The best time to examine your testicles is after a hot bath or shower, when the scrotum is most relaxed. Place your index and middle fingers under each testicle and the thumb on top, and roll the testicle between the thumb and fingers. If you feel a small, hard, usually painless lump or swelling, or anything unusual, consult a urologist.

cancerous growths, men should perform monthly testicular self-exams, as shown in Figure 10-9. Often the first sign of this cancer is a slight enlargement of one testicle. There also may be a change in the way it feels when touched. Sometimes men with testicular cancer report a dull ache in the lower abdomen or groin, along with a sense of heaviness or sluggishness. Lumps on the testicles also may indicate cancer.

Leukemia

Risk factors for this cancer of the blood include Down syndrome and other inherited abnormalities and excessive exposure to radiation or certain chemicals, such as benzene. Leukemia can be difficult to detect early because its symptoms are often similar to those of less serious conditions, such as influenza. Diagnosis is based on blood tests and a bone-marrow biopsy. Treatment may involve chemotherapy, drugs, blood transfusions, and bone-marrow transplants.

Lung Cancer

Cigarettes cause most cases of lung cancer, which is the leading cause of cancer deaths in women and the second leading cause in men. Risk factors include smoking for 20 or more years; exposure to certain industrial substances, particularly asbestos; passive smoking; radiation exposure; and radon exposure. A smoker's risk of developing lung cancer drops almost to that of a nonsmoker within 10 years after his or her last cigarette, although the lungs may still be damaged.

Lung cancer is very difficult to detect early. Warning signs include a persistent cough, sputum streaked with blood, chest pain, recurring bronchitis, or pneumonia. Diagnosis is based on a chest X ray, sputum cytology (cell) testing, and fiber-optic bronchoscopy (direct examination of the lungs by means of a specially lighted tube). Treatment generally involves surgery, chemotherapy, and/or radiation.

Oral Cancer

Heavy smoking of cigarettes, cigars, or pipes; excessive drinking; and the use of chewing tobacco increase the risk of oral cancer. Those who drink as well as smoke are particularly vulnerable. Early signs include a mouth sore that bleeds easily and doesn't heal; a lump or thickening; a reddish or whitish patch; and difficulty chewing, swallowing, or moving the tongue or jaws. Regular exams by your dentist or primary care physician can detect oral cancers. Surgery and radiation are the standard treatments.

New Hope Against Cancer

Because of advances in diagnosis and treatment, cancer is no longer a death sentence. Cancer survivors make up one of the fastest growing groups in the United States. Many have had no evidence of cancer for 5 years. Others survive in remission, a state in which patients have no symptoms, and the spread of cancerous cells is assumed to be temporarily stopped.

Cancer Therapy

The following are the primary forms of treatment for cancer:

- *Surgery* to remove a tumor and surrounding cells. The oldest and most widely used approach, surgery is most effective for small localized cancers.

- *Radiation therapy*, which exposes the involved area of the body to powerful radiation, which destroys cancer cells. Radiation therapy is sometimes used as an adjuvant, or supplementary, treatment along with surgery or chemotherapy.

- *Chemotherapy*, which uses powerful drugs or hormones, taken orally or through injection, to interfere with the reproduction of fast-multiplying cancer cells.

- *Immunotherapy*, which stimulates the body's own immune system to attack cancer cells.

Another treatment, **bone-marrow transplantation**, involves extremely high doses of radiation or, increasingly, chemotherapy to kill cancer cells; however, the marrow in the patient's body is also destroyed. The patient then receives healthy bone-marrow cells, either his or her own (which may have undergone treatment in a laboratory) or a carefully matched donor's. *Autologous* transplants (those using the person's own blood) have produced long-term survival rates of more than 50% for certain leukemias and lymphomas (cancer of the immune system). They're also being used experimentally in treating other cancers, including breast and ovarian tumors.

Other Chronic Diseases

Other noninfectious diseases besides heart disease and cancer have a debilitating effect on many people. But most of the diseases in this section can be controlled, if not cured.

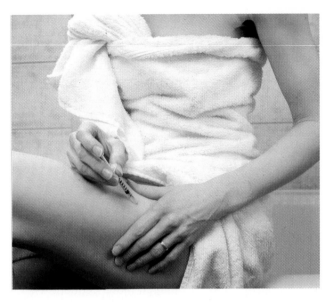

Many diabetics control their disease by injecting themselves with insulin.

Diabetes Mellitus

About 14 million Americans have **diabetes mellitus,** a disease in which the pancreas doesn't produce or respond properly to insulin, the hormone that regulates carbohydrate and fat metabolism. Without insulin, the glucose in the blood is unable to enter most body cells, so the cells' energy needs are not met.

In those with *insulin-dependent diabetes* (Type 1), insulin secretion is nonexistent. This form of diabetes usually occurs in childhood or young adulthood, and it requires the administration of insulin for life. *Non-insulin-dependent diabetes* (Type 2) usually occurs in people over age 30. Those at highest risk include relatives of diabetics and obese people. This form of diabetes can often be controlled with changes in diet and exercise, along with medication. The early signs of diabetes are frequent urination, excessive thirst, weakness, and a craving for sweets and starches.

Before the development of insulin injections, diabetes was a fatal illness. Today diabetics usually have normal lifespans. However, both types of diabetes can lead to serious complications, including increased risk of heart attack or stroke, kidney failure, blindness, and lack of circulation to the extremities. Diabetes claims more than 100,000 women's lives a year—more than the number who succumb to breast cancer.[41] Several minority groups, especially African Americans, Native Americans, and Latinos, are at especially high risk of developing diabetes.

Asthma

Some 14 to 15 million Americans, including 4.8 million children, suffer from **asthma**, a disease characterized by constriction of the breathing passages.[42] Asthma rates have skyrocketed in the last two decades. The problem is especially severe in inner cities, where emergency room visits and asthma mortality rates run as high as eight times the national average.[43] Symptoms of asthma include wheezing, coughing, shortness of breath, and chest tightness.

The two main approaches to asthma treatment are control of the underlying inflammation by means of anti-inflammatory drugs and short-term relief of symptoms with bronchodilators, which expand breathing passages. In its most recent guidelines, the National Heart, Lung, and Blood Institute encouraged more frequent use of inhaled steroids and less reliance on bronchodilators, which have little effect on the underlying inflammation.

Disorders of the Liver

Cirrhosis is characterized by significant loss of liver cells and the formation of scar tissue that can interfere with circulation in the liver. A major cause of cirrhosis is chronic alcoholism. Each year, about 30,000 Americans die of alcohol-related liver disorders.

Early signs of liver damage include an enlarged liver (which your doctor can feel during a physical exam) and tiny, spiderlike blood vessels visible on the surface of the skin. Cirrhosis symptoms, which occur only in the advanced stages of the disease, include yellow discoloration of the skin and eyes (jaundice), accumulation of fluid in the abdomen, and mental confusion. Liver transplants are the only hope for those with advanced liver disease.

Digestive Diseases

According to the National Digestive Diseases Advisory Board, almost half of the U.S. population suffers a digestive problem at some time in their lives. Some of the most common digestive diseases are:

● *Ulcers:* Open sores that develop in the lining of the stomach or the first part of the small intestine are called **ulcers**. The major symptom is a burning pain felt throughout the upper abdomen. The pain may come and go, and it may begin either right after eating or several hours later. Risk factors include heavy use of cigarettes, alcohol, or caffeine; frequent use of aspirin or ibuprofen; and advanced age. Treat-

ments include self-help measures, drug therapy, or surgery.

● *Inflammatory Bowel Disease (IBD).* As many as 2 million Americans—many in the prime of life—suffer from one of the two forms of **inflammatory bowel disease (IBD)**: Crohn's disease, which causes inflammation anywhere in the digestive tract, and ulcerative colitis, which creates ulcers in the inner lining of the colon and rectum. Both illnesses can trigger frequent and intense diarrhea, abdominal pain, gas, fever, and rectal bleeding. Treatment for IBD consists primarily of drugs, but surgery may also be needed.

● *Irritable Bowel Syndrome.* **Irritable bowel syndrome** is a common problem caused by intestinal spasms. The muscular contractions that move waste material through the intestines become irregular and uncoordinated, causing frequent feelings of a need to defecate, nausea, cramping, pain, and gas. There is no standard medical treatment for irritable bowel syndrome; some physicians may prescribe drugs or suggest changes in diet.

● *Gallstones.* An estimated 10% of the American population have **gallstones**: clumps of solid material, usually cholesterol, that form in the gallbladder. One-third to one-half of all gallstones produce no symptoms. However some get stuck in the bile duct and cause intense pain that lasts for several hours. Gallstones may be treated with long-term drug treatment or with surgery.

Disorders of the Muscles, Joints, and Bones

More than 17 million Americans suffer from some form of **arthritis**, an inflammatory disease of the joints that takes over 100 forms. Rheumatoid arthritis is an autoimmune disease in which the body attacks its own connective tissue; it's fairly common among younger people. Degenerative arthritis, or osteoarthritis, is characterized by changes in bone tissue and cartilage at the joints. It seems to be a result of normal wear and tear; women are generally affected more often than men. Drugs can relieve arthritis pain and reduce inflammation. Surgical treatments, including joint replacement, may also be used.

Back pain, another bone and joint disorder, eventually afflicts seven of every ten adults. Risk factors for a debilitating back injury include increasing age; tense, injured, or weak muscles; extra weight; and poor lifting techniques. The lower, or lumbar, part of the spine is most vulnerable to back strain. Some back problems are caused by the protrusion (or herniation) of the soft center of a vertebral disc or by structural defects such as osteoporosis or scoliosis.

Bed rest, supplemented by moist heat or other muscle relaxants and anti-inflammatory drugs, eases most backaches. However, the days when doctors recommended 2 weeks of bed rest for a bad back are gone. After 2 or 3 days, most back patients are urged to resume walking and light activity.

Strategies for Prevention

Preventing Back Problems

✔ When standing, shift your weight from one foot to the other. If possible, place one foot on a stool, step, or railing 4 to 6 inches off the ground. Hold in your stomach, tilt your pelvis toward your back, and tuck in your buttocks to provide crucial support for the lower back.

✔ Because sitting places more stress on the lower back than standing, try to get up from your seat at least once an hour to stretch or walk around. Whenever possible, sit in a straight chair with a firm back. Avoid slouching in overstuffed chairs or dangling your legs in midair. When driving, keep the seat forward so that your knees are raised to hip level; your right leg should not be fully extended. A small pillow or towel can help support your lower back.

✔ Sleep on a flat, firm mattress. The best sleep position is on your side, with one or both knees bent at right angles to your torso. The pillow should keep your head in line with your body so that your neck isn't bent forward or to the side.

✔ When lifting, bend at the knees, not from the waist. Get close to the load. Tighten your stomach muscles, but don't hold your breath. Let your leg muscles do the work.

✔ Always warm up and stretch before a workout. Exercise regularly, but don't push yourself too hard. The activities that are easiest on the back are swimming, cycling (in an upright position), walking, and jogging (preferably not on concrete). Activities that demand sudden stops and turns (such as tennis and other racket sports) or that involve a good chance of falling (such as downhill skiing) are most likely to spell trouble for your back—and you.

✔ Don't smoke. Smoking may interfere with circulation to the lower back; and a chronic smoker's cough can be so irritating that it provokes a back spasm.

Making This Chapter Work for You
Understanding Chronic Diseases

■ Factors predisposing an individual to heart disease or stroke include risks you can control, such as lack of exercise, cigarette smoking, obesity, high blood pressure, and high cholesterol levels. Other predisposing factors include diabetes mellitus, a family history of heart disease, age, race, and to a certain degree, gender.

■ The most common form of coronary artery disease is atherosclerosis, in which blood flow is impaired as the arteries narrow and lose their ability to dilate and contract because of plaque deposits inside the arteries. A blocked artery can cause a heart attack or stroke.

■ Some people suffer from chest pains, or angina pectoris, caused by periodic and temporarily inadequate blood flow to the heart. Chest pain may also be a result of coronary artery spasms.

■ Myocardial infarction, or heart attack, occurs when heart muscle tissue in the myocardium begins to die because its supply of oxygen and other nutrients has been cut off by the blocked artery. The damage caused by a heart attack can be reduced with early treatment, including the use of clot-dissolving drugs or tiny balloons to unclog arteries (a procedure called angioplasty).

■ Other heart problems include heartbeat irregularities, or arrhythmias, congestive heart failure, and congenital defects.

■ Doctors can evaluate the heart's condition through such procedures as electrocardiography, angiography, nuclear scanning, and through various types of imaging procedures. Hypertension, heart failure, angina, and arrhythmias can be treated with drugs. Surgical treatments include coronary bypass operation and angioplasty.

■ A stroke, or cerebrovascular accident, occurs when the blood supply to the brain is restricted or blocked. Risk factors for stroke are similar to those for heart disease.

Health Online

An Introduction to Skin Cancer
http://www.maui.net/~southsky/introto.html

Did you know that it is estimated that one in seven Americans will get skin cancer at some point in their lives? This page is dedicated to skin cancer, its causes, determining personal risk, prevention, and treatment. There are many special features, like a daily UV forecast for thirty cities across the country.

Think about it ...

• What are your personal risk factors for skin cancer? What could you do to lower your chances of getting this disease?

• Check out today's UV forecast for the city nearest where you live. What does it mean? What precautions should you take, if any?

• Skin cancer cases are on the rise in the United States. Can you think of three possible reasons for this?

■ In cancer, changes in the genetic material in the cells cause normal cells to turn into abnormal cells and multiply to form malignant tumors, or neoplasms. Benign tumors are not normally life-threatening. Heredity, viral, chemical, and physical factors can cause malignant tumors.

■ Prevention is the best approach to cancer. Lifestyle changes, including not smoking, limiting sun exposure, restricting alcohol intake, eating a high-fiber, low-fat diet, and exercising, can reduce the risk of developing cancer.

■ Some common sites of cancer include the lungs, skin, breasts, female reproductive tract, prostate, colon and rectum, blood, and mouth.

■ Having regular checkups, knowing the warning signs of cancer, and performing periodic self-exams can help identify potentially cancerous changes early so treatment can begin.

■ Cancer treatment often includes chemotherapy (drug treatment), surgery, and radiation.

■ Other major chronic diseases include diabetes mellitus, asthma, liver disease, digestive diseases, and disorders of the muscles, joints, and bones such as arthritis.

Key Terms

The terms listed here are used within the chapter. Page numbers are included for each term.
A definition of each term is given in the green Glossary pages at the end of this book.

angina pectoris *198*
angioplasty *201*
antioxidants *192*
aorta *191*
arteriosclerosis *197*
arthritis *214*

asthma *214*
atherosclerosis *197*
atrium *191*
bone-marrow transplantation *213*
capillary *191*

carcinogen *206*
cardiopulmonary resuscitation (CPR) *198*
chemoprevention *206*
cholesterol *193*
cirrhosis *214*

congestive heart failure *200*
coronary angiography *201*
coronary bypass *201*
diabetes mellitus *213*
diastole *191*
electrocardiogram (ECG, EKG) *201*
gallstones *214*
hypertension *193*
infiltration *203*
inflammatory bowel disease (IBD) *214*
irritable bowel syndrome *214*
lipoproteins *193*
lumpectomy *210*
mammography *210*
mastectomy *210*
metastasize *203*
myocardial infarction (MI) *198*
neoplasm *202*
percutaneous transluminal coronary angioplasty (PTCA) *201*
quadrantectomy *210*
stroke *201*
systole *191*
thallium scintigraphy *201*
triglyceride *193*
ulcer *214*
ventricle *191*

Review Questions

1. What are the uncontrollable risk factors for cardiovascular disease? Which risk factors are controllable? What preventive steps can you take to minimize these risks?
2. What are some health effects associated with hypertension? High cholesterol? List the risk factors and any effective treatments for each.
3. What is cancer? What warning signs should a person look for?
4. What factors put a person at greater risk of developing cancer? What can be done to reduce the risk of developing some of the more common types of cancer? What can be done to increase the likelihood of early detection of cancer?
5. What are some of the treatment options available to cancer patients?
6. Name some different types of noninfectious illnesses and describe the symptoms and risk factors for each of them.

Critical Thinking Questions

1. Have you had your blood pressure and cholesterol checked lately? If either reading was high, what steps are you now taking to help reduce them?
2. A friend of yours, Karen, discovered a small lump in her breast during a routine self-examination. When she mentions it, you ask if she has seen a doctor. She tells you that she hasn't had time to schedule an appointment; besides, she isn't sure it is the kind of lump one has to worry about. What advice would you give her?
3. Because of advances in antirejection treatment, organ transplants have proven highly successful in helping many people who might otherwise have died. However, because the demand for organs to transplant greatly exceeds the supply, health experts have debated how to set priorities. Should a 30-year-old be placed higher on the waiting list than a 70-year-old? Should a nurse who contracted hepatitis on the job get priority over an alcoholic whose liver has been destroyed by cirrhosis? Who, if anyone, should make such decisions? Would a lottery system be more equitable?

Connections to Personal Health Interactive

*To enhance your understanding of the material covered in this chapter, check out the following study aids on the **Personal Health Interactive CD-ROM**.*

- Personal Insights: Is Your Heart Happy?
- Personal Insights: What Is Your Risk for Cancer?
- Heart Disease and Preventative Behavior
- **Online Research:** Heart Health
- **Online Research:** Reducing the Risk of Cancer
- Glossary & Key Term Review

References

1. Frost, R. "Cardiovascular Risk Modification in the College Student: Knowledge, Attitude, and Behaviors." *Journal of General Internal Medicine*, May–June 1992.

2. Blair, Steven, et al. "Changes in Physical Fitness and All-Cause Mortality: A Prospective Study of Healthy and Unhealthy Men." *Journal of the American Medical Association*, Vol. 273, No. 14, April 12, 1995. Lee, I-Min, et al. "Exercise Intensity and Longevity in Men: The Harvard Alumni Health Study." *Journal of the American Medical Association*, Vol. 273, No. 14, April 12, 1995.

3. Hodis, Harold, et al. "Serial Coronary Angiographic Evidence That Antioxidant Vitamin Intake Reduces Progression of Coronary Artery Atherosclerosis." *Journal of the American Medical Association*, Vol. 273, No. 23, June 21, 1995.

4. Werner, Rachel, and Thomas Pearson. "What's So Passive About Passive Smoking?" *Journal of the American Medical Association*, Vol. 278, No. 2, January 14, 1998.

5. Moore, Peter. "Passive Smoking Changes Lipid Profiles in At-Risk Children." *Lancet*, Vol. 350, No. 9070, September 6, 1997.

6. Howard, George, et al. "Cigarette Smoking and Progression of Atherosclerosis." *Journal of the American Medical Association*, Vol. 278, No. 2, January 14, 1998.

7. Manson, JoAnn, et al. "A Prospective Study of Obesity and Risk of Coronary Heart Disease in Women." *New England Journal of Medicine*, March 29, 1990.

8. Murray, Robert. "Skin Color and Blood Pressure." *Journal of the American Medical Association*, February 6, 1991.

9. National Institute on Aging, Hearts, and Arteries. *What Scientists Are Learning About Age and the Cardiovascular System*. Gaithersburg, MD: NIA Information Center, 1995.

10. Quilligan, Edward. "Obstetrics and Gynecology." *Journal of the American Medical Association*, Vol. 273, No. 21, June 7, 1995.

11. Katzenstein, Larry. "Good News About Heart Disease." *American Health*, December 1994. Hoffman, Carolyn, and Theresa Turner. "Strategies for Using University Health Services for Cholesterol Screening." *Journal of American College Health*, Vol. 43, No. 2, September 1994.

12. Katzenstein, Larry. "Reversing Heart Disease." *American Health*, November 1994.

13. "People with Heart Disease." *American Health*, June 1995.

14. Gore, Joel, and James Dalen. "Cardiovascular Disease." *Journal of the American Medical Association*, Vol. 274, No. 7, August 16, 1995.

15. "Systolic Blood Pressure." *American Health*, June 1995.

16. Dienstrey, Harris. "What Makes the Heart Healthy? A Talk with Dean Ornish." *Advances: The Journal of Mind Body Health*, Spring 1992.

17. American Heart Association.

18. McBride, Gail. "Stroke: A Prevention and Survival Kit." *American Health*, January–February 1995.

19. Henry, Brian. "Hispanics Face Higher Risk for Bleeding Strokes Than Whites, Native Americans." American Heart Association, December 1997.

20. American Cancer Society.

21. National Cancer Institute.

22. Burtness, Barbara. "Oncology and Hematology." *Journal of the American Medical Association*, Vol. 273, No. 21, June 7, 1995.

23. Miller, Jeff. "Cancer Clues." *UCSF Magazine*, Vol. 15, No. 2, November 1994.

24. National Cancer Institute. "Human Papillomavirus." *Cancer Facts*. Bethesda, MD: National Institutes of Health.

25. Osborne, Michael, et al. "Cancer Prevention." *Lancet*, Vol. 349, No. 9063, May 17, 1997. Hong, Wan Ki and Michael Sporn. "Recent Advances in Chemoprevention of Cancer." *Science*, Vol. 278, No. 5340, November 7, 1997.

26. Miller, A. B., et al. "Diet in the Aetiology of Cancer: A Review." *European Journal of Cancer*, Vol. 30A, No. 2, 1994.

27. Harnack, Lisa, et al. "Association of Cancer Prevention-Related Nutrition Knowledge, Beliefs and Attitudes to Cancer Prevention Dietary Behavior." *Journal of the American Dietetic Association*, Vol. 97, No. 7, September 1997.

28. "Food Choices May Lower Risk for Ovarian Cancer." *Tufts University Diet & Nutrition Letter,* Vol. 12, No. 11, January 1995.

29. Robinson, John, and Tibbett Speer. "The Air We Breathe." *American Demographics*, Vol. 17, No. 6, June 1995.

30. Naylor, Mark. "The Case for Sunscreens." *Journal of the American Medical Association*, Vol. 278, No. 21, December 3, 1997.

31. Marwick, Charles. "New Light on Skin Cancer Mechanisms." *Journal of the American Medical Association*, Vol. 274, No. 6, August 9, 1995. *Melanoma Research Report*. Bethesda, MD: National Institutes of Health. National Cancer Institute. *Skin Cancers: Basal Cell and Squamous Cell Carcinomas, Research Report*. Bethesda, MD: National Institutes of Health, 1994.

32. "Assessing the Odds." *Lancet*, Vol. 350, No. 9091, November 29, 1997.

33. Runowicz, Carolyn. "Breast Cancer Genes and What They Mean." *New England Journal of Medicine Health News*, June 18, 1997.

34. Colditz, G., et al. "The Use of Estrogens and Progestins and the Risk of Breast Cancer in Postmenopausal Women." *New England Journal of Medicine*, Vol. 332, May 15, 1995. Stanford, Janet, et al. "Combined Estrogen and Progestin Hormone Replacement Therapy in Relation to Risk of Breast Cancer in Middle-Aged Women." *Journal of the American Medical Association*, Vol. 274, No. 2, July 12, 1995. Adami, Hans-Olov, and Ingemar Persson. "Hormone Replacement and Breast Cancer: A Remaining Controversy?" *Journal of the American Medical Association*, Vol. 274, No. 2, July 12, 1995.

35. Woolf, Steven, and Robert Lawrence. "Lessons from the Consensus Panel on Mammography Screening." *Journal*

of the American Medical Association, Vol. 278, No. 23, December 17, 1997.

36. National Cancer Institute. *What You Need to Know About Breast Cancer*. Bethesda, MD: National Institutes of Health.

37. National Cancer Institute. *What You Need to Know About Cervical Cancer*. Bethesda, MD: National Institutes of Health.

38. Newcomb, Polly. *Journal of the National Cancer Institute*, July 19, 1995. National Cancer Institute. *What You Need to Know About Cancer of the Colon and Rectum*. Bethesda, MD: National Institutes of Health.

39. American Cancer Society.

40. "Action Proposal on Prostate Cancer in African Americans Is Issued by the American Cancer Society." American Cancer Society news release, January 13, 1998.

41. Miller, Elizabeth. "Diabetes, a Greater Death Threat to Women Than Breast Cancer." American Diabetes Association National Service Center, June 11, 1995.

42. Voelker, Rebecca. "Taking Asthma Seriously." *Journal of the American Medical Association*, Vol. 278, No. 1, July 2, 1997.

43. "Asthma Hospitalization and Readmissions Among Children and Young Adults." *Morbidity & Mortality Weekly Report*, Vol. 46, No. 1, August 8, 1997.

Chapter 11

Drug Use, Misuse, and Abuse

After studying the material in this chapter, you should be able to:

- **Explain** factors affecting drug dependence.
- **Describe** the effects of cocaine and crack abuse.
- **Describe** the common forms and effects of amphetamines, depressants, cannabis products, psychedelics and hallucinogens, and narcotic drugs.
- **Describe** the issues affecting the treatment of drug dependence.
- **Define** addiction and **explain** the addictive process.

Although drug use has declined in the last two decades, the rates of drug abuse and drug-related problems remain high. About half of American adults surveyed report having used an illicit drug at some time in their lives; 15% say they did so in the preceding 12 months.[1]

This chapter provides information on the nature and effects of drugs, the impact of drugs on individuals and society, and the drugs Americans most commonly use, misuse, and abuse.

Understanding Drugs and Their Effects

A **drug** is a chemical substance that affects the way you feel and function. In some circumstances, taking a drug can help the body heal or relieve physical and mental distress. In other circumstances, taking a drug can distort reality, undermine well-being, and threaten survival. No drug is completely safe; all drugs have multiple effects that vary greatly in different people at different times. Knowing how drugs affect the brain, body, and behavior is crucial to understanding their impact and making responsible decisions about their use.

Drug misuse is the taking of a drug for a purpose or by a person other than that for which it was medically intended. Borrowing a friend's prescription for penicillin when your throat feels scratchy is an example of drug misuse. The World Health Organization defines **drug abuse** as excessive drug use that's inconsistent with accepted medical practice. Taking anabolic steroids, discussed later in this chapter, to look more muscular is an example of drug abuse.

There are risks involved with all forms of drug use. Even medications that help cure illnesses or soothe symptoms have side effects and can be misused. Some substances that millions of people use every day, such as caffeine, pose some health risks. Others—like the most commonly used drugs in our society, alcohol and tobacco—can lead to potentially life-threatening problems. With some illicit drugs, any form of use can be dangerous.

Many factors determine the effects a drug has on an individual. These include how the drug enters the body, the dosage, drug action, and presence of other drugs in the body—as well as the physical and psychological makeup of the person taking the drug and the setting in which the drug is used.

Routes of Administration

Drugs can enter the body in a number of ways (see Figure 11-1). The most common way of taking a drug is by swallowing a tablet, capsule, or liquid. However, drugs taken orally don't reach the bloodstream as quickly as drugs introduced into the body by other means. A drug taken orally may not have any effect for 30 minutes or more.

Drugs can enter the body through the lungs either by inhaling smoke, for example, from marijuana, or by inhaling gases, aerosol sprays, or fumes from solvents or other compounds that evaporate quickly. Drugs can also be injected with a syringe subcutaneously (beneath the skin), intramuscularly (into muscle tissue, which is richly supplied with blood vessels), or intravenously (directly into a vein). **Intravenous** (IV) injection gets the drug into the bloodstream immediately (within seconds in most cases); **intramuscular** injection is moderately fast (within a few minutes); and **subcutaneous** injection works more slowly (within 10 minutes).

Approximately 1.5 million Americans use illegal IV drugs. This practice is extremely dangerous because many diseases, including hepatitis and infection with human immunodeficiency virus (HIV), can be transmitted by sharing contaminated needles. Indeed, an estimated 250,000 to 300,000 of the nation's IV drug users are HIV-positive; they are the chief source of transmission of HIV among heterosexuals. About 70% of the

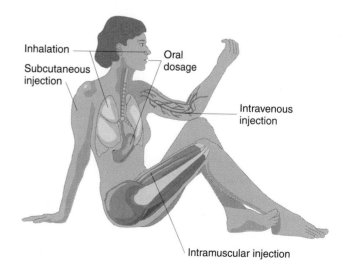

Figure 11-1

Routes of administration of drugs.

AIDS cases in women and children are linked directly or indirectly to IV drug use.

Dosage

The effects of any drug depend on the amount an individual takes. Increasing the dose usually intensifies the effects produced by smaller doses. Also, there may be a change in the kind of effect at different dose levels. For example, low doses of barbiturates may relieve anxiety, while higher doses can induce sleep, loss of sensation, even coma and death.

Individual Differences

Each person responds differently to different drugs, depending on circumstances or setting. The enzymes in our bodies reduce the levels of drugs in our bloodstream; because there can be eighty variants of each enzyme, every person's body may react differently.

Often drugs intensify the emotional state a person is in. If you're feeling depressed, a drug may make you feel more depressed. A generalized physical problem, such as having the flu, may make your body more vulnerable to the effects of a drug. Genetic differences among individuals also may account for varying reactions.

Personality and psychological attitude also play a role in drug effects, so that one person may have a frighteningly bad trip on the same LSD dosage on which another person has a positive experience. To a certain extent, this depends on each user's **set** (or mind-set)—his or her expectations or preconceptions about using the drug. Someone who snorts cocaine to enhance sexual pleasure may feel more stimulated simply because that's what he or she expects. The setting for drug use also influences its effects. Passing around a joint of marijuana at a friend's is not a healthy or safe behavior, but the experience of going to a crack house is very different—and entails greater dangers.

Types of Action

A drug can act *locally,* as Novocain does to deaden pain in a tooth; *generally,* throughout a body system, as barbiturates do on the central nervous system; or *selectively,* as a drug does when it has a greater effect on one specific organ or system than on others, such as a spinal anesthetic. A drug that accumulates in the body because it's taken in faster than it can be metabolized and excreted is called *cumulative;* alcohol is such a drug.

The danger of mixing alcohol with other drugs cannot be emphasized too strongly. Alcohol and marijuana intensify each other's effects, making driving and many other activities extremely dangerous. Some people have mixed sedatives or tranquilizers with alcohol and never regained consciousness.

Medications

Many of the medications and pharmaceutical products available in this country do indeed relieve symptoms and help cure various illnesses. However, every year thousands of Americans are hospitalized because of complications caused by medications. Because drugs are powerful, it's important to know how to use them appropriately.

Over-the-Counter (OTC) Drugs

More than half a million health products—remedies for everything from bad breath to bunions—are readily available without a doctor's prescription. This doesn't mean, however, that they're necessarily safe or effective. Indeed, many widely used **over-the-counter (OTC) drugs** pose unsuspected hazards. Among the most potentially dangerous is aspirin, the "wonder drug" in practically everyone's home pharmacy. When taken by someone who's been drinking (often to prevent or relieve hangover symptoms), for instance, aspirin increases blood-alcohol concentrations.[2] Along with other nonsteroidal anti-inflammatory drugs, such as ibuprofen (brand names include Advil and Nuprin), aspirin can damage the lining of the stomach and lead to ulcers in those who take large daily doses for arthritis or other problems. Kidney problems have also been traced to some pain relievers.

Like other drugs, OTC medications can be used improperly, often simply because of a lack of education about proper use. Among those most often misused are the following:

• *Nasal sprays.* Nasal sprays relieve congestion by shrinking blood vessels in the nose. If they are used too often or for too many days in a row, however, the blood vessels widen instead of contracting and the surrounding tissues become swollen, causing more congestion. To make the vessels shrink again, many people use more spray more often. The result can be permanent damage to nasal membranes, bleeding, infection, and partial or complete loss of smell.

- *Laxatives.* Believing that they must have one bowel movement a day (a common misconception), many people rely on laxatives. Brands that contain phenolphthalein imitate the lining of the intestines and cause muscles to contract or tighten, often making constipation worse rather than better. Bulk laxatives are less dangerous, but regular use is not advised. A high-fiber diet and more exercise are safer and more effective remedies for constipation.

- *Eye drops.* Eye drops make the blood vessels of the eye contract. However, as in the case of nasal sprays, with overuse (several times a day for several weeks), the blood vessels expand, making the eye look redder than before.

- *Sleep aids.* Although over-the-counter sleeping pills are widely used, there has been little research on their use and possible risks.[3]

Prescription Drugs

Medications are a big business in this country. However, the latest, most expensive drugs aren't necessarily the best. Each year the Food and Drug Administration (FDA) approves about twenty new drugs, yet no more than four are rated as truly meaningful advances. The others often are no better or worse than what's already on the market.

Many prescribed medications aren't taken the way they should be; millions simply aren't taken at all. The dangers of **noncompliance** (not taking prescription drugs properly) include recurrent infections, serious medical complications, and emergency hospital treatment. The drugs most likely to be taken incorrectly are those that treat problems with no obvious symptoms (such as high blood pressure), that require complex dosage schedules, that treat psychiatric disorders, or that have unpleasant side effects.

Side Effects

Most medications, taken correctly, cause only minor complications. However, no drug is entirely without side effects for all individuals taking it. Allergic reactions to drugs are common. The drugs that most often provoke allergic responses are penicillin and other antibiotics (drugs used to treat infection). Aspirin, sulfa drugs, barbiturates, anticonvulsants, insulin, and local anesthetics can also provoke allergic responses. Allergic reactions range from mild rashes to hives to a life-threatening constriction of the airways and sudden drop of blood pressure.

Strategies for Prevention

Ensuring Drug Safety

✔ Always ask about possible side effects of a drug. Find out if any other medicines might be just as effective with fewer side effects.

✔ Inform your physician of any other medicines that you take regularly, including birth control pills and over-the-counter preparations, such as sleeping pills.

✔ Report exactly how much alcohol and caffeine you consume every day. Find out how these substances might interact with the medications you're taking. Don't hesitate to ask a pharmacist about drug interactions.

✔ Check on timing. For example, drugs with sedative effects shouldn't be taken during the day, while those with stimulant effects shouldn't be taken at bedtime. If you're taking several medicines, take out 1-day's supply of pills at a time, make up a schedule for taking them, and check off each dose of each drug as you take it.

✔ If you've had a psychiatric problem, such as depression, in the past, or if you've ever experienced psychiatric side effects from drugs, tell your doctor.

✔ If you suspect that a medication is affecting your mind or behavior, tell your doctor exactly how you feel. Find out if you can switch to a lower dose or an alternative medication. If your physician says that there are no other options, consult a psychiatrist.

✔ Don't suddenly stop taking any medication on your own. You may endanger your physical well-being and end up feeling much greater anxiety, depression, or confusion.

Dozens of drugs—both over-the-counter and prescription—can cause changes in the way people think, feel, and behave. Unfortunately, neither patients nor their physicians usually connect such symptoms with medications. Doctors may not even mention potential mental and emotional problems because they don't want to scare patients away from what otherwise may be a very effective treatment. But what you don't know about a drug's effects on your mind can hurt you.

Drug Interactions

OTC and prescription drugs can interact in a variety of ways. For example, mixing some cold medications with tranquilizers can cause drowsiness and coordination problems, thus making driving dangerous. Moreover, what you eat or drink can impair or completely wipe out the effectiveness of drugs or lead to unexpected effects on the body. For instance, aspirin takes five to ten times as long to be absorbed when taken with food or shortly after a meal than when taken on an empty stomach. Or if tetracyclines encounter calcium in the stomach, they bind together and cancel each other out.

To avoid potentially dangerous interactions, check the label(s) for any instructions on how or when to take a medication, such as "with a meal" (see Figure 11-2). If the directions say that you should take a drug on an empty stomach, do it at least 1 hour before eating or 2 or 3 hours after eating. Don't drink a hot beverage with a medication, because the temperature may interfere with the effectiveness of the drug. Don't open, crush, or dissolve tablets or capsules without checking first with your physician or pharmacist.

Whenever you take a drug, be especially careful of your intake of alcohol, which can change the rate of metabolism and the effects of many different drugs. Because it dilates the blood vessels, alcohol can add to the dizziness sometimes caused by drugs for high blood pressure, angina, or depression. Also, its irritating effects on the stomach can worsen stomach upset from aspirin, ibuprofen, and other anti-inflammatory drugs.

Caffeine Use and Misuse

Caffeine, which has been drunk, chewed, or swallowed since the Stone Age, is the most widely used **psy-**chotropic (mind-affecting) drug in the world. Eighty percent of Americans drink coffee, our principal caffeine source—an average of 3.5 cups a day. Coffee contains 100 to 150 mg of caffeine per cup; tea, 40 to 100 mg; cola, about 45 mg. Most medications that contain caffeine are one-third to one-half the strength of a cup of coffee. However, some, such as Excedrin, are very high in caffeine.

The effects of caffeine vary. Because it is a **stimulant**, it relieves drowsiness, helps in the performance of repetitive tasks, and improves capacity for work. Some athletes feel that caffeine gives them an extra boost that allows them to go farther and longer in endurance events. However, consumption of caffeine can also lead to dependence, anxiety, insomnia, faster breathing, upset stomach and bowels, and dizziness.[4]

Caffeine withdrawal for those dependent on this substance can cause headaches. Those who must cut back should taper off gradually. One approach is to mix regular and decaffeinated coffee, gradually decreasing the quantity of the former.

Substance Use Disorders

People have been using mind-altering, or **psychoactive**, chemicals for centuries. Citizens of ancient Mesopotamia and Egypt used opium. More than 3000 years ago Hindus included cannabis products in religious ceremonies. For centuries the Inca Indians in South America have chewed the leaves of the coca bush. Yet while drugs existed in most societies, their use was usually limited to small groups. Today millions of Americans regularly turn to drugs to pick them up, bring them down, alter perceptions, or ease psychological pain.

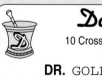

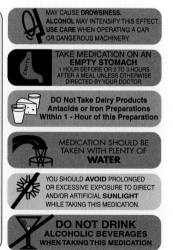

Figure 11-2

Drug interactions can alter the effectiveness of your medication. When you take a prescription medication, be sure to read warning labels about interactions, possible side effects, and whether the medication interacts with certain foods.

Pulsepoints

Ten Ways to Tell If Someone Is Abusing Drugs

1. An abrupt change in attitude. Individuals may lose interest in activities they once enjoyed or in being with friends they once valued.

2. Mood swings. Drug users may often seem withdrawn or "out of it," or they may display unusual temper flareups.

3. A decline in performance. Students may start skipping classes, stop studying, or not complete assignments; their grades may plummet.

4. Increased sensitivity. Individuals may react intensely to any criticism or become easily frustrated or angered.

5. Secrecy. Drug users may make furtive telephone calls or demand greater privacy concerning their personal possessions or their whereabouts.

6. Physical changes. Individuals using drugs may change their pattern of sleep, spending more time in bed or sleeping at odd hours. They also may change their eating habits and lose weight.

7. Money problems. Drug users may constantly borrow money, seem short of cash, or begin stealing.

8. Changes in appearance. As they become more involved with drugs, users often lose regard for their personal appearance and look disheveled.

9. Defiance of restrictions. Individuals may ignore or deliberately refuse to comply with deadlines, curfews, or other regulations.

10. Changes in relationships. Drug users may quarrel more frequently with family members or old friends and develop new, strong allegiances with new acquaintances, including other drug users.

The word **addiction** has moved out of the realm of scientific terminology and into the mainstream of American life. Among laypeople, addiction refers to the habitual use of substances, such as alcohol, psychoactive drugs, and nicotine, and also to compulsive behaviors, such as overeating. Like drugs, these activities can be used repeatedly to numb pain or enhance pleasure; some may alter a person's brain chemistry or create cravings; all can lead to a loss of internal control.

Today chemical addiction is viewed as a lifelong, chronic illness that affects mind, body, and spirit. Its key characteristics are repeated drug use, loss of control over how much or how often a person takes a drug, and continued use despite harmful consequences. Because addiction is considered too broad and judgmental a term for scientific use, mental health professionals describe drug-related problems in terms of dependence and abuse. However, they agree that there are four characteristic symptoms of addiction: compulsion to use the substance, loss of control, negative consequences, and denial.

Dependence

Individuals may develop **psychological dependence** and feel a strong craving for a drug because it produces pleasurable feelings or relieves stress or anxiety. **Physical dependence** occurs when a person develops *tolerance* to the effects of a drug and needs larger and larger doses to achieve intoxication or another desired effect. Individuals who are physically dependent and have a high tolerance to a drug may take amounts many times those that would produce intoxication or an overdose in someone who was not a regular user.

Individuals with drug dependence become intoxicated or high on a regular basis—whether every day, every weekend, or several binges a year. They may try repeatedly to stop using a drug and yet fail—even though they realize that their drug use is interfering with their health, family life, relationships, and work.

Abuse

Some drug users do not develop the symptoms of tolerance and withdrawal that characterize dependence, yet they use drugs in ways that clearly have a harmful effect. These individuals are diagnosed as having a *psychoactive substance abuse disorder*. They continue to use drugs despite their awareness of persistent or repeated social, occupational, psychological, or physical problems related to drug use, or they use drugs in dangerous ways or situations (before driving, for instance). (See Pulsepoints: "Ten Ways to Tell If Someone Is Abusing Drugs.")

Intoxication and Withdrawal

Intoxication refers to maladaptive behavioral, psychological, and physiologic changes that occur as a result of substance use. **Withdrawal** is the development of symptoms that cause significant psychological and physical distress when an individual reduces or stops drug use. (Intoxication and withdrawal from specific drugs are discussed later in this chapter.)

Polyabuse

Most users prefer a certain type of drug but also use several others; this behavior is called **polyabuse**. The average user who enters treatment is on five different drugs. The more drugs anyone uses, the greater the chance of side effects, complications, and possibly life-threatening interactions.

The Toll of Drugs

Drugs affect a person's physical, psychological, and social health; their effects can be *acute* (resulting from a single dose or series of doses) or *chronic* (resulting from long-term use). Acute effects vary with different drugs. Stimulants may trigger unpredictable rage; an overdose of heroin may lead to respiratory depression, a breathing impairment that can be fatal.

Over time, chronic drug users may feel fatigued, cough constantly, lose weight, become malnourished,

and ache from head to toe. They may suffer blackouts, flashbacks, and episodes of increasingly bizarre behavior, often triggered by escalating paranoia. Their risk of overdose rises steadily, and they must live with constant stress: the fear of getting busted for possession or of losing a job if they test positive for drugs, the worry of getting enough money for their next fix, the dangers of associating with dealers and other users.

The toll of drug use can be especially great on teenagers. Teenage drug use disrupts many critical developmental tasks of adolescence and young adulthood. Use of drugs during the teen years can lead to drug-related crime (including stealing), poor achievement in high school or college, and job instability.

Drugs in America

Drug abuse has remained a major problem in the 1990s, even though by late 1997, drug use among teenagers

Strategies for Prevention

Preventing Temptation

You can take steps to protect yourself from the temptation to use drugs. Among them are the following:

✔ *Learn how to cope with stress.* Try some of the coping techniques, such as exercise, guided imagery, or meditation, described in Chapter 2.

✔ *Strengthen your self-esteem.* Take pride in your achievements, particularly when setbacks bruise your confidence.

✔ *Develop a range of interests.* Get into the habit of finding pleasure in swimming, dancing, playing an instrument, doing volunteer work, or taking long walks.

✔ *Practice assertiveness.* Cultivate the art of speaking up and voicing your opinion—regardless of the subject or circumstances.

seemed to be leveling off. The estimated medical and social costs of drug abuse are believed to exceed $240 billion. Addiction to drugs, alcohol, or tobacco accounts for a third of all hospital admissions and a quarter of all deaths.[5]

There is no typical drug user. High school students, professional athletes, business executives, inner-city teenagers, rock musicians, doctors, truckers, teachers, and many others of different ages and ethnic groups use drugs regularly. However, we all pay a price for living in a drug-using society, including the costs of medical care, treatment, and imprisonment for addicts and drug traffickers. Other hidden costs include accidents caused by drug-using drivers and workers, drug-related violence and crime, and care for babies born to drug-dependent mothers.

In the last 20 years, the United States has spent nearly $70 billion fighting drugs. But victory is nowhere in sight. Criminal organizations in Latin America and Asia have increased production and become more sophisticated in distributing cocaine and heroin. Illicit drugs have become more available in more countries and at lower prices than ever before.

Critics of the nation's drug policy argue that the war is being fought on the wrong front. Currently, about two-thirds of federal spending for drug control goes toward law enforcement and only one-third toward pre-

vention and treatment. Many contend that more should be spent on antidrug education for children, on treatment for addicts, and on researching drugs that could help in overcoming drug dependence.

There is evidence that prevention can and does work. According to the National Clearinghouse for Alcohol and Drug Information, each month prevention efforts keep approximately 3.5 million youngsters from drinking alcohol and 24 million young adults from using illicit drugs.[6]

Student Drug Use

On college campuses, alcohol is the number-one drug of abuse, while marijuana remains the most commonly used illegal drug. As indicated in the Campus Focus: "College Students and Illegal Drug Use," about half of college students have tried marijuana, although the percentage of current users is much lower: 11.6% of women and 17.1% of men. About 14% of college students have tried cocaine.[7]

Various factors influence which students use drugs:

- *Gender.* Men are more likely to use drugs than are women, but the differences are not large.

- *Race/ethnicity.* In general, white students have higher levels of alcohol and drug use than do African-American students.

- *Perception of risk.* Students seem most likely to try substances they perceive as being "safe," or low-risk. Of these, the top three are caffeine, alcohol, and tobacco; marijuana is listed fourth in terms of perceived safety. Other agents—barbiturates, heroin, cocaine, PCP, speed, LSD, crack, and inhalants—are viewed as about equally risky and are used much less often.

- *Environment.* As with alcohol use, students are influenced by their friends, their residence, and the general public's attitude toward drug use.[8] Increasingly, college health officials are realizing that, rather than simply trying to change students' substance abuse, they also must change the environment to promote healthier lifestyle choices.

Common Drugs of Abuse

The psychoactive substances most often associated with both abuse and dependence include alcohol, amphetamines, cocaine, cannabis (marijuana), hallucinogens,

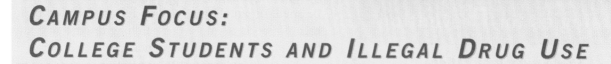

CAMPUS FOCUS:
COLLEGE STUDENTS AND ILLEGAL DRUG USE

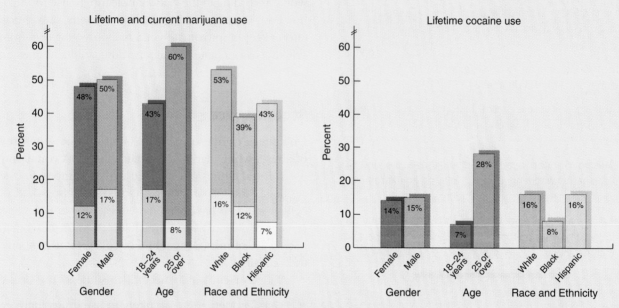

SOURCE: Douglas, Kathy, et al. "Results from the 1995 National College Health Risk Behavior Survey." *Journal of American College Health*, Vol. 46, September 1997.

inhalants, opioids, phencyclidine (PCP), and sedative-hypnotic or anxiolytic (antianxiety) drugs (see Table 11-1).

Amphetamines

Amphetamines, stimulants that were once widely prescribed for weight control because they suppress appetite, have emerged as a global danger. In 1997, the United Nations reported a worldwide surge in amphetamine abuse and described this trend as "more dangerous than heroin and cocaine." They trigger the release of epinephrine (adrenalin), which stimulates the central nervous system. Amphetamines are sold under a variety of names: amphetamine (brand name Benzedrine, street-name "bennies"), dextroamphetamine (Dexedrine, or "dex"), methamphetamine (Methedrine, or "meth" or "speed"), and Desoxyn ("copilots"). Related *uppers* include the prescription drugs methylphenidate (Ritalin), pemoline (Cylert), and phenmetrazine (Preludin).

Amphetamines are available in tablet or capsule form. Abusers may grind and sniff the capsules or make a solution and inject the drug. "Ice" is a smokable form of methamphetamine that is highly addictive and produces an intense physical and psychological high that can last from 4 to 14 hours. *Crank* is the street term for another central nervous system stimulant, propylexedrine, which is less potent than amphetamine. Abusers often extract the drug from the cotton plug of decongestant inhalants and inject it intravenously.

How Users Feel

Amphetamines produce a state of hyper-alertness and energy. Users feel confident in their ability to think clearly and to perform any task exceptionally well—although amphetamines do not, in fact, significantly boost performance or thinking. Higher doses make them feel "wired": talkative, excited, restless, irritable, anxious, moody.

If taken intravenously, amphetamines produce a characteristic "rush" of elation and confidence, as well as adverse effects, including confusion, rambling or incoherent speech, anxiety, headache, and palpitations. Individuals may become paranoid; be convinced they are having "profound" thoughts; feel increased sexual

TABLE 11-1 THE EFFECTS OF DRUGS

Drugs	What They Do	Health Effects	Major Risks
Amphetamines	Speed up physical and mental processes; create sense of heightened energy and confidence.	Loss of appetite, blurred vision, headache, dizziness, sweating, sleeplessness, trembling, anxiety, nausea or vomiting, suspiciousness, delusions, hallucinations, confusion, palpitations, jitteriness or agitation, unusual perceptions (such as a ringing in the ears or a sensation of insects crawling on the skin), increased heart rate, elevated blood pressure, muscular weakness, impaired breathing, movements, or muscle tone.	Dependence, chest pain, heart arrhythmias (disruption of heart rhythm), seizures, malnutrition, skin disorders, ulcers, lack of sleep, depression, paranoia, vitamin deficiencies, brain damage, sexual dysfunction, stroke, high fever, heart failure, violent behavior, coma, fatal overdose.
Cannabis (marijuana and hashish)	Relax the mind and body, alter mood, heighten perceptions.	Faster heartbeat and pulse, dry mouth and throat, impaired perception and reactions, lethargy, nausea, possible hallucinations, panic attacks, decreased motivation.	Psychological dependence; impaired thinking, perception, memory, and coordination; increased heart rate and blood pressure; impaired fertility; dampened immunity; bronchitis, emphysema, lung cancer.
Cocaine and crack	Speed up physical and mental processes; create sense of heightened energy and confidence.	Headaches, exhaustion, shaking, sweating, chills, blurred vision, nausea or vomiting, seizures, loss of appetite, impaired judgment, hyperactivity, babbling, speeding up or slowing down of physical activity, impaired breathing, chest pain, impaired movements or muscle tone.	Dependence; extreme suspiciousness; violence; damage to nose (if snorted), blood vessels, and heart; blood pressure irregularities; loss of sexual desire; impotence; seizures; chest pain; arrhythmias; heart attack; disruptions in heart rhythm; intracranial hemorrhage; damage to liver and lungs (if smoked); hepatitis, HIV infection, skin infections, inflammation of the arteries, and infection of the lining of the heart (if injected).
Hallucinogens (LSD, mescaline)	Alter perceptions and produce hallucinations, which may be frightening or pleasurable.	Increased heart rate, blood pressure, and body temperature; headache, nausea, sweating, trembling, heart palpitations, blurring of vision, tremors, poor coordination; "bad trips" and irrational acts on LSD.	With LSD, disturbing flashbacks, psychological dependence, delusional disorder.
Inhalants	Produce hallucinations and temporary feelings of well-being and giddiness.	Dizziness, involuntary eye movements, poor coordination, slurred speech, unsteady gait, lethargy, depressed reflexes, slowed-down movements, tremors, general muscle weakness, blurred vision, nausea, sneezing, coughing, nosebleeds, lack of coordination, loss of appetite,	Hepatitis, liver failure, kidney failure, respiratory impairment, blood abnormalities, irregular heart beat, heart failure, destruction of bone marrow and skeletal muscles, stupor, or coma.

(continued)

TABLE 11-1 CONTINUED

Drugs	What They Do	Health Effects	Major Risks
		decreased heart and breathing rates, loss of consciousness, aggressiveness, impulsiveness, impaired judgment, increased risk of accidents or injuries.	
Opioids (opium, morphine, heroin, or synthetic narcotics)	Relax the central nervous system, relieve pain, produce temporary sense of well-being.	Restlessness, nausea, vomiting, slowed breathing, weight loss, lethargy, loss of sex drive, mood swings, slurred speech, sweating, impaired judgment, drowsiness, impaired attention or memory.	Dependence, malnutrition, lower immunity, infections of the heart lining and valves, skin abscesses, congested lungs, hepatitis, tetanus, liver disease; if injected, infections of the heart lining and valves, and HIV transmission; depression of central nervous system; coma; fatal overdose.
Phencyclidine (PCP)	Produce changes in perceptions, including hallucinations, and distorted feelings, including delusions of great strength and invulnerability.	Increased heart rate and blood pressure, flushing, sweating, dizziness, painful sensitivity to sound, numbness, diminished sensitivity to pain, impaired coordination and speech, stupor.	Psychosis; increased danger of injury or harm to others because of impulsivity, aggressiveness, and violence; coma, convulsions, heart and lung failure, ruptured blood vessels in the brain, suicide, death.
Sedative-hypnotics and anxiolytic (antianxiety) drugs (including benzodiazepines and barbiturates)	Slow down the central nervous system; reduce or relieve tension; induce relaxation, drowsiness, or sleep; decrease alertness.	Drowsiness, impaired judgment, poor coordination, slowed breathing, weak and rapid heart beat, disrupted sleep, dangerously impaired vision, unsteady gait, sleepiness, confusion, irritability.	Dependence, stupor, coma, fatal overdose, or reaction to sudden withdrawal.

interest; and experience unusual perceptions, such as ringing in the ears, a sensation of insects crawling on their skin, or hearing their name called. Crank users may feel high and sleepy or may hallucinate and lose contact with reality.

Risks

Dependence on amphetamines can develop with episodic or daily use. Users typically take amphetamines in large doses to prevent crashing. "Binging"—taking high doses over a period of several days—can lead to an extremely intense and unpleasant crash—characterized by a craving for the drug, shakiness, irritablity, anxiety, and depression—that requires 2 or more days for recuperation.

The long-term effects of amphetamine abuse include malnutrition, skin disorders, ulcers, insomnia, depression, vitamin deficiencies, and in some cases,

brain damage that results in speech and thought disturbances. Sexual dysfunction and impaired concentration or memory also may occur. Abusers who inject may develop infected veins, and if they share needles, they risk infection with human immunodeficiency virus (HIV), which causes AIDS.

Cannabis Products

Marijuana ("pot") and **hashish**—the most widely used illegal drugs—are derived from the *cannabis* plant. The major psychoactive ingredient in both is *THC (delta-9-tetrahydrocannabinol)*. Nearly one of every three Americans over age 12 has tried marijuana at least once. Some 12 million Americans use it; more than 1 million cannot control this use. Marijuana has been used therapeutically, primarily to ease the nausea of chemother-

TABLE 11-2 ANNUAL PREVALENCE OF USE FOR VARIOUS TYPES OF DRUGS, 1995

Type of drug	Full-Time college students	Others
Any illicit drug	33.5%	34.0%
Marijuana	31.2	28.7
Inhalants	3.9	3.1
Hallucinogens	8.2	7.9
LSD	6.9	6.8
Cocaine	3.6	4.5
Crack	1.1	1.5
MDMA ("Ecstasy")	2.4	1.9
Heroin	0.3	0.7
Other opiates	3.8	4.0
Stimulants	5.4	7.5
"Ice"	1.1	2.2
Barbiturates	2.0	4.0
Tranquilizers	2.9	4.4
Alcohol	83.2	80.8
Cigarettes	39.3	47.7

SOURCE: National Survey Results on Drug Abuse from the Monitoring the Future Study, National Institute on Drug Abuse, 1995.

How Users Feel

In low to moderate doses, marijuana typically creates a mild sense of euphoria, a sense of slowed time (5 minutes may feel like an hour), a dreamy sort of self-absorption, and some impairment in thinking and communicating. Users report heightened sensations of color, sound, and other stimuli, relaxation, and increased confidence. The sense of being "stoned" peaks within half an hour and usually lasts about 3 hours. Even when alterations in perception seem slight, as noted earlier, it is not safe to drive a car for as long as 4 to 6 hours after smoking a single joint. Some users—particularly those smoking marijuana for the first time or taking a high dose in an unpleasant or unfamiliar setting—experience acute anxiety, which may be accompanied by a panicky fear of losing control. They may believe that their companions are ridiculing or threatening them and experience a panic attack, a state of intense terror.

The immediate physical effects of marijuana include increased pulse rate, bloodshot eyes, dry mouth and throat, slowed reaction times, impaired motor skills, increased appetite, and diminished short-term memory (see Figure 11-3). High doses reduce the ability to perceive and to react; all the reactions experienced with low doses are intensified, leading to sensory distortion

apy, and some researchers urge further study of its potential benefits.[9] However, "compassionate" use has been limited by law because some believe it undercuts government opposition to drug use.[10]

Different types of marijuana have different percentages of THC. Because of careful cultivation, the strength of today's marijuana is much greater than that of the pot used in the 1970s; the physical and mental effects are therefore greater. Usually, marijuana is smoked in a cigarette ("joint") or pipe; it may also be eaten as an ingredient in other foods (as when baked in brownies), though with a less predictable effect. The drug high is enhanced by holding the marijuana smoke in the lungs, and experienced smokers learn to hold the smoke for longer periods to increase the amount of drug diffused into the bloodstream. The circumstances in which marijuana is smoked, the communal aspects of its use, and the user's experience all can affect the way a pot-induced high feels.

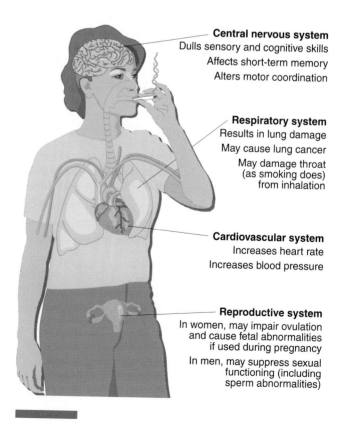

Central nervous system
Dulls sensory and cognitive skills
Affects short-term memory
Alters motor coordination

Respiratory system
Results in lung damage
May cause lung cancer
May damage throat
(as smoking does)
from inhalation

Cardiovascular system
Increases heart rate
Increases blood pressure

Reproductive system
In women, may impair ovulation
and cause fetal abnormalities
if used during pregnancy
In men, may suppress sexual
functioning (including
sperm abnormalities)

Figure 11-3

Some effects of long-term marijuana use on the body.

and—in the case of hashish—vivid hallucinations and LSD-like psychedelic reactions. The drug remains in the body's fat cells 50 hours or more, so people may experience psychoactive effects for several days after use. Drug tests may produce positive results for days or weeks after last use.

Risks

Dependence or abuse usually develops with repeated use over a long period of time. Typically, individuals smoke more often rather than smoking a larger amount. With chronic heavy use, users may feel a lessening or loss of the pleasurable effect and may develop lethargy, a loss of pleasure in activities, and persistent attention and memory problems. Chronic marijuana use seems to impair thinking, reading comprehension, verbal and mathematical skills, coordination, and short-term memory. Teenagers who smoke pot regularly often lose interest in school and do not remember what they learned when they were high. Some long-term regular users of marijuana may experience *burnout*, a dulling of their senses and responses termed *amotivational syndrome*.

Chronic use can also lead to bronchitis, emphysema, and lung cancer. Smoking a single joint can be as damaging to the lungs as smoking five tobacco cigarettes. Marijuana may suppress ovulation and alter hormone levels in female users and may impair the fertility of male users. Frequent use of marijuana during pregnancy can lower birth weight and cause abnormalities in the fetus similar to those of fetal alcohol syndrome.

Cocaine

Cocaine ("coke," "snow," "lady") is a white crystalline powder extracted from the leaves of the South American coca plant. Usually mixed with various sugars and local anesthetics like lidocaine and procaine, cocaine powder is generally inhaled. When sniffed or snorted, cocaine anesthetizes the nerve endings in the nose and relaxes the lung's bronchial muscles.

Cocaine can be dissolved in water and injected intravenously. The drug is rapidly metabolized by the liver, so the high is relatively brief, typically lasting only about 20 minutes. This means that users will commonly inject the drug repeatedly, increasing the risk of infection and damage to their veins.

Cocaine alkaloid—or *freebase*—is obtained by removing the hydrocholoride salt from cocaine powder. "Freebasing" is smoking the fumes of the alkaloid form of cocaine. *Crack*, pharmacologically identical to free-

base, is a cheap, easy-to-use, widely available, smokeable and potent form of cocaine named for the popping sound it makes when burned. Because it is absorbed rapidly into the bloodstream and large doses reach the brain very quickly, it is particularly dangerous. However, its low price and easy availability have made it a common drug of abuse in poor urban areas.[11]

How Users Feel

A powerful stimulant to the central nervous system, cocaine produces feelings of soaring well-being and boundless energy. Users feel that they have enormous physical and mental ability, yet are also restless and anxious. After a brief period of euphoria, users slump into a depression. They often go on cocaine binges, lasting from a few hours to several days, and consume large quantities of cocaine.

With crack, dependence develops quickly. As soon as crack users come down from one high, they want more crack. Whereas heroin addicts may shoot up several times a day, crack addicts need another hit within minutes. Thus, a crack habit can quickly become more expensive than heroin addiction. Some "crackheads" have $1000-a-day habits.

With continuing use, cocaine users experience less pleasure and more unpleasant effects. Eventually they may reach a point at which they no longer experience euphoric effects and crave the drug simply to alleviate their persistent hunger for it.

Risks

Cocaine dependence is an easy habit to acquire. With repeated use, the brain becomes tolerant of the drug's stimulant effects, and users must take more of it to get high. Its grip is strong. Those who smoke or inject cocaine can develop dependence within weeks. Those who sniff cocaine may not become dependent on the drug for months or years. It is thought that 5% to 20% of all coke users—a group as large as the estimated total number of heroin addicts—are dependent on the drug.

The physical effects of acute cocaine intoxication include dilated pupils, elevated blood pressure, perspiration or chills, nausea or vomiting, speeding up or slowing down of physical activity, muscular weakness, impaired breathing, chest pain, and impaired movements or muscle tone.

Cocaine use can cause blood vessels in the brain to clamp shut and can trigger a stroke, bleeding in the brain, and potentially fatal brain seizures. Cocaine users can also develop psychiatric or neurological complications (Figure 11-4). Repeated or high doses of cocaine can lead to impaired judgment, hyperactivity, nonstop babbling, feelings of suspicion and paranoia, and violent behavior. The brain never learns to tolerate cocaine's negative effects; users may become incoherent and paranoid and may experience unusual sensations, such as ringing in their ears, feeling insects crawling on the skin, or hearing their name called.

Cocaine causes the heart rate to speed up and blood pressure to rise suddenly. Its use is associated with many cardiac complications, including arrhythmia (disruption of heart rhythm), angina (chest pain), and acute myocardial infarction (heart attack). These cardiac complications can lead to sudden death.

Cocaine users who inject the drug and share needles put themselves at risk for another potentially lethal problem: HIV infection. Other complications of injecting cocaine include skin infections, hepatitis, inflammation of the arteries, and infection of the lining of the heart.

The most common ways of dying from cocaine use are persistent seizures that result in respiratory collapse, cardiac arrest from arrhythmias, myocardial infarction, and intracranial hemorrhage or stroke. The combination of alcohol and cocaine is particularly lethal. Alcohol and cocaine together are second only to the combination of heroin and alcohol in causing deaths related to substance abuse.

Cocaine is dangerous for pregnant women and their babies, causing miscarriages, developmental disorders, and life-threatening complications during birth. Women who use the drug while pregnant are more likely to miscarry in the first 3 months of pregnancy than women who do not use drugs or who use heroin and other opioids. When used early in pregnancy, cocaine can reduce the fetal oxygen supply, possibly interfering with the development of the fetus's nervous system. Infants born to cocaine and crack users can suffer withdrawal and may have major complications or permanent disabilities.

Hallucinogens

The drugs known as **hallucinogens** produce vivid and unusual changes in thought, feeling, and perception. The most widely used in the United States is *LSD (lysergic acid diethylamide*, or "acid"), which was initially developed as a tool to explore mental illness. It became popular in the 1960s and resurfaced among teenagers in the 1990s. LSD is taken orally, either blotted onto pieces of paper which are held in the mouth or chewed along with another substance, such as a sugar cube. Much less commonly used in this country is *peyote* (whose active ingredient is *mescaline*).

How Users Feel

Agents such as LSD produce hallucinations, including bright colors and altered perceptions of reality. Effects from a single dose begin within 30 to 60 minutes and last 10 to 12 hours. During this time, there are slight increases in body temperature, heart rate, and blood pressure; sweating, chills and goose pimples appear. Some users develop headache and nausea.

The effects of hallucinogens depend greatly on the dose, the individual's expectations and personality, and the setting for drug use. Many users report religious or mystical imagery and thoughts; some feel they are experiencing profound insights. Usually the user realizes that perceptual changes are caused by the hallucinogen, but some become convinced that they have lost their minds. Drugs sold as hallucinogens are frequently mixed with other drugs, such as PCP and amphetamines, which can produce unexpected and frightening effects.

Risks

Physical symptoms include dilated pupils, rapid heart rate, sweating, heart palpitations, blurring of vision, tremors, and poor coordination. These effects may last 8

Central nervous system
Repeated use or high dosages may cause severe psychological problems
Suppresses desire for food, sex, and sleep
Can cause strokes, seizures, and neurological damage

Nose
Damages mucous membrane

Cardiovascular system
Increases blood pressure by constricting blood vessels
Causes irregular heartbeat
Damages heart tissue

Respiratory system
Freebasing causes lung damage
Overdose can lead to respiratory arrest

Reproductive system
In men, affects ability to maintain erections and ejaculate; also causes sperm abnormalities
In women, may affect ability to carry pregnancy to term

Figure 11-4

Some effects of cocaine on the body.

to 12 hours. Hallucinogen intoxication also produces changes in emotions and mood, such as anxiety, depression, fear of losing one's mind, and impaired judgment.

LSD can trigger irrational acts. LSD users have injured or killed themselves by jumping out of windows, swimming out to sea, or throwing themselves in front of cars. Some individuals develop a delusional disorder, in which they become convinced that their distorted perceptions and thoughts are real. They may experience flashbacks (reexperiencing of symptoms felt while intoxicated), which include geometric hallucinations, flashes of color, halos around objects, and other perceptual changes.

Inhalants

Inhalants or **deleriants** are chemicals that produce vapors with psychoactive effects. The most commonly abused inhalants are solvents, aerosols, model-airplane glue, cleaning fluids, and petroleum products like kerosene and butane. Some anesthetics and nitrous oxide (laughing gas) are also abused. Almost 20% of eighth graders surveyed have used household products, such as glue, solvents, and aerosols, to get high.[12]

To inhale intoxicating vapors, individuals soak a rag in the substance, place it against the mouth and nose, and inhale; or inhale fumes from a substance placed in a paper or plastic bag; or inhale vapors directly from their containers. Young people, especially those who may not have money for or access to other drugs, are most likely to try inhalants. Children aged 9 to 13 tend to use inhalants with a group of peers who are likely to use alcohol and marijuana as well. Users are in all racial, socioeconomic, and gender groups, but the incidence of use is higher among poor minority youth. Many users come from families that have separated or been affected by alcohol or drug problems; they often have school difficulties, such as truancy and poor grades, or problems adjusting to work.[13]

How Users Feel

Inhalants reach the lungs, bloodstream, and other parts of the body very rapidly. At low doses, users may feel slightly stimulated; at higher doses, they may feel less inhibited. Intoxication often occurs within 5 minutes and can last more than an hour. Inhalant users do not report the intense rush associated with other drugs, nor do they experience the perceptual changes associated with LSD. However, inhalants interfere with thinking and impulse control, so users may act in dangerous or destructive ways.

Often there are visible external signs of use: a rash around the nose and mouth; breath odors; residue on face, hands, and clothing; redness, swelling, and tearing of the eyes; and irritation of throat, lungs, and nose that leads to coughing and gagging. Nausea and headache also may occur.

Risks

Regular use of inhalants leads to tolerance, so that the sniffer needs more and more to attain the desired effects. Younger children who use inhalants several times a week may develop dependence. Older users who become dependent may use the drugs many times a day.

Although some young people believe inhalants are safe to use, this is far from true. Inhalation of butane from cigarette lighters displaces oxygen in the lungs, causing suffocation. Users also can suffocate while covering their heads with a plastic bag to inhale the substance or from inhaling vomit into their lungs while high. According to the International Institute on Inhalant Abuse, the effects of inhalants are unpredictable, and even a single episode could trigger asphyxiation or cardiac arrhythmia, leading to disability or death. Abusers also can develop difficulties with memory, with abstract reasoning, problems with coordination, and with uncontrollable movements of the extremities.

Opioids

The **opioids** include *opium* and its derivatives (*morphine, codeine,* and *heroin*) and nonopioid synthetic

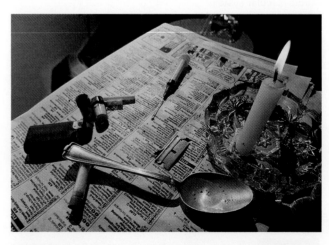

Opioid drugs, made from the Asian poppy, come in both legal and illegal forms. In any form, these substances can readily become addictive.

drugs that have similar sleep-inducing and pain-relieving properties. The opioids come from a resin taken from the seed pod of the Asian poppy. **Nonopioids**, such as *meperidine* (Demerol), *methadone*, and *propoxyphene* (Darvon), are chemically synthesized. These drugs are powerful narcotics, or painkillers.

Heroin, the most widely abused opioid, is illegal in this country. In other nations it is used as a potent painkiller for conditions such as terminal cancer. There are an estimated 400,000 to 600,000 heroin addicts in the United States, with men outnumbering women addicts by three to one. Purer forms of heroin, available in many cities, can be snorted; this has led to a surge in the drug's popularity, especially among middle- and upper-class users.

Morphine, used as a painkiller and anesthetic, acts primarily on the central nervous system, eyes, and digestive tract and masks pain by producing mental clouding, drowsiness, and euphoria. It does not decrease the physical sensation of pain as much as it alters a person's awareness of the pain; in effect, he or she no longer cares about it. Codeine is a weaker painkiller and sedative than morphine. It is an ingredient prescribed in liquid products for relieving coughs and in tablet and injectable form for relieving pain.

Prescription opioids are taken orally in pill form but can also be injected intravenously. Heroin users typically inject the drug into their veins. However, individuals who experiment with whatever recreational drug is new and trendy often prefer *skin-popping* (subcutaneous injection) rather than *mainlining* (intravenous injection); they also may snort heroin as a powder or dissolve it and inhale the vapors. To try to avoid addiction, some users begin by *chipping*, taking small or intermittent doses. Regardless of the method of administration, tolerance can develop rapidly.

How Users Feel

All the opioids relax the user. When injected, they can produce an immediate "rush," or high, that lasts 10 to 30 minutes. For 2 to 6 hours thereafter, users may feel indifferent, lethargic, and drowsy; they may slur their speech and have problems paying attention, remembering, and going about their normal routine. The primary attractions of heroin ("horse," "junk," "smack," or "downtown") are the euphoria and pain relief it produces. However, some people experience very unpleasant feelings, such as anxiety and fear. Other effects include a sensation of warmth or heaviness, dry mouth, facial flushing, and nausea and vomiting (particularly in first-time users).

Risks

Addiction is common. Almost all regular users of opioids rapidly develop drug dependence, which can lead to lethargy, weight loss, loss of sex drive, and the continual effort to avoid withdrawal symptoms through repeated drug administration. In addition, they experience anxiety, insomnia, restlessness, and craving for the drug. Users continue taking opioids as much to avoid the discomfort of withdrawal—a classic sign of addiction—as to experience pleasure.

Opioid intoxication is characterized by changes in mood and behavior, such as initial euphoria followed by apathy or discontent and impaired judgment. Physical symptoms include constricted pupils (although pupils may dilate from a severe overdose), drowsiness, slurred speech, and impaired attention or memory. Morphine affects blood pressure, heart rate, and blood circulation in the brain. Both morphine and heroin slow down—depress—the respiratory system; overdoses can cause fatal respiratory arrest.

Opioid poisoning or overdose causes shock, coma, and depressed respiration and can be fatal. Emergency medical treatment is critical, often with drugs called narcotic antagonists that rapidly reverse the effects of opioids when administered intravenously.

Over time, users who inject opioids may develop infections of the heart lining and valves, skin abscesses, and lung congestion. Infections from unsterile solutions, syringes, and shared needles can lead to hepatitis, tetanus, liver disease, and HIV transmission. The annual death rate among those dependent on opioids is twenty times higher than among other young people, primarily because of physical complications, overdose, suicide, and the violent lifestyle of many users.

Phencyclidine (PCP)

PCP (phencyclidine) (brand name Sernyl; street names "angel dust," "peace pill," "lovely," and "green") is an illicit drug manufactured as a tablet, capsule, liquid, flake, spray, or crystal-like white powder that can be swallowed, smoked, sniffed, or injected. Sometimes it is sprinkled on crack, marijuana, tobacco, or parsley and smoked. A fine-powdered form of PCP can be snorted or injected. Once PCP was thought to have medicinal value as an anesthetic, but its side effects, including delirium and hallucinations, made it unacceptable for medical use.

How Users Feel

The effects of PCP are utterly unpredictable. It may trigger violent behavior or irreversible psychosis the first time it is used, the twentieth time, or never. In low doses, PCP produces changes—from hallucinations to euphoria to feelings of emptiness or numbness—similar to those produced by other psychoactive drugs. Higher doses may produce a stupor that lasts several days, increased heart rate and blood pressure, flushing, sweating, dizziness, and numbness.

Risks

Some first-time users feel PCP is too unpredictable and do not try it again. Others quickly become heavy users. Many go on PCP binges or runs that can last several days. Some people use it daily, often along with alcohol and marijuana. It takes only a short period of occasional use for dependence or abuse to develop.

The behavioral changes associated with PCP intoxication, which can develop within minutes, include belligerence, aggressiveness, impulsiveness, unpredictability, agitation, poor judgment, and impaired functioning at work or in social situations. The physical symptoms of PCP intoxication include involuntary eye movements, increased blood pressure or heart rate, numbness or diminished responsiveness to pain, impaired coordination and speech, muscle rigidity, seizures, and a painful sensitivity to sound. Some people experience repetitive motor movements, such as facial grimacing, hallucinations, and paranoia. Suicide is a definite risk. Intoxication typically lasts 4 to 6 hours, but some effects can linger for several days. Delirium may occur within 24 hours of taking PCP or after recovery from an overdose and can last as much as a week.

Sedative-Hypnotics or Anxiolytic (Antianxiety) Drugs

These drugs depress the central nervous system, reduce activity, and induce relaxation, drowsiness, or sleep. They include the benzodiazepines and the barbiturates.

The **benzodiazepines**—the most widely used drugs in this category—are commonly prescribed for tension, muscular strain, sleep problems, anxiety, panic attacks, anesthesia, and in the treatment of alcohol withdrawal. They include such drugs as *chlordiazepoxide* (Librium), *diazepam* (Valium), *oxazepam* (Serax), *lorazepam* (Ativan), *flurazepam* (Dalmane), and *alprazolam* (Xanax).

Benzodiazepine sleeping pills have largely replaced the **barbiturates**, which were used medically in the past for inducing relaxation and sleep, relieving tension, and treating epileptic seizures. These drugs are usually taken by mouth in tablet, capsule, or liquid form. When used as

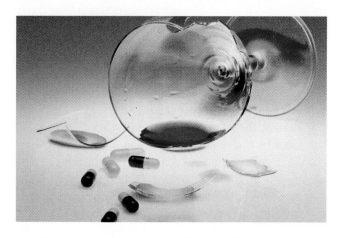

Sedating drugs react dangerously with alcohol.

a general anesthetic, they are administered intravenously. Barbiturates such as *pentobarbital* (brand name Nembutal, or "yellow jackets"), *secobarbital* (Seconal, or "reds"), and *thiopental* (Pentothal) are short-acting and rapidly absorbed into the brain. The longer acting barbiturates, such as *amobarbital* (brand name Amytal, or "blues" or "downers") and *phenobarbital* (Luminal, or "phennies"), which usually are taken orally and absorbed slowly into the bloodstream, take a while to reach the brain and have an effect for several days.

How Users Feel

The lower doses of these drugs may reduce or relieve tension, but increasing doses can cause a loosening of sexual or aggressive inhibitions. Individuals using this class of drugs may experience rapid mood changes, impaired judgment, and impaired social or occupational functioning. High doses produce slurred speech, drowsiness, and stupor.

Risks

All the sedative-hypnotic and anxiolytic drugs can produce physical and psychological dependence within 2 to 4 weeks. A complication specific to sedatives is *cross-tolerance*—or cross-addiction—which occurs when users develop tolerance for one sedative or become dependent on it and develop tolerance for other sedatives as well. Individuals with a prior history of substance abuse are at greatly increased risk of abusing this class of drugs if they are prescribed by a physician. However, those who have not abused drugs or alcohol in the past rarely develop a substance-abuse problem from these medications when they are prescribed for legitimate psychiatric disorders, such as panic disorder or generalized anxiety disorder.

Intoxication with these drugs can produce changes in mood or behavior, such as inappropriate sexual or aggressive acts, mood swings, and impaired judgment. Physical signs include slurred speech, poor coordination, unsteady gait, involuntary eye movements, impaired attention or memory, and stupor or coma.

Taken in combination with alcohol, these drugs have a synergistic effect that can be dangerous or even lethal. For example, an individual's driving ability, already impaired by alcohol, will be made even worse, increasing the risk of an accident. Alcohol in combination with sedative-hypnotics leads to respiratory depression and may result in respiratory arrest and death. Regular users of any of these drugs who become physically dependent should not try to cut down or quit on their own. If they try to quit suddenly, they run the risk of seizures, coma, and death.

Sedative-hypnotic and anxiolytic drugs can easily cross through the placenta and cause birth defects and behavioral problems. Babies born to women who used these drugs during pregnancy may be physically dependent on the drugs and may develop breathing problems, feeding difficulties, disturbed sleep, sweating, irritability, and fever.

Anabolic Steroids

Anabolic steroids, synthetic derivatives of the male hormone testosterone, are powerful compounds prescribed for the treatment of burns and injuries. An estimated 1 million Americans, half of them adolescents (many of whom started steroid use before age 16), use

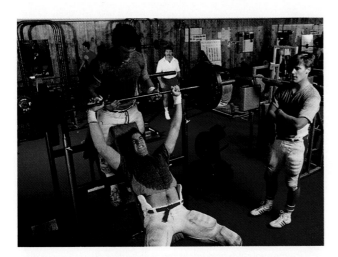

Pumping up. Steroids are an attractive—and highly dangerous—route to a muscular body. They are also illegal, and the side effects range from signs of mental illness to serious heart and liver damage.

illicit steroids. Nonmedical distribution of steroids is a federal offense punishable by 5 years in prison.

The potential side effects of anabolic steroids include an increased risk of heart disease, stroke, or obstructed blood vessels; liver tumors and jaundice; acne; transmission, through shared needles, of HIV; breast enlargement, atrophy of the testicles, and impotence in men; and deepened voice, breast reduction, and beard growth in women. Even a brief period of use in childhood or adolescence can have lasting effects on brain and body chemistry. Steroids may increase the risk of heart disease by lowering levels of high-density lipoproteins (HDL), the "good" blood fat believed to remove deposits from artery walls.[14] Steroids can also create the same problems with dependence and withdrawal as cocaine.

Designer Drugs

Designer drugs ("Adam," "Eve," "China White") are produced in chemical laboratories and sold illegally. Easy to manufacture from available raw materials, the drugs themselves were once technically legal because the law had to specify the exact chemical structure of an illicit drug. However, a law now bans all chemical "cousins" of illegal drugs.

Some of the drugs that emerged as dangers in the 1990s are legal and have legitimate medical uses. They include gamma hydroxybutyrate, or GHB or Liquid X, a depressant with potential benefits for people with narcolepsy, and Rohypnol, a tranquilizer used overseas. Both are better known as date-rape or "easy-lay" drugs that are slipped into women's drinks to knock them out and cause short-term amnesia. Since the drugs are odorless and tasteless, a woman has no way of knowing whether her drink has been tampered with; the subsequent loss of memory leaves her with no explanation for where she's been or what's happened in the hours before she regains consciousness.[15]

Another new drug of abuse is "K," or ketamine, an anesthetic used by veterinarians. When cooked, dried, and ground into a powder for snorting, K blocks chemical messengers in the brain that carry sensory input. As a result, the brain fills the void with hallucinations. Too much K can cause such massive sensory deprivation that researchers compare the impact to a near-death experience. Ketamine is illegal in several states, but the federal government has not yet deemed it a controlled substance—a step that would substantially increase penalties for its use.[16]

Another synthetic, developed by college students in Pennsylvania in the early 1990s, is *methcathinone*, or "cat," a powerful synthetic stimulant that can produce a high that lasts up to 6 days. Cat usually contains a mix of chemicals along with small doses of Drano or battery acid, which act as a catalyst.[17]

MDMA (*methylene dioxymethylamphetamine*, commonly called "ecstasy") is somewhat related to mescaline and amphetamine. An estimated 500,000 to 4 million people—mostly college-age Americans—use the drug, which creates feelings of warmth and openness. The use of ecstasy has increased greatly on campus, with almost one of every four students at some universities reporting its use.[18]

Users can develop insomnia, loss of appetite, muscle aches or stiffness, nausea, fatigue, and problems concentrating. MDMA destroys brain cells in animals; in humans it may damage the nerve cells that produce serotonin, a neurotransmitter involved in regulating responses to stress and pain, appetite, and sexual behavior. According to a 1995 report from Johns Hopkins University, the damage produced by ecstasy may do lasting harm by causing key nerve cells in the brain to grow back abnormally.[19]

Treating Drug Dependence and Abuse

The most difficult step for a drug user is to admit that he or she *is* in fact an addict. If they are not forced to deal with their problem through some unexpected trauma, such as being fired or going bankrupt, those who care—family, friends, coworkers, doctors—may have to confront them and insist that they do something about their addiction. Often this intervention can be the turning point for addicts and their families.

Treatment may take place in an outpatient setting, a residential facility, or a hospital. Increasingly, treatment thereafter is tailored to address coexisting or dual diagnoses. A personal treatment plan may consist of individual psychotherapy, marital and family therapy, medication, and behavior therapy. Once an individual has made the decision to seek help for substance abuse, the first step usually is detoxification, which involves clearing the drug from the body. An exception is methadone maintenance, which does not rely on complete detoxification.

Controlled and supervised withdrawal within a medical or psychiatric hospital may be recommended if an individual has not been able to stop using drugs as an outpatient or in a residential treatment program. Detoxification is most likely to be complicated when a person is a polysubstance abuser and may require close monitoring and treatment of potentially fatal withdrawal symptoms.

Outpatient programs for substance abuse, offered by freestanding centers, hospitals, and community mental health centers, often run 4 or 5 nights a week for 4 to 8 weeks, or in daily 8-hour sessions for 7 to 8 days, followed by weekly group therapy. These outpatient programs allow recovering drug users to go on with their daily lives and learn to deal with day-to-day work and family stresses. Mental health professionals in private practice also offer individually structured outpatient treatment.

Twelve-Step Programs

Since its founding in 1935, Alcoholics Anonymous (AA)—the oldest, largest, and most successful self-help program in the world—has spawned a movement (see Chapter 12). As many as 200 different recovery programs are based on the spiritual **twelve-step program** of AA. Participation in twelve-step programs for drug abusers, such as Substance Anonymous, Narcotics Anonymous, and Cocaine Anonymous, is of fundamental importance in promoting and maintaining long-term abstinence.[20]

Strategies for Change

Getting the Most Out of a Twelve-Step Program

✔ Try out different groups until you find one you like and in which you feel comfortable.

✔ Once you find a group in which you feel comfortable, go back several times (some recommend a minimum of six meetings) before making a final decision on whether to continue.

✔ Keep an open mind. Listen to other people's stories and ask yourself if you've had similar feelings or experiences.

✔ Accept whatever feels right to you and ignore the rest. One common saying in twelve-step programs is, "Take what you like and leave the rest."

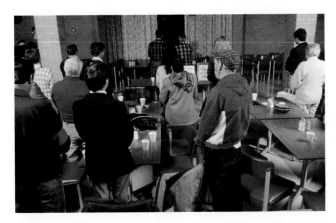

Twelve-step programs, based on the Alcoholics Anonymous model, have helped many people overcome behavioral addictions and addictions to alcohol, food, and drugs. The one requirement for membership is a desire to stop living out a pattern of addictive behavior.

The basic precept of twelve-step programs is that members have been powerless when it comes to controlling their addictive behavior on their own. These programs don't recruit members. The desire to stop must come from the individual, who can call the number of a twelve-step program, listed in the telephone book, and find out when and where the next nearby meeting will be held. A representative may offer to send someone to the caller's house to talk about the problem and to escort him or her to the next meeting.

Meetings of various twelve-step programs are held daily in almost every city in the country. (Some chapters, whose members often include the disabled or those in remote areas, "meet" via electronic bulletin boards on their personal computers.) There are no dues or fees for membership. Many individuals belong to several programs because they have several problems, such as alcoholism, substance abuse, and pathological gambling. All have only one requirement for membership: a desire to stop an addictive behavior.

Relapse Prevention

The most common clinical course for substance abuse disorders involves a pattern of multiple relapses over the course of a lifespan. It is important for individuals with these problems and their families to recognize this fact. When relapses do occur, they should be viewed as neither a mark of defeat nor evidence of moral weakness. While painful, they do not erase the progress that has been achieved and ultimately may strengthen self-

Strategies for Change

If Someone You Love Has a Drug Problem

✔ Get as much information as you can so that you understand what you—and your loved one—are up against. Also get some intervention training. Specially trained counselors work at most chemical-dependence units; some offer advice by phone.

✔ Confront the user. Along with other loved ones and, if possible, a professional counselor, detail incident after incident in which the drug abuse affected or hurt you, other members of your family, or the user.

✔ Don't expect a drug abuser to quit without help. Chemical dependence is a medical and psychological disorder that requires professional treatment. Offer your support, but make it clear that you expect your loved one to undergo therapy.

✔ If your loved one agrees to treatment, make sure that the program is based on a complete evaluation, checking for medical and emotional problems, as well as chemical dependence.

✔ Don't believe abusers who say they've learned to control their drug use. Abstinence is a cornerstone of any good rehabilitation program.

✔ Encourage a user to attend support groups, such as Cocaine Anonymous or Narcotics Anonymous, for at least 1 year after rehabilitation. Get help for yourself. Most hospitals and chemical-dependence programs offer educational programs for codependents.

understanding. They can serve as reminders of potential pitfalls to avoid in the future.

One key to preventing relapse is learning to avoid obvious cues and associations that can set off intense cravings. This means staying away from the people and places linked with past drug use.

Another important lesson that therapists emphasize is that every "lapse" does not have to lead to a full-blown relapse. Users can turn to the skills acquired in treatment—calling people for support or going to meetings—to avoid a major relapse. Ultimately, users must learn much more than how to avoid temptation; they must examine their entire view of the world and learn new ways to live in it without turning to drugs. This is the underlying goal of the recovery process.

Health Online

Dapa-PC Drug Abuse Screening   http://www.danya.com/middle5.htm

Are you at risk for drug abuse? Take this online screening test and find out. The anonymous assessment looks at your drug-taking behavior, its effects on your life, and other physical, mental, emotional, and social risk factors for drug abuse.

Think about it ...

- According to this assessment, do you have any risk factors for drug abuse? What are they and how might you avoid them?

- Have you ever misused a drug, even caffeine, or an over-the-counter medication? If so, why? What was the experience like?

- Do you think that there are situations in which it is okay to use an illegal psychoactive drug? Do you think using these drugs to enhance performance or as a recreational activity is legitimate? Why or why not?

Making This Chapter Work for You
Working Toward a Drug-Free Future

- Drugs—chemical substances that alter physiological or psychological processes—can be misused (used for a purpose—or person—other than that for which they were medically intended) or abused (used excessively or inappropriately). The misuse or abuse of psychoactive drugs can lead to physical and psychological dependence.

- Physical dependence occurs when physiological changes in the body caused by a drug result in an intense need for the drug. Psychological dependence occurs when users crave a drug for the emotional or mental changes it produces.

- Over-the-counter (OTC) drugs and prescription drugs can be misused or abused. The OTCs most often abused include painkillers and nasal inhalants. Prescription medications are often misused despite serious physical risks.

- Caffeine, though habit-forming and implicated in various health problems, doesn't seem to present any clear health threat if used in moderation.

- Amphetamine abusers may suffer from tremors, irregular heartbeat, loss of coordination, psychosis and paranoia, malnutrition, skin disorders, ulcers, depression, brain damage, and heart failure. A form of smokeable methamphetamine, known as ice or glass, increases heart rate and blood pressure; high doses can cause permanent damage to blood vessels in the brain. Crank (propylhexedrine) produces effects similar to those of amphetamines.

- THC, the primary psychoactive ingredient in marijuana and hashish, can produce an increased heart rate, dry mouth and throat, and altered perception; high doses may result in distorted perception, hallucinations, and acute panic attacks. Long-term marijuana use may result in psychological dependence; lung damage; impairment of the central nervous system, reproductive system, and immune system; use of other drugs; mental and emotional dulling; loss of drive; and legal consequences.

- Cocaine, which produces feelings of high energy, may be snorted as a powder, smoked (or freebased) in a form called crack or rock, or dissolved in a solution that's then injected. The effects of cocaine use include impaired judgment, psychological disorders (including psychosis), headache, nausea, damaged nasal membranes in snorters, weight loss, liver damage, heart attack, stroke, brain seizure or hemorrhage, complications during pregnancy, and mental and physical damage to infants born to cocaine users.

- Sedative-hypnotics and antianxiety agents turn down the central nervous system. Barbiturate use can result in physical dependence, and because the addict needs increasingly larger doses, the risk of fatal overdose is high. Antianxiety medications, such as Valium and Xanax, can produce dependence, drowsiness, and slurred speech; withdrawal can produce coma, psychosis, and even death.

■ Hallucinogens, including peyote and its active ingredient, mescaline; lysergic acid diethylamide (LSD); psilocybin; and phencyclidine (PCP) can produce hallucinations and, in some users, panic, paranoia, and psychotic episodes. PCP is a dangerous psychoactive drug because of its effects on behavior.

■ The opiates, including opium, morphine, heroin, and codeine, may lead to infections of the heart, skin abscesses, and congested lungs, as well as tetanus, liver disease, hepatitis, and HIV infection from the use of unsterile syringes and needles.

■ Inhalants can lead to serious complications. Designer drugs are illegally manufactured drugs that are far more potent than natural substances.

■ Treatment for drug dependence usually includes a combination of approaches, including detoxification in a hospital or as an outpatient, admission to a residential therapeutic community, or treatment in an outpatient drug-counseling program.

▶ Key Terms

The terms listed here are used within the chapter. Page numbers are included for each term. A definition of each term is given in the green Glossary pages at the end of this book.

▶ Review Questions

1. What does it mean to be drug dependent? What are the contributing factors? How can you tell if someone is abusing drugs?

2. What is an amphetamine? What are some common forms of amphetamines? Describe the uses of amphetamines and their effects on the user.

3. What are sedatives, hypnotics, and antianxiety drugs? What are some common forms of these drugs? Describe their uses and the effects on the user.

4. List some methods of treatment for drug dependence. What are some of the issues affecting treatment?

▶ Critical Thinking Questions

1. New testing procedures have been developed that allow one to detect the presence of drugs, such as marijuana, simply by using a sample of the drug user's hair. Parents could presumably use this test to determine if their children have been taking drugs. How do you feel about this? Is it fair? Would you use such a test on your children? What would you say if your parents used the test on you?

2. Alan has experimented with cocaine on a few occasions, and he talks about his experience in glowing terms. In fact, as your best friend, he'd like you to try it with him sometime. When you question him about the dangers of addiction, he says, "Are you crazy? I don't do this more than once a month. I'm not addicted!" How would you respond to Alan?

3. Sheila was doing spring cleaning when she came across a brown bag at the back of the linen closet.

That evening she confronted her roommate about keeping an illegal substance in the apartment. Meg's response was, "Oh, I forgot that little bit of weed was even there. Besides, no one would *ever* find it. What are you so uptight about?" Sheila insisted, "I don't care if it's just a little—it's still illegal, and I don't want it here." How would you resolve their dispute?

 ## Connections to Personal Health Interactive

To enhance your understanding of the material covered in this chapter, check out the following study aids on the **Personal Health Interactive CD-ROM** .

- Personal Insights: How Do You Feel About Drugs?
- **Online Research:** Drugs, Alcohol, and Tobacco

- Study Page: Drug Effects
- Glossary & Key Term Review

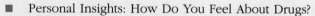 ## References

1. Warner, Lynn, et al. "Prevalence and Correlates of Drug Use and Dependence in the United States: Results from the National Comorbidity Survey." *Archives of General Psychiatry*, Vol. 52, March 1995.
2. "Aspirin." *Remedy*, Summer 1995.
3. Pilliteri, Janine, et al. "Over-the-Counter Sleep Aids: Widely Used but Rarely Studied." *Journal of Substance Abuse*, Vol. 6, No. 3, 1994.
4. "Caffeine's Hook." *Current Health*, Vol. 2, No. 24, January 1998.
5. Wren, Christopher. "Survey Suggests Leveling Off in Use of Drugs by Students." *New York Times*, December 21, 1997.
6. Eigen, Lewis, and David Rowden. "The Success of Alcohol, Tobacco and Other Drug Prevention: A White Paper." National Clearinghouse for Alcohol and Drug Information, Rockville, MD, 1993.
7. Douglas, Kathy, et al. "Results from the 1995 National College Health Risk Behavior Survey." *Journal of American College Health*, Vol. 46, September 1997.
8. Urberg, Kathryn, et al. "Close Friend and Group Influence on Adolescent Cigarette Smoking and Alcohol Use." *Developmental Psychology*, Vol. 130, No. 5, September 1997.
9. Lehrman, Sally. "Make Marijuana Research Easier, Panel Urges NIH." *Nature*, Vol. 388, No. 6643, August 14, 1997.

10. Grinspoon, Lester, and James Bakalar. "Marijuana As Medicine." *Journal of the American Medical Association*, Vol. 273, No. 23, June 21, 1995.
11. Brownsberger, William. "Prevalence of Frequent Cocaine Use in Urban Poverty Areas." *Contemporary Drug Problems*, Vol. 24, No. 2, Summer 1997.
12. Chrebet, Jennifer. "Getting High on Household Products." *American Health*, November 1994.
13. International Institute on Inhalant Abuse, 450 West Jefferson Ave., Englewood, CO 80110.
14. Sachtleben, Thomas, et al. "Serum Lipoprotein Patterns in Long-term Anabolic Steroid Users." *Research Quarterly for Exercise & Sport*, Vol. 68, No. 1, March 1997.
15. Gorman, Christine. "Liquid X." *Time*, September 30, 1996.
16. Cloud, John. "Is Your Kid on K?" *Time*, October 20, 1997.
17. Monroe, Judy. "Designer Drugs: Cat & LSD." *Current Health*, Vol. 21, No. 1, September 1994.
18. Cuomo, Michael, et al. "Increasing Use of 'Ecstasy' (MDMA) and Other Hallucinogens on a College Campus." *Journal of American College Health*, Vol. 42, No. 6, May 1994.
19. Ricaurte, George, et al. "Street Drug Ecstasy May Cause Lasting Brain Damage." *Journal of Neuroscience*, August 1995.
20. Lurtz, Linda. "Recovery, the 12-step Movement, and Politics." *Social Work*, Vol. 42, No. 14, July 1997.

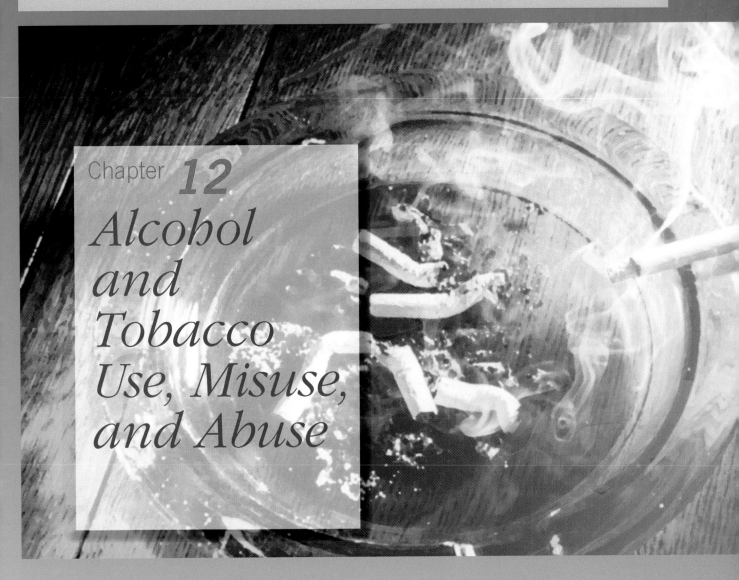

Chapter 12
Alcohol and Tobacco Use, Misuse, and Abuse

After studying the material in this chapter, you should be able to:

- **Describe** the effects of alcohol on the body, behavior, and thought.
- **Define** alcohol abuse, dependence, and alcoholism and **list** their symptoms.
- **List** the negative consequences to individuals and to our society from alcohol abuse.
- **List** the health effects of smoking tobacco and using smokeless tobacco.
- **Describe** the social impact of individuals' tobacco use.
- **List** the health effects of environmental tobacco smoke.

*D*o you want to live to a healthy old age? Keep this in mind: The biggest causes of premature death and disability are alcohol- and tobacco-related problems. Together, their toll on society, families, and individual lives is incalculable. This chapter provides information about alcohol and tobacco, their impact on the body, brain, behavior, and society, patterns of use, and ways people can stop using these substances.

Alcohol and Its Effects

Pure alcohol is a colorless liquid obtained through the fermentation of a liquid containing sugar. **Ethyl alcohol**, or *ethanol*, is the type of alcohol in alcoholic beverages. Another type—methyl, or wood, alcohol—is a poison that should never be drunk. Any liquid containing 0.5% to 80% ethyl alcohol by volume is an alcoholic beverage. However, different drinks contain different amounts of alcohol (see Figure 12-1).

One drink can be any of the following:

- One bottle or can (12 ounces) of beer, which is 5% alcohol.

- One glass (4 ounces) of table wine, such as burgundy, which is 12% alcohol.

- One small glass (2½ ounces) of fortified wine, such as sherry, which is 20% alcohol.

- One shot (1 ounce) of distilled spirits, such as whiskey, vodka, or rum, which is 50% alcohol.

All of these drinks contain close to the same amount of alcohol—that is, if the number of ounces in each drink is multiplied by the percentage of alcohol, each drink contains the equivalent of approximately ½ ounce of 100% ethyl alcohol. With distilled spirits (such as bourbon, scotch, vodka, gin, and rum), alcohol content is expressed in terms of **proof**, a number that is *twice* the percentage of alcohol: 100-proof bourbon is 50% alcohol; 80-proof gin is 40% alcohol.

But the words "bottle" and "glass" can be deceiving in this context. Drinking a 16-ounce bottle of malt liquor, which is 6.4% alcohol, is *not* the same as drinking a 12-ounce glass of 3.2% beer.

As with other substance-use disorders, prevention is the best approach to alcohol problems. According to public health officials, if Americans drank less, the rates of alcohol dependence and abuse could be cut almost in half—from the current 15.5% of the population to 8.2%.[1]

How Much Can You Drink?

The best way to figure how much you can drink safely is to determine the amount of alcohol in your blood at any given time, or your **blood-alcohol concentration (BAC)**. BAC is expressed in terms of the percentage of alcohol in the blood and is often measured from breath or urine samples. Law enforcement officers use BAC to determine whether a driver is legally drunk. The Federal Department of Transportation has called on states to set 0.08% as the threshold at which a person can be cited for drunk driving. In the past, 0.1% was often the legal limit (see Figure 12-2).

A BAC of 0.05% indicates approximately 5 parts alcohol to 10,000 parts other blood components. Most people reach this level after consuming one or two drinks and experience all the positive sensations of drinking—relaxation, euphoria, and well-being—without feeling intoxicated. If they continue to drink past the 0.05% BAC level, they start feeling worse rather than better, gradually losing control of speech, balance, and emotions (see Table 12-1). At a BAC of 0.2%, they may pass

Figure 12-1

The alcohol content of different drinks.

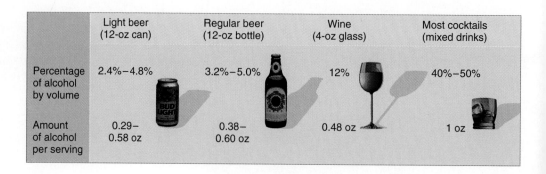

	Light beer (12-oz can)	Regular beer (12-oz bottle)	Wine (4-oz glass)	Most cocktails (mixed drinks)
Percentage of alcohol by volume	2.4%–4.8%	3.2%–5.0%	12%	40%–50%
Amount of alcohol per serving	0.29–0.58 oz	0.38–0.60 oz	0.48 oz	1 oz

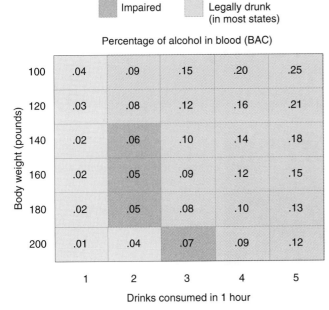

Figure 12-2

Blood-alcohol concentration and body weight. How fast one's BAC level rises depends on body weight and on how many drinks one has in a given amount of time. One drink is 12 ounces of beer, 4 ounces of wine, or 1½ ounces of 80-proof liquor.

out. At a BAC of 0.3%, they could lapse into a coma; at 0.4%, they could die.

How You Respond to Alcohol

Many factors affect an individual's BAC and response to alcohol, including the following:

- *How much and how quickly you drink.* The more alcohol you put into your body, the higher your BAC. If you chug drink after drink, your liver, which metabolizes about 1/2 ounce of alcohol an hour, won't be able to keep up—and your BAC will soar.

- *What you're drinking.* The stronger the drink, the faster and harder the alcohol hits. Straight shots of liquor and cocktails such as martinis get alcohol into your bloodstream faster than beer or table wine. Beer and wine not only contain lower concentrations of alcohol, but they also contain nonalcoholic substances that slow the rate of **absorption** (passage of the alcohol into your body tissues). If the drink contains water, juice, or milk, the rate of absorption will be slowed. However, carbon dioxide—whether in champagne, ginger ale, or a cola—whisks alcohol into your bloodstream. Also, the alcohol in warm drinks—such as a hot rum toddy or warmed sake—moves into your bloodstream more quickly than the alcohol in chilled wine or scotch on the rocks.

- *Your size.* If you're a large person (whether due to fat or to muscle), you'll get drunk more slowly than someone smaller who's drinking the same amount of alcohol at the same rate. Heavier individuals have a larger water volume, which dilutes the alcohol they drink.

- *Your gender.* Women have lower quantities of a stomach enzyme that neutralizes alcohol, so one drink for a woman has the impact that two drinks have for a man.

- *Your age.* The same amount of alcohol produces higher BACs in older drinkers, who have lower volumes of body water to dilute the alcohol than younger drinkers do.

- *Your race.* Many members of certain ethnic groups, including Asians and Native Americans, are unable to break down alcohol as quickly as Caucasians. This can result in higher BACs, as well as uncomfortable reactions, such as flushing and nausea, when they drink. (See Spotlight on Diversity: "Drinking and Ethnic Groups.")

TABLE 12-1 RECOGNIZING THE WARNING SIGNS OF ALCOHOLISM

• Experiencing the following symptoms after drinking: frequent headaches, nausea, stomach pain, heartburn, gas, fatigue, weakness, muscle cramps, or irregular or rapid heartbeats. • Needing a drink in the morning to start the day.	• Denying any problem with alcohol. • Doing things while drinking that are regretted afterward. • Dramatic mood swings, from anger to laughter to anxiety. • Sleep problems.	• Depression and paranoia. • Forgetting what happened during a drinking episode. • Changing brands or going on the wagon to control drinking. • Having five or more drinks a day.

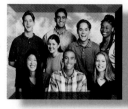

Spotlight on Diversity
Drinking and Ethnic Groups

Individuals in any racial and ethnic group can develop drinking problems, but certain groups suffer disproportionately high rates of alcohol dependence and abuse and related illnesses. These groups include African Americans, Latinos, and Native Americans. In addition, alcohol presents other concerns for Asians and Asian Americans.

• **The African-American Community** Overall, African Americans consume less alcohol per person than whites, yet twice as many blacks die of cirrhosis of the liver each year. In some cities, the rate of cirrhosis is ten times higher among African-American than white men. Alcohol also contributes to high rates of hypertension, esophageal cancer, and homicide among African-American men.

• **The Latino Community** Latino societies discourage any drinking by women but encourage heavy drinking by men as part of their machismo, or feelings of manhood. According to the Department of Health and Human Services, Latino men have higher rates of alcohol use and abuse than the general population and suffer a high rate of cirrhosis. Moreover, American-born Latino men drink more than those born in other countries.

• **The Native-American Community** Not all Native Americans drink, and not all who drink do so to excess. However, they have three times the general population's rate of alcohol-related injury and illness. Moreover, cirrhosis of the liver is the fourth leading cause of death among this cultural group. While many Native-American women don't drink, those who do have high rates of alcohol-related

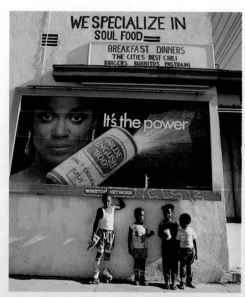

The makers of alcoholic beverages market their products aggressively in poor urban neighborhoods, where liquor stores and bars are common.

problems, which affect both them and their children. Their rate of cirrhosis of the liver is thirty-six times that of white women. In some tribes, 10.5 out of every 1000 newborns have fetal alcohol syndrome, compared with 1–3 out of 1000 in the general population (see Figure 12-4).

Both a biological predisposition and socioeconomic conditions may contribute to alcohol abuse by Native Americans. In addition, according to their cultural beliefs, alcoholism is not a physical disease but a spiritual disorder—making it less likely that they'll seek appropriate treatment.

• **The Asian-American Community** Asian Americans tend to drink very little or not at all, in part because of an inborn physiological reaction to alcohol that causes facial flushing, rapid heart rate, lowered blood pressure, nausea, vomiting, and other symptoms. A very high percentage of women of all Asian-American nationalities abstain completely. Some sociologists have expressed concern, however, that as Asian Americans become more assimilated into American culture, they'll drink more—and possibly suffer very adverse effects from alcohol.

SOURCES: Caetano, Raul. "Drinking and Alcohol-Related Problems Among Minority Women." *Alcohol Health & Research World*, Vol. 18, No. 3, Summer 1994. Atkinson, Donald, et al. "Mexican American and European American Ratings of Four Alcoholism Treatment Programs." *Hispanic Journal of Behavioral Sciences*, Vol. 16, No. 3, August 1994. Higuchi, Susumu, and Hiroaki KoNo. "Early Diagnosis and Treatment of Alcoholism: The Japanese Experience." *Alcohol & Alcoholism*, Vol. 29, No. 4, July 1994.

• *Other drugs.* Some common medications—including aspirin, acetaminophen (Tylenol), and ulcer medications—can cause blood-alcohol levels to increase more rapidly. Individuals taking these drugs can be over the legal limit for blood-alcohol concentration after as little as a single drink.[2]

• *Family history of alcoholism.* Some children of alcoholics don't develop any of the usual behavioral

symptoms that indicate someone is drinking too much. It's not known whether this behavior is genetically caused or is a result of growing up with an alcoholic.

• *Eating.* Food slows the absorption of alcohol by diluting it, by covering some of the membranes through which alcohol would be absorbed, and by prolonging the time the stomach takes to empty.

- *Expectations.* In various experiments, volunteers who believed they were given alcoholic beverages but were actually given nonalcoholic drinks acted as if they were guzzling the real thing and became more talkative, relaxed, and sexually stimulated.[3]

- *Physical tolerance.* If you drink regularly, your brain becomes accustomed to a certain level of alcohol. You may be able to look and behave in a seemingly normal fashion, even though you drink as much as would normally intoxicate someone your size. However, your driving ability and judgment will still be impaired.

Once you develop tolerance, you may drink more to get the desired effects from alcohol. In some people, this can lead to abuse and alcoholism. On the other hand, after years of drinking, some people become exquisitely sensitive to alcohol. Such reverse tolerance means that they can become intoxicated after drinking only a small amount of alcohol.

How Much Is Too Much?

Unlike many other drugs of abuse, including tobacco, any and all amounts of alcohol are not toxic. According to a 1997 study of nearly 500,000 people from ages 35 to 69, one drink a day can in fact be good for health. Those who had one serving (see Figure 12-1) of wine, beer, or hard liquor had a death rate 20% lower than nondrinkers over a 5-year period. Nearly all of the benefit came from a reduction in the risk of heart disease. However, the researchers cautioned that for women, a drink a day—while lowering the overall risk of deaths—increased by 30% the chance of dying from breast cancer.[4]

Federal health authorities at the National Institute of Alcohol and Alcohol Abuse (NIAAA) recommend that men have no more than two drinks a day and women no more than one. Some people—such as women who are pregnant or trying to conceive; individuals with problems, such as ulcers, that might be aggravated by alcohol; those taking medications such as sleeping pills or antidepressants; and those driving or operating any motorized equipment—shouldn't drink at all.

The dangers of alcohol increase along with the amount you drink. Heavy drinking destroys the liver, weakens the heart, elevates blood pressure, damages the brain, and increases the risk of cancer. Individuals who drink heavily have a higher mortality rate than those who have two or fewer drinks a day. However, the boundary between safe and dangerous drinking isn't the same for everyone. For some people, the

upper limit of safety is zero: Once they start, they can't stop.

Intoxication

If you drink too much, the immediate consequence is that you get drunk—or, more precisely, intoxicated. According to the American Psychiatric Association's *Diagnostic and Statistical Manual of Mental Disorders,* 4th edition *(DSM-IV),* **intoxication** consists of "clinically significant maladaptive behavioral or psychological changes," such as inappropriate sexual or aggressive behavior, mood changes, and impaired judgment and social and occupational functioning.[5] Alcohol intoxication, which can range from mild inebriation to loss of consciousness, is characterized by at least one of the following signs: slurred speech, poor coordination, unsteady gait, abnormal eye movements, impaired attention or memory, stupor, or coma. Medical risks of intoxication include falls, hypothermia in cold climates, and increased risk of infections because of suppressed immune function.

Time and a protective environment are the recommended treatments for alcohol intoxication. Anyone who passes out after drinking heavily should be monitored regularly to ensure that vomiting (the result of excess alcohol irritating the stomach) doesn't block the

Strategies for Change

How to Promote Responsible Drinking

✔ When preparing drinks for guests, measure the amount of alcohol you use and figure out how many ounces your wine and beer glasses hold. Avoid pushing drinks on guests and refilling glasses quickly.

✔ Always serve food when serving drinks—but not the salty nuts, chips, and pretzels bars serve to increase thirst. Stop serving alcohol 1 hour before the evening is to end.

✔ Make sure nonalcoholic alternatives are available.

✔ Never serve alcohol to a guest who seems intoxicated.

✔ Never let an intoxicated person drive home. You could be legally, as well as morally, responsible in the event of an accident. Call a taxi or have a friend who hasn't been drinking drive the person home. As a last resort, call the police. In many communities, they'll drive an intoxicated person home as a public service.

breathing airway. Always make sure that an unconscious drinker is lying on his or her side, with the head lower than the body. Intoxicated drinkers can slip into shock, a potentially life-threatening condition characterized by a weak pulse, irregular breathing, and skin-color changes. This is an emergency, and professional medical care should be sought immediately.

The Impact of Alcohol

Unlike drugs in tablet form or food, alcohol is directly and quickly absorbed into the bloodstream through the stomach walls and upper intestine. The alcohol in a typical drink reaches the bloodstream in 15 minutes and rises to its peak concentration in about an hour. The bloodstream carries the alcohol to the liver, heart, and brain (see Figure 12-3).

Alcohol is a *diuretic*, a drug that speeds up the elimination of fluid from the body. Most of the alcohol you drink can leave your body only after metabolism by the liver, which converts about 95% of the alcohol to carbon dioxide and water. The other 5% is excreted unchanged, mainly through urination, respiration, and perspiration. Alcohol lowers body temperature, so you should never drink to get or stay warm.

Digestive System

Alcohol reaches the stomach first, where it is partially broken down. The remaining alcohol is absorbed easily through the stomach tissue into the bloodstream. When it's in the stomach, alcohol triggers the secretion of acids in the stomach, which irritate its lining. Excessive drinking at one sitting may result in nausea; chronic drinking may result in peptic ulcers (breaks in the stomach lining) and bleeding from the stomach lining.

The alcohol in the bloodstream eventually reaches the liver. The liver, which bears the major responsibility of fat metabolism in the body, converts this excess alcohol to fat. After a few weeks of four or five drinks a day, liver cells start to accumulate fat. Alcohol also stimulates

Figure 12-3

The effects of alcohol abuse on the body.

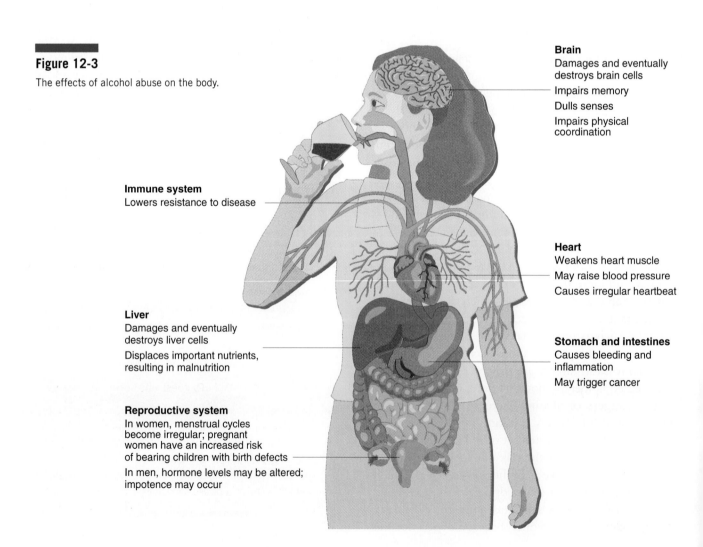

Immune system
Lowers resistance to disease

Liver
Damages and eventually destroys liver cells

Displaces important nutrients, resulting in malnutrition

Reproductive system
In women, menstrual cycles become irregular; pregnant women have an increased risk of bearing children with birth defects

In men, hormone levels may be altered; impotence may occur

Brain
Damages and eventually destroys brain cells
Impairs memory
Dulls senses
Impairs physical coordination

Heart
Weakens heart muscle
May raise blood pressure
Causes irregular heartbeat

Stomach and intestines
Causes bleeding and inflammation
May trigger cancer

liver cells to attract white blood cells, which normally travel throughout the bloodstream engulfing harmful substances and wastes. If white blood cells begin to invade body tissue, such as the liver, they can cause irreversible damage.

Cardiovascular System

Alcohol gets mixed reviews regarding its effects on the cardiovascular system. Moderate drinkers have healthier hearts, suffer fewer heart attacks, have less buildup of cholesterol in their arteries, and are less likely to die of heart disease than heavy drinkers or teetotalers.

Excessive drinking can clearly endanger the heart's health. Alcohol use can weaken the heart muscle directly, causing a disorder called cardiomyopathy.[6] The combined use of alcohol and other drugs, including tobacco and cocaine, greatly increases the likelihood of damage to the heart.

Immune System

Chronic alcohol use can inhibit the production of both white blood cells, which fight off infections, and red blood cells, which carry oxygen to all the organs and tissues of the body. Alcohol may increase the risk of infection with human immunodeficiency virus (HIV) by altering the judgment of users so that they more readily engage in activities, such as unsafe sexual practices, that put them in danger. If you drink when you have a cold or the flu, alcohol interferes with the body's ability to recover. It also increases the chance of bacterial pneumonia in flu sufferers.

Brain and Behavior

At first, when you drink, you feel up. In low dosages, alcohol affects the regions of the brain that inhibit or control behavior, so you feel looser and act in ways you might not otherwise. However, you also experience losses of concentration, memory, judgment, and fine motor control, and you have mood swings and emotional outbursts. Moderate and heavy drinkers have shown signs of impaired intelligence, slowed-down reflexes, and difficulty remembering.[7]

Interaction with Other Drugs

Alcohol can interact with other drugs—prescription and nonprescription, legal and illegal. Of the 100 most frequently prescribed drugs, more than half contain at least one ingredient that interacts adversely with alcohol. Because alcohol and other psychoactive drugs may work on the same areas of the brain, their combination can produce an effect much greater than that expected of either drug by itself. The consequences of this synergistic interaction can be fatal. Alcohol is particularly dangerous when combined with depressants and antianxiety medications.

Increased Risk of Dying

Alcohol kills. The mortality rate for alcoholics is two and a half times higher than for nonalcoholics of the same age. The leading alcohol-related cause of death is injury, chiefly auto accidents involving a drunk driver. Alcohol is associated with at least half of all traffic fatalities, half of all homicides, and a quarter of all suicides.

The second leading cause of alcohol-related deaths is digestive disease, including *cirrhosis* of the liver, a chronic disease that causes extensive scarring and irreversible damage. In addition, as many as half of the patients admitted to hospitals and 15% of those making office visits seek or need medical care because of the direct or indirect effects of alcohol.[8]

Young drinkers—teens and those in their early twenties—are at highest risk of dying from injuries, mostly car accidents. Older drinkers over age 50 face the greatest danger of premature death from cirrhosis of the liver, hepatitis, and other alcohol-linked illnesses.

Drinking in America

According to a survey of 47,485 households sponsored by the NIAAA, about half (52%) of American adults drink.[9] The survey showed little variation among the races with respect to quantity, frequency, and amount of alcohol consumed, although whites were more likely to be classified as daily or nearly daily drinkers than non-whites. A greater percentage of females than males reported a lifetime pattern of infrequent drinking (less than twelve drinks a year).[10] Men and women are most likely to drink between the ages of 21 and 34. Drinking typically declines with age.

The National Council on Alcoholism describes alcohol as the number-one drug problem among the nation's youth, with boys and girls experimenting with alcohol at younger ages than in previous decades. According to NIAAA statistics, the average age at which children take their first drink is now just under 13, and 40% have tasted alcohol by the age of 10. About 30% of teenagers experience negative consequences of alcohol abuse, including alcohol-related accidents, arrests, or impaired health or school performance.[11]

Pulsepoints

Ten Steps to Responsible Drinking

1. Don't drink alone. Cultivate friendships with nondrinkers and responsible moderate drinkers.

2. Don't use alcohol as a medicine. Rather than reaching for a drink to put you to sleep, help you relax, or relieve tension, develop alternative means of unwinding, such as exercise, meditation, or listening to music.

3. Develop a party plan. Set a limit on how many drinks you'll have before you go out—and stick to it.

4. Alternate alcoholic and nonalcoholic drinks. At a social occasion, have a nonalcoholic beverage to quench your thirst.

5. Drink slowly. Never have more than one drink an hour.

6. Eat before and while drinking. Choose foods high in protein (cheese, meat, eggs, or milk) rather than salty foods (peanuts or chips) that increase thirst.

7. Be wary of mixed drinks. Fizzy mixers, like club soda and ginger ale, speed alcohol to the blood and brain.

8. Don't make drinking the primary focus of any get-together. Cultivate other interests and activities that you can enjoy on your own or with friends.

9. Learn to say no. A simple "Thank you, but I've had enough" will do.

10. Stay safe. During or after drinking, avoid any tasks, including driving, that could be affected by alcohol.

Why People Drink

The most common reason people drink alcohol is to relax. Because it depresses the central nervous system, alcohol can make people feel less tense. Other motivations for drinking include the following:

- *Celebration.* Unless alcohol use violates family, ethnic, or religious values, people raise their glasses together on life's important occasions—births, graduations, weddings, promotions.

- *Friendship.* When friends visit, you may have a drink, or you may meet friends somewhere for a drink. Young people are much more likely to experiment with alcohol if their friends drink.[12]

- *Social ease.* When we use alcohol, we may seem bolder, wittier, sexier. At the same time, the people drinking with us become more relaxed and seem to enjoy our company more. Because alcohol lowers inhibitions, some people see it as a prelude to seduction.

- *Self-medication.* Like other drugs, alcohol may be the means some people use to treat—or escape from— painful feelings or bad moods.

- *Role models.* Athletes, some of the most admired celebrities in our country, have a long history of appearing in commercials for alcohol. Many advertisements feature glamorous women holding or sipping alcoholic beverages.

- *Advertising.* Brewers and beer distributors spend $15–$20 million a year promoting their products to college students. Their message: If you want to have fun, have a drink. Adolescents may be especially responsive to such sales pitches.

Drinking on Campus

Colleges today have been described as among the nation's "most alcohol-drenched institutions." Every year America's 12 million undergraduates drink 4 billion cans of beer, averaging fifty-five six-packs apiece, and spending $446 on alcoholic beverages—more than they spend on soft drinks and textbooks combined.[13]

Despite these figures, fewer students drink than in the past. In 1980, 9.5% of college students nationwide said they abstained from alcohol; by 1996, 17% did. According to the University of Michigan's Institute for Social Research, the percentage of students reported drinking daily also declined: from 6.5% in 1980 to 3.2%—as did those reporting binge drinking—from 44% to 38%. The National College Health Risk Behavior Survey, as shown in Campus Focus: "College Students and Alcohol Use," found that 6.6% of men and 2.2% of women reported "frequent" alcohol use, while a much

CAMPUS FOCUS: COLLEGE STUDENTS AND ALCOHOL USE

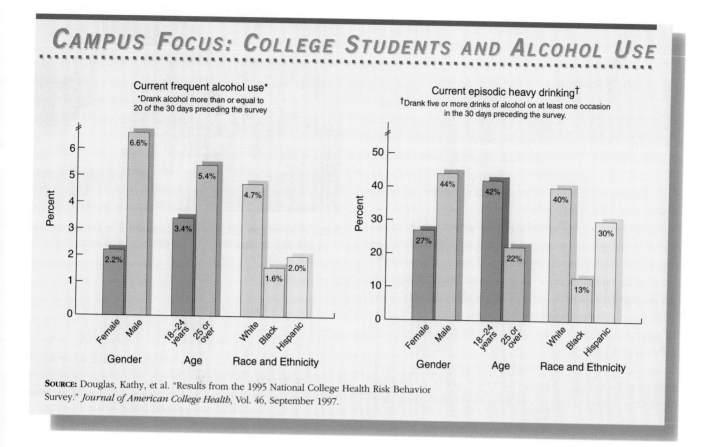

Current frequent alcohol use*
*Drank alcohol more than or equal to 20 of the 30 days preceding the survey

Current episodic heavy drinking†
†Drank five or more drinks of alcohol on at least one occasion in the 30 days preceding the survey.

SOURCE: Douglas, Kathy, et al. "Results from the 1995 National College Health Risk Behavior Survey." *Journal of American College Health*, Vol. 46, September 1997.

higher percentage—43.8% of men and 27% of women—reported episodic heavy drinking.[14]

Why College Students Drink

Most college students drink for the same reasons undergraduates have always turned to alcohol. Away from home, often for the first time, many are both excited by and apprehensive about their newfound independence. When new pressures seem overwhelming, when they feel awkward or insecure, when they just want to let loose and have a good time, they reach for a drink.

Some students, however, seem especially vulnerable to problem drinking. In one new study, undergraduates who felt unable to cope with bad moods and had low expectations of their ability to handle emotional or other difficulties were more prone to problems with alcohol. Rather than rely on coping strategies that would enable them to meet problems head on, they turned to alcohol.[15]

Students may be especially vulnerable to dangerous drinking in their freshman year as they struggle to adapt to an often bewildering new world. In a study of freshmen at a medium-sized state university and at a small,

predominantly African-American university who were nondrinkers as high school seniors, almost half (46.5%) started to drink in college. They were less likely to do so if they had friends who discouraged them from drinking.

Other studies have also linked alcohol consumption with where students live on campus and what they perceive as the norm for acceptable drinking. Members of sororities and fraternities rated all drinking norms as more extreme and perceived fraternity drinking as particularly heavy—but these beliefs existed even before college.

The most dramatic increases in college drinking have been among women: 86% of female undergraduates say they drink; 37%—compared with only 14% in 1977—say they get drunk one to three times in a month. While men tend to drink as a way of partying, women on campus may drink for other reasons. Psychologists have theorized that college women may drink as a way of being with and relating to others, seeking acceptance from peers, and numbing the pain that comes from relationships that don't work.[16]

Among both men and women, those with alcoholic parents and dysfunctional families are at greater risk of substance abuse. By some estimates, one of five college students comes from an alcoholic home and may be at increased risk of developing a drinking problem.[17]

Dangerous Drinking

Binge drinking has emerged as a serious threat to the health and lives of college students. In a single month—November 1997—five college students died in alcohol-related accidents in the state of Virginia alone. At the University of Virginia, a survey found that 25% of students had participated in binge drinking three or more times in the previous 2 weeks.[18]

College students who binge on alcohol face other dangers: They are seven to ten times more likely to engage in unplanned or unprotected sex, to have problems with campus police, or to get hurt. Although female students drink less and less dangerously than men, female binge drinkers are more likely to engage in sexual activity, including intercourse, under the influence of alcohol than women who never binge. Binge-drinking women also report engaging in sexual behaviors when they would otherwise not have and not practicing safe sex, thereby putting themselves at greater risk.

Binge drinkers create problems, not just for themselves, but for others (see Table 12-2). According to one survey, at schools where drinking was most popular,

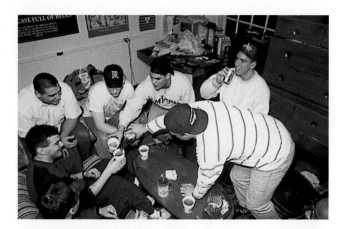

Binge drinkers can get into—and cause—trouble. Dangerously large amounts of alcohol can cause death, and heavy party drinking often results in violence.

two-thirds of students reported having their sleep or studies interrupted by drunken students; more than half had been forced to care for a drunk friend; and at least a fourth had suffered an unwanted sexual advance.[19]

The American College Health Association estimates that drinking accounts for almost two-thirds of all violence on campus and about one-third of all emotional and academic problems among students. Alcohol may play a role in 90% of rapes and sexual assaults.[20] Drinking also claims the lives of many students each year,

---

TABLE 12-2 THE TROUBLES THAT "FREQUENT BINGE DRINKERS" CREATE FOR ...

Themselves*	(% of those surveyed who admitted having had the problem)	And Others†	(% of those surveyed who had been affected)
Missed a class	61%	Had study or sleep interrupted	68%
Forgot where they were or what they did	54%	Had to care for drunken student	54%
Engaged in unplanned sex	41%	Been insulted or humiliated	34%
Got hurt	23%	Experienced unwanted sexual advances	26%
Had unprotected sex	22%	Had serious argument	20%
Damaged property	22%	Had property damaged	15%
Got into trouble with campus or local police	11%	Been pushed or assaulted	13%
Had five or more alcohol-related problems in school year	47%	Had at least one of the above problems	87%

* "Frequent binge drinkers" were defined as those who had had at least four or five drinks at one time on at least three occasions in the previous 2 weeks.

† These figures are from colleges where at least 50% of students are binge drinkers.

SOURCE: Survey of 140 U.S. colleges by the Harvard School of Public Health.

sometimes because of car accidents and sometimes because of drinking games, in which individuals consume dangerously large quantities of alcohol.

Even though students report concern about alcohol, few seek counseling or other services.[21] Colleges are working to improve screening for alcohol problems among students and to educate students about responsible drinking.[22] At some schools, underage students caught drinking must attend a course that introduces the concepts of abstinence and controlled drinking.[23]

Students also are taking steps to ban drunkenness on campus. In addition, there's been an increase in on-campus chapters of national support groups such as AA, Al-Anon, Adult Children of Alcoholics, and a peer-education program called BACCHUS: Boost Alcohol Consciousness Concerning the Health of University Students.

Women and Alcohol

About half of women drink: Of these, 45% are light drinkers; 3%, moderate drinkers; 2%, heavy drinkers; and 21%, binge drinkers.[24] According to the NIAAA, almost 4 million women suffer from alcohol abuse or dependence. But women who drink have different risk factors, potential dangers, and drinking patterns than men.

Problems directly related to a woman's alcohol use range from the consequences of risky sexual behavior after alcohol consumption (such as unwanted pregnancy or STDs) to severe physiological problems related to fertility and pregnancy.[25] Because they have far smaller quantities of a protective enzyme in the stomach to break down alcohol before it's absorbed into the bloodstream, women absorb about 30% more alcohol into their bloodstream than men do.

Among the other health dangers that alcohol holds for women are:

- *Gynecologic problems.* Moderate to heavy drinking may contribute to infertility, menstrual problems, sexual dysfunction, and premenstrual syndrome.[26]

- *Pregnancy and fetal alcohol syndrome (FAS).* When a woman drinks during pregnancy, her unborn child drinks, too. According to Centers for Disease Control (CDC) estimates, more than 8000 alcohol-damaged babies are born every year. One out of every 750 newborns has a cluster of physical and mental defects called **fetal alcohol syndrome (FAS)**: small head, abnormal facial features (see Figure 12-4), jitters, poor muscle tone, sleep disorders, sluggish

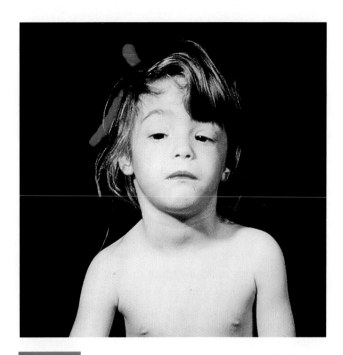

Figure 12-4

A child with fetal alcohol syndrome (FAS) has distinctive facial characteristics that vary with the severity of the disease, including droopy eyelids, a thin upper lip, and a wide space between the nose and upper lip.

motor development, failure to thrive, short stature, delayed speech, mental retardation, or hyperactivity. Many more babies suffer **fetal alcohol effects (FAE)**: low birth weight, irritability as newborns, and permanent mental impairment as a result of their mothers' alcohol consumption.

- Labels on alcoholic beverages have had a proven but modest effect on reducing drinking in pregnancy, while community-based education efforts have been much more effective. Drug and alcohol abuse also can affect the quality of a woman's mothering.[27]

- *Breast cancer.* Numerous studies have suggested an increased risk of breast cancer among women who drink, and many physicians feel that those at high risk for breast cancer should stop, or at least reduce, their consumption of alcohol.

- *Osteoporosis.* As women become older, their risk of osteoporosis, a condition characterized by calcium loss and bone thinning, increases. Alcohol can block the absorption of many nutrients, including calcium, and heavy drinking may worsen the deterioration of bone tissue.

- *Heart disease.* Women who are very heavy drinkers are more at risk of developing irreversible heart disease than are men who drink even more. A 121-pound woman who drinks about 9 ounces of 86-proof liquor or about a liter of wine a day for 20 years puts herself at risk for cardiomyopathy—a disease relatively uncommon among women in general.[28]

Drinking and Driving

Drunk driving is the most frequently committed crime in the United States. In the last two decades, families of the victims of drunk drivers have organized to change the way America treats its drunk drivers. Because of the efforts of MADD (Mothers Against Drunk Driving), SADD (Students Against Driving Drunk), and other lobbying groups, cities, counties, and states are cracking down on drivers who drink. An increasing number of states have toughened their enforcement of drunk-driving penalties. Some suspend a driver's license for several months for a first offense; repeat offenders can lose their licenses for a year or more.

These tougher policies seem to be working. Drunken-driving deaths have declined 31% since 1982.[29] However, they still account for more than 40% of automobile fatalities. According to studies by the National Highway Safety Administration, chronic drunk drivers continue to be a major safety threat. People with prior convictions for drunk driving represent fewer than 2% of all adults, yet they cause up to 60% of all alcohol-related deaths and injuries on U.S. roads.[30]

The National Commission Against Drunk Driving defines chronic drunk drivers as individuals who frequently drive with blood-alcohol levels of 0.15 or higher. These drivers tend to be single men between the ages of 25 and 45, with high school educations or less, blue-collar jobs, and a preference for beer rather than wine or hard liquor. They typically drive intoxicated four times a week, or 200 times a year.[31]

Strategies for Prevention

How to Prevent Drunk Driving

✔ When going out in a group, always designate one person who won't drink at all to serve as the driver.

✔ Never get behind the wheel if you've had more than 2 drinks within 2 hours, especially if you haven't eaten.

✔ Never let intoxicated friends drive home. Call a taxi, drive them yourself, or arrange for them to spend the night in a safe place.

Alcohol-Related Problems

Alcohol abuse, as defined by the American Psychiatric Association's *Diagnostic and Statistical Manual of Mental Disorders,* 4th edition *(DSM-IV),* involves continued use of alcohol despite awareness of social, occupational, psychological, or physical problems related to drinking, or drinking in dangerous ways or situations (before driving, for instance).[32]

Alcohol dependence is a separate disorder, in which individuals develop a strong craving for alcohol because it produces pleasurable feelings or relieves stress or anxiety. Over time they experience physiological changes that lead to *tolerance* of its effects; this means that they must consume larger and larger amounts to achieve intoxication. If they abruptly stop drinking, they suffer *withdrawal,* a state of acute physical and psychological discomfort.[33]

Alcoholism, as defined by the National Council on Alcoholism and Drug Dependence and the American Society of Addiction, is a primary, chronic disease in which genetic, psychosocial, and environmental factors influence its development and manifestations. The disease is often progressive and fatal. Its characteristics include impaired control of drinking, a preoccupation with alcohol, continued use of alcohol despite adverse consequences, and distorted thinking, most notably denial. Like other diseases, alcoholism is not simply a matter of insufficient willpower, but a complex problem that causes many symptoms, can have serious consequences, yet can improve with treatment.

According to the NIAAA, 9% of adults meet the criteria for alcohol abuse or dependence. White males 18 to 29 years old have 2.4 times greater prevalence of abuse and dependence than nonwhites. Among those over age 64, nonwhites have a prevalence rate of abuse and dependence 28.4% higher than whites.[34]

Probably fewer than 5% of alcoholics and problem drinkers are "skid-row drunks." The other 95% are all around us, every day. Alcoholism generally first appears between the ages of 20 and 40, although even children and young teenagers can become alcoholics. It takes 5 to 15 years of heavy drinking for an adult to become alcoholic, but just 6 to 18 months for an adolescent to develop the disease.

Although the exact cause of alcohol dependence and abuse is not known, certain factors—including biochemical imbalances in the brain, heredity, cultural acceptability, and stress—all seem to play a role.

Medical Complications of Alcohol Abuse and Dependence

Excessive alcohol use adversely affects virtually every organ system in the body, including the brain, the digestive tract, the heart, muscles, blood, and hormones. In addition, because alcohol interacts with many drugs, it can increase the risk of potentially lethal overdoses and harmful interactions. Among the major risks and complications are:

- *Liver disease.* Chronic heavy drinking can lead to alcoholic hepatitis (inflammation and destruction of liver cells) and, in the 15% of people who continue drinking beyond this stage, cirrhosis (irreversible scarring and destruction of liver cells). The liver eventually may fail completely, resulting in coma and death.

- *Cardiovascular system.* Heavy drinking can weaken the heart muscle (causing cardiac myopathy), elevate blood pressure, and increase the risk of stroke.

- *Cancer.* Heavy alcohol use may contribute to cancer of the liver, stomach, and colon, as well as malignant melanoma, a deadly form of skin cancer.

- *Brain damage.* Chronic brain damage resulting from alcohol consumption is second only to Alzheimer's disease as a cause of cognitive deterioration in adults.

- *Vitamin deficiencies.* Alcoholics often tend to have very poor nutrition. Alcoholism is associated with vitamin deficiencies, especially of thiamine (B-1), which may be responsible for certain diseases of the neurological, digestive, muscular, and cardiovascular systems.

- *Digestive problems.* Chronic drinking may result in peptic ulcers (breaks in the stomach lining) and bleeding from the stomach lining.

- *Reproductive and sexual dysfunction.* Alcohol interferes with male and female sexual function and fertility through direct effects on hormones and the sex organs.

- *Fetal alcohol syndrome.* Because no one knows how much—if any—alcohol is safe during pregnancy, the National Institute of Alcohol Abuse and Alcoholism recommends that pregnant women not drink at all.[35]

- *Accidents and injuries.* Alcohol may contribute to almost half of the deaths caused by car accidents, burns, falls, and choking.

- *Higher mortality.* The mortality rate for alcoholics is two to three times higher than that for nonalcoholics of the same age.

Alcohol Treatments

The first phase of treatment for alcohol dependence focuses on **detoxification**, the gradual withdrawal of alcohol from the body. For 90% to 95% of alcoholics, withdrawal symptoms are mild to moderate. Those who have drunk heavily for a prolonged period may develop more severe symptoms, including seizures or alcohol withdrawal delirium, commonly known as **delirium tremens**, or **DTs**, characterized by agitated behavior, delusions, rapid heart rate, sweating, vivid hallucinations, trembling hands, and fever.

In the past, 28-day treatment programs in a medical or psychiatric hospital or a residential facility were the cornerstone of early recovery treatment. According to outcome studies, inpatient treatment was effective, with as many as 70% of "graduates" remaining abstinent or stable nonproblem drinkers for 5 years after. However, because of cost pressures from the insurance industry, the length of stay has been reduced, and there's been increasing emphasis on outpatient care.

Outpatient treatment may involve group therapy, individual supportive therapy, marital or family therapy, regular attendance at Alcoholics Anonymous (AA) or another support group, brief interventions, and relapse prevention. According to outcome studies, intensive outpatient treatment at a day hospital (with individuals returning home every evening) is as effective as inpatient care.[36] Outpatient therapy continues for at least a year, but many individuals continue to participate in outpatient programs for the rest of their lives.

The best-known and most commonly used self-help program for alcohol problems is Alcoholics Anonymous (AA), which was founded more than 60 years ago and has grown into an international organization that includes 2 million members and 185,000 groups worldwide. Acknowledging the power of alcohol, AA offers support from others struggling with the same illness,

Strategies for Prevention

Preventing Relapses

✔ Exercise, which provides an outlet for aggression, enhances self-image and reduces mild depression.

✔ Lifestyle changes, including developing a network of non-drinking friends; removing alcohol from the house; and avoiding high-risk situations, such as stopping at a bar.

✔ Refusal training; rehearsing various ways of saying no.

✔ Stress reduction to ease the desire to drink; learning to live with craving.

from a sponsor available at any time of the day or night, and from fellowship meetings that are held every day of the year. Because anonymity is a key part of AA, it has been difficult for researchers to study its success, but it is generally believed to be a highly effective means of overcoming alcoholism and maintaining abstinence. Its twelve steps, which emphasize honesty, sobriety, and acknowledgment of a "higher power," have become the model for self-help groups for other addictive behaviors, including drug abuse and compulsive eating.

The Impact on Relationships

Alcoholism shatters families and creates unhealthy patterns of communicating and relating. Separation and divorce rates are high among alcoholics. Another common occurrence is **codependence**, a term used to describe the behavior of close family members or friends who act in ways that enable their spouses, parents, or friends to continue their self-destructive behavior.

Codependent spouses of alcoholics follow a predictable pattern of behavior: While trying to control the drinkers, they act in ways that enable the drinkers to keep drinking. If an alcoholic finds it hard to get up in the morning, his wife wakes him up, pulls him out of bed and into the shower, and drops him off at work. If he is late, she makes excuses to his boss. By helping him evade his responsibilities, his wife is helping him continue drinking. Indeed, he might not be able to keep up his habit without her cooperation.

Growing up with an alcoholic parent can have a long-lasting effect. Adult children of alcoholics are at risk for many problems. Some try to fill the emptiness inside with alcohol, drugs, or addictive habits. Others find themselves caught up in destructive relationships that repeat the patterns of their childhood. They are likely to have difficulty solving problems, identifying and expressing their feelings, trusting others, and being intimate. In addition to their own increased risk of addictive behavior, they are likely to marry individuals with some form of addiction and keep on playing out the roles of their childhood. They may feel inadequate, not know how to set limits or recognize normal behavior, be perfectionistic, and want to control all aspects of their lives. However, not all adult children are alike or necessarily suffer from psychological problems or face an increased risk of substance abuse themselves.[37]

Because the impact of alcoholism can be so enduring, support groups—such as Adult Children of Alcoholics, Children of Alcoholics, and Adult Children of

Strategies for Change

Recognizing Signs of Codependence

If you're involved with someone with an addictive behavior, read through the following list of characteristics of codependence. If you identify with some of the statements, you may wish to visit a self-help group in your area:

✔ "Covering" for another person's alcohol or drug use, eating disorders, gambling, sexual escapades, or general behavior.

✔ Spending a great deal of time talking about—and worrying about—other people's behavior/problems/future instead of living your own life.

✔ Marking or counting bottles, searching for a hidden "stash," or in other ways monitoring someone else's behavior.

✔ Taking on more responsibility at home or in a relationship—even when you resent it.

✔ Ignoring your own needs in favor of meeting someone else's.

✔ Worrying that if you leave a relationship, the other person will fall apart.

✔ Self-esteem that depends on what others say and think.

✔ Growing up in a family where there was little communication, where expressing feelings was not acceptable, and where there were either rigid rules or none at all.

Dysfunctional Families—have spread throughout the country in the last decade. These organizations provide adult children of alcoholics a mutually supportive group setting to discuss their childhood experiences with alcoholic parents and the emotional consequences they carry into adult life. Through such groups or other forms of therapy, individuals may learn to move beyond anger and blame, see the part they themselves play in their current state of unhappiness, and create a future that is healthier and happier than their past.

Tobacco and Its Effects

Tobacco, an herb that can be smoked or chewed, directly affects the brain. While its primary active ingredient is nicotine, there are almost 400 other compounds and chemicals in tobacco smoke, including gases, liquids, particles, tar, carbon monoxide, cadmium, pyridine, nitrogen dioxide, ammonia, benzene, phenol, acrolein, hydrogen cyanide, formaldehyde, and hydrogen sulfide. See Figure 12-5 for a summary of their physiological effects.

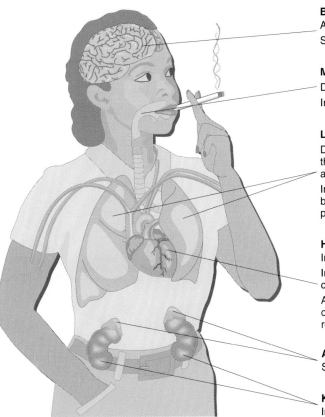

Brain
Alters mood-regulating chemicals
Stimulates cravings for more nicotine

Mouth and throat
Dulls taste buds
Irritates the membranes

Lungs
Damages the air sacs, which affects the lungs' ability to bring in oxygen and remove carbon dioxide
Increases mucus secretion in the bronchial tubes, which narrows air passages

Heart
Increases heart rate
Increases blood pressure by constricting blood vessels
Affects the oxygen-carrying ability of hemoglobin so less oxygen reaches the heart

Adrenal glands
Stimulates adrenaline production

Kidneys
Inhibits formation of urine

Figure 12-5

Some effects of smoking on the body.

Nicotine, Tar, and Carbon Monoxide

A colorless, oily compound, **nicotine** is poisonous in concentrated amounts. If you inhale while smoking, 90% of the nicotine in the smoke is absorbed into your body. Even if you draw smoke only into your mouth and not into your lungs, you still absorb 25% to 30% of the nicotine. The FDA has concluded that nicotine is a dangerous, addictive drug that should be regulated.

Nicotine stimulates the cerebral cortex, the outer layer of the brain that controls complex behavior and mental activity and enhances mood and alertness. It also stimulates the adrenal glands to produce adrenaline, a hormone that increases blood pressure, speeds up the heart rate by fifteen to twenty beats a minute, and constricts blood vessels (especially in the skin). Nicotine inhibits the formation of urine, dampens hunger, irritates the membranes in the mouth and throat, and dulls the taste buds, so foods don't taste as good as they would otherwise. Nicotine is a major contributor to heart and respiratory diseases.

As it burns, tobacco produces **tar**, a thick, sticky dark fluid made up of several hundred different chemicals—many of them poisonous, some of them *carcinogenic* (enhancing the growth of cancerous cells). As you inhale tobacco smoke, tar and other particles settle in the forks of the branchlike bronchial tubes in your lungs, where precancerous changes are apt to occur. In addition, tar and smoke damage the mucus and the cilia in the bronchial tubes, which normally remove irritating foreign materials from your lungs.

Smoke from cigarettes, cigars, and pipes also contains **carbon monoxide**, the deadly gas that comes out of the exhaust pipes of cars, in levels 400 times those considered safe in industry. Carbon monoxide interferes with the ability of the hemoglobin in the blood to carry oxygen, impairs normal functioning of the nervous system, and is at least partly responsible for the increased risk of heart attack and strokes in smokers.

The Impact of Tobacco

Smoking tobacco is the largest and most preventable cause of mortality in the United States, causing more than 430,000 deaths among smokers and another 50,000 deaths among nonsmokers exposed to environmental tobacco smoke.[38] Americans who die of smoking-related causes before age 65 lose a total of 949,924 years of potential life. Moreover, smoking-related diseases account for $22 billion in health-care costs and $43 billion in lost productivity each year.[39]

Health Effects of Cigarette Smoking

Tobacco is the ultimate underlying cause of nearly one of every five deaths in the United States every year.[40] If you're a smoker who inhales deeply and started smoking before the age of 15, you're trading a minute of future life for every minute you now spend smoking (see Figure 12-6).

Heart Disease and Stroke

Although a great deal of publicity has been given to the link between cigarettes and lung cancer, heart attack is actually the leading cause of death for smokers. Smoking doubles the risk of heart disease, and smokers who suffer heart attacks have only a 50% chance of recovering. Smokers have a 70% higher death rate from heart disease than do nonsmokers, and those who smoke heavily have a 200% higher death rate. Even aerobic exercise, which generally protects the heart's health, cannot overcome the negative effects of smoking, especially on cholesterol levels.[41]

Even people who have smoked for decades can reduce their risk of heart attack if they quit smoking. However, recent studies indicate some irreversible dam-

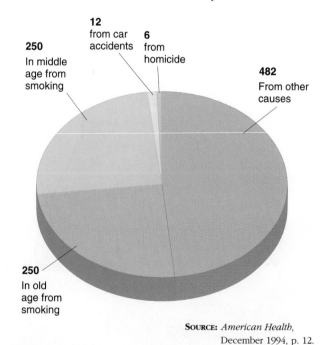

HOW SMOKERS WILL DIE

For every 1000 20-year-olds who smoke, here's a look ahead at how they will die:

12 from car accidents

6 from homicide

250 In middle age from smoking

482 From other causes

250 In old age from smoking

SOURCE: *American Health,* December 1994, p. 12.

Figure 12-6

age to blood vessels. Progression of atherosclerosis—hardening of the arteries—among past smokers continues at a faster pace than among those who never smoked.[42]

In addition to contributing to heart attacks, cigarette smoking increases the risk of stroke two to three times in men and women, even after other risk factors are taken into account. According to one study of middle-aged men, giving up smoking leads to a considerable decrease in the risk of stroke within 5 years of quitting, particularly in smokers of less than twenty cigarettes a day. Those with hypertension show the greatest benefit. The risk for heavy smokers declines but never reverts back to that of men who never smoked.[43]

Cancer

The American Cancer Society estimates that tobacco smoking is the cause of 28% of all deaths from cancer and the cause of more than 85% to 90% of all cases of lung cancer. The more people smoke, the longer they smoke, and the earlier they start smoking, the more likely they are to develop lung cancer.

Smokers of two or more packs a day have lung cancer mortality rates fifteen to twenty-five times greater than nonsmokers. If smokers stop smoking before cancer has started, their lung tissue tends to repair itself, even if there were already precancerous changes. Former smokers who haven't smoked for 15 or more years have lung cancer mortality rates only somewhat above those for nonsmokers.

Despite some advances in treating lung cancer, the prognosis for sufferers is not good. Even with vigorous therapy, fewer than 10% survive for 5 years after diagnosis. This is one of the lowest survival rates of any type of cancer. And if the cancer has spread from the lungs to other parts of the body, only 1% survive for 5 years after diagnosis.

Respiratory Diseases

Smoking quickly impairs the respiratory system. Even some teenaged smokers show signs of respiratory difficulty—breathlessness, chronic cough, excess phlegm production—when compared with nonsmokers of the same age. Cigarette smokers are up to eighteen times more likely than are nonsmokers to die of noncancerous diseases of the lungs.

Cigarette smoking is the major cause of chronic obstructive lung disease (COLD), which includes emphysema and chronic bronchitis, in men and women. COLD is characterized by progressive limitation of the flow of air into and out of the lungs. In chronic bronchi-

tis, the bronchial tubes in the lungs become inflamed, thickening the walls of the bronchi, and the production of mucus increases. The result is a narrowing of the air passages.

Other Smoking-Related Problems

Smokers are more likely than nonsmokers to develop gum disease, and they lose significantly more teeth. Even those who quit have worse gum problems than people who never smoked at all. Smoking may also contribute to the loss of teeth and teeth supporting bone, even in individuals with good oral hygiene.

Cigarette smoking is associated with stomach and duodenal ulcers; mouth, throat, and other types of cancer; and cirrhosis of the liver. Smoking may worsen the symptoms or complications of allergies, diabetes, hypertension, peptic ulcers, and disorders of the lungs or blood vessels. Some men who smoke ten cigarettes or more a day may experience sexual impotence. Cigarette smokers also tend to miss work one-third more often than do nonsmokers, primarily because of respiratory illnesses. In addition, each year cigarette-ignited fires claim thousands of lives.

The Financial Cost of Smoking

The total costs of cigarette smoking to American society include greater work absenteeism, higher insurance

---

Strategies for Prevention

Why Not to Light Up

Before you start smoking—before you ever face the challenge of quitting—think of what you have to gain by not smoking:

✔ A significantly reduced risk of cancer of the larynx, mouth, esophagus, pancreas, and bladder.

✔ Half the risk of heart disease that smokers face.

✔ A lower risk of stroke, chronic obstructive lung disease (COLD), influenza, ulcers, and pneumonia.

✔ A lower risk of having a low-birth-weight baby.

✔ A longer life span.

✔ Potential savings of tens of thousands of dollars that you would otherwise spend on tobacco products and medical care.

CAMPUS FOCUS: COLLEGE STUDENTS AND SMOKING

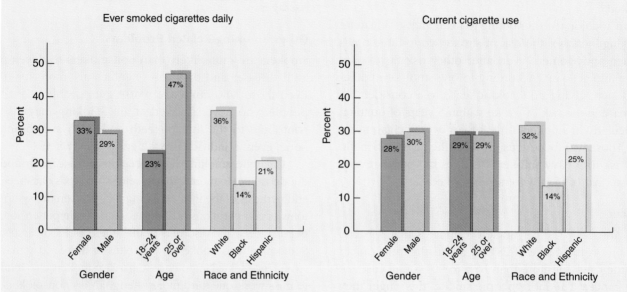

SOURCE: Douglas, Kathy, et al. "Results from the 1995 National College Health Risk Behavior Survey." *Journal of American College Health*, Vol. 46, 1997.

premiums, disability payments, and training costs to replace employees who die prematurely from smoking. In the course of a lifetime, the average smoker can expect to spend $10,000 to $20,000 on cigarettes—but that's only the beginning. The potential costs for medical services for a man between the ages of 35 and 39 who smokes heavily may be as high as $60,000. But the greatest toll—the pain and suffering of cancer victims and their loved ones—obviously cannot be measured in dollars and cents.

Smoking in America

Tobacco use remains the most serious and widespread addictive behavior in the world and the major cause of preventable deaths in our society. Although smoking by adults has declined, many young teenagers—particularly white girls—are smoking as much or more than young teenagers 10 years ago.

Why People Start Smoking

The two main factors linked with the onset of a smoking habit are age and education. The vast majority of white

men (93%) with less than a high school education are current or former daily cigarette smokers. Women and Latinos with a similar educational background are also very likely to smoke or to have smoked every day. And most adults who smoke started in the teen years or earlier, at an average age of 12.2 years, and most were regular smokers by age 14.[44] Some other risk factors are:

- *Heredity.* Researchers speculate that genes may account for about 50% of smoking behavior.

- *Parental role models.* The majority of children who smoke have parents who smoke.

- *Adolescent experimentation and rebellion.* Many young people try smoking out of curiosity or because they want to defy adults.

- *Weight control.* Young women, especially, may start smoking in an attempt to control their weight.

- *Aggressive marketing.* Cigarette companies spend billions each year on advertising, often targeting teens, minorities, women, and the poor.

- *Stress.* An individual with a high stress level is about fifteen times as likely to be a smoker as a person with a low stress level.

Women and Smoking: Special Risks

The World Health Organization (WHO) reports that 20% to 30% of women in wealthy nations smoke, compared with 2% to 10% of women in the developing nations. In the United States, 26% of women smoke, and more young women than men are starting the habit. This is a troubling trend because, once women start, they often find it difficult to quit, in part because they fear gaining weight.[45]

Lung cancer now claims more women's lives than breast cancer. The risk of heart attack in women who smoke twenty-five or more cigarettes a day is more than 500% greater than the risk in women who don't smoke. Even smoking just one to four cigarettes a day doubles the risk. Women who smoke low-nicotine cigarettes are four times more likely to have a first heart attack than women who don't smoke—the same risk as for those who smoke high-nicotine cigarettes.

Smoking directly affects women's reproductive organs and processes. Women who smoke are less fertile and experience menopause 1 or 2 years earlier than women who don't smoke. Smoking also boosts a woman's likelihood of developing cervical cancer and greatly increases the possible risks associated with taking oral contraceptives. Older women who smoke are weaker, have poorer balance, and are at greater risk of physical disability than nonsmokers.[46]

Women who smoke also are more likely to develop osteoporosis. They tend to be thin, which is a risk factor for osteoporosis, and they enter menopause earlier, thus extending the period of jeopardy from estrogen loss.

An estimated 19% to 27% of women smoke during pregnancy, thereby increasing their risk of miscarriage and pregnancy complications, including bleeding, premature delivery, and birth defects such as cleft lip or palate.[47] Women who smoke are twice as likely to have an ectopic pregnancy (in which a fertilized egg develops in the fallopian tube rather than in the uterus) and to have babies of low birth weight as those who have never smoked. However, women who stop smoking before pregnancy reduce their risk of having a low-birth-weight baby to that of women who don't smoke. Even those who quit 3 or 4 months into the pregnancy have babies with higher birth weights than those who continue smoking throughout pregnancy.

Other Forms of Tobacco

Other ways of ingesting tobacco may be less deadly than smoking cigarettes, but all are dangerous. Smoking clove cigarettes, cigars, and pipes, and chewing or sucking on smokeless tobacco all put the user at risk of cancer of the lip, tongue, mouth, and throat—as well as other diseases and ailments.

Clove Cigarettes

Sweeteners have long been mixed into tobacco, and clove, a spice, is the latest ingredient to be added to the recipe for cigarettes. Clove cigarettes typically contain two-thirds tobacco and one-third cloves. Consumers of these cigarettes are primarily teenagers and young adults.

Clove cigarettes may actually be more harmful than conventional cigarettes. Puff for puff, they deliver twice as much nicotine, tar, and carbon monoxide as moderate-tar American brands. Moreover, eugenol, the active ingredient in cloves (which dentists have used as an anesthetic for years), deadens sensation in the throat, allowing smokers to inhale more deeply and hold smoke in their lungs for a longer time. Close chemical relatives of eugenol can produce the kind of damage to cells that may eventually lead to cancer.

Cigars

Cigar smoking has become a widespread fad, particularly among men. Total cigar consumption in the United States totals approximately 4.5 billion cigars, and consumption of larger cigars increased by 44.5% from 1993 to 1996.

Many cigar smokers of all ages assume that because they do not inhale the smoke, they are not at risk for heart disease or lung cancer. This has not been proven. And it has been shown that cigars, like cigarettes, greatly increase the risk of cancer of the mouth, larynx, throat, and esophagus.[48]

Pipes

Many cigarette smokers switch to pipes to reduce their risk of health problems. But former cigarette smokers may continue to inhale, even though pipe smoke is more irritating to the respiratory system than cigarette smoke. People who have only smoked pipes and who do not inhale are much less likely to develop lung and heart disease than are cigarette smokers. However, they are as likely as cigarette smokers to develop—and die of—cancer of the mouth, larynx, throat, and esophagus.

Smokeless Tobacco

Other tobacco products may be taking the place of cigarettes in the mouths of Americans. The sale and consumption of smokeless tobacco products are rising, particularly among young males. These substances include snuff, finely ground tobacco that can be sniffed or placed inside the cheek and sucked, and chewing tobacco, which consists of tobacco leaves mixed with flavoring agents such as molasses. With both, nicotine is absorbed through the mucous membranes of the nose or mouth.

Although not as deadly as cigarette smoking, the use of smokeless tobacco is dangerous. It can cause cancer and noncancerous oral conditions and lead to nicotine addiction and dependence. Smokeless tobacco users are more likely than nonusers to become cigarette smokers.[49] Cancers of the lip, pharynx, larynx, and esophagus have all been linked to smokeless tobacco.

Environmental Tobacco Smoke

Maybe you don't smoke—never have, never will. That doesn't mean you don't have to worry about the dangers of smoking, especially if you live or work with people who smoke. **Environmental tobacco smoke**, or secondhand cigarette smoke, the most hazardous form of indoor air pollution, ranks behind cigarette smoking and alcohol as the third-leading preventable cause of death. Its annual toll in lives lost: 53,000.[50]

Mainstream and Sidestream Smoke

On the average, a smoker inhales what is known as **mainstream smoke** eight or nine times with each cigarette, for a total of about 24 seconds. However, the cigarette burns for about 12 minutes, and everyone in the room (including the smoker) breathes in what is known as **sidestream smoke**.

According to the American Lung Association, incomplete combustion from the lower temperatures of a smoldering cigarette makes sidestream smoke dirtier and chemically different from mainstream smoke. It has twice as much tar and nicotine, five times as much carbon monoxide, and fifty times as much ammonia. And because the particles in sidestream smoke are small, this mixture of irritating gases and carcinogenic tar reaches deeper into the lungs. If you're a nonsmoker sitting next to someone smoking seven cigarettes an hour, even in a ventilated room, you'll take in almost twice the maximum amount of carbon monoxide set for air pollution in industry—and it will take hours for the carbon monoxide to leave your body.

New research indicates that environmental tobacco smoke is even more dangerous than previously thought. According to the Centers for Disease Control and Prevention (CDC), every year environmental tobacco smoke causes 3000 deaths from lung cancer.[51] In a Harvard University study that tracked 10,000 healthy women who never smoked over 10 years, regular exposure to other people's smoke at home or work almost doubled the risk of heart disease. On the basis of their findings, the researchers estimated that up to 50,000 Americans may die of heart attacks from environmental tobacco smoke every year, while 3000 to 4000 die of other forms of heart disease.[52]

The Politics of Tobacco

More than three decades after government health authorities began to warn of the dangers of cigarette smoking, tobacco remains a politically hot topic. In 1997 the tobacco industry and attorneys general from nearly 40 states reached a historic settlement. Major tobacco companies agreed to pay $368.5 billion to settle smoking-related lawsuits filed by states, to finance antismoking campaigns, to restrict marketing, to permit federal regulation of tobacco, and to pay fines if tobacco use by minors does not decline. In return, the industry would be protected against most tobacco-related lawsuits and the awarding of punitive damages. The Food and Drug Administration (FDA) would have regulatory control over the way cigarettes are manufactured and packaged.

In the course of congressional hearings on this settlement, investigators discovered documents indicating that tobacco manufacturers had been aware of nicotine's addictive potential and had deliberately directed advertising campaigns at adolescents and at African Americans. In November 1998, a team of attorneys general announced a settlement that mandates the largest financial recovery in the nation's history. Under the proposal, tobacco companies would agree to significant curbs on their advertising and marketing campaigns, fund a $1.5 billion antismoking campaign, and disband industry trade groups that concealed damaging research.

The Fight for Clean Air

Nonsmokers, realizing that their health is being jeopardized by environmental tobacco smoke, have increasingly turned to legislative and administrative measures

people's smoke can cause headaches or hoarseness and may pose more serious health hazards. In addition, smokers jeopardize nonsmokers by increasing the danger of fire.

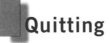

Quitting

Tobacco dependence may be the toughest addiction to overcome. One-third of smokers try to quit annually, but fewer than 10% succeed. Most people who eventually quit on their own have already tried other methods. According to therapists, quitting usually isn't a one-time event but a "dynamic process" that may take several years and four to ten attempts. The good news is that half of all living Americans who ever smoked have managed to quit. And thanks to new products and programs, it may be easier now than ever before to become an ex-smoker.

Quitting on Your Own

More than 90% of former smokers quit on their own—by throwing away all their cigarettes, by gradually cutting down, or by first switching to a less potent brand. One characteristic of successful quitters is that they see themselves as active participants in health maintenance and take personal responsibility for their own health.[54] Often they experiment with a variety of strategies, such as learning relaxation techniques. In women, exercise has proven

to clear the air and protect their rights (see Figure 12-7). More than 1000 cities, towns, and counties now restrict smoking in public places or regulate the sale of tobacco to minors.[53]

Supporters of smoking restrictions argue that no one should be subjected involuntarily to the dangers of environmental tobacco smoke. They point out that other

Figure 12-7

Nonsmoker's bill of rights.

Nonsmoker's Bill of Rights

Nonsmokers Help Protect the Health, Comfort, and Safety of Everyone by Insisting on the Following Rights:

The Right to Breathe Clean Air

Nonsmokers have the right to breathe clean air, free from harmful and irritating tobacco smoke. This right supersedes the right to smoke when the two conflict.

The Right to Speak Out

Nonsmokers have the right to express — firmly but politely — their discomfort and adverse reactions to tobacco smoke. They have the right to voice their objections when smokers light up without asking permission.

The Right to Act

Nonsmokers have the right to take action through legislative means — as individuals or in groups — to prevent or discourage smokers from polluting the atmosphere and to seek the restriction of smoking in public places.

especially effective for quitting and avoiding weight gain.[55] (See Pulsepoints: "Ten Ways to Kick the Habit" for tips on how to smoke less—and less dangerously.)

Stop-Smoking Groups

Joining a support group doubles your chances of quitting for good. The American Cancer Society's FreshStart Program runs about 1500 stop-smoking clinics, each with about eight to eighteen members meeting for eight 2-hour sessions over 4 weeks. Instructors explain the risks of smoking, encourage individuals to think about why they smoke, and suggest ways of unlearning their smoking habit. A quitting day is set for the third or fourth session.

The American Lung Association's Freedom from Smoking Program consists of eight 1- to 2-hour sessions over 7 weeks. The approach is similar to the American Cancer Society's, but smokers keep diaries and team up with buddies. Ex-smokers serve as advisers on quitting day. Both groups estimate that 27% or 28% of their participants successfully stop smoking.

Nicotine Replacement Therapy

This approach uses a variety of products that supply low doses of nicotine in a way that allows smokers to taper off gradually over a period of months. They include nicotine gum (available in two doses) and slow-release skin patches (Figure 12-8). Although still experimental, a nasal spray also has shown promise.[56]

In research studies, nicotine replacement is the only treatment for nicotine addiction that has proven clearly beneficial. When measured against a look-alike placebo treatment, nicotine gum and patches have doubled the initial quitting rate and the numbers of smokers who remain abstinent 6 months to 1 year later. However, even with these approaches, only about one smoker in four quits completely; about half of these remain abstinent over the long term. Sales of nicotine patches, which rose rapidly after their introduction in 1992 to $600 million, have declined to $200 million annually.[57]

Making This Chapter Work for You
Thinking About Alcohol and Tobacco Use

■ When comparing amounts and types of alcohol, assume that one drink contains the equivalent of ½ ounce of 100% ethyl alcohol. A person's blood alcohol concentration (BAC) is the measurement used by

---

Pulsepoints

Ten Ways to Kick the Habit

1. Use delaying tactics. Have your first cigarette of the day 15 minutes later than usual, then 15 minutes later than that the next day, and so on.

2. Distract yourself. When you feel a craving for a cigarette, talk to someone, drink a glass of water, or get up and move around.

3. Establish nonsmoking hours. Instead of lighting up at the end of a meal, for instance, get up immediately, brush your teeth, wash your hands, or take a walk.

4. Never smoke two packs of the same brand in a row. Buy cigarettes only by the pack, not by the carton.

5. Make it harder to get to your cigarettes. Lock them in a drawer, wrap them in paper, or leave them in your coat or car.

6. Change the way you smoke. Smoke with the hand you don't usually use. Smoke only half of each cigarette.

7. Keep daily records. Chart your daily cigarette tally to see what progress you're making.

8. Stop completely for just 1 day at a time. Promise yourself 24 hours of freedom from cigarettes; when the day's over, make the same commitment for one more day. At the end of any 24-

hour period, you can go back to smoking and not feel guilty.

9. Spend more time in places where you can't smoke. Take up bike-riding or swimming. Shower often. Go to movies or other places where smoking isn't allowed.

10. Go cold turkey. If you're a heavily addicted smoker, try a decisive and complete break. Smokers who quit completely are less likely to light up again than those who gradually decrease their daily cigarette consumption, switch to low-tar and low-nicotine brands, or use special filters and holders.

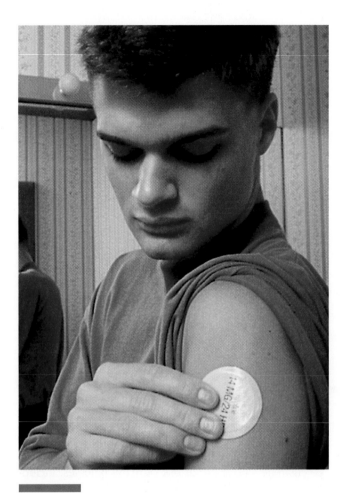

Figure 12-8
A nicotine patch releases nicotine transdermally (through the skin) in measured amounts, which are gradually decreased over time.

law enforcement officers to determine whether someone is legally drunk.

■ The rate of alcohol absorption depends on many factors: the strength of the drink; the drinker's size, age, and race; family history of alcoholism; whether there is food in the drinker's stomach; and the drinker's tolerance for alcohol.

■ Moderate amounts of alcohol may have a positive effect on the cardiovascular system. In excess, however, alcohol can weaken the heart muscle and increase the risk of cardiovascular disease.

■ Alcohol, a central nervous system depressant, also impairs thinking, vision, motor skills, hearing, smell and taste, sense of time and space, speech, and sexual response and performance. When combined with other drugs, alcohol can have serious adverse effects.

■ Alcohol is the substance most commonly abused by college students. Drinking by college women and binge drinking have increased on campuses. Alcohol abuse by students has led to violence, sexual assaults, and other dangers.

■ Women drink for different reasons and in different ways than men. They feel its impact more quickly and severely and face special risks from abuse, such as breast cancer, infertility, and osteoporosis.

■ Although there has been a successful campaign against drunk driving, this dangerous crime continues to kill thousands of Americans.

■ There is a spectrum of alcohol problems that range from problem drinking to alcohol dependence or abuse to alcoholism. The difference is one of degree and of loss of control over one's craving for alcohol.

■ Chronic heavy drinking can cause severe liver damage, vitamin deficiency, brain damage, cardiovascular disease, and some types of cancer.

■ Treatment for alcohol problems includes detoxification, inpatient or outpatient care, or self-help groups such as Alcoholics Anonymous.

■ Loved ones of alcoholics are at a risk for dysfunctional relationships that do not promote healthy communication, honesty, and intimacy.

■ Many people have stopped smoking because of the health risks associated with tobacco use and because, as a social behavior, smoking has become unpopular. However, smoking is increasing among young white teens.

■ Nicotine affects mood, hunger, blood pressure, and the performance of certain mental tasks. It also contributes to heart and respiratory diseases. The tar and carbon monoxide in cigarettes are carcinogenic and can damage the respiratory system.

■ The incidence of heart attack is high among smokers. In the United States, more people die from lung cancer, usually caused by smoking, than of any other type of cancer. Smoking also contributes to the development of other cancers, lung disease, ulcers, and liver and gum disease.

■ Women who smoke face the additional risk of developing reproductive disorders such as cervical cancer. A pregnant woman who smokes has a high risk of miscarriage, premature birth, and having an underweight baby.

Health Online

The Quitnet   http://www.quitnet.org

This site is dedicated to helping smokers kick the habit. It contains many interactive exercises, including quizzes to determine why you smoke and where you are in the quitting process. There are also features to help you set a quit date, make a behavior change plan, and an online support forum to allow you to chat with others who are trying to stop smoking. If you want further references on tobacco use, turn to the library, links, or news features.

Think about it ...

* If you are currently a smoker, would this Web site make it easier for you to quit?
  What features would be most helpful to you?

* Do you have any friends or family members who are smokers?
  How do you feel about their smoking? Do you know if they have ever tried to quit?

* What strategies does this site offer that might apply to other behaviors you would
  like to change in your life?

■ Clove cigarettes, cigars, pipes, and smokeless to-bacco are also harmful and increase the risk of teeth and gum conditions and cancer of the mouth and throat.

■ Environmental, or secondhand, smoke is a dangerous carcinogen. Nonsmokers constantly exposed to cigarette smoke are at risk of many illnesses, including lung cancer and heart disease.

■ Approaches to quitting cigarettes include quitting on one's own, stop-smoking groups, and nicotine replacement therapy.

Key Terms

The terms listed here are used within the chapter. Page numbers are included for each term.
A definition of each term is given in the green Glossary pages at the end of this book.

absorption *245*
alcohol abuse *254*
alcohol dependence *254*
alcoholism *254*
**blood-alcohol concentration
  (BAC)** *244*
carbon monoxide *258*
codependence *256*

delirium tremens (DTs) *255*
detoxification *255*
environmental tobacco smoke
  262
ethyl alcohol *244*
fetal alcohol effects (FAE) *253*
fetal alcohol syndrome (FAS)
  253

intoxication *247*
mainstream smoke *262*
nicotine *258*
proof *244*
sidestream smoke *262*
tar *258*

Review Questions

1. How does alcohol affect the body's various systems?
2. What are the negative consequences of being an alcoholic?
3. How is BAC relevant to the drunk-driving laws in your state? At what BAC level are you considered legally drunk?

4. Who is likely to be today's tobacco smoker? Why do young people start to smoke?
5. How does smoking tobacco affect a person's health? What health problems can be prevented by quitting smoking?
6. What is environmental tobacco smoke? How does it affect the health of nonsmokers?

Critical Thinking Questions

1. Driving home from a party, 18-year-old Rick has had too much to drink. As he crosses the dividing line of the road, the driver of an oncoming car—a young mother—swerves to avoid an accident. She hits a concrete wall and dies instantly. Rick has no record of drunk driving. Should he go to prison? Is he guilty of manslaughter? How would you feel if you were the victim's husband? If you were Rick's friend?
2. What effects have alcohol use had in your life? Try making a list of the positive and negative effects

your own alcohol use has had. Be specific. If you continue to drink at your current rate, what effects will it have on your future? What effects have other people's drinking had on your life?
3. Has smoking become unpopular among your friends or family? What social activities continue to be associated with smoking? Are you exposed to environmental tobacco smoke often?

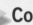

Connections to Personal Health Interactive

To enhance your understanding of the material covered in this chapter, check out the following study aids on the **Personal Health Interactive CD-ROM**.

- Personal Insights: How Do You Feel About Alcohol?
- Personal Insights: How Do You Feel About Tobacco?

- Alcohol and Its Effects on the Body
- **Online Research:** Drugs, Alcohol, and Tobacco
- Glossary & Key Term Review

References

1. Archer, Loran, et al. "What If Americans Drank Less? The Potential Effect on the Prevalence of Alcohol Abuse and Dependence." *American Journal of Public Health*, Vol. 85, No. 1, January 1995.
2. Whitcomb, David, and Geoffrey Block. "Association of Acetaminophen Hepatotoxicity with Fasting and Ethanol Use." *Journal of the American Medical Association,* Vol. 272, No. 23, December 21, 1994. Sherlock, Sheila. "Alcoholic Liver Disease." *Lancet,* Vol. 345, No. 8944, January 28, 1995.
3. Johnson, Patrick. "Alcohol Expectancies and Reaction Expectancies: Their Impact on Student Drinking." *Journal of Alcohol & Drug Education,* Vol. 40, No. 1, Fall 1994. de Boer, Mieke, et al. "The Effects of Alcohol, Expectancy, and Alcohol Beliefs on Anxiety and Self-Disclosure in Women: Do Beliefs Moderate Alcohol Effects?" *Addictive Behaviors,* Vol. 19, No. 5, September–October 1994.

4. Thun, Michael, et al. "Alcohol Consumption and Mortality Among Middle-aged and Elderly U.S. Adults." *New England Journal of Medicine*, Vol. 337, No. 24, December 11, 1997.
5. American Psychiatric Association. *Diagnostic and Statistical Manual of Mental Disorders*, 4th edition *(DSM-IV)*. Washington, DC: American Psychiatric Press, 1994.
6. Urbano-Marquez, Alvaro, et al. "The Greater Risk of Alcoholic Cardiomyopathy and Myopathy in Women Compared with Men." *Journal of the American Medical Association,* Vol. 274, No. 2, July 12, 1995.
7. Tracy, Joseph, and Marsha Bates. "Models of Functional Organization As a Method for Detecting Cognitive Deficits: Data from a Sample of Social Drinkers." *Journal of Studies on Alcohol*, Vol. 55, No. 6, November 1994.
8. Skelly, Flora Johnson. "The Drinking Diagnosis." *American Medical News*, May 11, 1992.

9. "Bibulous America: Over Half of All Adults Are Drinkers." *Dialogue*, Vol. 5, No. 1, February 1995.

10. Centers for Disease Control and Prevention. "Frequent Alcohol Consumption Among Women of Childbearing Age." *Journal of the American Medical Association*, Vol. 271, No. 23, June 15, 1994.

11. "Bibulous America."

12. Urberg, Kathryn, et al. "Close Friend and Group Influence on Adolescent Cigarette Smoking and Alcohol Use." *Developmental Psychology*, Vol. 130, No. 5, September 1997.

13. Cohen, Adam. "Battle of the Binge." *Time*, September 8, 1997.

14. Douglas, Kathy, et al. "Results from the 1995 National College Health Risk Behavior Survey." *Journal of American College Health*, Vol. 46, September 1997.

15. Kassel, Jon. Presentation, Association for the Advancement of Behavior Therapy, November 1997.

16. Gleason, Nancy. "College Women and Alcohol: A Relational Perspective." *Journal of American College Health*, Vol. 42, No. 6, May 1994.

17. Wright, Deborah, and Paul Heppner. "Examining the Wellbeing of Nonclinical College Students: Is Knowledge of the Presence of Parental Alcoholism Useful?" *Journal of Counseling Psychology*, Vol. 40, No. 3, July 1993.

18. Winerip, Michael. "Binge Nights: The Emergency on Campus." *New York Times Education Life*, January 4, 1998.

19. *Time,* December 19, 1994.

20. Rivinus, Timothy, and Mary Larimer. "Violence, Alcohol, Other Drugs, and the College Student." *Journal of College Student Psychotherapy*, Vol. 8, No. 1–2, 1993.

21. Nathan, Peter. "Unanswered Questions About Distressed Faculty, Staff and Students: Why Won't They Let Us Help Them?" In *Alcohol Use and Misuse by Young Adults*. Notre Dame, IN: University of Notre Dame Press, 1994. Kinney, Jean. "A Model Comprehensive Alcohol Program for Universities." In *Alcohol Use and Misuse by Young Adults*. Notre Dame, IN: University of Notre Dame Press, 1994.

22. Ross, Helen, and Gordon Tisdall. "Identification of Alcohol Disorders at a University Medical Health Center Using the CAGE." *Journal of Alcohol & Drug Education*, Vol. 39, No. 3, Spring 1994. Presley, Cheryl, et al. "Development of the Core Alcohol and Drug Survey: Initial Findings and Future Directions." *Journal of American College Health*, Vol. 42, No. 6, May 1994.

23. Gose, Ben. "Colleges Try to Curb Excessive Drinking by Saying Moderation Is Okay." *Chronicle of Higher Education*, Vol. 44, No. 9, October 24, 1997. Piombo, Maria, and Melinda Piles. "The Relationship Between College Females' Drinking and Their Sexual Behavior." *Women's Health Issues*, Vol. 6, No. 4, July–August 1996. Wilsnack, Sharon, et al. "Childhood Sexual Abuse and Women's Substance Abuse." *Journal of Studies on Alcohol*, Vol. 58, No. 5, May 1997.

24. Centers for Disease Control and Prevention. "Frequent Alcohol Consumption Among Women of Childbearing Age." *Journal of the American Medical Association,* Vol. 271, No. 23, June 15, 1994.

25. Thorp, John, and Susanne Hiller-Sturumhofel. "The Obstetrician/Gynecologist." *Alcohol Health & Research World*, Vol. 18, No. 2, 1994.

26. Grodstein, Francine, et al. "Infertility in Women and Moderate Alcohol Use." *American Journal of Public Health*, Vol. 84, No. 9, September 1994.

27. Stewart, Donna, and David Streiner. "Alcohol Drinking in Pregnancy." *General Hospital Psychiatry*, Vol. 16, No. 6, November 1994. Drug and alcohol abuse also can affect a woman's mothering. See Eliason, Michele, and Anne Skinstad. "Drug/Alcohol Addictions and Mothering." *Alcoholism Treatment Quarterly*, Vol. 12, No. 1, 1995.

28. Urbano-Marquez. "The Greater Risk of Alcoholic Cardiomyopathy and Myopathy in Women Compared with Men."

29. National Highway Safety Administration.

30. Castaneda, Carol, and Paul Hoversten. "War of Attrition on Drunken Driving." *USA Today*, May 23, 1997.

31. Hoversten, Paul. "Most Repeat Offenders Are Beer-Drinking Men." *USA Today*, May 23, 1997.

32. American Psychiatric Association.

33. Ibid.

34. "Bibulous America."

35. Hankin, Janet. "FAS Prevention Strategies: Passive and Active Measures." *Alcohol Health & Research World*, Vol. 18, No. 1, 1994.

36. McCaul, Mary, and Janice Furst. "Alcoholism Treatment in the United States." *Alcohol Health & Research World*, Vol. 18, No. 4, 1994.

37. Mintz, Laurie, et al. "Relations Among Parental Alcoholism, Eating Disorders, and Substance Abuse in Non Clinical College Women: Additional Evidence Against the Uniformity Myth." *Journal of Counseling Psychology*, Vol. 42, No. 1, January 1995.

38. "New APA Position Statement Urges Action to Reduce High Rates of Nicotine Dependence." *Psychiatric Services*, Vol. 46, No. 2, February 1995.

39. American Cancer Society.

40. Koop, C. Everett, et al. "Reinventing American Tobacco Policy." *Journal of the American Medical Association*, Vol. 279, No. 7, February 18, 1998.

41. "Smoking Found to Snuff Out the Benefits of Exercise." *American Medical News*, April 6, 1992.

42. Howard, George, et al. "Cigarette Smoking and Progression of Atherosclerosis." *Journal of the American Medical Association*, Vol. 279, No. 2, January 14, 1998.

43. Wannamethee, S. Goya, et al. "Smoking Cessation and the Risk of Stroke in Middle-Aged Men." *Journal of the American Medical Association*, Vol. 274, No. 2, July 12, 1995.

44. Kemper, Vicki. "Where the Action Is." *Common Cause Magazine*, Vol. 21, No. 1, Spring 1995. Spector, Rosanne. "White Men with Limited Education Almost Certain to Smoke; Hispanics Less Likely." Stanford University Medical Center, August 8, 1995.

45. "Nicotine Addiction in Female Smokers." *American Family Physician*, Vol. 51, No. 7, May 15, 1994.

46. Helson, Heidi, et al. "Smoking, Alcohol and Neuromuscular and Physical Function of Older Women." *Journal of*

the American Medical Association, Vol. 272, No. 23, December 21, 1994.

47. Morbidity and Mortality Weekly Report (MMWR). "Medical Care Expenditures Attributable to Cigarette Smoking During Pregnancy." *Journal of the American Medical Association*, Vol. 278, No. 23, December 17, 1997.

48. Cowley, Geoffrey. "Are Stogies Safer Than Cigarettes?" *Newsweek*, July 21, 1997.

49. Federal Trade Commission. *Smokeless Tobacco Report 1997.*

50. Glantz, Stanton, and William Parmley. "Passive Smoking and Heart Disease." *Journal of the American Medical Association*, Vol. 273, No. 13, April 5, 1995.

51. Centers for Disease Control and Prevention (CDC). "State-specific Prevalence of Cigarette Smoking Among Adults, and Children's and Adolescents' Exposure to Environmental Tobacco Smoke." *Journal of the American Medical Association*, Vol. 278, No. 23, December 17, 1997.

52. Grady, Denise. "Study Finds Second-hand Smoke Doubles Heart Disease." *New York Times*, May 2, 1997.

53. Meier, Barry. "Data on Tobacco Show a Strategy Aimed at Blacks." *New York Times*, February 6, 1998.

54. Siegel, Michael, et al. "Preemption in Tobacco Control." *Journal of the American Medical Association*, Vol. 278, No. 10, September 10, 1997.

55. Cooper, Thomas. *New Hope for Heavy Smokers.* Lexington, KY: SBC, 1992.

56. Marcus, Bess, et al. "Exercise Enhances the Maintenance of Smoking Cessation in Women." *Addictive Behaviors*, Vol. 20, No. 1, January–February 1995.

57. Apgar, Barbara, et al. "Effect of Nicotine Nasal Spray on Smoking Cessation." *Archives of Internal Medicine*, November 28, 1994.

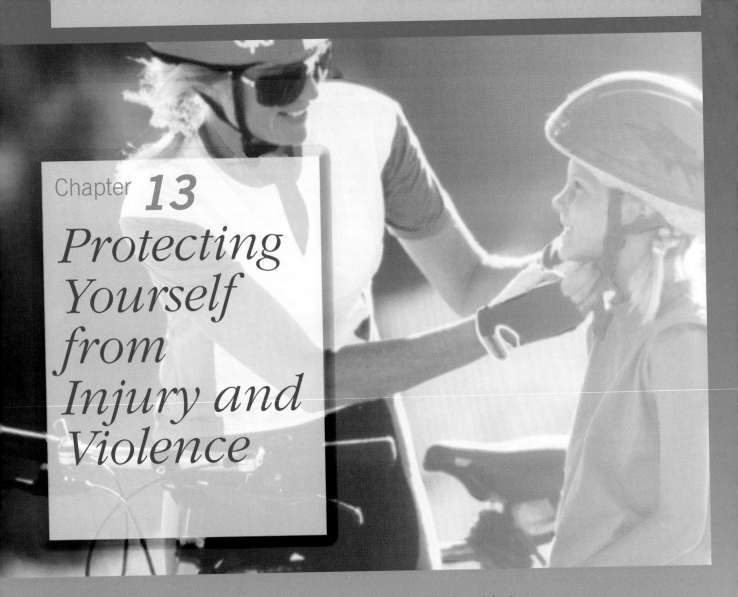

Chapter **13**

Protecting Yourself from Injury and Violence

After studying the material in this chapter, you should be able to:

- **Describe** safety procedures for road, residential, worksite, and outdoor safety.
- **Define** sexual victimization, sexual harassment, and sexual coercion and **explain** how each can develop.
- **Describe** recommended actions for preventing rape.
- **Explain** the consequences of sexual violence and **describe** how they can be treated.
- **Describe** the abuse pattern and **explain** how it relates to child abuse and partner abuse.

The major threats to the well-being of most college students aren't illnesses but injuries and violence. This chapter is a primer in self-protection that could help safeguard—perhaps even save—your life. Included are recommendations for common sense safety on the road, at home, outdoors, and on the job. This chapter also explores other serious threats to personal safety in our society—violence, both public and domestic, and sexual victimization.

Unintentional Injury: Why Accidents Happen

You may assume that most accidents happen without any warning. Yet often an accident is the unfortunate result of a series or combination of events. The more you know about the factors that increase the likelihood of an accident or injury, the more you can do to prevent it.

Where do you feel safest? Chances are you'll answer by naming the places that are most familiar to you: your room, your home, your car. Yet that's where you're most likely to have an accident—often because you let your guard down. While listening to the morning news, you may forget to shut off a burner on the stove. Since there usually isn't much traffic on your street, you may back out of your driveway without looking both ways. Most of the time you, or someone with you, is able to correct such dangerous situations before a fire or collision occurs. But you can't count on always being so lucky.

Keep in mind that *feeling* safe is not the same as *being* safe. Away from home, unsafe attitudes can set the stage for unsafe behaviors. If you're overly confident in your driving skills, you may speed on a winding or wet road. If you're daydreaming, you may trip and fall as you hike. Keeping your wits about you is essential to keeping yourself safe.

Safety on the Road

Although the number of deaths and injuries from car crashes has declined in recent years, motor-vehicle accidents remain the leading cause of death among Ameri-

cans aged 1 to 34 and the third most significant cause of lost years of potential life (after heart disease and cancer). As shown in Campus Focus: "College Students and Road Safety," many college students also take risks on the road: 12.3% of men and 6.6% of women rarely or never buckle up; 33.2% of men and 22.8% of women have driven after drinking; among those who rode motorcycles in the previous year, 31.1% of men and 37% of the women rarely or never wore helmets.[1]

Defensive Driving

Basic precautions can greatly increase your odds of reaching a destination alive. Number one is not driving after drinking. In recent years, there has been a decline

---

Strategies for Prevention

How to Drive Safely

Don't drive while under the influence of alcohol or other drugs, including medications that may impair your reflexes, cause drowsiness, or affect your judgment. Never get into a car if you suspect the driver may be intoxicated or affected by a drug.

✔ Remain calm when dealing with drivers who are reckless or rude. Be alert and anticipate possible hazards. Don't let yourself be distracted by conversations, children's questions, arguments, food or drink, or scenic views. If you become exhausted, pull over and rest.

✔ Don't get too comfortable. Alertness matters. Use the rearview mirror often. Don't let passengers or packages obstruct your view. Use the turn signals when changing lanes or making a turn. If someone cuts you off, back off to a safe distance. When you can, drive so that you have enough space around you.

✔ Make sure small children are in safety seats. Unless pets are trained to ride quietly in a car, keep them in carrying cases.

✔ Drive more slowly if weather conditions are bad. Avoid driving at all during heavy rain, snow, or other conditions that affect visibility and road conditions.

✔ Maintain your car properly, replacing windshield wipers, tires, and brakes when necessary. Keep flares and a fire extinguisher in your car for use in emergencies.

✔ To avoid a head-on collision, generally veer to the right—onto a shoulder, lawn, or open space.

CAMPUS FOCUS: COLLEGE STUDENTS AND ROAD SAFETY

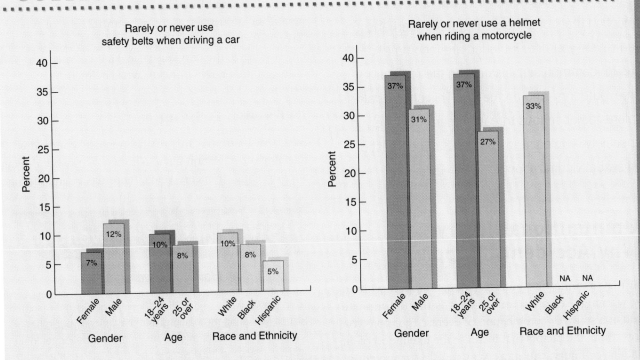

SOURCE: Douglas, Kathy, et al. "Results from the 1995 National College Health Risk Behavior Survey," *Journal of American College Health*, Vol. 46, September 1997.

in the number of fatalities caused by drunk driving, particularly among young people. The National Highway Traffic Safety Administration attributes this decline to increases in the drinking age from 18 to 21 in all 50 states and the District of Columbia, to educational programs aimed at reducing and driving by teens, to the formation of Students Against Driving Drunk (SADD) and similar groups, and to changes in state laws that penalize drivers younger than age 21 for driving with even lower blood-alcohol concentration levels than were previously acceptable (from 0.01% to 0.05%).

Falling asleep at the wheel is second only to alcohol as a cause of serious motor-vehicle accidents. According to the National Commission on Sleep Disorders Research, each year 200,000 sleep-related motor-vehicle accidents claim more than 5000 lives, cause hundreds of thousands of injuries, and lead to billions of dollars in indirect costs.

The best lifesavers for drivers and passengers are seatbelts, which are now required for children and adults in many states. Because of changes in federal law, beginning with 1998 models, all new cars will be equipped with air bags. Safety officials recommend that people shopping for a new car invest in vehicles with dual air bags in front and lap-shoulder belts for the rear as well as the front seats.

Although air bags can save adults' lives, they may be hazardous to infants and young children. In 1998, the National Highway Traffic Safety Administration gave automobile owners permission to deactivate air bags. However, the American Academy of Pediatrics, which has argued that deactivation may pose an even greater risk by jeopardizing the safety of older children, teenagers, and adult passengers, has recommended that children be placed in the backseat, whether or not the car is equipped with an air bag.[2]

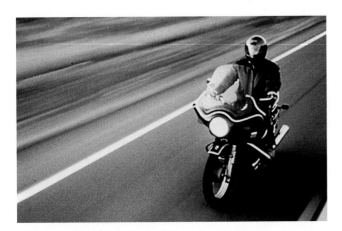

Use your head. Head trauma is the most common motorcycle injury—and one of the most preventable.

Safe Cycling

Mile for mile, motorcycling is far riskier than automobile driving. The most common motorcycle injury is head trauma, which can lead to physical disability, including paralysis and general weakness, as well as problems reading and thinking. Complete recovery from head trauma can take 4 to 6 years, and the costs can be staggering. Head injury can also result in permanent disability, coma, and death. To prevent head trauma, motorcycle helmets are required in most states. Federal law dictates that a certain percentage of highway construction funds be reallocated for safety programs in states that don't require motorcycle helmets.

Bicycling injuries cause almost 200,000 head injuries each year; they account for 70% to 80% of all bicycle fatalities. According to CDC estimates, safety helmets—now required by law in some states—reduce the risk of head injury by 85% and could prevent one death every day and one head injury every 4 minutes.[3]

In addition to wearing helmets, cyclists should know and follow traffic rules: Yield right of way appropriately, signal turns properly, obey stop signs, and so on. They should use bike lanes if they're available and avoid weaving in and out of traffic or riding in the center of the street or against the flow of traffic. Bikes should have reflectors on the front, back, and both wheels, as well as taillights and headlights for night use.

Safety at Home and on the Job

Every year home accidents claim more than 24,000 lives and cause nearly 25 million injuries. Common dangers

are poisoning, falls, and burns. Half a million children swallow poisonous materials each year; 90% are under age 5. Adults may also be poisoned by mistakenly taking someone else's prescription drugs or taking medicines in the dark and swallowing the wrong one. In most cities, you can call a poison control center for advice.

Falls

Falls are the leading cause of fatal accidents at home. High heels or worn footgear, poor lighting, slippery or uneven walkways, broken stairs and handrails, loose or worn rugs, or objects left where people walk all increase the likelihood of a slip. Falls are an especially serious health risk for the elderly. Each year about one-third of all people 65 years of age or older who live at home fall; 6% to 10% of these falls result in injury, including fractures, muscle injuries, sprains, lacerations, and dislocations. Fearing another fall, older people may limit their activity, becoming less independent and fit.

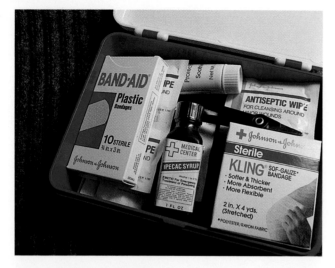

Your home first-aid kit should include (at minimum) bandages, sterile gauze pads, adhesive tape, scissors, cotton, antibiotic ointment, a needle, safety pins, calamine lotion, syrup of ipecac to induce vomiting, and a thermometer.

Fires

You can prevent fires from occurring by making sure that the three ingredients of fire—fuel, a heat source, and oxygen—don't get a chance to mix. Almost any-

Strategies for Prevention

Staying Safe from Fires

✔ Keep gasoline, paint, oily rags, newspapers, plastics, glues, and lightweight materials away from pilot lights, heaters, and other sources of heat. Store flammables in metal cans. Clean up grease on stoves.

✔ Don't overload electrical circuits, use worn wiring, or use portable heaters that have no cutoff feature if they tip over.

✔ Keep matches and cigarette lighters out of children's reach. Don't smoke in bed.

✔ Check to see that at least one smoke detector has been installed on each floor of your dorm or home. Make sure that you have a multipurpose fire extinguisher available to put out small fires.

✔ Close bedroom doors when you sleep. Closed doors slow the spread of fire. Keep a flashlight by each bedside to light the way out at night.[4]

thing can act as fuel for fire, including paper, wood, and, of course, flammable liquids such as oils, gasoline, and some paints. A heat source can be a spark from a lighted match, pilot light, or an electrical wire. Oxygen is necessary for the chemical reaction between the fuel and heat source that causes combustion.

If a fire starts and it's small, you may be able to put it out with a portable fire extinguisher before it spreads. However, if the fire does get out of control, you might have only 2 to 5 minutes to get out of the house or building alive. A fire-escape plan can save time and lives. Sketch a plan of your house, apartment building, dormitory, or fraternity or sorority house. Identify two ways out of each room or apartment. Make sure everyone is familiar with these escape routes. Designate an area outside where all family members or dorm residents should meet after escaping from a fire.

If a fire breaks out in your dorm room, get out as quickly as possible, but don't run. Before opening a room door, place your hand on it. If it's hot, don't open it. If the door feels cool, open it slightly to check for smoke. If there's none, leave by your planned escape route. If you're on an upper floor and your escape routes are blocked, open a window (top and bottom, if possible) and wait or signal from the window for help. Never try to use an elevator in a fire.

If you can't leave your room safely during a fire, call for help and turn off the air-conditioning or heating systems. To block smoke, press sheets and towels (wet, if possible) around and under the door. Keep as close to the floor as possible (where there's likely to be more oxygen) and place a wet washcloth over your face to filter out smoke particles.

Working with Computers

A new concern among many workers is **repetitive motion injury (RMI)**, which has surpassed back and neck injuries as the number-one claim for workers compensation injuries. Repeated motions—such as the hand and arm movements made while using a computer keyboard—all day, every day, can result in muscle and tendon strain and inflammation. Symptoms include pain, swelling, and numbness and weakness in the hands or the arms. If these problems are identified early, permanent damage can generally be avoided by altering the work environment and allowing for more breaks during the day. If you work at a computer, good posture and correct positioning of the computer screen and keyboard can help prevent repetitive motion injuries, eye-

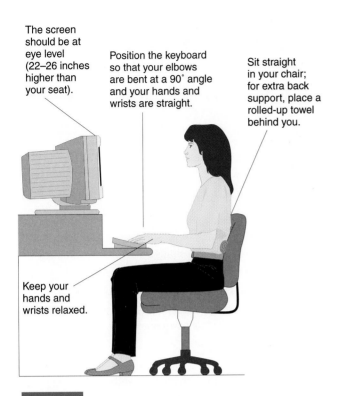

The screen should be at eye level (22–26 inches higher than your seat).

Position the keyboard so that your elbows are bent at a 90° angle and your hands and wrists are straight.

Sit straight in your chair; for extra back support, place a rolled-up towel behind you.

Keep your hands and wrists relaxed.

Figure 13-1

Safe computing. By paying attention to your posture and your computer's position, you can help protect yourself from repetitive motion injury, back strain, and eyestrain.

strain, and back strain (see Figure 13-1). Here are some additional tips:

- Place the keyboard so that your elbows are bent at a 90° angle and you don't have to bend your wrists to type.

- Use a chair that provides ample back support. Keep your thighs parallel to the floor and your feet on the floor. If your feet don't reach the floor, use a footrest.

- If you experience neck strain, place a document holder next to your screen so that you can view the materials you are typing more easily.

- Every 15 minutes take a 30-second break, stretch your arms, and walk around the office. Take a 15-minute break at least once every 2 hours.

Recreational Safety

When you want to take a break, exercise, or simply enjoy yourself, you probably go outside. But if you aren't careful, even a simple stroll or swim can turn into a hazardous event. According to a study by the Johns

Hopkins School of Public Health, every year 750,000 Americans are injured during recreational activities such as horseback riding, skiing, sledding, snowboarding, skating, and playground activities; 82,000 suffer head injuries requiring emergency room or hospital treatment. Two dangers on the increase are in-line skating (rollerblading) and skateboarding. Public health experts urge helmet use for sports such as rollerblading and skateboarding because such activities combine high speeds with exposure to traffic.[5]

Heat and Cold

Each year as many as 1000 Americans die from heat-caused illnesses that are almost always preventable. Two common heat-related maladies are **heat cramps** and **heat stress**. Heat cramps are caused by hard work and heavy sweating in the heat. Heat stress may occur simultaneously or afterward, as the blood vessels try to keep body temperature down. **Heat exhaustion**, a third such malady, is the result of prolonged sweating with inadequate fluid replacement.

The first step in treating these conditions is to stop exercising, move to a cool place, and drink plenty of water. Don't resume work or activity until all the symptoms have disappeared; see a doctor if you're suffering from heat exhaustion. **Heat stroke** is a life-threatening medical emergency caused by the breakdown of the body's mechanism for cooling itself. The treatment is to cool the body down: Move to a cooler environment; sponge down with cool water and apply ice to the back of the neck, armpits, and groin. Immersion in cold water could cause shock. Get medical help immediately.

The tips of the toes, fingers, ears, nose, chin, and cheeks are most vulnerable to exposure to high wind speeds and low temperatures, which can result in **frostbite**. There are two types of frostbite, *superficial* and *deep*. Superficial frostbite, the freezing of the skin and tissues just below the skin, is characterized by a waxy look and firmness of the skin, although the tissue below is soft. Initial treatment should be to slowly rewarm the area. As the area thaws, it will be numb and bluish or purple, and blisters may form. Cover the area with a dry, sterile dressing and protect the skin from further exposure to cold. See a doctor for further treatment. Deep frostbite, the freezing of skin, muscle, and even bone, requires medical treatment. It usually involves the tissues of the hands and feet, which appear pale and feel frozen. Keep the victim dry and as warm as possible on the way to a medical facility. Cover the frostbitten area with a dry, sterile dressing.

The gradual cooling of the center of the body may occur at temperatures above, as well as below, freezing—usually in wet, windy weather. When body temperature falls below 95°F, the body is incapable of rewarming itself because of the breakdown of the internal system that regulates its temperature. This state is known as **hypothermia**. The first sign of hypothermia is severe shivering. Then the victim becomes uncoordinated, drowsy, listless, confused, and is unable to speak properly. Symptoms become more severe as body temperature continues to drop, and coma or death can result.

Hypothermia requires emergency medical treatment. Try to prevent any further heat loss: Move the victim to a warm place, cover him or her with blankets, remove wet clothing, and replace it with dry garments. If the victim is conscious, administer warm liquids, not alcohol.

Drowning

Drowning claims more than 6000 lives a year, according to the National Safety Council. Toddlers under age 4 and teenage boys between 15 and 19 are at greatest risk. Among young children, 90% of drownings occur in residential swimming pools.[6]

The causes of drowning, in order of frequency, are becoming exhausted, being swept into deep water, losing support, becoming trapped or entangled, having a cramp or other attack, and striking an underwater object. Many drowning victims were strong swimmers. Most drownings occur at unorganized facilities, such as ponds or pools with no lifeguard present. Health officials believe that pool fencing alone, along with ade-

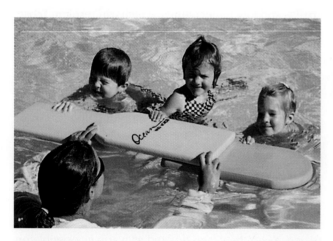

Water safety training can begin in early childhood. Swimming, treading water, and engaging in safe water practices are important to preventing drownings.

Strategies for Prevention

How to Enjoy the Water Safely

✔ Learn "drownproofing," or ways of treading water or moving with minimal output of energy. Know your limits as a swimmer and don't try to swim beyond your depth or capability.

✔ Don't swim after drinking.

✔ Don't swim in the dark, especially in the ocean. Find out about currents, undertows, or sharp underwater rocks before swimming in a strange place. Never dive before knowing the depth of the water below you.

✔ Always use a buddy system, even when swimming with a group. Even a strong swimmer can suffer a cramp or another problem that can jeopardize his or her ability to stay afloat.

✔ Don't swim in boating or fishing areas. If thrown from a boat or canoe, stay with the craft and use it for support. Wear a personal flotation device whenever you're boating, rafting, or canoeing.

✔ Be careful when diving into waves and pay attention to the undertow, which could pull you out to sea.

quate gates and latches, could prevent as many as half of all drownings or near-drownings of children.

Alcohol increases the dangers of swimming and boating accidents. Among the college students who reported swimming or boating in the previous year, 30.5% had used alcohol before going into or on the water. More than a third of the men—35.2%—said they had drunk alcohol when boating or swimming.[7]

Intentional Injury: Violence in America

Crime in the United States has declined throughout the 1990s. Experts cite many reasons: an improved economy, an older population, more police, longer prison sentences, a decline in the use of crack cocaine and other drugs.[8] But crime still touches many people's lives. For every 1000 persons age 12 or older, the public experiences two rapes or attempted rapes, two assaults with serious injury, and five robberies. According to the Bureau of Justice Statistics, U.S. residents age 12 or older experience approximately 39.6 million crimes a year. About 29 million are property crimes, 9.9 million are crimes of violence, and 396,000 are personal thefts. In the mid-1990s, the violent crime rate declined about 10% a year, and property crimes continued a 16-year decline.[9]

The Roots of Aggression and Violence

While anger is considered a normal, sometimes inevitable emotion, aggression—behavior with the intent to control or dominate—is a threat to individuals and to society. Angry people may want to push or punch someone; aggressive people carry through on such impulses and become violent. Why? The reasons, discussed in the following sections, are complex.

Biological Causes

Traumatic brain injury, which can lead to violent outbursts of explosive anger, is one of many medical factors associated with violence. As many as 70% of those who suffer head injuries report some degree of irritability or explosive rage. The use of alcohol or drugs before or after a head injury may increase the likelihood of such problems. Illnesses that affect the brain—stroke and neurologic diseases, brain tumors, infectious illnesses, epilepsy, metabolic disorders (such as hyperthyroidism or hypothyroidism), multiple sclerosis, and systemic lupus erythematosus—can also lead to aggressive behavior.[10]

Developmental Factors

Many developmental factors—childrearing practices, parental discipline, relations to peers, sex-role socialization, economic inequality, lack of opportunity, and media influences—contribute to violence. Parents who reject their youngsters, who are physically abusive, or who have a criminal history are most likely to have children with early signs of aggressive behavior. As discussed later in this chapter, violence in the home, especially when it is experienced at a young age, breeds more violence. Brutalized children learn to be brutal themselves. The reason for this may be that such children haven't learned effective ways to relate to others, or they may suffer from emotional and cognitive disorders.

Violence in the Media

The media's portrayal of aggressive acts can stimulate violence. A riot, cross-burning, or grisly television mur-

---

Strategies for Prevention

Ways to Stop Violence

✔ Object to jokes about racism, women, rape, minorities, or nationalities.

✔ Watch your own anger—talk it out, write it out, sing it out—but don't act on it.

✔ Refuse to hate.

✔ Don't retaliate.

✔ Volunteer at a shelter for battered women or runaway youths.

✔ Write a letter protesting a violent movie or television program.

✔ Support a tax on guns and ammunition that would help pay for health care.

✔ Avoid a conflict. It's usually not worth it to argue.

✔ Be charitable toward rude people—they don't know better.

✔ Don't get discouraged. Hope grows the way a path does in the country. As more people walk it, it turns into a road.

---

der sometimes triggers similar forms of violence. The average American youth is exposed to 40,000 deaths and hundreds of thousands of incidents of other mayhem while growing up. Researchers estimate that, if television had never been invented, there would be 10,000 fewer murders, 70,000 fewer rapes, and 700,000 fewer assaults each year in the United States.

Guns

Almost half of all homes in the United States contain at least one firearm, which may be kept for self-defense, hunting, target shooting, or collecting. An estimated 3 to 4 million handguns are circulating in the United States; an estimated 100,000 students carry a gun to school.[11] In eight states, firearms kill more people than motor-vehicle accidents. Across the country, they are quickly becoming the leading cause of traumatic brain injury and traumatic death.[12] For each fatal shooting, there are an estimated 2.6 injuries. The price tag for treating firearms-related injuries has been estimated at $20 billion a year.[13]

Social Factors

Extreme poverty, deprivation, unemployment, prejudice, discrimination, involvement with gangs, and repeated exposure to actual violence all contribute to aggressive and violent behavior. The risk of violence increases for those who can find few, if any, economic and social opportunities in mainstream society. Violence is most common among the poor, regardless of race. Most people of color, including those who grow up with poverty, discrimination, and family disruptions, do not engage in violence and are more likely to be victims of violent crime than white Americans.

Crime on Campus

Once considered havens from the meanness of America's streets, colleges and universities have seen a dramatic rise in crime in recent years. In a survey of more than 2400 schools, there were 30 murders, almost 1000 rapes, and more than 1800 robberies, along with 32,127 burglaries and 8981 car thefts.[14] Under the Federal Student Right to Know and Campus Security Act, all colleges and universities receiving federal funds must publish and make readily available the number of campus killings, assaults, sexual assaults, robberies, burglaries and other crimes, and their security policies.[15]

As the national College Health Risk Behavior Survey found, the majority of college students are not violent. Yet a not-significant minority—14.2% of the men—reported being involved in at least one physical fight during the previous year, and 13.8% of the men said they had carried a weapon (gun, knife, or club) at least once during the preceding 30 days.[16]

Because of concerns about safety on campus, more schools are taking tougher stands on student behavior. Many have established codes of conduct barring the use of alcohol and drugs, fighting, and sexual harassment. Many also have instituted policies requiring suspension or expulsion of students who violate this code.[17]

Many campuses have set up public safety programs, which include late-night shuttle buses and escorts, student bicycle patrols, outdoor emergency phones, and increased numbers of police and security guards. Sexual-assaults services provide counseling, crisis intervention, and educational programs. Students are urged to walk in groups, lock doors and windows, and limit alcohol consumption. Freshman orientation often includes mandatory sessions on campus safety and sexual assault.[18]

Domestic Violence

Violence doesn't stop at the front doors of America's homes. According to the Federal Bureau of Investigation, the most common and least reported violent crimes are attacks in which the victim and the perpetrator knew each other at the time of or before the incident. One-third of all murders occur within families. Physical violence may occur in 20% to 30% of all American households.[19]

Partner Abuse

Every 9 seconds a woman is battered by her partner. During their lifetime, at least one of every five women will be assaulted by a partner or ex-partner. Domestic violence is the single most common cause of injury to women—more common than car accidents, muggings, and rapes combined—and accounts for 42% of female murders.[20]

The primary factors contributing to physical abuse are the degree of frustration and stress a man is under, his use of alcohol (involved in up to 60% of battering cases), and whether he was raised in an abusive home. Only one in twenty men who beat their partners is violent outside the home; nine in ten refuse to admit that they have a problem. In homes where a wife is beaten, children also may be abused. The primary risk factors for domestic murder are poverty and household crowding; the lower a family's socioeconomic status—regardless of its racial or ethnic background—the greater the risk of deadly violence.[21]

Abused wives and children are often trapped in terror. Wives may stay with abusive husbands because of love, financial dependence, shame, guilt, fear of being pursued, harmed, or killed if they leave, or a sense of responsibility to their children. The incidence of alcoholism, substance abuse, depression, and suicide attempts is higher in battered women than others.

Child Abuse

Severe child abuse occurs an estimated 1.7 million times each year and claims the lives of as many as 5000 children a year. Parents in every economic, social, educational, religious, and racial group abuse children, but poverty is a significant factor in abuse. Mistreatment is seven times more likely in families with incomes under $15,000.

Abuse can take many forms: physical, psychological, or sexual. Physical abuse often leaves visible marks. However, emotional abuse—rejection, verbal cruelty such as constant berating and belittling, serious threats of harm, frequent tension in the home, and violent arguments with parents—can be just as devastating to a child.

Sexual abuse of children involves *any* sexual contact, whether it is sexually suggestive conversation, prolonged kissing, petting, oral sex, or intercourse, between an adult and child. Because children are not intellectually or emotionally mature enough to consent to sexual involvement, any such action is illegal and a violation of a child's rights.

Pedophilia, or child molestation, refers to abuse by individuals—teachers, babysitters, neighbors, and so on—who are not related to the child. **Incest** is sexual contact between two people who are closely related, including siblings as well as children and parents, grandparents, uncles, and aunts. Abuse—emotional, physical, or sexual—can affect every aspect of a child's life. Youngsters may develop physical symptoms, such as headaches, stomachaches, and sleep problems, and run into academic and social difficulties in school. Since children often blame themselves for whatever happened and assume they are responsible, they may develop a sense of hopelessness, shame, and pessimism. Some become clinically depressed or develop other mental or emotional problems that may continue into adolescence and adulthood, including more reports of headaches, depression, insomnia, obesity, and fatigue.

Many abusive families can be helped with appropriate treatment. Usually, this involves counseling for the entire family. Within the family structure, the abusive parent must learn to trust, to establish healthy intimate relationships, and to ask for help when it's needed. Parents must learn to view their children realistically; their children must realize that it's permissible to act like children.

The effects of any form of child abuse can be lifelong. Sexual abuse survivors suffer deep psychological wounds, including a profound sense of betrayal and loss. As adults, many find it hard to form intimate adult relationships and experience sexual difficulties. Other common problems include depression, feelings of guilt or shame, inability to trust, drug and alcohol abuse, and a vulnerability to other forms of victimization.[22]

Sexual Victimization and Violence

Sexual victimization refers to any situation in which a person is deprived of free choice and forced to comply with sexual acts. It is not only a woman's issue; in fact, men are also victimized. In recent years, researchers have come to view acts of sexual victimization along a continuum, ranging from behaviors such as street hassling, grabbing, and obscene telephone calls to rape, battering, and incest.

While obscene comments or calls may seem minor annoyances compared with acts of sexual violence, all forms of sexual victimization attack a person's integrity. The roots of this problem extend beyond individuals to our society and the beliefs and assumptions—many of them false—that it engenders:

- *Acceptance of myths about sexual conduct.* Our culture, consciously and unconsciously, teaches women not to make sexual advances and to limit sexual intimacy to love relationships. At the same time, men are encouraged to pursue sexual encounters with numerous partners and to view sex as an achievement. Men who accept these gender roles—particularly those who admit to using force or deception to obtain sex—may believe that women who say no really mean yes, and that women like to lead men on. They may also feel that coercion is legitimate in certain situations—for example, if a woman asks a man out or comes to his apartment or home.[23]

- *Acceptance of male aggression.* Boys in our culture learn at early ages that "real men" are aggressive and powerful and are expected to make sexual conquests.

- *The uncontrollable male sex drive.* Both men and women often believe—erroneously—that young men, once stimulated, cannot control their sexual appetites. Yet, as educators have pointed out, any college-age man would be able to stop immediately if his partner's parents walked into the room. A related myth is that stopping sexual activity is in some way harmful to a male; it isn't.

- *Blaming the victim.* Although victims of thefts, carjackings, and other crimes aren't blamed for what happened to them, women are often held responsible for "provoking" sexual attacks by wearing tight clothing, flirting, or going to a bar alone.

- *Trivializing.* Many acts of sexual victimization, such as the use of verbal slurs when talking about women's bodies, are treated as jokes or pranks rather than serious offenses. This makes such behaviors seem acceptable and denies the very real distress they cause.

- *Exposure to sexually violent material.* Repeated exposure to magazines, books, movies, and videos that link sex and violence may desensitize men to violence toward women so that they come to think of it as normal and acceptable.

Sexual Harassment

All forms of sexual harassment or unwanted sexual attention—from the display of pornographic photos to the use of sexual obscenities to a demand for sex by anyone in a position of power or authority—are illegal. (See Pulsepoints: "Ten Ways to Prevent Sexual Victimization.")

Sexual Harassment on the Job

As defined by the Equal Employment Opportunity Commission, sexual harassment takes two basic forms: In **quid pro quo** harassment, a person in power or authority makes unwanted sexual advances as a condition for receiving a job, a promotion, or another type of favor; in harassment by means of a **hostile or offensive environment**, supervisors or coworkers engage in persistent inappropriate behaviors that make the workplace hostile, abusive, or otherwise unbearable.

"There's a spectrum of verbal, nonverbal and physical acts, ranging from making off-color remarks to grabbing someone's breast or buttocks," says consultant Susan L. Webb of Seattle, author of *Step Forward: Sexual Harassment in the Workplace.* "But sexual harassment always involves behavior that is related to or based on sex, that is deliberate or repeated, and that is not welcome, not asked for, and not returned."[24] Sexual com-

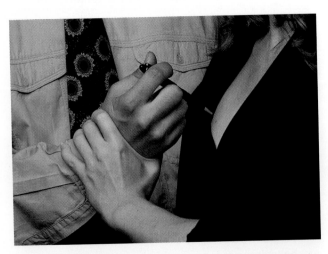

Sexual harassment on the job can take many forms, from remarks, unwelcome attention, and violations of personal space to the extreme of sexual assault.

Strategies for Change

Gender Etiquette on the Job

✔ Be polite and respectful. Whenever possible, rely on courtesy rather than contact. Offer a handshake instead of a hug; an encouraging word, not a pat on the back.

✔ Use the same-sex standard. If you're not sure whether a comment is appropriate, think of what you would do with a colleague of the same sex.

✔ Give compliments based on merit, not appearance. "Men will compliment a woman on what she's wearing, rather than the report she wrote," says Webb. "This puts her gender and looks above her status as a coworker."

✔ Think of how a loved one would react. If you're a man, before making a comment or telling a joke, imagine how your mother, sister, or daughter would respond. If you're a woman, think of the impact your words might have on your father, brother, or son.

✔ Speak up. If you don't like your boss to rub your neck or you don't appreciate tasteless jokes on your e-mail, say, "I find your behavior offensive, and I'd appreciate your stopping it." Focus on the behavior, not the person, to take the emotion out of the interaction.

ments, propositions, dirty jokes, suggestive looks or remarks, displays of pinups or pornography, "accidental" touches, pats, squeezes, pinches, fondling and ogling are all potentially offensive.[25]

Workers who feel victimized by sexual harassment should document their complaints by writing down specific incidents (including dates, times, places, and what happened). It sometimes helps initially to confront the harasser, either in person or by writing a note, and state that you're not interested in his or her attention. Many companies have established grievance procedures for handling sexual harassment complaints. The courts have awarded substantial payments of both punitive and compensatory damage to victims of physical and verbal harassment and have held companies liable for failing to halt offensive actions.

Sexual Harassment on Campus

As many as a third to a half of female undergraduates and 20% of males have experienced some form of sexual harassment. Professors or supervisors may pressure students into sexual involvement for the sake of a grade,

Pulsepoints

Ten Ways to Prevent Sexual Victimization

1. Challenge gender stereotypes. Just because you're male doesn't mean you have to act in a macho, sexually aggressive way. Just because you're female doesn't mean you have to be passive and accepting of male behavior.

2. Don't tolerate inappropriate language or behavior. If you find someone's sexually crude language offensive, say so. If you don't like to be touched by casual acquaintances, back away and keep your distance.

3. Be careful of your sexual signals. Men often assume that women who smile, make conversation, and flirt are signaling sexual availability. Women typically think they're just being friendly. Make sure you know the message you want to send—and don't assume you can tell what someone else is trying to signal.

4. Choose safe settings. If you're going out with someone you don't know well or have reservations about being alone with, suggest meeting in a public place or participating in a group activity.

5. Think about your sexual expectations for a relationship. What are you willing to do? How much sexual activity is enough? Where do you want to draw the line? Remember, your partner will be making decisions about the same things.

6. Talk about sex. Using the communication guidelines in Chapter 7, bring up the topic of sexual involvement. Let your date know from the beginning how you feel about sexual activity on first, second, third, or twentieth dates.

7. Think ahead. Rather than letting yourself get carried away by passion, anticipate what could happen if, for instance, you agree to go to your date's apartment for a drink or park in an isolated spot. State your feelings clearly.

8. Say "no" clearly when you mean it and accept "no" when you hear it. If you're the one saying no, use a firm, even loud voice, and back up what you say with body language. If you're on the receiving end of a no, pay attention. A no—even if said quietly and shyly—still means no.

9. Keep your wits about you. Alcohol and other drugs can affect your judgment and inhibitions. You may become more sexually aggressive under their influence, or you may greatly increase your risk of being victimized.

10. Call it like it is. If you're the target of sexual taunts or unwanted propositions on campus or at work, say, "What you're doing is sexual harassment, and I'm going to report it." If a date or acquaintance won't respect your limits, one of the most effective defensive tactics is saying, "This is rape, and I'm calling the cops."

recommendation, or special opportunity. If a student tries to end a sexual relationship, they may threaten reprisals. Most harassment comes from male faculty members, but both men and women report having been harassed by either male or female faculty (see Figure 13-2). Overall, 94% of female students reportedly had been harassed by men and 15% by women; 79% of male students reportedly had been harassed by women and 55% by men.

Sexual harassment can undermine students' well-being and academic performance. Its effects include diminished ambition and self-confidence, reduced ability to concentrate, sleeplessness, depression, physical aches, and ailments. Some students avoid classes or work with certain faculty members because of the risk of sexual advances. However, few file official grievances.

Because college administrations can be held legally responsible for allowing a hostile or offensive sexual environment, many schools have set up committees to handle such student reports and to take action against

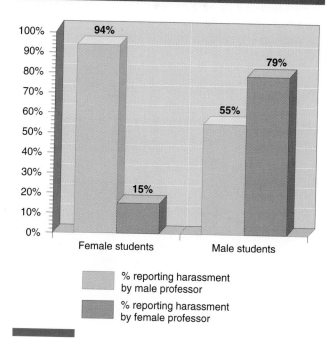

Figure 13-2

Sexual harassment does happen on campus, to both women and men. Such harassment can affect self-esteem and academic performance.

faculty members. Universities also are discouraging and, in some cases, restricting consensual relationships between teachers and students, especially any dating of students by their academic professors or advisers. Although such relationships may seem consensual, in reality they may not be, because of the power faculty members have to determine students' grades and futures. In some cases, students have sued their universities for failing to protect them from professors who pressured them into sexual liaisons.

If you encounter sexual harassment as a student, report it to the department chair or dean. If you don't feel that you're getting an adequate response to your complaint, talk with the campus representatives who handle matters involving affirmative action or civil rights. Federal guidelines prevent any discrimination against you in terms of grades or the loss of a job or scholarship if you report harassment. Schools that do not take measures to remedy harassment could lose federal funds.

Sexual Coercion and Rape

At a bar on a weekend night, a group of intoxicated young men grab a woman and squeeze her breasts as she struggles to get free. At a party, a man offers his date drugs and alcohol in the hope of lowering her resistance to sex. Although some people don't realize it, such actions are forms of sexual coercion (forced sexual activity), which is very common, on and off college campuses.

Sexual coercion can take many forms, including exerting peer pressure, taking advantage of one's desire for popularity, threatening an end to a relationship, getting someone intoxicated, stimulating a partner against

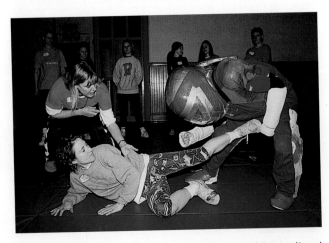

Model mugging courses train women to actively resist assault and rape.

Strategies for Prevention

Reducing the Risk of Stranger Rape

Rape prevention consists primarily of making it as difficult as possible for a rapist to make you his victim:

✔ Don't advertise that you're a woman living alone. Use initials on your mailbox and in the phone book; even add a fictitious name.

✔ Install and use secure locks on doors and windows, changing door locks after losing keys or moving into a new residence. A peephole in your front door can be particularly helpful.

✔ Don't open your door to strangers. If a repairman or public official is at your door, ask him to identify himself and call his office to verify that he is a reputable person on legitimate business.

✔ In public, demonstrate self-confidence through your body language and speech to communicate that you won't be intimidated. Rapists often select as victims women who exhibit passivity and submissiveness.

✔ Lock your car when it's parked and drive with locked car doors. Should your car break down, attach a white cloth to the antenna and lock yourself in. If someone other than a uniformed officer stops to offer help, ask this person to call the police or a garage but do not open your locked car door.

✔ Avoid dark and deserted areas, and be aware of the surroundings where you're walking. This may help if you need an opportunity to escape. Should a driver ask for directions when you're a pedestrian, avoid approaching his car. Instead, call out your reply from a safe distance.

✔ Have house or car keys in hand before coming to the door, and check the back seat before getting into your car.

✔ Wherever you go, it can be very helpful to carry a device for making a loud noise, like a whistle or, even better, a small compressed air horn available in many sporting goods and boat supply stores. Sound the noise alarm at the first sign of danger.

✔ Take a self-defense class to learn techniques of physical resistance that can injure the attacker or distract him long enough for you to escape.

his or her wishes, or insinuating an obligation based on the time or money one has expended. Men may feel that they need to live up to the sexual stereotype of taking advantage of every opportunity for sex. Women are far more likely than men to encounter physical force.

Rape refers to sexual intercourse with an unconsenting partner under actual or threatened force. Sexual intercourse between a male over the age of 16 and a female under the "age of consent" (which ranges from 12 to 21 in different states) is called *statutory* rape. In *acquaintance* rape, or *date* rape, discussed in depth later in this chapter, the victim knows the rapist; in stranger rape, the rapist is an unknown assailant. Both stranger and acquaintance rape are serious crimes that can have a devastating impact on their victims.

Acquaintance or Date Rape

Most rapes are committed by someone who is known to the victim. Both women and men report having been forced into sexual activity by someone they know. Many college students are in the age group most likely to face this threat: women aged 16 to 25 and men under 25. Women are most vulnerable and men are most likely to commit assaults during their senior year of high school and their first year of college. In several surveys of college students, 79.7% to 97.5% of the women and 62.1% to 93.5% of the men reported that they had been coerced into some unwanted sexual behavior.[26]

The same factors that lead to other forms of sexual victimization can set the stage for date rape. Socialization into an aggressive role, acceptance of rape myths, and a view that force is justified in certain situations increase the likelihood of a man's committing date rape. Other factors can also play a role, including the following:

- *Personality and early sexual experiences.* Psychological studies haven't found that date rapists are more disturbed than other men. However, certain factors may predispose individuals to sexual aggression, including first sexual experience at a very young age, earlier and more frequent than usual childhood sexual experiences (both forced and voluntary), hostility toward women, irresponsibility, lack of social consciousness, and a need to dominate sexual partners.

- *Situational variables (what happens during the date).* Men who initiate a date, pay all expenses, and provide transportation are more likely to be sexually aggressive, perhaps because they feel that they can call all the shots.

Strategies for Prevention

Preventing Date Rape

For men:

✔ Remember that it's okay not to "score" on a date.

✔ Be aware of your partner's actions. If she pulls away or tries to get up, understand that she's sending you a message—one you should acknowledge and respect.

✔ Don't assume that a sexy dress or casual flirting is an invitation to sex.

✔ Be aware of drinking, drug use, or other behaviors (such as hanging out with a group known to be sexually aggressive in certain situations) that could affect your judgment and ability to act responsibly.

✔ Think of the way you'd want your sister or a close woman friend to be treated by her date. Behave in the same manner.

For women:

✔ Be wary if the man calls all the shots (ordering for you at restaurants, planning what to do on your date); he may do the same when it comes to sex.

✔ Back away from a man who pressures you into other activities you don't want to engage in on a date, such as chugging beer or drag racing with his friends.

✔ Avoid misleading messages and avoid behavior that may be interpreted as sexual teasing.

✔ If, despite direct communication about your intentions, your date behaves in a sexually coercive manner, use a strategy of escalating forcefulness—direct refusal, vehement verbal refusal, and if necessary, physical force.

✔ Avoid using alcohol or other drugs when you definitely do not wish to be sexually intimate with your date.

- *Acceptance of sexual coercion.* Some social groups, such as fraternities or athletic teams, may encourage the use of alcohol, reinforce stereotypes about masculinity, and emphasize violence, force, and competition.

- *Drinking.* Alcohol use is one of the strongest predictors of acquaintance rape. Men who've been drinking may not react to subtle signals, may misinterpret a woman's behavior as come-ons, and may feel more sexually aroused. At the same time, drinking may impair a woman's ability to communicate her wishes effectively and to cope with a man's aggressiveness.

- *Date rape drugs.* At least two drugs—Rohypnol and gammahydroxybutrate (GHB)—have been implicated in cases of acquaintance or date rape.

- *Gender differences in interpreting sexual cues.* In research comparing college men and women, men typically overestimated women's sexual availability and interest, seeing friendliness, revealing clothing, and attractiveness as deliberately seductive.

Male Rape

No one knows how common male rape is because men are less likely to report such assaults than women. However, in recent years, there have been more frequent reports of male rape by both other men and by women. Researchers estimate that the victims in about 10% of acquaintance rape cases are men. These "hidden victims" often keep silent because of embarrassment, shame, or humiliation and their own feelings and fears about homosexuality and conforming to conventional sex roles.

Although many people think that men who rape other men are always homosexuals, most male rapists consider themselves to be heterosexual. Young boys aren't the only victims. The average age of male rape victims is 24. Rape is a serious problem in prison, where men may experience brutal assaults by men who usually resume sexual relations with women once they're released.

What to Do in Case of Rape

If a woman has been raped, she will have to decide whether to report the attack to the police. Even an unsuccessful rape attempt should be reported because the information a woman provides about the attack—the assaulter's physical characteristics, voice, clothes, car, even an unusual smell—may prevent another woman from being raped. A woman shouldn't bathe or change her clothes before calling the police. Semen, hair, and material under her fingernails or on her apparel all may be useful in identifying the man who raped her. Many rape victims find it very helpful to contact a rape crisis center, where qualified staff members assist in dealing with the trauma. Many colleges, universities, and large urban communities in the United States have such programs. Friends and family members should remember that many women will mistakenly blame themselves

Strategies for Prevention

What to Do in Threatening Situations Involving Strangers

When a woman is approached by a man or men who may intend to rape her, she will have to decide what to do. Each situation, assailant, and woman is unique. There are no absolute rules, but the following can serve as guides:

✔ Run away if you can.

✔ Resist if you can't run. Make it difficult for the rapist. Many men, upon locating a potential victim, test her to see if she's easily intimidated. Shout, kick, create a scene, run away, fight back.

✔ Ordinary rules of behavior do not apply. Vomiting, screaming, or acting crazy—whatever you're willing to try—can be appropriate responses to an attempted rape.

✔ Stall to give yourself a chance to devise an escape plan or another strategy. Get the attacker to start talking ("What has happened to make you so angry?") or to negotiate ("Let's take time to talk about this").

✔ Remain alert for an opportunity to escape—for example, if a passerby approaches.

for the rape. However, the victim hasn't committed a crime—the man who raped her has.

Halting Sexual Violence: Prevention Efforts

Sexual violence has its roots in social attitudes and beliefs that demean women and condone aggression. As colleges and universities have become more aware of the different forms of sexual danger, many have taken the lead in setting up primary prevention programs (including newspaper articles; seminars in dormitories, fraternities, and sororities; and lectures) to help students examine their attitudes and values, understand cultural influences, and develop skills for avoiding or escaping from dangerous situations. All men and women should understand the impact of socialization on their willingness to tolerate or participate in sexual victimization, recognize misleading rape myths, and develop effective

Health Online

Rate Your Risk http://www.Nashville.Net/~police/risk/

This site, courtesy of the Nashville Police Department, will allow you to rate your chances of becoming a crime victim. There are detailed questionnaires that measure your risk of being raped, assaulted, murdered, or burglarized, including feedback on what your risk factors are and how you might change them.

Think about it ...

● According to these quizzes, are you at high risk for becoming a victim of a crime? If so, what steps could you take to lower your risk?

● Can you list five risk factors for violence that a person could change (e.g., varying their daily routine) and five that couldn't be easily changed (e.g., living in an urban area)?

● What special risks might college students face for becoming victims of crime?

ways of communicating to avoid misinterpretation of sexual cues. Students should also know where they can turn to learn more about and seek help for sexual victimization: counselors, campus police, deans of student

All-male workshops can generate discussion about gender roles, violence, and other societal ideas. These discussions may also provide positive pressure against rape and other forms of aggression against women.

affairs, fraternity or sorority representatives, campus ministers, and so on.

In addition, practical institutional steps—such as providing adequate lighting, escort services, and clear policies against both violence and drug and alcohol abuse—can help. Some campuses offer self-defense classes, which teach women how to avoid becoming victims either by escaping or protecting themselves. Individuals who advocate such training believe that it can strengthen women's physical capacities and encourage them to be less passive in encounters with potential victimizers.

Campuses are also providing "secondary prevention" by getting help to victims of sexual violence as soon as possible through rape crisis teams and emergency mental-health services. "Tertiary prevention" works with victims to ameliorate the long-term effects of their experience through psychotherapy, educational services, and medical care.

Making This Chapter Work for You
Staying Alive and Healthy

■ The most common causes of fatal accidents for Americans are motor-vehicle injuries. Using seat belts, practicing defensive driving, being extra cautious, and wearing a helmet when on a motorcycle or bicycle increase your odds of staying safe on the road.

- The risk of accidents is greatest in the home and at work. Falls are a common cause of injury, particularly for the elderly. Fires, another serious threat, can often be prevented by eliminating hazards, using caution with flammable materials, and knowing the proper way to use and maintain electrical appliances.

- Recreational safety demands common sense and proper planning. Anyone who exercises or spends a great deal of time outdoors should be aware of the early warning signs of problems related to temperature—whether they're caused by excess heat or extreme cold. Even strong swimmers are at risk of drowning, especially if they drink before diving into the water or ignore safety precautions.

- Many factors contribute to aggression and violence: biological causes, such as traumatic brain injury, certain medications, and the abuse of drugs or alcohol; developmental factors, such as harsh parental discipline, relations to peers, sex-role socialization, economic inequality, and lack of opportunity; exposure to violence in the media; the widespread availability of guns; and social factors, such as extreme poverty, deprivation, unemployment, prejudice, discrimination, involvement with gangs, and repeated exposure to actual violence.

- There has been a dramatic increase in crime on college and university campuses. Federal law requires disclosure of school crime statistics and security policies. Many campuses have set up safety programs, which include late-night shuttle buses and escorts, patrols, outdoor emergency phones, and increased numbers of guards.

- Physical violence may occur in 20% to 30% of all American households. Domestic violence is the single most common cause of injury to women—more common than car accidents, muggings, and rapes combined. Severe child abuse occurs an estimated 1.7 million times each year and claims the lives of as many as 5000 children.

- Sexual victimization refers to any situation in which a person is deprived of free choice and is forced to comply with sexual acts. At its root are false beliefs and callous attitudes that stem from myths about sexual conduct, acceptance of male aggression, trivialization of the impact of sexual misconduct, blame of the victim, and exposure to sexually violent material.

- Any unwanted sexual attention by a teacher, counselor, boss, coworker, or other authority figure constitutes sexual harassment and is illegal. The two basic forms are "quid pro quo" harassment, in which a person in power or authority makes unwanted sexual advances as a condition for receiving a job, a promotion, or another type of favor, and creation or tolerance of a "hostile or offensive environment," in which supervisors or coworkers engage in persistent inappropriate behaviors that make the workplace hostile, abusive, or otherwise unbearable.

- Sexual coercion (forced sexual activity) is common on college campuses. Both men and women report that they have performed sexual acts because of peer pressure, a desire for popularity, a threatened end to a relationship, intoxication, obligation, or unwanted physical stimulation.

- Rape refers to sexual intercourse with an unconsenting partner, who may be a stranger or an acquaintance, under actual or threatened force.

- Date or acquaintance rape, usually committed for the sake of sexual gratification, stems from the same factors that lead to other forms of sexual victimization, including male socialization into an aggressive role, widespread acceptance of rape myths, early sexual experiences (both forced and voluntary), the acceptance of sexual coercion, drinking, and gender differences in interpreting verbal and nonverbal sexual cues.

▶ Key Terms

The terms listed here are used within the chapter. Page numbers are included for each term.
A definition of each term is given in the green Glossary pages at the end of this book.

frostbite *275*	hostile or offensive	quid pro quo *280*
heat cramps *275*	environment *280*	rape *283*
heat exhaustion *275*	hypothermia *276*	repetitive motion injury
heat stress *275*	incest *279*	(RMI) *274*
heat stroke *275*	pedophilia *279*	sexual coercion *282*

Review Questions

1. What can you do to increase safety on the road, at home, outdoors, and at work?
2. What is sexual victimization? Why does it occur? What are the consequences?
3. What is sexual harassment? How can it be prevented or discouraged?

4. Describe the typical pattern of abuse. How does it apply to partners and to children?
5. What are the characteristics of date rape? What should a person do if she or he is raped? Where can someone who has been raped seek help?

 # Critical Thinking Questions

1. Can you name two risk factors in your daily life that might increase the likelihood of accidental injury? What actions have you taken to keep yourself safe? Are there any additional risk factors you haven't taken action to minimize or eliminate? What might you do about them?
2. A friend of yours, Eric, frequently makes crude or derogatory comments about women. When you finally call him on it, his response is, "I didn't say anything wrong. I like women." What might you say to him?

3. At one college, women raped by acquaintances or dates scrawled the names of their assailants on the walls of women's rest rooms on campus. Several young men whose names appeared on the list objected, protesting that they were innocent and were being unfairly accused. How do you feel about this method of fighting back against date rape? Do you think it violates the rights of men? How do you feel about naming in news reports women who've been raped?

 # Connections to Personal Health Interactive

*To enhance your understanding of the material covered in this chapter, check out the following study aids on the **Personal Health Interactive CD-ROM**.*

- Personal Insights: How Well Are You Protected?
- **Online Research:** Violence and Health
- Glossary & Key Term Review

 # References

1. Douglas, Kathy, et al. "Results from the 1995 National College Health Risk Behavior Survey." *Journal of American College Health*, Vol. 46, September 1997.
2. National Highway Traffic Safety Administration, American Academy of Pediatrics.
3. "Bicycle Helmets Policy." *Pediatrics*, April 1995.
4. National Safety Council.
5. National Safe Kids Campaign. "Skate Smart and Safeboard Safe." May 1995. "Skateboard Injuries." *Pediatrics*, April 1995.
6. National Safety Council.
7. Douglas, et al., "Results from the 1995 National College Health Risk Behavior Survey."
8. Butterfield, Fox. "Drop in Homicide Rate Linked to Crack's Decline." *New York Times*, October 27, 1997.
9. Bureau of Justice Statistics.
10. Yudofsky, Stuart, and Robert Hales. *Textbook of Neuropsychiatry*. 2nd ed. Washington, DC: American Psychiatric Press, 1994.
11. Kellerman, Arthur, et al. "Weapon Involvement in Home Invasion Crimes." *Journal of the American Medical Association*, Vol. 273, No. 22, June 14, 1995.
12. Marwick, Charles. "A Public Health Approach to Making Guns Safer." *Journal of the American Medical Association*, Vol. 273, No. 22, June 14, 1995. Sosin, Daniel, et al. "Trends in Death Associated with Traumatic Brain Injury, 1979 Through 1992." *Journal of the American Medical Association*, Vol. 273, No. 22, June 14, 1995.
13. Annest, Joseph, et al. "National Estimates of Nonfatal Firearm-Related Injuries." *Journal of the American Medical Association*, Vol. 273, No. 22, June 14, 1995.
14. McLarin, Kimberly. "Fear Prompts Self-Defense As Crime Comes to College." *New York Times*, September 7, 1994.
15. Kirtley, Jane. "Shedding Light on Campus Crime," *American Journalism Review*, Vol. 19, No. 6, July–August 1997.
16. Douglas, et al., "Results from the 1995 National College Health Risk Behavior Survey."

17. Lewin, Tamar. "Schools Are Moving to Police Students' Off-Campus Lives." *New York Times*, February 6, 1998.

18. Whitaker, Leighton, and Jeffrey Pollard. "Campus Violence: Kinds, Causes and Cures." *Journal of American College Health*, Vol. 43, No. 2, September 1994.

19. Hyman, Ariela, et al. "Laws Mandating Reporting of Domestic Violence." *Journal of the American Medical Association*, Vol. 273, No. 22, June 14, 1995. McAfee, Robert. "Physicians and Domestic Violence." *Journal of the American Medical Association*, Vol. 273, No. 22, June 14, 1995.

20. Correia, Felicia Collins. "Domestic Violence Can Be Cured." *USA Today* (*Magazine*), Vol. 126, No. 2630, November 1997.

21. Centerwall, Brandon. "Race, Socioeconomic Status, and Domestic Homicide." *Journal of the American Medical Association*, Vol. 273, No. 22, June 14, 1995.

22. Leidig, Marjorie Whittaker. "The Continuum of Violence Against Women: Psychological and Physical Consequences." *Journal of American College Health*, January 1992.

23. Berkowitz, Alan. "College Men As Perpetrators of Acquaintance Rape and Sexual Assault: A Review of Recent Research." *Journal of American College Health*, January 1992.

24. Fisher, Anne. "After All This Time, Why Don't People Know What Sexual Harassment Means?" *Fortune*, Vol. 137, No. 1, January 12, 1998.

25. Webb, Susan. Personal interview.

26. Crooks, Robert, and Carla Baur. *Human Sexuality*. 7th ed. Pacific Grove, CA: Brooks/Cole, 1999.

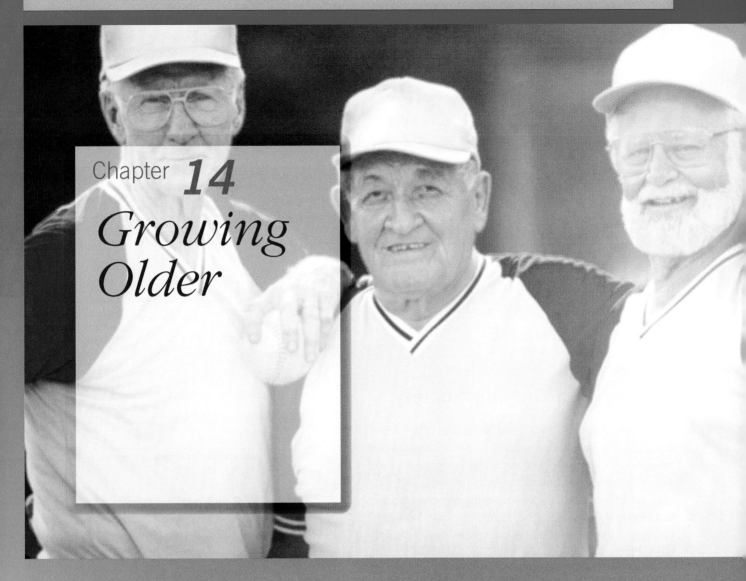

Chapter **14**

Growing Older

After studying the material in this chapter, you should be able to:

■ **Explain** the impact of aging on major body systems and on mental health.

■ **List** and **explain** major health-related problems faced by older people in our society.

■ **Define** death and **explain** the stages of emotional reaction experienced in facing death.

■ **Describe** the impact of death on the grieving survivors.

Although the process of aging is inevitable, you can do a great deal to influence the impact that the passage of time has on you. As a result of the preventive steps you take now, you can expand your "health span"—your years of health and vitality—as well as possibly expand your lifespan. This chapter gives you a preview of the changes age brings, the steps you can take to age healthfully, and ways to make the most of all the years of your life. We'll also explore the meaning of death and its effects on survivors.

Living in a Graying Society

In the last 100 years, the United States and other developed nations have experienced a greater increase in life expectancy than in all of recorded history prior to 1900. Today the elderly account for 13% of the American population.[1] The ranks of the elderly will grow even more in the next few decades, as the 75 million "baby boomers" conceived from 1946 to 1964 pass their sixty-fifth birthdays (Figure 14-1).

Regardless of your age, you will be affected by this "graying" of the American population. This is one reason why it's important to bridge the gap in understanding and information between younger and older Americans.

Strategies for Prevention

How to Live to Be 100 Years Old

The Committee for an Extended Lifespan, in San Marcos, California, collected information on 100 men and women who lived 100 years or more. Here's what they can teach us about how to survive for a century:

✔ *Do nothing in excess.* The centenarians who drink do so in moderation. Few are fat. They aren't given to binges of any kind.

✔ *Get up early.* The centenarians are early risers. Usually, this means they go to bed early, too.

✔ *Have faith in some higher power.* A high proportion have led what they consider a spiritual life.

✔ *Keep busy.* Few are dreamers or loungers. The majority attribute their long survival to hard work.

✔ *Take care of yourself.* Centenarians are as self-sufficient as possible.

A survey of 1200 men and women by the American Association of Retired Persons (AARP) revealed many misconceptions: 46% of respondents said that most older people could not adapt to change; 65% felt that most older people are lonely; 71% thought that one of every ten elderly Americans lives in an institution (the actual percentage, according to the AARP, is one in twenty).[2] Such negative assumptions may reflect **ageism**, a form

Figure 14-1

Tracking the baby-boom generation in the United States.

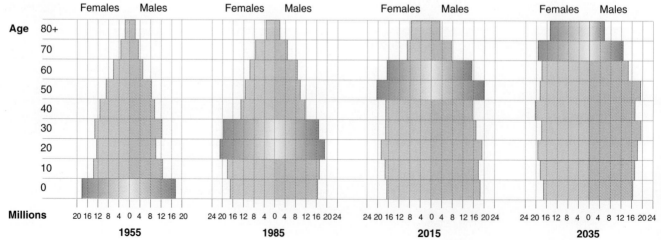

Sources: Population Reference Bureau and U.S. Census Bureau

of discrimination based on myths about aging and the elderly. As with other forms of discrimination, the best way to confront ageism is to seek accurate information, challenge stereotypes, and get involved in overcoming barriers to understanding.

As Time Goes By

For years, **gerontologists**—specialists in the interdisciplinary field that studies aging—viewed the process of getting older only in terms of deterioration, frailty, the grinding away of time. Today, instead of focusing on the minority of the elderly who go into a steady decline, they are studying the majority of men and women who remain vital and resilient in their later years. The term *optimal aging* refers to the new focus on ways to enhance the well-being and preserve the abilities of older people. Its goal is to enable people to live through old age with the best possible quality of life and the least possible premature disability.

The Impact of Age

From a purely physiological standpoint, the body's finest years come in youth, when lung capacity is greatest, grip is firmest, motor responses are quickest, and physical endurance is longest. After age 30, the body's powers gradually decline. Between the ages of 20 and 80, the percentage of body fat typically increases from 15% to 35% or 40% in men and from 20% to 40% in women.

After age 30, the heart's ability to pump blood decreases about 1% each year. At age 30, your heart pumps 3.6 quarts of blood per minute, but at age 70, only 2.6 quarts per minute. Blood pressure rises; circulation slows. These changes simply mean that the average 70-year-old can't compete with a 30-year-old in wrestling or running, but has sufficient energy and stamina for day-to-day functioning (see Figure 14-2).

Figure 14-2

The effects of aging on the body.

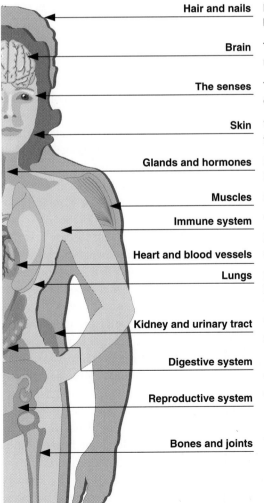

Hair and nails	Hair often turns gray and thins out. Men may go bald. Fingernails can thicken.
Brain	The brain shrinks, but it is not known if that affects mental functions.
The senses	The sensitiviy of hearing, sight, taste, and smell can all decline with age.
Skin	Wrinkles occur as the skin thins and the underlying fat shrinks, and age spots often crop up.
Glands and hormones	Levels of many hormones drop, or the body becomes less responsive to them.
Muscles	Strength usually peaks in the twenties, then declines.
Immune system	The body becomes less able to resist some pathogens.
Heart and blood vessels	Cardiovascular problems become more common.
Lungs	It doesn't just seem harder to climb those stairs; lung capacity drops.
Kidney and urinary tract	The kidneys become less efficient. The bladder can't hold as much, so urination is more frequent.
Digestive system	Digestion slows down as the secretion of digestive enzymes decreases.
Reproductive system	Women go through menopause, and testosterone levels drop for men.
Bones and joints	Wear and tear can lead to arthritic joints, and osteoporosis is common, especially in women.

Aerobic capacity—the amount of oxygen the body can use and the best measure of ability to do work—declines with age. By age 75, a man's aerobic capacity is less than half what it was at age 17; a woman's is about one-third what it was in her twenties.

Strength also diminishes slowly. Between the ages of 30 and 70, muscle strength declines about 12% to 15%, and the speed of muscle contraction and coordination drops 25%. Each decade after age 25, men and women lose 3% to 5% of their muscle mass, which often is replaced by fatty tissue.

As you get older, bones lose minerals and become softer and shorter. Your muscles weaken and your back slumps. The disks between the bones of the spine also deteriorate, moving those bones closer together. As a result, after 30, both men and women shrink by as much as half an inch in total height with each decade. Basal metabolism—the fundamental chemical process of living—slows down because the aging body requires less upkeep. The rate at which the body turns food into energy declines about 3% every 10 years.[3]

As we age, the brain becomes smaller, but mental abilities do not diminish. Aging nerve cells, however, result in slower reaction times and slower movement, and we process information more slowly. A grandfather playing a video game with his 14-year-old grandson will lose every time. However, on tests that involve real-life experience and acquired knowledge, he has the edge.

How Men and Women Age

People of both genders go through numerous physiological changes at midlife. Men experience a decrease in the level of the male sex hormone testosterone, leading to a slowing of the sexual response. Changes in the prostate gland also cause increased urinary urgency, particularly at night (the condition may be alleviated with foods rich in zinc, such as whole grains and milk); the risk of developing prostate cancer grows.

For women, the changes at midlife, especially physical ones, can be even more profound. The period from the mid-forties through the mid-sixties is called the *climacteric;* its most obvious change is the onset of *menopause,* the end of ovulation and menstruation.

An estimated 10% to 15% of women sail through menopause without any significant complaints. At the other end of the spectrum, a similar percentage develop symptoms that make it difficult, if not impossible, for them to function as usual. The majority of women—70% to 80%—are somewhere in between. Most can take advantage of new insight into the processes involved in menopause and new approaches to relieving its symptoms.

The most serious health hazard associated with menopause is an increased risk of heart disease. Throughout a woman's reproductive years, estrogen keeps her arteries supple, prevents blood clots, boosts levels of beneficial high-density lipoproteins (HDL), and decreases harmful low-density lipoproteins (LDL). As estrogen falls at menopause, a woman's heart becomes as vulnerable as a man's. Her HDL slumps; her LDL increases; her risk of blood clots grows; atherosclerotic plaque builds up in her arteries. After age 45, one in nine women has a least one symptom of heart disease. By 65, this figure rises to one in three.

Also at risk are a woman's bones. Although the process of bone loss begins in a woman's thirties, it speeds up to as much at 2% to 5% annually in the first 5 years after menopause. Women with small bones, smokers, and those with a family history of bone problems are at increased risk of fractures and the bone-thinning disease known as osteoporosis, which strikes more than a third of older women (discussed later in this chapter).

Hormone replacement therapy (HRT) is synthetic estrogen, often combined with progesterone, which is given in the form of a pill or a patch to postmenopausal women. It often relieves symptoms of menopause and provides health benefits. The most compelling reason to take replacement hormones is to protect the heart. "Regardless of when a postmenopausal woman starts HRT or for how long she takes it, there is an association with lower incidence of coronary artery disease," says Marianne Legato, M.D., the director of the Partnership for Women's Health at Columbia University. "If a woman has coronary artery disease, HRT may extend her lifespan by 2½ years. If she doesn't have heart disease, estrogen won't prolong her life, but it will lower her risk of developing cardiovascular problems."[4] HRT also protects a woman's bones. However, the benefits last only as long as the woman takes estrogen, and doctors are still debating whether it's best to start HRT immediately after menopause or later in life.

In addition to these long-term benefits, replacement estrogen relieves hot flashes, improves sleep, alleviates sexual symptoms, makes intercourse more comfortable, and lessens urinary tract problems. Women on HRT report that they think better, remember more, and feel more energetic. They're less prone to many age-related problems, such as tooth loss and driving accidents (possibly a consequence of improved concentration). They also live longer. Compared with women who never used replacement hormones, women who take HRT are less likely to die of what researchers call "all-cause mortality" (that is, for any and every reason). In one analysis of 40,000 postmenopausal women followed for 16 years, the risk of death in those taking estrogen was 37% lower than those who had never taken HRT. The risk of fatal heart disease was 53% lower.[5]

The number-one reason women are wary of HRT is the risk of breast cancer. Although there have been contradictory findings, breast cancer rates generally increase among women who take replacement hormones for prolonged periods. (In various studies, these have extended for 5, 7, or 10 or more years.)[6] Based on this evidence, physicians may advise against HRT for women who've had breast cancer or who are at high risk for this disease. But for other women, the potential benefits of HRT may outweigh the dangers. Even among those at high risk of breast cancer, the presence of even one risk factor for heart disease tips the balance in favor of HRT.[7] "Women are ten times more likely to die of heart disease than breast cancer," notes Legato. "For many, the risks of not taking HRT are far greater than its use."

Good News About Getting Older

The key to staying vital and healthy in old age is maintaining healthful behaviors throughout life. As many as half of the losses linked to age may be the result not of time's passage but of disuse. "If you don't use it, you lose it," says Dr. James Fries, a Stanford University professor who's done extensive research on aging.

Heredity's Role

Genes aren't destiny, but they have a continuing impact throughout the lifespan. Yet even individuals with genes that contribute to fast aging can modify their impact. What you do to stop the genes that speed up aging is less important than what you do to cooperate with the genes that slow it down. (See Pulsepoints: "Ten Ways to Live Longer.")

Exercise: An Antiaging Pill

Staying in bed for 3 weeks has the same effect on fitness as aging 30 years. At any age, the unexercised body—though free of the symptoms of illness—will rust out long before it could ever wear out. Inactivity can make anyone old before his or her time. Just as inactivity accelerates aging, activity slows it down. The effects of ongoing activity are so profound that gerontologists sometimes refer to exercise as "the closest thing to an antiaging pill." Exercise can reverse many of the changes that occur with age, including increases in body fat and decreases in muscle strength. The bottom line: What you *don't* do may matter more than what you do do.

Pulsepoints

Ten Ways to Live Longer

1. Exercise regularly. By improving blood flow, staving off depression, warding off heart disease, and enhancing well-being, regular workouts help keep mind and body in top form.

2. Don't smoke. Every cigarette you puff can snuff out 7 minutes of your life, according to the Centers for Disease Control and Prevention.

3. Watch your weight and blood pressure. Increases in these vital statistics can increase your risk of hypertension, cardiovascular disease, and other health problems.

4. Eat more fruits and vegetables. These foods, rich in vitamins and protective antioxidants, can reduce your risk of cancer and damage from destructive free radicals.

5. Cut down on fat. Fatty foods can clog the arteries and contribute to various cancers.

6. Limit drinking. Alcohol can undermine physical health and sabotage mental acuity.

7. Cultivate stimulating interests. Elderly individuals with complex and interesting lifestyles are most likely to retain sharp minds and memories beyond age 70.

8. Don't worry; be happy. At any age, emotional turmoil can undermine well-being. Relaxation techniques, such as meditation, help by reducing stress.

9. Reach out. Try to keep in contact with other people of all ages and experiences. Make the effort to invite them to your home or go out with them. On a regular basis, do something to help another person.

10. Make the most of your time. Greet each day with a specific goal—to take a walk, write letters, visit a friend.

The Aging Brain

Mental ability does not decline along with physical vigor. Researchers have been able to reverse the supposedly normal intellectual declines of 60 to 80 year olds by tutoring them in problem solving. Reaction time, intellectual speed and efficiency, nonverbal intelligence, and maximum work rate for short periods may diminish by age 75. However, understanding, vocabulary, ability to remember key information, and verbal intelligence remain about the same.

Mental Health

Optimal aging demands a redefinition of who a person is and what makes his or her life worthwhile. Some sources of satisfaction, such as physical challenges or professional achievements, diminish later in life. Yet older people in general feel psychologically better than young people, with fewer worries about themselves and how they look to other people, higher self-esteem, and less loneliness.[8]

The secret of emotional well-being in old age doesn't seem to be professional success or a happy marriage but the ability to cope with life's setbacks without blame or bitterness. In general, psychiatric disorders do not occur more frequently in the elderly. Even depression—which is not uncommon among the elderly—strikes less often in old age than at earlier stages of the life cycle. Those most likely to become depressed often have lost a spouse and have few social supports. The social ties of the elderly are most likely to fray as they retire, move, or lose spouses and close friends.[9]

Intimacy and Sexual Activity

Sexual activity typically decreases in the elderly, but it doesn't end. According to a 1995 national survey by Mark Clements Research, Inc., about 55% of those between ages 65 and 69 remain sexually active. This percentage declines with age—to 48% of those between 70 and 74, 28% of those 75 to 79, 21% of those 80 to 84, and 13% of those over age 85.[10]

Aging does cause some changes in sexual response: Women produce less vaginal lubrication, and it takes longer for an older man to achieve an erection or orgasm and longer to attain another erection after ejaculating. Both men and women experience fewer contractions during orgasm. However, none of these changes reduces sexual pleasure or desire.

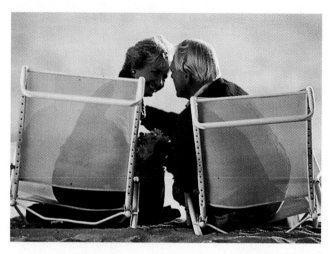

Many senior citizens remain sexually active. Affection and sexual intimacy may increase as the pressures of child-raising and careers ease.

Problems of the Elderly

Sadly, life's final decades aren't always golden. Senior citizens may face physical, economic, social, and psychological challenges during what one therapist describes as "the season of loss." They may have to give up many things: gratifying work, cherished friendships, financial and physical independence. Millions are economically vulnerable: A serious illness, the loss of their home in a fire or flood, or other unexpected catastrophes could easily plunge them into poverty. A lack of money limits the options of the elderly and can impair their health. They may not be able to afford nutritious food, regular health checkups, new eyeglasses or hearing aids, or the small pleasures that make life enjoyable. The cumulative impact of such challenges, one often following the other before individuals have a chance to adjust or cope, can take a toll on physical and emotional well-being.

Physical Problems

With the passage of time, many people develop serious diseases such as arthritis, atherosclerosis, and cancer. In the past, elderly men and women often were not treated as aggressively for some conditions, such as cancer, as younger patients. But research has shown that older patients can respond well to aggressive therapeutic approaches and benefit just as much as younger individuals.[11]

Nutritional Needs

Among the elderly, nutritional deficiencies are a serious problem; being underweight can be as great a health risk as being overweight. About 16% of Americans over age 65 consume fewer than 1000 calories a day—too little to provide an adequate supply of vitamins and minerals. Common causes of malnutrition in old age include medications, emotional depression, loss of teeth, swallowing and absorption disorders, lack of money, and difficulties shopping and preparing food. Many nutritionists recommend multivitamin and mineral supplements for the elderly, although they caution against overdosing or taking any single vitamin or mineral without medical supervision.

Osteoporosis

One common problem, especially among elderly women, is **osteoporosis**, a condition in which losses in bone density become so severe that a bone will break after even slight trauma or injury (see Figure 14-3). Among those who live to age 90, 32% of women and 19% of men will suffer a hip fracture as a result of osteoporosis.[12] Women, who have smaller skeletons, are more vulnerable than men; in extreme cases, their spines may become so fragile that just bending causes severe pain.

Osteoporosis doesn't begin in old age. In fact, the best time for preventive action is early in life. Increased calcium intake, particularly during childhood and the growth spurt of adolescence, can produce a heavier, denser skeleton and reduce the risk of the complications of bone loss later in life. College-age women also can strengthen their bones and reduce their risk of osteoporosis by increasing their calcium intake and physical activity. Adequate dietary calcium in adulthood can help maintain bone density for years.

Various factors can increase a woman's risk of developing osteoporosis, including family history (a mother, grandmother, or sister with osteoporosis, fractures, height loss, or humped shoulders); petite body structure; white or Asian background; menopause before age 40; smoking; heavy alcohol consumption; loss of ovarian function through chemotherapy, radiation, or hysterectomy; low calcium intake; and a sedentary lifestyle.

Substance Misuse and Abuse

Misuse and abuse of prescription and over-the-counter medications occur frequently among the elderly. In part this is because people over age 65 consume one-quarter of all drugs prescribed in the United States. Moreover, many older people have multiple health problems, requiring several medications at the same time. The drugs may interact and cause a confusing array of symptoms and reactions.

Alcohol abuse can be particularly harmful for older men and women because it increases the likelihood of malnutrition, liver disease, heart damage, digestive problems, cognitive impairment, and dementia. Depending on the severity of the problem, older individuals may require close supervision in a hospital during withdrawal.

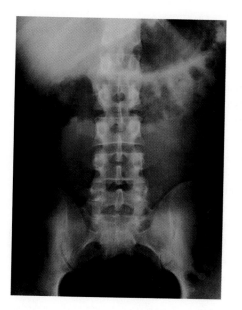
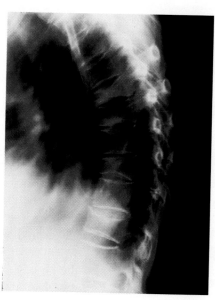

Figure 14-3

Comparison of a normal backbone (left) to one with osteoporosis (right).

Psychological Problems

As men and women end their careers, and as friends and loved ones become ill or die, loneliness can become a chronic problem. Women, who generally outlive their husbands, are most likely to find themselves living alone. Whereas seven out of ten men age 75 or older are still married and living with their spouses, seven out of ten women in that age group are widowed. "We have our children and grandchildren and friends," says one woman in her eighties who lives in an apartment complex for elderly widows. "But we do miss our men."

Depression

According to a report by the National Institutes of Health Consensus Development Panel on Depression in Later Life, about 15% of men and women over 65 living in the community experience depression. In nursing homes, the rate is higher: 15% to 25%. Moreover, recurrences are common, with 40% of older persons suffering repeat bouts with depression.[13]

Late-life depression can be particularly hard to spot because older men and women often do not display the typical symptoms, or their symptoms are mistaken for normal signs of aging.[14] Elderly people with physical problems are most prone to depression. Some classic signs of depression—appetite changes, a gain or loss of 5% of body weight in a month, insomnia or excessive sleep, fidgeting or extremely slow movements or speech, fatigue, or loss of energy—may be attributed to

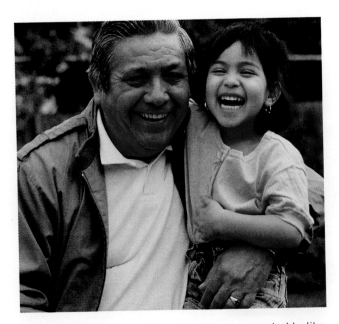

Family ties are extremely important to young and old alike.

medical problems, medications, or old age itself. Depression that develops following an illness or injury, if not identified and treated, can hinder recovery.

The consequences of not recognizing and treating depression late in life can be tragic. Older Americans have the highest suicide rates in our society, with some 8500 elderly persons killing themselves every year. The suicide rate is five times higher for those aged 65 or older than for younger individuals. And depressed older men and women are also more likely to die of other causes. However, late-life depression can be overcome. With treatment, more than 70% of the depressed elderly improve dramatically.

Mental Deterioration

About 15% of older Americans lose previous mental capabilities, a brain disorder called **dementia**. Sixty percent of these—a total of 4 million men and women over age 65—suffer from the type of dementia called **Alzheimer's disease**, a progressive deterioration of brain cells and mental capacity.

Women are more likely to develop Alzheimer's than men. By age 85, as many as 28% to 30% of women suffer from Alzheimer's, and women with this form of dementia perform significantly worse than men in various visual, spatial, and memory tests. Estrogen replacement—despite the risks and concerns discussed earlier—may help keep women's brains healthy as they age, particularly for those at high genetic risk for Alzheimer's. In various studies of postmenopausal women, those taking replacement hormones were up to 40% less likely to develop Alzheimer's. And women who do develop Alzheimer's show less mental deterioration if they are taking estrogen.[15]

Often the illness progresses slowly, stealing bits of a person's mind and memory a little at a time. Its victims may withdraw into a world of their own, become quarrelsome or irritable, and say or do inappropriate things. The personalities of individuals with Alzheimer's often change. Some become more stubborn or impulsive; others may become increasingly apathetic, withdrawn, irritable, or suspicious, accusing others of thefts, betrayal, or plotting against them. As cognitive impairment worsens, inhibitions often loosen; they may masturbate or take off their clothes in public. Some become aggressive or violent. Eventually, individuals may forget the names of their close relatives, their own occupations, occasionally even their own names.[16]

Even though no one can restore a brain that is in the process of being destroyed by an organic brain disease like Alzheimer's, medications can control difficult behavioral symptoms and enhance or partially restore cognitive ability. Often physicians find other medical or psychiatric problems, such as depression, in these patients; recognizing and treating these conditions can have a dramatic impact. Most people with Alzheimer's do best in consistent, familiar surroundings, with daily routines, prominently displayed clocks and calendars, nightlights, checklists, and diaries.

Nursing Homes

Many older people need help from another person in performing some daily living activity, such as dressing, walking, bathing, or shopping. In the past, aging parents tended to live with their children's families. That's changed dramatically—not only because children live farther away, or may be separated or divorced, but also because the older parents seem to prefer their independence. Problems can develop, however, when declining health or increasing disability makes it more difficult for the elderly to manage on their own. Home-care services, day care, and foster homes help growing numbers of the elderly by filling the gap between living at home and entering a nursing home.

More than 1.5 million elderly Americans currently live in nursing homes, and their numbers are certain to grow in the coming decades. But such care is expensive and can be substandard, if not abusive. Families of elderly patients mistreated in nursing homes have successfully sued the homes, not for acts that led to death or disability, but for neglect, such as leaving residents in a smelly room or not bathing them or verbal abuse.[17]

Understanding the Meaning of Death

In our society, death isn't a part of everyday life, as it once was. Because machines can now keep alive people who, in the past, would have died, the definition of death has become more complex. Death has been broken down into the following categories:

- *Functional death*. The end of all vital functions, such as heartbeat and respiration.

- *Cellular death*. The gradual death of body cells after the heart stops beating. If placed in a tissue culture or, as is the case with various organs, transplanted to another body, some cells can remain alive indefinitely.

- *Cardiac death*. The moment when the heart stops beating.

- *Brain death*. The end of all brain activity, indicated by an absence of electrical activity (confirmed by an *electroencephalogram,* or *EEG*) and a lack of reflexes.

- *Spiritual death*. The moment when the soul, as defined by many religions, leaves the body.

Emotional Responses to Death

Elisabeth Kübler-Ross has identified five typical stages of reaction that a person goes through when facing death:

1. *Denial ("No, not me")*. At first knowledge that death is coming, a terminally ill patient rejects the news. The denial overcomes the initial shock and allows the person to begin to gather together his or her resources. Denial, at this point, is a healthy defense mechanism. It can become distressful, however, if it's reinforced by the relatives and friends of the dying patient.

2. *Anger ("Why me?")*. In the second stage, the dying person begins to feel resentment and rage regarding imminent death. The anger may be directed at God or at the patient's family and caregivers, who can do little but try to endure any expressions of anger, provide comfort, and help the patient on to the next stage.

3. *Bargaining ("Yes, me, but...")*. In this stage, a patient may try to bargain, usually with God, for a way to reverse, or at least postpone, dying. The patient may promise, in exchange for recovery, to do good works or to see family members more often. Alternatively, the patient may say, "Let me live long enough to see my grandchild born" or "to see the spring again."

4. *Depression ("Yes, it's me")*. In the fourth stage, the patient gradually realizes the full consequences of his or her condition. This may begin as grieving for health that has been lost and then become anticipatory grieving for the loss that is to come of friends, loved ones, and life itself. This is perhaps the most difficult time: The dying person should not be left alone during this period. Neither should one try to cheer the patient, however, who must be allowed to grieve.

5. *Acceptance ("Yes, me; and I'm ready")*. In this last stage, the person has accepted the reality of death: The moment looms as neither frightening nor painful, neither sad nor happy—only inevitable. The person who waits for the end of life may ask to see fewer visitors, to separate from other people, or perhaps to turn to just one person for support.

Several stages may occur at the same time and some may happen out of sequence. Each stage may take days

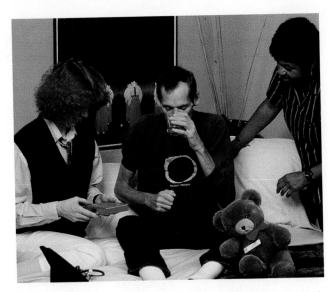

Humanitarian caregiving for both critically ill patients and their loved ones can help take some of the fear out of death.

or only hours or minutes. Throughout, denial may come back to assert itself unexpectedly—and hope for a medical breakthrough or a miraculous recovery is forever present.

Some experts dispute Kübler-Ross's basic five-stage theory as too simplistic and argue that not all people go through such well-defined stages in the dying process. The way a person faces death is often a mirror of the way he or she has faced other major stresses in life: Those who have had the most trouble adjusting to other crises will have the most trouble adjusting to the news of their impending death.

Ethical Dilemmas

Modern medicine can do more to delay or defeat death than was once thought possible. However, the ability to sustain life in patients with no hope of recovery has created wrenching medical and moral dilemmas. Increasingly, lawyers, ethicists, and consumer advocates are arguing that health-care providers must recognize a fundamental right of patients: the right to die.

Health economists, noting that more than half of U.S. health-care dollars are spent in the last year of life, have questioned "heroic" measures to prolong the life of chronically ill elderly patients or those with fatal diseases. Policies on such aggressive measures vary from hospital to hospital and state to state. Some health-care facilities require that staff members try to resuscitate any patient whose heart stops unless a do-not-resuscitate (DNR) order has been written, usually with the

family's permission. In other cases, physicians may decide against resuscitation despite the family's wishes if they think that treatment would be futile and that the family's objections are not based on the patient's values or best interests. However, the wishes of dying patients often go unheeded. Even when patients have specified that they do not want high-tech treatments or life support, physicians may continue to order such care.[18]

Preparing for Death

Throughout this book we have stressed the ways in which you can determine how well and how long you live. You can also make decisions about the end of your life, particularly its impact on other people.

Advance Directives and Living Wills

Every state and the District of Columbia have laws authorizing the use of **advance directives** to specify the kind of medical treatment individuals want in case of a medical crisis. However, only 4% to 24% of the people in America have any type of advance directive. These documents are important because, without clear indications of a person's preferences, hospitals and other institutions often make decisions on an individual's behalf, particularly if family members are not available or disagree.[19]

A *health-care proxy* is an advance directive that gives someone else the power to make decisions on your behalf. People typically name a relative or close friend as their agent. Let family and friends know your thoughts about treatments and life-support. You also should let your primary physician know about the type of care you would or wouldn't want to receive in various circumstances, such as an accident that results in an irreversible coma, but you should not designate your doctor as your agent. Many states prohibit this. Even when allowed, it is not a good idea because your doctor's primary responsibility is to administer care.

Living wills aren't just for people who don't want to be kept alive by artificial means. Individuals can also use these advance directives to indicate that they want all possible medical treatments and technology used to prolong their lives. Most states recognize living wills as legally binding, and a growing number of health-care professionals and facilities are offering patients help in drafting living wills. You can obtain state-specific forms

UNIFORM DONOR CARD

OF _____

Print or type name of donor

In the hope that I may help others, I hereby make this anatomical gift, if medically acceptable, to take effect upon my death. The words and marks below indicate my desires.

I give   (a) ___ any needed organs or parts

I give   (b) ___ only the following organs or parts

_____

Specifiy the organ(s) or part(s)

for the purposes of transplantation, therapy, medical research, or education:

I give   (c) ___ my body for anatomical study if needed

Limitations or
special wishes. if any _____

Figure 14-4

Example of a uniform donor card.

for living wills and health-care proxies free from an organization called Choice in Dying (1-800-989-WILL). Computer software for preparing such documents also is available.

The Gift of Life

If you're at least 18 years old, you can fill out a donor card (see Figure 14-4), agreeing to designate, in the event of your death, any organs or tissues needed for transplantation. Corneas may help a blind person see, for example. Kidneys, or even a heart, may be transplanted. The donation takes effect upon your death and is a generous way of giving others the possibilities for life that you have had yourself. The card should be filled out and signed; some must be signed in the presence of two witnesses. Attach the donor card to the back of your driver's license or I.D. card. (Whole-body donations may require other arrangements.)

Funeral Arrangements

Memorial societies are voluntary groups that help people plan in advance for death. They obtain services at moderate cost, keep the arrangements simple and dignified, and—most important, perhaps—ease the emotional and financial burden on the rest of the family when death finally does come.

A body can be either buried or cremated. Burial requires the purchase of a cemetery plot, which many families do decades before death. If the body is to be cremated, you must comply with some additional formalities, with which the funeral director can help you.

After a cremation (incineration of the remains), you can either collect the ashes to keep, bury, or scatter yourself, or ask the crematorium to dispose of them.

The tradition of a funeral may help survivors come to terms with the death, enabling them both to mourn their loss and to celebrate the dead person's life. Alternatively, the body may be disposed of immediately, through burial, cremation, or bequeathal to a medical school, and a memorial service held later.

Funerals are usually held 2 to 4 days after the death. Many have two parts: a religious ceremony at a church or funeral home and a burial ceremony at the grave site. In a memorial service, the body is not present, which may change the focus of the service from the person's death to his or her life.

Grief

An estimated 8 million Americans lose a member of their immediate families each year. The death of a loved one may be the single most upsetting and feared event in a person's life.

The death of a family member produces a wide range of reactions, including anxiety, guilt, anger, and financial concern. Many see the death of an old person as less tragic (usually) than the death of a child or young person. A sudden death is more of a shock than one following a long illness. A suicide can be particularly devastating, because family members may wonder whether they could have done anything to prevent it. The cause of death can also affect the reactions of friends and acquaintances.

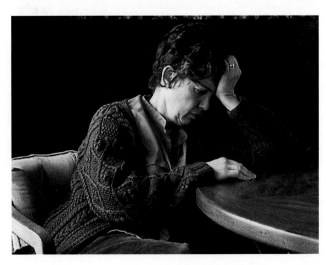

Grief can take an enormous physical and psychological toll on family members and loved ones.

Some people express less sympathy and support when individuals are murdered or take their own lives.

All grieving people continue to need support for many months. The anniversary of a death or the first several holidays spent alone can be particularly difficult. (See Pulsepoints: "Ten Ways to Cope with Grief.") For individuals who remain intensely distressed, or whose grief does not ease over time, therapy and medication may be enormously helpful—and potentially life-saving. Grieving parents, partners, or adult children are at increased risk of serious physical and mental illness, suicide, and premature death. The family members of a suicide victim are especially likely to need, and benefit from, professional help in sorting out their feelings of failure, anger, and sorrow.

The Effects of Grief

Men and women who lose partners, parents, or children endure so much stress that they're at increased risk of serious physical and mental illness, and even of premature death. Studies of the health effects of grief have found the following:

- Grief produces changes in the respiratory, hormonal, and central nervous systems and may affect functions of the heart, blood, and immune systems.

- Grieving adults may experience mood swings between sadness and anger, guilt and anxiety. They may feel physically sick, lose their appetites, sleep poorly, or fear that they're going crazy because they "see" the deceased person in different places.

- Friends and remarriage offer the greatest protection against health problems.

- Some widows may have increased rates of depression, suicide, and death from cirrhosis of the liver. The greatest risk factors are poor previous mental and physical health and a lack of social support.[20]

Grief is a psychological necessity, not self-indulgence. Psychotherapists refer to grief as work, and it is—slow, tedious, and painful. Yet only by working through grief, by dealing with feelings of anger and despair, and adjusting emotionally and intellectually to the loss can bereaved individuals make their way back to the living world of hope and love.[21]

Helping Survivors

Although we grieve for the dead, the living are the ones who need our help. Bereavement is such an intense state that survivors may be too numb or too stunned to ask for help. Family and friends must take the initiative and spend time with them, even if that means sitting together silently. Offer empathy and support, and let the grieving person know with verbal and nonverbal expressions that you care and wish to help. Simply being there is enough to let your friend know you care.

Pulsepoints Ten Ways to Cope with Grief

1. Accept your feelings—sorrow, fear, emptiness, whatever—as normal.

2. Don't try to deny emotions such as anger, guilt, despair, or relief.

3. Let others help you—by bringing you food, by taking care of daily necessities, by providing companionship and comfort. (It will make them feel better, too.)

4. Express your feelings—through tears, recollections, and talking with others—so that you can accept the loss.

5. Don't feel that you must be strong and brave and silent, though you have every right to keep your grief private.

6. Face each day as it comes. Let yourself live in the here-and-now until you're ready to face the future.

7. Give yourself time—perhaps more than you ever imagined—for the pain to ebb, the scars to heal, and your life to move on.

8. Commemorate. A funeral or memorial service can help you come to terms with a loved one's death and provides an opportunity to celebrate the dead person's life.

9. Don't think there's a right or wrong way to grieve. Mourning takes many forms, and there's no set timetable for working through the various stages of grief.

10. Seek professional counseling if you remain intensely distressed for more than 6 months or your grief does not ease over time. Therapy can be enormously helpful—and can help prevent potentially serious physical and psychological problems.

You may also wish to write a simple note expressing your sympathy. A phrase, such as "I want to let you know I'm thinking of you and praying for you," can mean a great deal. A small gift, such as a book or plant, is also thoughtful. Or you can invite your friend to do something with you. Choose something you know your friend might enjoy—a walk in the country or a concert. And don't just give your help over the first few days or weeks and then withdraw. Grieving people continue to need support for many months. The first anniversary of a death or the first holiday spent alone can be particularly difficult.

Most bereaved people don't need professional psychological counseling. In most instances, sharing their feelings with friends is all that's needed. However, you should urge a friend or relative to seek help if he or she shows no sign of grieving or exhibits as much distress a year after the loss as during the first months. The family members of a suicide victim are those most likely to need, and benefit from, professional help in sorting out their feelings of failure, anger, and sorrow.

Making This Chapter Work for You
Growing Older

■ Life expectancies for Americans are growing. Although the process of aging is inevitable, individuals can do a great deal to influence the impact of the passage of time.

■ Whether or not we can add years to our lives, we can add life to our years. The key to optimal aging—living through old age with the best possible quality of life and the least possible premature disability—is maintaining good health habits throughout life.

■ Many of the physical changes that accompany aging—such as the decline in heart and lung functioning, slowing of circulation and metabolism, loss of muscular strength, and slowing of reaction time—can be delayed by regular exercise and a nutritious diet.

■ Most intellectual abilities don't diminish with age, although some, such as the ability to remember names and newly learned information, do decline. Sexual interest need not fade with age, although sexual activity may decrease.

■ The elderly face physical and psychological challenges, including a greater likelihood of illness and disability. Osteoporosis, a major health problem for elderly people, can be prevented by exercise and increased calcium intake. Depression, which is not uncommon in the elderly, responds well to treatment.

■ One of the greatest fears about aging is that we will lose our memories and our minds. Diminished mental capacity can be the result of any of a number of physical disorders, including Alzheimer's disease, a progressive condition in which the mind slowly deteriorates Although there are no cures for

Health Online

Family Caregiver Alliance http://www.caregiver.org/

This site provides information and support to those who care for older family members or friends. It includes information on finding in-home help, selecting an assisted living or residential care facility, respite resources, balancing work, family, and caregiving, medical information, online support, and much more.

Think about it ...

• Have you or your parents ever been called on to help care for an older person? What kinds of decisions were involved? What was the impact of caregiving on your family?

• What kinds of decisions could you or your parents make now that will make growing older easier on your family?

• If you are called on to help care for an older relative, what resources do you have to help you? Consider friends and family and community, government, financial, and technological resources. What personal qualities do you have that you could bring to the situation?

this form of dementia, treatments can sometimes relieve symptoms and enhance mental abilities.

■ There are a variety of ways to define death. But while death itself is an end, dying can be a long, complicated process.

■ Individuals with fatal illnesses may go through various emotional stages: denial, anger, bargaining, depression, and acceptance.

■ The ability to sustain life by artificial means has created agonizing dilemmas for health-care professionals and families. The courts have upheld an individual's right to refuse treatment and have allowed patients with no hope of recovery to be removed from ventilators and feeding tubes.

■ You can assure that your wishes concerning heroic treatments are heeded by several means, including advance directives, such as health-care proxies and living wills.

■ People over 18 years of age can designate that, in the event of their death, their organs be donated to others.

■ When a loved one dies, individuals must deal with many practical matters, including funeral and burial or cremation arrangements.

■ Grief encompasses many feelings, including sadness, anger, guilt, despair, confusion, relief, and fear, and has a profound effect on the body. Individuals mourn in different ways.

Key Terms

The terms listed here are used within the chapter. Page numbers are included for each term. A definition of each term is given in the green Glossary pages at the end of this book.

advance directives *298*
ageism *290*
Alzheimer's disease *296*
dementia *296*

gerontologists *291*
hormone replacement therapy (HRT) *292*
living wills *298*

osteoporosis *295*

Review Questions

1. What kinds of physical changes take place as you age?
2. What are some health problems faced by the elderly? How can these problems be alleviated or prevented?
3. What are the effects of aging on mental faculties? What can be done to lower the chances of mental decline with age?

4. How is death defined?
5. What are the five stages of a person's emotional reaction to a terminal illness, as described by Elisabeth Kübler-Ross?
6. How does death affect the survivor? Can you name some strategies for dealing with grief?

Critical Thinking Questions

1. If you had to choose between an extremely long life and an extremely satisfying or happy one, which would you choose? What can you do now to ensure that you will live as long or as well as you'd like?
2. For years, your parents fed, sheltered, clothed, and nurtured you. Someday, they may need this care from you as much as you once needed it from them. Think ahead to the time when your parents will be 75, 85, or even older. What if they need

constant care? What would be your responsibility? What options will you have? Can you do anything now to prepare for your parents' later years?

3. Do you think that coming to terms with mortality allows an individual to live each day to its fullest, rather than putting off what he or she would like to do until tomorrow? How does this concept affect your own life? Explain. Do you believe in a next life or a greater reality? If so, how does this affect your view of life and death?

Connections to Personal Health Interactive

To enhance your understanding of the material covered in this chapter, check out the following study aids on the **Personal Health Interactive CD-ROM**.

- Personal Insights: How Do You Feel About Death?
- Personal Insights: How Long Do You Think You Are Going to Live?

- U.S. Population Patterns
- Glossary & Key Term Review

References

1. Steel, Knight. "Research on Aging: An Agenda for All Nations Individually and Collectively." *Journal of the American Medical Association,* Vol. 278, No. 16, October 22/29, 1997.
2. Stock, Robert. "Senior Class." *New York Times,* June 1, 1995.
3. "Can You Live Longer?" *American Health,* August 1994.
4. Legato, Marianne. Personal interview.
5. Stewart, Donna, and Gail Robinson. *A Clinician's Guide to Menopause.* Washington, DC: Health Press, 1997.
6. "Breast Cancer and Hormone Replacement Therapy: Collaborative Reanalysis of Data from 51 Epidemiological Studies of 52,705 Women with Breast Cancer and 108,411 Women Without Breast Cancer." *Lancet,* Vol. 350, No. 9084, October 11, 1997.
7. LaCroix, Andrea, and Wylie Burke. "Breast Cancer and Hormone Replacement Therapy." *Lancet,* Vol. 350, No. 9084, October 11, 1997.
8. Sheehy, Gail. *New Passages.* New York: Random House, 1995.
9. Hales, Dianne, and Robert Hales. *Caring for the Mind.* New York: Bantam Books, 1995.
10. Mark Clements Research, Inc. "Sex over 65 Survey." August 1995.
11. American Cancer Society. Doll, R., et al. (eds.). *Trends in Cancer Incidence and Mortality.* Plainview, NY: Cold Spring Harbor Laboratory Press, 1994. Skolnick, Andrew. "Leader in War on Cancer Looks Ahead: Talking with Vincent T. DeVita, Jr., M.D." *Journal of the American Medical Association,* Vol. 273, No. 7, February 15, 1995.
12. Krall, Elizabeth, et al. "Bone Mineral Density and Biochemical Markers of Bone Turnover in Healthy Elderly Men and Women." *Journal of Gerontology,* Vol. 52, No. 2, March 1997.
13. Blazer, Dan. "Depression in Late Life." *Health in Mind & Body,* Vol. 2, No. 1, January 1998.
14. Valan, N. M., and D. M. Hilty. "Depression in the Elderly Not Always What It May Seem." *Health in Mind & Body,* Vol. 2, No. 1, January 1998.
15. Gilman, Sid. "Alzheimer's Disease." *Perspectives in Biology & Medicine,* Vol. 40, No. 2, Winter 1997.
16. Lawlor, Brian. *Behavioral Complications in Alzheimer's Disease.* Washington, DC: American Psychiatric Press, 1995.
17. "New Census Report Details Graying of U.S." *HealthSpan,* Vol. 6, No. 1, Summer 1995. Kane, Robert. "Improving the Quality of Long-Term Care." *Journal of the American Medical Association,* Vol. 273, No. 17, May 3, 1995.
18. Lo, Bernard. "Improving Care near the End of Life: Why Is It So Hard?" *Journal of the American Medical Association,* Vol. 274, No. 20, November 22–29, 1995. SUPPORT Principal Investigators. "A Controlled Trial to Improve Care for Seriously Ill Hospitalized Patients." *Journal of the American Medical Association,* Vol. 274, No. 20, November 22–29, 1995.
19. Carney, Maria, and Sean R. Morrison. "Advance Directives: When, Why, and How to Start Talking." *Geriatrics,* Vol. 52, No. 4, April 1997.
20. Prigerson, Holly, et al. "Complicated Grief and Bereavement-Related Depression As Distinct Disorders." *American Journal of Psychiatry,* Vol. 152, No. 1, January 1995.
21. Smith-Stoner, Marilyn, and Amy Lynn Frost. "Coping with Grief and Loss: Bringing Your Shadow Self into the Light." *Nursing,* Vol. 28, No. 2, February 1998.

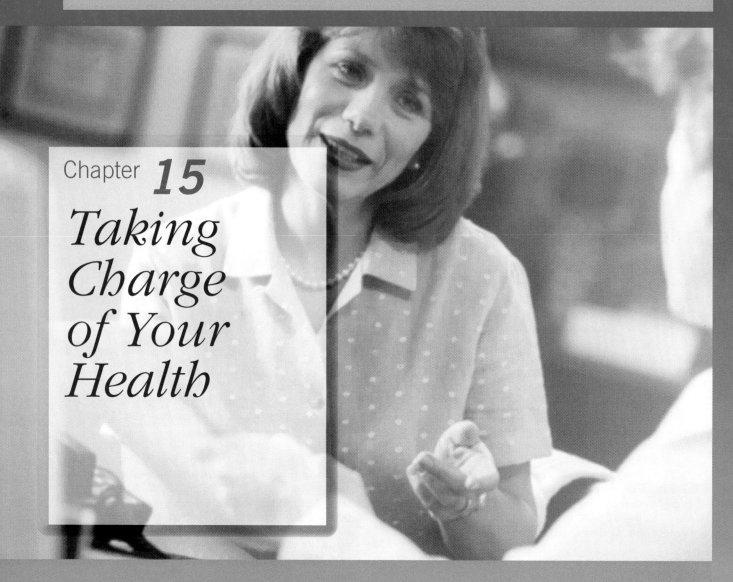

Chapter **15**

Taking Charge of Your Health

After studying the material in this chapter, you should be able to:

■ **Define** *self-care* and **describe** appropriate self-care actions.

■ **Describe** different types of health-care professionals and explain what to consider in selecting a health-care professional.

■ **Describe** the different types of health-care facilities.

■ **Explain** how medical treatments are evaluated.

■ **Discuss** the issues facing the U.S. health-care system today.

■ **List** and **explain** the most common methods of paying for medical care.

■ **Describe** alternative forms of therapy.

*B*ecause of the dramatic changes in the American health-care system described in this chapter, now more than ever you have to be a savvy, informed, and involved health-care consumer. The reason for learning how to take charge of your health care is simple: No one cares more about your health than you do, and no one will do more on your behalf.

Personal Health Care

Knowing how to spot health problems, what to expect from health-care professionals, and where to turn for appropriate treatment can help you keep your own costs down while ensuring the best possible care.

Self-Care

Most people do treat themselves. You probably prescribe aspirin for a headache, chicken soup or orange juice for a cold, or a weekend trip to unwind from stress. At the very least, you should know what your **vital signs** are and how they compare against normal readings (see Figure 15-1).

Some simple tests, such as examinations of the skin, breasts, and testicles for changes that might be an early indication of cancer, require no special equipment and should be part of your normal health routine. Other tests require diagnostic equipment, such as digital blood pressure cuffs that inflate automatically and print out the reading, date, and time; ovulation predictors; and home pregnancy tests. Home testing can be useful, but it is not a substitute for medical evaluation. An essential part of taking good care of yourself is knowing when to seek professional care.

Self-care also can mean getting involved in the self-help movement, which has grown into a major national

Figure 15-1

What's normal? How to check your vital signs.

WHAT'S NORMAL?

Vital Sign	Normal Measurement[a]
Temperature	98.9°F in the morning and 99.9°F overall is the upper limit of normal oral temperature in individuals 40 years old or younger. Normal temperatures can range from 96°F to 99.9°F, typically rising from a low point in early morning to a peak between 4:00 and 6:00p.m. Women's temperatures are slightly higher than men's; African Americans' are slightly higher than white Americans'.
Blood pressure	120/70 to 140/90, depending on age and sex
Pulse rate	72 beats per minute
Respiration rate	15–20 breaths per minute

Temperature

Pulse rate
(taken at carotid artery in the neck, or at the wrist)
Respiration rate
(rate of breathing)

Blood pressure
(check your local drugstore to purchase a blood pressure cuff or digital blood pressure monitor)

[a]You can measure your temperature (with a thermometer), pulse rate, and respiration rate yourself. If you want to invest in the equipment, you can monitor your blood pressure as well. Home blood pressure readings are one way of monitoring your health so that you know when to seek medical advice and treatment.

[b]Mackowiak, Philip, et al. "A Critical Appraisal of 98.6°F, the Upper Limit of the Normal Body Temperature, and Other Legacies of Carl Reinhold August Wunderlich." *Journal of the American Medical Association*, September 23-30, 1992.

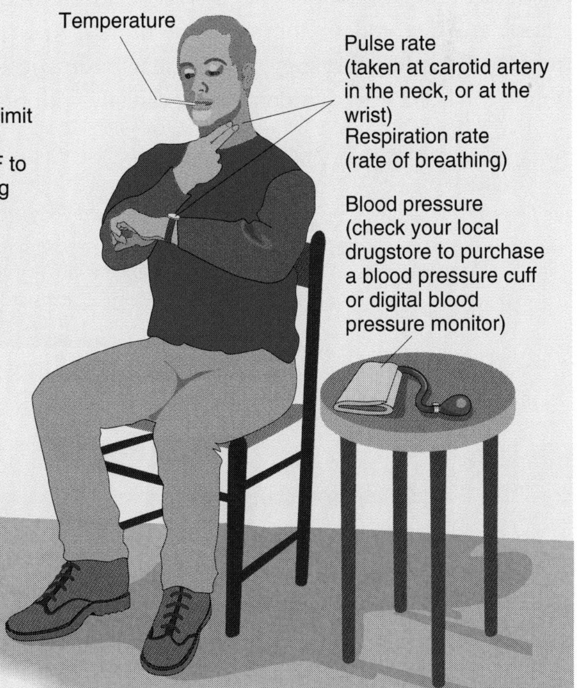

trend involving an estimated 25 million Americans. Initially criticized for implicitly blaming victims rather than changing society, many self-help groups have become more politicized and are working not just to address specific needs of individuals, but to transform social structures.

The Internet has had a tremendous impact. According to some experts, it "may represent the most powerful new element in self-help's future," primarily by providing person-to-person communication and support.[1] For example, an estimated 40,000 people with diabetes share information and experience via chat rooms and other Web sites.

Health-Care Practitioners

Fewer than 10% of health-care practitioners are physicians; other types of health professionals are assuming more important roles in delivering primary, or basic, health services. As a consumer, you should be aware of the range and special skills of the most common types of health-care providers.

Physicians

A medical doctor (M.D.) trained in American medical schools usually takes at least 3 years of premedical college courses (with an emphasis on biology, chemistry, and physics) and then completes 4 (but sometimes 3 or 5) years of medical school. The first 2 years of medical school are devoted to the study of human anatomy, embryology, pharmacology, and similar basic subjects. During the last 2 years, students work directly with physi-

cians in hospitals. Medical students who pass a series of national board examinations then enter a 1-year internship in a hospital, followed by another 2 to 5 years of residency (depending on their specialty), which leads to certification in a particular field, or specialty (Figure 15-2).

Nurses

A registered nurse (R.N.) graduates from a school of nursing approved by a state board and passes a state board examination. R.N.s may have a bachelor's or an associate degree and may specialize in certain areas, such as intensive care or nurse-midwifery. Nurse practitioners (R.N.s with advanced training and experience) may run community clinics or provide screening and preventive care at group medical practices. Some have independent practices.

Licensed practical nurses (L.P.N.s), also called licensed vocational nurses, are licensed by the state. After graduating from state-approved schools of practical nursing, they must take a board exam. They work under the supervision of R.N.s or physicians. Nursing aides and orderlies assist registered and practical nurses in providing services directly related to the comfort and well-being of hospitalized patients.

Specialized and Allied-Health Practitioners

More than sixty different types of health practitioners work with physicians and nurses in providing medical services. Some, such as *occupational therapists,* have at least a bachelor's degree. Allied-health professionals may specialize in a variety of fields. *Clinical psychologists,* for example, have graduate degrees and provide a

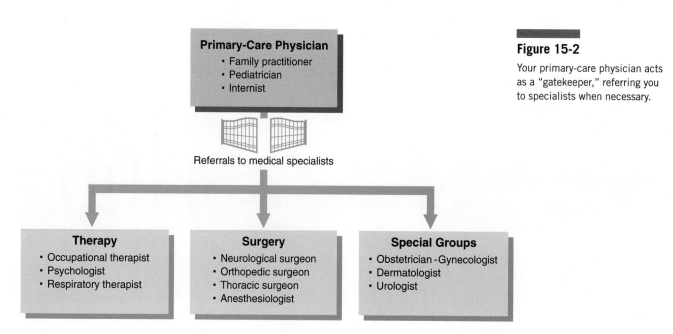

Figure 15-2

Your primary-care physician acts as a "gatekeeper," referring you to specialists when necessary.

Primary-Care Physician
- Family practitioner
- Pediatrician
- Internist

Referrals to medical specialists

Therapy
- Occupational therapist
- Psychologist
- Respiratory therapist

Surgery
- Neurological surgeon
- Orthopedic surgeon
- Thoracic surgeon
- Anesthesiologist

Special Groups
- Obstetrician-Gynecologist
- Dermatologist
- Urologist

wide range of mental health services but don't prescribe medications, as *psychiatrists* do. *Optometrists*, trained in special schools of optometry, diagnose visual abnormalities and prescribe lenses or visual aids; however, they don't prescribe drugs, diagnose or treat eye diseases, or perform surgery—functions performed by *ophthalmologists*. *Podiatrists* are specially trained, licensed health-care professionals who specialize in problems of the feet.

Dentists

Most dental students earn a bachelor's degree and then complete 2 more years of training in the basic sciences and 2 years of clinical work before graduating with a degree of Doctor of Dental Surgery (D.D.S.) or Doctor of Medical Dentistry (D.M.D.). To qualify for a license, graduates must pass both a written and a clinical examination. Dentists may work in general practice or choose a specialty, such as *orthodontics* (straightening teeth).

Chiropractors

Chiropractors hold the degree of Doctor of Chiropractic (D.C.), which signifies that they have had 2 years of college-level training plus 4 years in a health-care school specializing in **chiropractic**, a method of treatment based on the theory that most human diseases are caused by misalignment of the bones *(subluxation)*. In particular, chiropractic theory holds that the misalignment of individual vertebrae in the backbone leads to pressure on nerve tissue, which in turn affects other parts of the body. Chiropractors emphasize wellness and healing without drugs or surgery. Although chiropractors may use X rays in making diagnoses, chiropractic treatment consists solely of the manipulation of bones. Spinal manipulation has proven effective in relieving certain types of lower back pain.

Health-Care Facilities

As a prospective patient, you can choose from various options: a physician's office, a clinic, an emergency room, or a hospital. Most **primary care**—also referred to as ambulatory or outpatient care—is provided by a physician in an office, emergency room, or clinic. *Secondary care* usually is provided by specialists or subspecialists in either an outpatient or inpatient (hospital) setting. *Tertiary care*, available at university-affiliated hospitals and regional referral centers, includes special procedures such as kidney dialysis, open-heart surgery, and organ transplants.

College Health Centers

The American College Health Association estimates that about 1500 institutions of higher learning provide direct health services. Student health centers range in size from small dispensaries staffed by nurses to large-scale, multispecialty clinics that provide both inpatient and outpatient care and are fully accredited by the Joint Commission on Accreditation of Healthcare Organizations (JCAH). Some serve only students; others provide services for faculty, staff, and family members.

On some campuses, health educators work with the student health centers to provide counseling on such topics as nutrition; tobacco, drug, and alcohol abuse; exercise and fitness; sexuality; and contraception. Some college health centers provide psychological counseling, as well as dental, pharmacy, and optometric services. Some campuses also provide sports-medicine services for student athletes. Services are paid for by various combinations of prepaid health fees, general university funds, fee-for-service charges, and health-insurance reimbursements.

Outpatient Treatment Centers

Increasingly, procedures that once required hospitalization, such as simple surgery, are being performed at outpatient centers, which may be freestanding or affiliated with a medical center. Patients have any necessary tests performed beforehand, undergo surgery or receive treatment, and return home after a few hours to recuperate. Outpatient centers can handle many common surgical procedures, including cataract removal, tonsillectomy, breast biopsy, dilation and curettage (D and C), vasectomy, and face-lifts.

Hospitals and Medical Centers

Different types of hospitals offer different types of care. The most common type of hospital is the *private*, or community, *hospital*, which may be run on a profit or a nonprofit basis. It generally contains 50 to 400 beds and provides more personalized care than public hospitals do. The quality of care individual patients receive depends mostly on the physicians themselves. *Public hospitals* include city, county, public health service, military, and Veterans Administration hospitals. The quality of patient care depends on the overall quality of the institution.

Of the more than 6500 hospitals nationwide, about 300 are major *academic medical centers* or teaching hospitals. Affiliated with medical schools, they generally provide the most up-to-date and experienced care because staff physicians must stay current to teach their students. These centers, with the best equipment, researchers, and resources, have been described as representing "the high-technology care that many U.S. citizens associate with worldwide leadership in the quality of their medical care."[2]

The Joint Commission on the Accreditation of Healthcare Organizations reviews all hospitals every 3 years. Eighty percent of hospitals qualify for JCAH accreditation. If you have to enter a hospital and your health insurance or plan allows a choice, try to find out as much as you can about the alternatives available to you:

- Talk to your physician about a hospital and why he or she recommends it.

- As a cost-cutting strategy, many hospitals have cut back on the use of registered nurses. Check with the local nursing association about the ratio of patients to nurses and the ratio of R.N.s to licensed practical, or vocational, nurses.

- Find out room rates and charges for ancillary services, including tests, lab work, X rays, and medications. Check with your health plan to see whether you need preapproval for any of these costs and ask what you will be expected to pay.

- Ask how many times in the past year the hospital has performed the procedure recommended for you and what the success and complication rates have been. Ask about the hospital's nosocomial (hospital-caused) infection rate and accident rate. You also have the right to information on the number and types of malpractice claims filed against a hospital.

- If possible, go on a tour of the hospital. Does the setting seem comfortable? Is the staff courteous? Does the hospital seem clean and efficiently run?

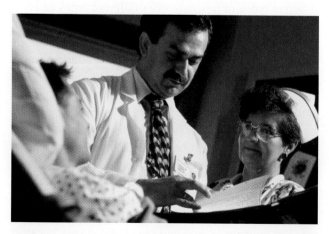

A healthy hospital stay. Read consent forms carefully and ask for more information if you don't understand. Talk to the staff and pay attention to your care routine.

Strategies for Prevention

How to Survive a Hospital Stay

✔ Make sure the name on your wristband is spelled correctly and clearly. Talk to everyone who brings you a pill or performs a test or procedure. Patient charts can get mixed up, and you don't want to undergo a treatment intended for someone else.

✔ Know which medicines you're supposed to get and what they look like. If you're uncertain that a medication is the right one for you, ask someone to double-check.

✔ Make sure the people caring for you wash their hands. A polite reminder won't offend good professionals—and could prevent infection.

✔ Be sure to bring along any recent test results or X rays that your physician feels may be helpful. You may be able to avoid some repeat testing.

✔ If you're asked to sign a consent form, read it carefully. If you want more information, ask before signing. Don't feel pressured to sign if you want to discuss something with your physician first.

The Doctor-Patient Relationship

Once the family doctor was indeed part of the family. The family doctor brought babies into the world, shepherded them through childhood, comforted and counseled them, stood by their bedside in their darkest hours. Patients entrusted the doctor with their cares, their confidences, their very lives. In the 20th century, with dramatic breakthroughs in diagnosing and treating illness, the focus in medicine shifted from the family physician to the specialist, from basic caring to high-tech medical care. Patients today are more likely to be cured of a vast array of illnesses than those of a century ago. However, they often complain of insensitive, uncaring physicians who focus on their diseases rather than on them as individuals.[3]

As more physicians have joined managed-care organizations (discussed later in this chapter), which emphasize efficiency, they sometimes feel pressure to see more patients a day, to spend less time with each, and to discourage expensive tests and treatments. Because physicians have less time and less autonomy, patients today must do more. Your first step should be learning more about your body, any medical conditions or problems you develop, and your options for treatment. You can find a great deal of information via computer online services (which often have discussion groups, or "chat rooms," dedicated to a particular medical topic), patient advocacy and support organizations, and libraries.

This information can help you know what questions to ask and how to evaluate what your doctor says. But you have to be willing to speak up. "Too many patients are so respectful of—and intimidated by—doctors that they don't realize that they have a right and an obligation to be assertive about their health situation," say Richard Podell, M.D., and William Proctor, authors of *When Your Doctor Doesn't Know Best*. Their advice: Be courageous.

"To be effective as a patient in the current health-care environment, you must have the guts to stand up to your doctor and ask pointed questions. The alert—and safe—patient is the one who can be assertive, even aggressive, with physicians. The goal isn't to pick a fight but to work instead toward an active collaboration. Done smartly and effectively, being an alert patient should improve, not harm, your relationship with your doctor."[4] (See Pulsepoints: "Ten Ways to Get Good Health Care.")

Your "Primary" Physician

The primary-care physicians who are playing increasingly important roles in American health care include family practitioners, general internists, and pediatricians. Obstetrician-gynecologists serve as the primary providers of health care for more than half of all women.[5] If you're a woman and your gynecologist is

---

Pulsepoints Ten Ways to Get Good Health Care

1. Trust your instincts. You know your body better than anyone else. If something is bothering you, it deserves medical attention. Don't let your health-care provider—or your health-plan administrator—dismiss it without a thorough evaluation.

2. Inform yourself. Go to the library or an online information service and find articles that describe what you're experiencing. The more you know about possible causes of your symptoms, the more likely you are to be taken seriously.

3. Find a good primary-care physician who listens carefully and responds to your concerns. Look for a family doctor or general internist who takes a careful history, performs a thorough exam, and listens and responds to your concerns.

4. See your doctor regularly. If you're in your twenties or thirties, you may not need an annual exam, but it's important to get checkups at least every 2 or 3 years, not so much for the sake of finding hidden disease, but so you and your doctor can get to know each other and develop a trusting, mutually respectful relationship.

5. Get a second opinion. If you are uncertain of whether to undergo treatment or which therapy is best, see another physician and listen carefully for any doubts or hesitation about what you're considering.

6. Challenge medical judgments based on personal circumstances. Insist that your doctor base any diagnosis on a thorough medical evaluation, not on a value judgment about you or your lifestyle.

7. Seek support. Patient support and advocacy groups can offer emotional support, information on many common problems, and referral to knowledgeable

physicians. (See the Hales Health Directory at the back of the book for numbers and addresses.)

8. If your doctor cannot or will not respond to your concerns, get another one. Regardless of your health coverage, you have the right to replace a physician who is not meeting your health-care needs.

9. Speak up. If you don't understand, ask. If you feel that you're not being taken seriously or being treated with respect, say so. Sometimes the only difference between being a patient or becoming a victim is making sure your needs and rights are not forgotten or overlooked.

10. Bring your own advocate. If you become intimidated or anxious talking to physicians, ask a friend to accompany you, to ask questions on your behalf, and to take notes.

the only physician you see, make sure that he or she performs other tests, such as measuring your blood pressure, in addition to a pelvic and breast exam. If you develop other symptoms or health concerns, ask for an appropriate referral.

One key to making the health-care system work for you lies in choosing a good physician. After seeing your primary-care physician, ask yourself the following questions to evaluate the quality of care you are getting.

- Did your physician take a comprehensive history? Was the physical examination thorough?

- Did your physician explain what he or she was doing during the exam?

- Did he or she spend enough time with you?

- Did you feel free to ask questions? Did your physician give you straight answers? Did he or she reassure you when you were worried?

- Did your physician seem willing to admit that he or she doesn't know the answers to some questions?

- Did your physician hesitate to refer you to a specialist even when you have a complex problem that warrants such care?

Look back at your answers. If they make you feel uneasy, have a talk with your physician. Or find a physician or a health plan that provides better service.

Medical Exams and Tests

Most physicians believe that you don't need annual checkups if you're young and feel well. However, certain types of screening tests should be performed peri-

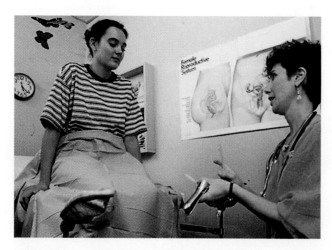

Many women choose female health-care practitioners to provide gynecologic services.

odically, particularly if you're 45 or older or if you are at a higher-than-average risk of developing a particular disease, such as high blood pressure or colon cancer.

Your physician will want a past medical history, including major illnesses, surgery, and treatments. Report any allergies you have, particularly to drugs, and the medications you take, including aspirin, antacids, sleeping pills, oral contraceptives, and recreational drugs, even if illegal. Your physician may also want to know about topics you consider private, such as sexually transmitted diseases. Remember that he or she is attempting to gather all the information needed to provide you with comprehensive treatment. Note, too, that a physician must report certain information—for example, certain sexually transmitted diseases—to health authorities.

After the physician has asked you questions about your complaints, medical history, and lifestyle, he or she will probably perform some standard tests. During the examination, point out any pains, lumps, or skin growths you've noticed. If you feel pain when the physician palpates (feels) any part of your body, say so.

The physician may order some laboratory and other tests, including the following:

- *Chest X ray.* A chest X ray can reveal abnormalities of the heart and lungs; if you're a smoker, the physician may insist on one.

- *Electrocardiogram.* The *electrocardiogram* is a test performed while you're at rest that records the electrical activity of your heart. It can show irregularities in heart rhythm or muscle damage, as well as hardening of the arteries.

- *Urinalysis.* Your urine may be analyzed by a medical laboratory. If sugar (glucose) is found in your urine, your physician may order a separate blood test to check for diabetes. The presence of blood cells may indicate infection of the bladder or kidneys. Abnormal amounts of albumin (protein) in the urine may also suggest kidney disease.

- *Blood tests.* The physician or laboratory technician may draw blood to do a blood cell count. An excess of white blood cells may be an indication of infection or, occasionally, leukemia. A deficiency of red blood cells may indicate anemia. A sample of your blood may also be analyzed to measure the levels of its various components. High levels of glucose may indicate diabetes, and high levels of uric acid may mean gout or kidney stones. A high cholesterol level may indicate cardiac risk.

Your Medical Rights

As a consumer, you have basic rights that help ensure that you know about any potential dangers, receive competent diagnosis and treatment, and retain control and dignity in your interactions with health-care professionals. Many hospitals publish a patient's bill of rights, including your rights to know whether a procedure is experimental; to refuse to undergo a specific treatment; to designate someone else to make decisions about your care if and when you cannot; and to leave the hospital, even against your physician's advice.

You have the right to be treated with respect and dignity, including being called "Mr." or "Ms." or whatever you wish, rather than by your first name. Make clear your preferences. If you feel that health-care professionals are being condescending or inconsiderate in any way, say so—in the same tone and manner that you would like others to use with you. If you're hospitalized, find out if there's a patient advocate or representative at your hospital. These individuals can help you communicate with physicians, make any special arrangements, and get answers to questions or complaints.

You have the right to give consent to donate an organ while alive or have your organs removed in the event of an accident, injury, or illness that leaves you brain-dead. However, you cannot agree to donate a body part for money or other compensation. Congress has prohibited the marketing of organs; any attempt to do so is a felony punishable by up to 5 years in jail and a $50,000 fine.

Your Right to Information

By law, a patient must give consent for hospitalization, surgery, and other major treatments. **Informed consent** is a right, not a privilege. Use this right to its fullest. Ask questions. Seek other opinions. Make sure that your expectations are realistic and that you understand the potential risks, as well as the possible benefits, of a prospective treatment. Informed consent is required for research studies, but patients often don't realize that they have the right not to participate and to get complete information on the purpose and nature of the study.

Your Medical Records

You have a right to know what is in your medical records. Some states have laws assuring patient access to records. Consumer advocates advise that you routine-ly request records from physicians, hospitals, and laboratories—first verbally, then in writing.

To protect your privacy, don't routinely fill out medical questionnaires or histories. Always ask the purpose and find out who will have access to it. Specifically ask if your history may be entered into a computer database.[6] Tell your physician or health-care group that you do not want your records to leave their offices without your approval. Put it in writing. When you do have to authorize the release of your records, limit the information to a specific condition, physician, and hospital rather than authorizing release of all your records.

The American Health-Care System: A Revolution in Progress

As technological breakthroughs have transformed modern medicine, subspecialists multiplied, and medical costs spiraled upward. Finally, in the 1990s, health policymakers and the employers that had footed the bills agreed that health costs, which had grown to almost 14% of the gross domestic product, had to be controlled.[7]

The first Clinton administration's plan to reform health-care failed to meet with congressional approval in 1994. However, other attempts to reduce health-care costs have continued, including the movement toward **managed care**, a new way of delivering and paying for health-care services. Managed-care organizations provide health-care or health-care insurance at lower costs to employers. The tradeoff for such savings is that a third party makes the final decision on when or if a medical visit or treatment is necessary.[8] This differs from traditional *fee-for-service* medicine, in which patients decide when to seek care and choose which physician to see (see Figure 15-3).

Both fee-for-service and managed-care systems have drawbacks. Fee-for-service medicine errs on the side of doing too much and providing unneeded tests and therapies. Managed-care organizations are more likely to do too little so they can keep costs low. "The more care you're given by a private physician, the more money he or she can make," note Richard Podell, M.D., and William Proctor, authors of *When Your Doctor Doesn't Know Best*. In some managed-care plans, by comparison, your primary-care doctor "may have funds deducted from his or her income each time you're referred to a specialist."[9]

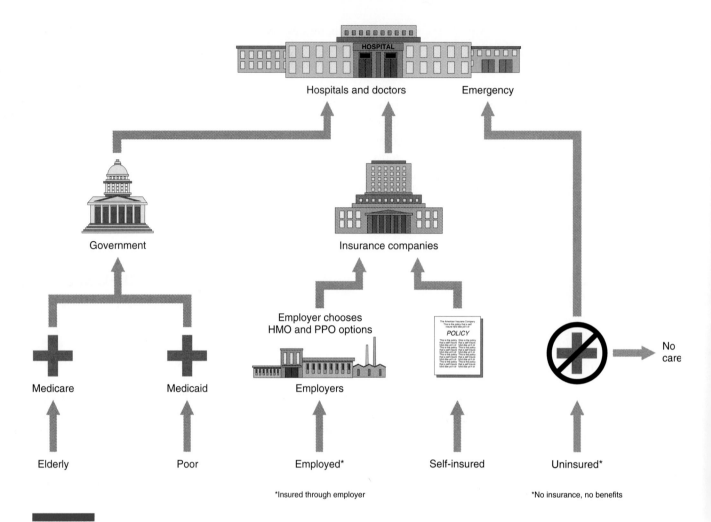

Hospitals and doctors   Emergency

Government   Insurance companies

Employer chooses
HMO and PPO options

POLICY

No care

Medicare   Medicaid   Employers   Self-insured   Uninsured*

Elderly   Poor   Employed*

*Insured through employer   *No insurance, no benefits

Figure 15-3

Medical coverage in the United States is complex; you and your doctor are connected through a bureaucracy of policies and agencies.

Traditional Health Insurance

In the past, most working Americans relied on conventional **indemnity** insurance policies to pay major medical expenses. Policyholders paid a percentage (generally 20%) of hospitalization costs and a deductible (a minimum paid out each year before the insurance company pays anything). While indemnity insurance gave patients freedom to choose physicians and hospitals, it often failed to cover routine physical exams and screening tests. Individuals with "preexisting" conditions often could not qualify for coverage or were not reimbursed for treatments related to these conditions. In the last decade, as health-care costs skyrocketed, insurers increasingly refused to pay claims, canceled groups with high medical bills, or denied coverage to people in high-risk occupations.

Managed Care

There has been a dramatic shift away from indemnity insurance to managed-care plans, which cost less but also offer less freedom and flexibility (see Table 15-1). Managed-care organizations, which take various forms, deliver care through a network of physicians, hospitals, and other health-care professionals who agree to provide their services at fixed or discounted rates.

Consumers in a managed-care group must follow certain procedures in advance of seeking care (for example, getting prior approval for a test or treatment) and must abide by a limit on reimbursement for certain services. Some procedures may be deemed unnecessary and not be covered at all. Patients who choose to see a physician who is not a participating member of

TABLE 15-1 THE GROWTH OF MANAGED CARE

Year	Managed Care	Fee-for-Service
1988	29%	71%
1992	55%	45%
1996	74%	26%

SOURCE: KPMG Peat Marwick LLP Survey of Employer Sponsored Health Benefits, 1996; 1995; 1994; 1993; 1992.

the medical-insurance coverage group may have to pay the entire fee themselves.[10]

Managed-care plans have been criticized for pressuring providers to "undertreat" patients—for example, sending them home from the hospital too soon or denying them costly tests or treatments. Some members complain of long waits, the need to switch primary physicians if their doctor leaves the plan, difficulty getting approval for needed services, and a sense that providers pay more attention to the bottom line than to their health needs. There have been increasing demands for government regulation of managed-care plans.[11]

Health maintenance organizations, or **HMOs**, are managed-care plans that emphasize routine care and prevention by providing complete medical services in exchange for a predetermined monthly payment. HMOs deliver health care to more than 25% of the population.[12] In a **preferred provider organization (PPO)**, a third party—a union, an insurance company, or a self-insured business—contracts with a group of physicians and hospitals to treat members at a discount. PPO members may choose any physician within the network, and usually pay a 10% copayment for care within the system and a higher percentage (20%–30%) for care elsewhere. PPOs generally require prior approval for expensive tests or major procedures.

Government-Financed Insurance Plans

The government provides two major forms of health financing: Medicare and Medicaid. Under Medicare, the federal government pays 80% of most medical bills, after a deductible fee, for people over age 65. Medicare doesn't cover drugs, eyeglasses, or dental work.

Medicaid, a federal and state insurance plan that protects people with very low or no incomes, is the chief source of coverage for the unemployed. However, many unemployed Americans don't qualify because their family incomes are above the poverty line. Publicly insured patients are more likely than those with private insurance to receive inadequate care and to experience adverse health outcomes.

The Uninsured

As many as 42 million Americans lack health insurance; many others are underinsured, meaning that they don't have adequate coverage (see Figure 15-4).[13] Uninsured patients have shorter hospital stays, cannot undergo costly therapies, and have a greater risk of dying in the hospital than insured patients. About 85% of uninsured Americans are from families in which the head of the family works but can't get insurance through his or her employer. Some of these people work part-time and do not qualify for insurance. Others work for businesses too small to qualify for group insurance. The availability of insurance affects both access to care and the way care is delivered.

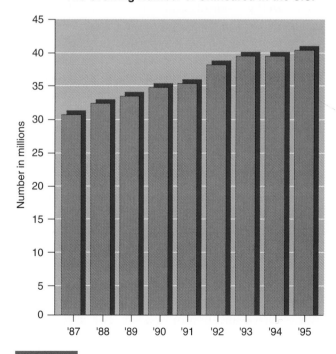

The Growing Number of Uninsured in the U.S.

Figure 15-4

Evaluating Health News and Online Medical Advice

Cure! Breakthrough! Medical miracle! These are the words headlines are made of. But remember that although medical breakthroughs and cures do occur, most scientific progress is made one small step at a time. And even though medicine is considered a science, some experts estimate that no more than 15% of medical interventions can be supported by reliable scientific evidence.[14]

Medical opinions invariably change over time, sometimes going from one extreme to another. For instance, several decades ago the treatment of choice for breast cancer was radical mastectomy—removal of the woman's breast, lymph nodes, and chest wall. Since then much less extensive surgery (lumpectomy), coupled with chemotherapy or radiation, or both, has proven equally effective. Once individuals who'd suffered heart attacks were advised to limit all physical activity. Today a progressive exercise program is a standard component of rehabilitation.

Health researchers are struggling to find better ways of assessing what they know and need to know to offer more complete and balanced information to consumers. However, sometimes the only certainty is uncertainty. Rather than putting your faith in the most recent report or the hottest trend, try to gather as much background information and as many opinions as you can. Weigh them carefully—ideally with a trusted physician—and make the decision that seems best for you.

In recent years the Internet has become a major source of health information—and misinformation. More than 10,000 health-related web sites offer ways for patients to educate themselves about medical problems and options for treatment and share experiences with other people with similar conditions. The Internet also permits ease of access to cutting-edge medical knowledge and bridges the communication gap created by high-tech medicine.

However, there also are serious drawbacks. There is no regulation of Web site accuracy or reliability. Many sites are used to promote products or people. Some chat rooms can lead to encounters with unpleasant people. Even when information is technically precise, laypeople may not know how to interpret it properly.[15]

Whenever using the Internet for medical guidance, always check the sponsor of a site. Is it a hospital, a research institute, a drug manufacturer, or a distributor of an herbal remedy? Look for references to peer-reviewed medical journals. Beware of endorsements of

Strategies for Change

How to Evaluate Health News

When reading a newspaper or magazine story or listening to a radio or television report about a medical advance, look for answers to the following questions:

✔ Who are the scientists involved? Are they recognized, legitimate health professionals? What are their credentials? Are they affiliated with respected medical or scientific institutions? Be wary of individuals whose degrees or affiliations are from institutions you've never heard of, and be sure that the person's educational background is in a discipline related to the area of research reported.

✔ Where did the scientists report their findings? The best research is published in peer-reviewed professional journals, such as the *New England Journal of Medicine*. Research developments also may be reported at meetings of professional societies.

✔ Is the information based on personal observations? Does the report include testimonials from cured patients or satisfied customers? If the answer to either question is yes, be wary.

✔ Does the article, report, or advertisement include words like *amazing*, *secret*, or *quick*? Does it claim to be something the public has never seen or been offered before? Such sensationalized language is often a tip-off to a dubious treatment.

✔ Is someone trying to sell you something? Manufacturers who cite studies to sell a product have been known to embellish the truth.

✔ Does the information defy all common sense? Be skeptical. If something sounds too good to be true, it probably is.

miracle products that claim to cure various diseases and flashy sites that may have little substance behind them. Always verify any information before you act on it with organizations such as the American Medical Association or the National Institutes of Health.

Alternative Forms of Therapy

Modern medicine, with its emphasis on technology and highly specialized treatments, is most successful in fighting disease rather than preventing illness or dealing with lifestyle problems such as stress, addiction, and obesity. As a consequence, as many as 50% of Americans have turned to alternative or nontraditional health-care approaches.[16]

Alternative therapies appeal to people for many reasons. They often cost less. They cause fewer side effects. Practitioners spend more time with and listen more attentively to patients. In addition, they often emphasize the connection between mind and body, and the body's own healing powers, thereby giving individuals a greater sense of control over their health. One danger, say their critics, is that people who turn to alternative therapies may ignore or refuse conventional medicines that could improve their health or even save their lives.

At present, alternative medicine is exactly that: an option to be considered as carefully as any more widely known and accepted medical therapy. If you're considering a nontraditional treatment, first compare what traditional medical science has to offer and what the alternatives claim. Avoid practitioners who insist that their brand of healing is the only effective approach. Check practitioners' credentials as carefully as possible. Some "doctors" in white coats have questionable degrees, often in fields that are not at all related to health. Remember that you are ultimately responsible for your well-being: Don't entrust it to anyone who doesn't deserve your trust.

The National Institutes of Health (NIH), noting that "treatments considered unconventional today may become conventional in the future," has begun investigating such practices, including those discussed in the following sections.[17] Although there has been some controversy in traditional scientific and medical circles about the NIH's move, there is increasing recognition of the need for such research.[18]

Acupuncture

An ancient Chinese form of medicine, **acupuncture** is based on the philosophy that a cycle of energy circulating through the body controls health. Pain and disease are the result of a disturbance in the energy flow, which can be corrected by inserting long, thin needles at specific points along longitudinal lines, or *meridians,* throughout the body. Each point controls a different corresponding part of the body. Once inserted, the needles are rotated gently back and forth or charged with a small electric current for a short time. Western scientists aren't sure exactly how acupuncture works, but some believe that the needles alter the functioning of the nervous system.

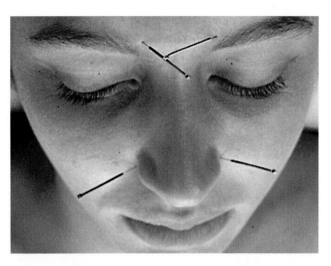

The ancient Chinese practice of acupuncture produces healing through the insertion and manipulation of needles at specific points throughout the body. The procedures are not painful.

In *acupressure,* the therapist uses his or her finger and thumb to stimulate certain points, relieve pain, and relax muscles. *Reflexology* is based on the theory that massaging certain points on the foot or hand relieves stress or pain in corresponding parts of the body. These methods seem most effective in easing chronic pain, arthritis, and withdrawal from nicotine, alcohol, or drugs.

An NIH consensus development panel that evaluated current research into acupuncture concluded that there is "clear evidence" that acupuncture can control nausea and vomiting in patients after surgery or while undergoing chemotherapy and relieve postoperative dental pain. The panel said that acupuncture is "probably" also effective in the control of nausea in early pregnancy and that there were "reasonable" studies showing that the use of acupuncture, by itself or as an adjunct to other therapies, resulted in satisfactory treatment of a number of other conditions, even though there was not "firm evidence of efficacy at this time." These conditions include addiction to illicit drugs and alcohol (but not to tobacco), stroke rehabilitation, headache, menstrual cramps, tennis elbow, general muscle pain, low back pain, carpal tunnel syndrome, and asthma.[19]

Ayurveda

Considered alternative here, **ayurveda** is a traditional form of medical treatment in India, where it has evolved over thousands of years. Its basic premise is that illness stems from incorrect mental attitudes, diet, and posture.

Practitioners use a discipline of exercise, meditation, herbal medication, and proper nutrition to cope with such stress-induced conditions as hypertension, the desire to smoke, and obesity. The best known advocate of ayurvedic medicine in the United States is Deepak Chopra, M.D., an endocrinologist (specialist in hormone-related disorders) who has written several books on ayurveda and the intimate relationship between consciousness and health.

Biofeedback

A marriage of technology and mysticism, biofeedback uses machines that measure temperature or skin responses and relays (or feeds back) this information to the subject. In this way, people can learn to control usually involuntary functions, such as circulation to the hands and feet, tension in the jaws, and heartbeat rates. Biofeedback has been used to treat dozens of ailments, including asthma, epilepsy, pain, and *Reynaud's disease* (a condition in which the fingers become painful and white when exposed to cold). Many health insurers now cover biofeedback treatments.

Bodywork

Numerous techniques focus on manipulation of the body. The *Alexander technique,* popular among actors and dancers, coaches people to improve their posture to relieve tension and pain. *Hellerwork* uses deep massage to eliminate pain and tension. Practitioners of *therapeutic touch* move their hands above the body; as they do, they sense blockages in a person's "life energy" and redirect energy to promote healing.

Herbal Medicine

Herbal medicine, or **herbology**, an ancient form of treatment, uses substances derived from trees, flowers, ferns, seaweeds, or lichens to treat disease. Many manufactured drugs are made from plants or are synthetic re-creations or modifications of naturally occurring substances. However, advocates of herbal medicine feel that herbs work differently on the body than purified drugs, with fewer side effects and faster healing.[20]

Herbal treatments have been developed for practically all known diseases from corns and callouses to anemia and hypertension. While plant extracts can be beneficial, many producers don't monitor the purity or potency of herbal products, which may contain insect parts, pollen, molds, and toxins such as lead and arsenic

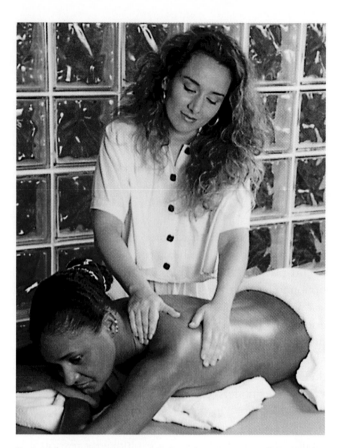

Bodywork practitioners use touch and massage to relieve tension and improve energy flow, thereby enhancing the body's own healing power.

acquired from the soil. Never use more than the recommended amounts, and don't continue to take an herbal remedy for prolonged periods of time or if you're pregnant or using a prescription drug. Watch out for allergic reactions to herbs, including herbal teas. And always seek medical care if symptoms persist or worsen over time.

Homeopathy

Homeopathy is based on three fundamental principles: Like cures like; treatment must always be individualized; and less is more—increasing dilution (lowering the dosage) can increase efficacy. By administering doses of animal, vegetable, or mineral substances to a large number of healthy people to see if they all develop the same symptoms, homeopaths determine which substances may be given, in small quantities, to alleviate the symptoms. Some of these substances are the same as those used in conventional medicine: nitroglycerin for certain heart conditions, for example, although the dose is minuscule.

The FDA hasn't demanded proof of efficacy for homeopathic remedies because they aren't considered harmful. However, some consumer groups are petitioning the FDA to require that homeopathic products be proven safe and effective before they're marketed. These products amount to about $250 million in annual sales; most popular are products for insomnia, coughs, and colds.[21]

Naturopathy

Naturopathic physicians (who are not M.D.s) emphasize natural remedies, such as sun, water, heat, and air, as the best treatments for disease. Therapies might include dietary changes (such as more vegetables and no salt or stimulants), steam baths, and exercise. Some work closely with medical doctors in helping patients.

Visualization

Carl Simonton, M.D., a cancer specialist, developed the technique of creative **visualization**, or imaging, to help heal cancer patients, including some diagnosed as terminally ill. On the premise that positive and negative beliefs and attitudes have a great deal to do with whether people get well or die of disease, patients imagine themselves getting well—they "see," for instance, their immune-system cells marching to conquer the cancer cells. Others use visualization in different ways—for example, to create a clear idea of what they want to achieve, whether the goal is weight loss or relaxation.

Quackery

Every year millions of Americans go searching for medical miracles that never happen. In all, they spend more than $10 billion on medical **quackery**, unproven health products and services. Those who lose only money are the lucky ones. Many also waste precious time, during which their conditions worsen. Some suffer needless pain, along with crushed expectations. Far too many risk their lives on a false hope—and lose.

The peddlers of such false hopes are quacks, who, by definition, promote for profit worthless or unproven treatments. A quack's greatest skill is telling people what they want to hear. Quackery's most recent disguise has been in the form of untested treatments for cancer, HIV infection and AIDS, and other life-threatening conditions. Many men and women who

---

Strategies for Prevention

Protecting Yourself Against Quackery

✔ Arm yourself with up-to-date information about your condition or disease from appropriate organizations, such as the American Cancer Society or the Arthritis Foundation, which keep track of unproven and ineffective methods of treatment.

✔ Ask for a written explanation of what a treatment does and why it works, evidence supporting all claims (not just testimonials), and published reports of the studies that have been done, including specifics on numbers treated, doses, and side effects. Be skeptical of self-styled "holistic practitioners," treatments supported by crusading groups, and endorsements from so-called authorities.

✔ Don't part with your money quickly. You need to be especially careful because insurance companies won't reimburse for unproven therapies.

✔ Don't discontinue your current treatment without your physician's approval. Many physicians encourage supportive therapies—such as relaxation exercises, meditation, or visualization—as a supplement to standard treatments.

---

aren't ill or in pain take various powders and extracts to enhance their health or delay aging. Some see lifestyle or self-care approaches, such as taking megadoses of vitamins or eating special foods, as a means of staying in control of their bodies and preventing disease or deterioration.

Sometimes individuals with certain diseases, such as arthritis or multiple sclerosis, who try unproven remedies do indeed improve. "If someone with arthritis starts feeling better the day after getting a copper bracelet, the bracelet will get the credit," says one physician. "Yet it's just coincidence." This is one reason scientists put little stock in enthusiastic testimonials from people who genuinely believe they have been helped by a new drug or treatment. Their heartfelt stories can be persuasive but are scientifically meaningless. The satisfied patient may not actually have had the disease in the first place, may have gotten other treatments too, or may be responding to a remedy that masks the symptoms without treating the disease.

Health Online

A Guide to Health-Care Reform for Young Americans
http://www.iuma.com/rtv/

The current health-care crisis is likely to affect younger Americans the most. This site, designed especially for this generation, outlines the issues that our health-care system faces and what you can do about it. There are stories about young people entangled with the system and how their plight illustrate larger social issues. In the Resources section, there are ideas for how you can write to your political representatives to urge them to make changes to the system.

Think about it ...

- Have you or a friend or family member ever faced a medical crisis without health insurance? Why wasn't this person insured?

- Do the stories told on this Web site make health-care issues seem more personal and urgent to you? What special health-care issues do young people face?

- If you were in charge of overhauling the American health-care system, what changes would you make?

Making This Chapter Work for You
Smart Health-Care Decisions

- The American health-care system, though considered among the best in the world, is complex and changing, and people must become savvy consumers to ensure that they get the best possible care.

- Self-care is an important aspect of maintaining good health and preventing disease. Home tests and equipment can identify any suspicious signs that require professional care.

- As a consumer, you may turn to physicians, nurses, and any number of specialists and allied-health professionals.

- Health-care facilities include student health centers, clinics, hospitals, outpatient surgery centers, and free-standing emergency centers.

- Most primary care is provided by a physician in an office, emergency room, or clinic. Secondary care usually is provided by specialists or subspecialists in either an outpatient or inpatient (hospital) setting. Tertiary care is available at university-affiliated hospitals and regional referral centers.

- A thorough medical evaluation includes a medical history and a physical examination that evaluates all systems of the body and includes appropriate screening and medical tests.

- As a consumer, you have the right of information about possible treatments, access to your records, respectful treatment, and safe, quality care.

- The effort to control health-care costs has led to dramatic changes in how we pay for health care. Fewer Americans now have conventional indemnity health insurance policies, which pay physicians and hospitals for the services they perform.

- Managed-care plans, which now dominate the health-care system, offer lower costs by providing services through an organized network of providers, who receive a fixed or discounted rate for their services.

- Health maintenance organizations, or HMOs, are managed-care groups that emphasize preventive health care. Preferred provider organizations, or PPOs, allow consumers to choose from a selected list of physicians and facilities.

- The government helps defray medical expenses through two programs: Medicare, for people over age 65, and Medicaid, for people unable to pay for health care.

■ Millions of Americans, often disillusioned by conventional therapists and therapies, have tried alternative forms of healing, which are undergoing assessment by the National Institutes of Health. Alternative therapies include acupuncture, biofeedback, homeopathy, naturopathy, visualization, and other approaches that stress the mind-body connection.

■ Quackery is worthless, fraudulent, or unproven treatment for incurable diseases, longer life, better health, or delayed aging.

 ## Key Terms

The terms listed here are used within the chapter. Page numbers are included for each term. A definition of each term is given in the green Glossary pages at the end of this book.

acupuncture *315*
ayurveda *315*
chiropractic *307*
health maintenance organizations (HMOs) *313*
herbal medicine *316*
herbology *316*

homeopathy *316*
indemnity *312*
informed consent *311*
managed care *311*
preferred provider organization (PPO) *313*
primary care *307*

quackery *317*
visualization *317*
vital signs *305*

Review Questions

1. What does self-care mean? What actions are involved in practicing self-care?
2. Name some different types of health-care professionals and their responsibilities. What criteria should you use in selecting a health-care professional?
3. Do medical patients have rights? If so, what are they?
4. What are the most common methods of payment for medical care?

Critical Thinking Questions

1. Think about an experience you've had with a medical practitioner. How did you feel during the physical examination? Did you trust the practitioner? Were you comfortable with the level of communication? Evaluate your experience and give your opinion of the value of the checkup.
2. What nontraditional or alternative approaches to health care are you aware of? How do you feel about alternative care? Do you feel confident in knowing the difference between alternative care and quackery?
3. What do you see as the solution to America's health-care crisis? What role should the government play? What should be done so that all Americans have access to necessary health services?

Connections to Personal Health Interactive

*To enhance your understanding of the material covered in this chapter, check out the following study aids on the **Personal Health Interactive CD-ROM**.*

■ Personal Insights: Are You in Control of Your Health?
■ Glossary & Key Term Review

References

1. "The Future of Self-Help." *Social Policy*, Vol. 27, No. 3, Spring 1997.
2. Epstein, Arnold. "U.S. Teaching Hospitals in the Evolving Health Care System." *Journal of the American Medical Association*, Vol. 273, No. 15, April 19, 1995.
3. Hathaway, Stacey. "The Intelligent Patient's Guide to the Doctor-Patient Relationship: Learning How to Talk So Your Doctor Will Listen." *Library Journal*, Vol. 122, No. 16, October 1, 1997.
4. Podell, Richard, and William Proctor. *When Your Doctor Doesn't Know Best*. New York: Simon & Schuster, 1995.
5. Hale, Ralph. "The Obstetrician and Gynecologist: Primary Care Physician or Specialist." *American Journal of Obstetrics & Gynecology*, Vol 171, No. 4, April 1995. Gerbie, Albert. "The Obstetrician-Gynecologist: Specialist and Primary Care Physician."*American Journal of Obstetrics & Gynecology*, Vol. 171, No. 4, April 1995.
6. Turkington, Richard. "Medical Record Confidentiality Law, Scientific Research, and Data Collection in the Information Age." *Journal of Law, Medicine & Ethics*, Vol. 25, No. 2–3, Summer–Fall 1997.
7. Lundberg, George. "The Failure of Organized Health System Reform—Now What?" *Journal of the American Medical Association*, Vol. 273, No. 19, May 17, 1995.
8. Barron, Bruce. "The Price of Managed Care." *Commentary*, Vol. 103, No. 5, May 1997.
9. Podell, Richard, and William Proctor. "Watching Out for Yourself." *Remedy*, March–April 1995. Vladeck, Bruce. "Managed Care and Quality." *Journal of the American Medical Association*, Vol. 273, No. 19, May 17, 1995. McCann, Karen. *Take Charge of Your Hospital Stay: A "Start Smart" Guide for Patients and Care Partners*. New York: Insight Books, Plenum Press, 1994.
10. Barron, "The Price of Managed Care."
11. Carey, Mary Agnes. "Managed Care Faces Showdown over Federal Regulation. *Congressional Quarterly Weekly Report*, Vol. 55, No. 46, November 22, 1997.
12. Evans, M. Stanton. "If You're in an HMO, Here's Why." *Consumer Research Magazine*, Vol. 80, No. 12, December 1997.
13. "Health Care Services." *Forbes*, Vol. 161, No. 1, January 12, 1998.
14. Nuland, Sherwin. "Medical Fads: Bran, Midwives and Leeches." *New York Times*, June 25, 1995. Richardson, W. Scott, et al. "Users' Guides to the Medical Literature." *Journal of the American Medical Association*, Vol. 273, No. 20, May 24–31, 1995.
15. Parrish, Michael. "On-Line Medical Advice." *American Health*, October 1996.
16. Elder, Nancy. "Use of Alternative Health Care by Family Practice Patients." *Journal of the American Medical Association*, Vol. 278, No. 1, July 2, 1997.
17. Wadman, Meredith. "Row over Alternative Medicine's Status at NIH." *Nature*, Vol. 389, No. 6652, October 16, 1997.
18. Micozzi, Marc. "The Need for Research on 'Complementary' Medicine." *Chronicle of Higher Education*, Vol. 44, No. 14, November 28, 1997.
19. Marwick, Charles. "Acceptance of Some Acupuncture Applications." *Journal of the American Medical Association*, Vol. 278, No. 231, December 3, 1997.
20. Tyler, Varro. "The Herbal Remedies Market." *Chemtech*, May 1997.
21. Katzenstein, Larry. "Protesting Homeopathic Products." *American Health*, May 1995.

ALMANAC

▷ **HEALTH INFORMATION ON THE INTERNET**

▶ **EMERGENCY!**

▶ **A CONSUMER'S GUIDE TO MEDICAL TESTS**

▶ **COUNTING YOUR CALORIES AND FAT**

▷ **YOUR HEALTH DIRECTORY**

HEALTH INFORMATION ON THE INTERNET

Using the Internet

The Internet: A Gateway to Health Information

What are the very latest statistics on the incidence of AIDS? Are any new drugs in the works for the treatment of diabetes? How can I get in touch with others who suffer from asthma? Is it possible to make a low-fat chocolate cake? These are the kinds of questions you can answer from your home or computer lab, with the help of the Internet. The Internet is a gold mine of information for the student of health. It can help you with research for your schoolwork, and also with personal questions and concerns about your own health. But the Internet is not comprehensively catalogued, and finding the information you need can be daunting. This guide will introduce you to health resources on the Internet and how to find them.

When you first start to explore the world of the Internet, it can seem overwhelming. What are the practical uses of the Internet for the student of health and the health care consumer?

- *Educational resources.* Most colleges and universities now have Internet hosts and World Wide Web sites. Faculty often post course information and syllabi on line, and some courses are even offered entirely on line. Some instructors require students to do tutorials or other projects on the Internet, or to do research using the Internet. In addition, you may be able to get general information about your school, its policies, programs, graduation requirements, and faculty on the Net.

- *Research.* The Internet is a repository for many health journals, government statistics, archives, and other sources of scholarly information. In addition, subscribing to a mailing list or posting to a newsgroup in an area of interest can yield new sources of information that would be hard to get elsewhere.

- *Graduate school and career information.* The Internet is a great resource for those interested in a career in a health-related field. Most graduate schools have Web sites that list their programs, entrance requirements, faculty profiles, and other information of interest to prospective students. And once you get that degree you can consult on line listings of jobs available in many areas of health care.

- *Self-help and support.* The Internet is a good way of providing information and support to people who might not otherwise have access to it. There are dozens of newsgroups and mailing lists that offer support and advice for people dealing with all kinds of health-related issues, from Alzheimer's caregivers to people with eating disorders to athletes comparing training programs.

- *Goods and services.* As many people have discovered, the Web can serve as an electronic shopping mall. For people with concerns about health it can be a place to order books, software, or journals of interest, sign up for classes or conferences, or even get online professional consultations (though we're not recommending that).

The World Wide Web

The World Wide Web is an information retrieval system designed to offer a user-friendly graphical interface with the Internet. You can surf the Web using any one of a number of different programs called browsers, such as Netscape or Microsoft Explorer. Many Web sites now offer exciting capabilities, such as audio, video, animation clips, and interactivity. Each Web site has its own unique address, or URL. URLs often begin with the characters http://. To go to a Web site, you can either type its URL into the box at the top of your browser, or click on a hyperlink from another page that will take you to the new site. Hyperlinks often appear as color or underlined text, and offer links to other Web sites that may be of interest.

There are thousands of sites related to health and wellness on the World Wide Web. As a starting point, you can try using any of the sources listed in the Resources section of this appendix. Or you can try to look for specific information by doing a Web search.

Bookmarks

When you find a website you will want to return to again in the future, you can "bookmark" it. To bookmark a site, go to that site and choose "bookmark" from your menu bar. Your browser will record the address of that site in your bookmark folder. Anytime you want to return to that site, you simply open the bookmark folder and click on the title of that website.

Tips for Using the World Wide Web

- *Be patient.* Accessing a Web site can take time depending on how elaborate the site is, how fast your modem can download the information, and what time of day you are surfing. You can speed things up a bit by turning off the "auto load image" option in your browser.

- *Keep in mind that glitches can occur in the transfer process.* Sometimes the server of the Web site you are trying to reach may be down, there may be a lot of activity on that site, or there may be line noise. Just try again to load the Web site, or try again later.

- *Because the Web is so dynamic, sites and links change every day.* You might find some links on Web pages that go nowhere, if the link has moved their pages to a new server or address.

- *Remember that while the Web is a great source of information, not everything on it is true.* It is up to you to evaluate the information you get from the Web; see the section on Thinking Critically about Health Information on the Internet.

Searching the Web

How do you go about finding Web sites that might interest you? One way is to use one of the popular directories on the Web called search engines. A search engine allows you to type in keywords on the topic that you are interested in, and it will retrieve sites that contain those words. Some of the larger and more popular search engines are:

- **Yahoo!**

  http://www.yahoo.com

- **Alta Vista**

  http://altavista.digital.com

- **Excite**

  http://www.excite.com

- **Hot Bot**

  http://www.hotbot.com

- **Lycos**

  http://www.lycos.com

- **Infoseek**

  http://www.infoseek.com

- **WebCrawler**

  http://webcrawler.com

To use a search engine, type in one of the URLs listed above. When the home page for the site comes up you will notice a "search" box in which you can type one or more key words or phrases. The engine will then search all the sites in its index and return a list to you, with hyperlinks and sometimes short descriptions, of those that contain your keywords.

There is no single search engine that contains all the contents of the Internet. After connecting to a search engine for the first time, it is a good idea to read the tool's description, search options, and rules and restrictions. Each engine offers a different "view" of the Web and you'll want to tailor your query to make the best use of that system. Some search engines contain indexes to huge amounts of online information, so it pays to make precise queries so you don't get thousands of sites returned to you. It is also possible to make queries that are too precise and retrieve no results.

The key to an effective search is picking the right keywords. Commonly used words make poor search keywords; try to find distinctive words or combinations of words. If you use several keywords, separate them with one of these three operators: AND, OR, and NOT. Using the word AND actually narrows the results you obtain in a search. For example, if you search for "pregnancy AND teen," you will get back only sites that contain both these keywords. The word "OR" broadens the search results. You may try searching "pregnancy AND teen OR adolescent," to find sites that refer to teen or adolescent pregnancy. To limit your results, you can use the word NOT. Searching for "pregnancy AND teen NOT United States" might help you find sites that deal with teen pregnancy in other countries.

Now that you have done your search, you may end up with hundreds or even thousands of results—or only a few. If you have more results than you can handle, try making the keywords in your search more precise. See if you can think of words that uniquely identify what you are looking for, and use several relevant keywords. If you have too few results, try another search engine, using synonyms or variations on your keywords, or be less specific in your query.

Newsgroups

Newsgroups are a way of discussing topics over the Internet with other people who share the same interests or concerns. They are a popular way to establish an online community, share information, and give and receive support. For example, a person suffering from a relatively rare disorder may not know anyone else with the same problems and concerns on campus or in town, but he or she can frequent a newsgroup specifically for people with that disorder to learn about other peoples' experiences, the latest treatments, and just to commiserate. Or a person who is trying to quit smoking can participate in a newsgroup to share frustrations, tips, and successes. But, as always, be aware that not everything posted to a newsgroup is necessarily true; you must be a critical thinker.

Many commercial online services offer members-only newsgroups to their subscribers, but there are many other newsgroups available to anyone. To find a newsgroup on a topic of interest to you, try looking on the Deja News Web page, http://www.dejanews.com, which lists hundreds of newsgroups. Some health-related newsgroups are listed in the Resources section of this appendix.

Newsgroup addresses are grouped into several broad categories called hierarchies. Listed below are some of the standard hierarchies that relate to health.

- **alt**

  groups generally alternative in nature (i.e., alt.sex)

- **bionet**

  groups discussing biology and biological sciences (i.e., bionet.immunology)

- **misc**

  groups that don't fit into other categories (i.e., misc.fitness)

- **rec**

  groups discussing hobbies, sports, music, and art (i.e., rec.food)

- **sci**

  groups discussing subjects related to science and scientific research (i.e., sci.epidemiology)

- **soc**

  groups discussing social issues including politics, social programs, etc. (i.e., soc.college)

- **talk**

  public debating forums on controversial issues (i.e., talk.abortion)

Before you make a posting to a newsgroup, you may want to "lurk" for awhile, that is, read the discussion without contributing your own posting. Lurking will give you a sense of the kinds of postings that are appropriate for that newsgroup and what the newsgroup culture is like. It is also a good idea to read the newsgroup's "FAQ," or list of answers to frequently asked questions.

Postings to many newsgroups are

updated frequently, so if an item is of interest to you, you should print it or save it to your computer since it may be gone the next day. After lurking for awhile, you can join in the discussion by posting a message to the newsgroup. You may also want to reply only to the originator of a certain message. You may want to join in on the discussion of an already-existing topic, or start your own "thread."

Mailing Lists

Mailing lists (or listservs) are groups of people who "get together" via e-mail to discuss a specific topic. Mailing lists offer a way to participate in lively discussions, stay up on current research, or find out answers to burning questions. There are mailing lists on nearly every topic imaginable. Mailing lists are similar to newsgroups in that they are forums for discussion, but the messages are delivered to your e-mail account instead of to a public bulletin board. Here's how it works:

- First, find a mailing list dealing with a subject you are interested in discussing with others (i.e., attention deficit disorder). A good list of health-related mailing lists can be found on the Good Health Web site, http://www.social.com/health/mlists. html.

- In order to get involved in a discussion group, you have to subscribe to it. To subscribe, send an e-mail to that mailing list's "subscribe" address with the word "subscribe" in the subject line and in the main body of the text. Also include your e-mail address.

- Usually, the listserv will then subscribe you to the list and send you instructions on how to "post" to the group. "Posting" means that you send out a comment to the entire mailing list that you have subscribed to.

- Every time any member posts to the listserv, all the subscribers get that posting as an e-mail message in their mailbox.

- Once you have subscribed you will begin to receive e-mail messages from the mailing list. Be careful though: some discussion groups have a large

following and you may find your mailbox filling up faster than you can read the messages.

- Again, evaluate carefully any information you get from a mailing list to make sure it is accurate.

Thinking Critically About Health Information on the Internet

Unlike information in most books and journals, anyone can post information or advice on the Internet. Some of this information can be misleading or downright harmful, so it is important to use your best critical thinking skills to evaluate health information you find on the Internet. When evaluating information on the Net, ask yourself the following questions.

- *Who is the author or sponsor of the information?* The author of the site is usually listed at the top or bottom of a site's home page. Be very wary of any anonymous site. Sites that are maintained by established schools or universities, government agencies, professional organizations, or other established organizations like the American Cancer Society are probably trustworthy. Sites created by individuals or other groups may or may not contain valid information; see if you can verify their information in other places. And keep in mind that many sites contain links to other pages which may be maintained by other less (or more) reliable sources.

- *Is it current?* Many sites post the date of their most recent modification. Look for sites where you can determine when the information was created or modified; many of the best sites are updated weekly or even daily.

- *What is the purpose of the site?* The hidden purpose of some health Web sites is to sell products or act as a vehicle for advertisements. Be wary of any site that tries to sell you things or get your money. Also beware of sites that seem to be trying to persuade you of things, promote "miracle cures" or anything that seems too good to be true. There are also people who use newsgroups and other chat forums to

sell or persuade. Be skeptical and use your common sense.

- *Who is the intended audience?* Some Internet information is intended for doctors and other health care professionals; although the information may be accurate, it may be too difficult for a layperson to interpret on his or her own. Other Web sites or Internet forums are targeted toward people with specific problems or disorders, students, or the general public.

- *Is the information verifiable?* To get a better perspective on information from the Internet, see if you can verify it with other sources. Before you follow any health advice you get from the Net, check it out with your physician.

Health Resources on the Internet

General Health Resources

Centers for Disease Control and Prevention
http://www.cdc.gov

National Health Information Center (NHIC)
http://nhic-nt.health.org/

Yahoo Health Directory
http://www.yahoo.com/health

Achoo Health Directory
http://www.achoo.com/

American Medical Association
http://www.ama-assn.org

Go Ask Alice
http://www.columbia.edu/cu/health-wise/all.html

Healthfinder
http://www.healthfinder.gov/

Health A to Z
http://www.HealthAtoZ.com

Duke University Diet and Fitness Center Home Page
http://dmi-www.mc.duke.edu/dfc/home.html

Healthy People 2000
http://odphp.osophs.dhhs.gov/pubs/hp2000/

Mental, Emotional, and Spiritual Health

National Institute of Mental Health (NIMH)
http://www.nimh.nih.gov/

Psych Central: Dr. John Grohol's Mental Health Page
http://www.coil.com/~grohol/

Internet Mental Health
http://www.mentalhealth.com/

American Psychological Association
http://www.apa.org

National Depressive/Manic-Depressive Association
http://www.ndmda.org/

Stress Management
http://www.ivf.com/stress.html

Stress Busters
http://stressrelease.com/strssbus.html

Stress, Depression, Anxiety, Sleep Problems, and Drug Use
http://www.teachhealth.com/

Trauma Info Pages
http://gladstone.uoregon.edu/~dvb/trauma.htm

The International Society for Traumatic Stress Studies
http://istss.com

Newsgroups
- alt.support.anxiety-panic
- alt.support.depression
- alt.support.loneliness
- alt.support.sleep-disorders
- soc.support.depression.crisis
- soc.support.dpression.family
- soc.support.depression.manic
- soc.support.depression.misc
- soc.support.depression.seasonal
- soc.support.depression.treatment
- alt.support.ocd
- alt.support.schizophrenia
- alt.support.shyness

Fitness

The Fitness Partner Connection Jumpsite
http://www.primusweb.com/fitnesspartner/

The Internet's Fitness Resource
http://www.netsweat.com

President's Council on Physical Fitness and Sports
http://phs.os.dhhs.gov/progorg/ophs/pcpfs.htm

Worldguide Online
http://www.worldguide.com/Fitness/

Stretching Information
http://www.enteract.com/~bradapp/docs/rec/stretching/stretching_1.html

American College of Sports Medicine (ACSM)
http://www.a1.com/sportsmed/

Newsgroups
- misc.fitness
- misc.fitness.aerobic
- rec.fitness

Nutrition and Eating Issues

FDA Center for Food Safety and Applied Nutrition
http://vm.cfsan.fda.gov/list.html

USDA Food and Nutrition Information Center
http://www.nal.usda.gov/fnic/

Diet Analysis Web Page
http://dawp.anet.com/

Fast Food Finder
http://www.olen.com/food/

Virtual Vegetarian
http://www.vegetariantimes.com/

Center for Science in the Public Interest
http://www.cspinet.org/

Meals Online
http://www.meals.com

The Overeaters Recovery Group
http://recovery.hiwaay.net/

Overeaters Anonymous
http://www.overeatersanonymous.org/

Cyberdiet
http://www.cyberdiet.com/

Light Cooking
http://www.lightliving.com/

Eating Disorders
http://www.something-fishy.org

Newsgroups
- sci.med.nutrition
- alt.support.diet
- alt.support.obesity
- alt.support.big-folks
- alt.support.eating-diord

Sexuality

Planned Parenthood
http://www.ppfa.org/ppfa/

Ultimate Birth Control Links Page
http://gynpages.com/ultimate/

Association of Voluntary and Safe Contraception International
http://www.avsc.org/avsc/

National Abortion Federation
http://www.prochoice.org/

National Abortion and Reproductive Rights League
http://www.naral.org/

National Right to Life Committee
http://www.nrlc.org/

Labor and Birth Resources
http://www.childbirth.org/articles/labor.html

International Council on Infertility Information Dissemination
http://www.inciid.org

Pregnancy, Reproduction, and Health Education
http://www.childbirth.org/

It's Just Another Baby
http://www.westnet.com/~crywalt/pregnancy/

The Kinsey Institute for Research in Sex, Gender, and Reproduction
http://www.indiana.edu/~kinsey/

The Institute for Advanced Study of Human Sexuality
http://www.netinc.ca/~sexorg/

Sexology Netline
http://www.netinc.ca/~sexorg/

Sexuality Information and Education Council of the United States (SIECUS)
http://www.siecus.org/

The Johns Hopkins University STD Page
http://www.med.jhu.edu/jhustd/

The Safer Sex Page
http://www.safersex.org/

American Social Health Association
http://metalab.unc.edu/ASHA/

Newsgroups
- sci.med.midwifery
- sci.med.obgyn
- alt.infertility.primary
- alt.infertility.secondary
- misc.health.infertility
- soc.support.pregnancy.loss
- alt.support.breastfeeding
- alt.support.childfree
- talk.abortion
- alt.support.abortion
- alt.support.herpes
- alt.sex.safe

Diseases and Disorders

CDC National AIDS Clearinghouse
http://www.cdcnac.org/

The CDC HIV/AIDS Page
http://www.cdc.gov/diseases/hivqa.html

Harvard AIDS Institute
http://www.hsph.harvard.edu/Organizations/hai/home_pg.html

UCSF AIDS Health Project
http://www.ucsf-ahp.org/

HIV Infoweb
http://carebase2.jri.org/infoweb/

Newsgroups
- sci.med.aids
- misc.health.aids
- clari.tw.health.aids
- alt.sex.safe

American Cancer Society
http://www.cancer.org

National Cancer Institute
http:www.nci.nih.gov/

Med Help International/Cancer Library
http://medhlp.netusa.net/general/cancer2/cancerpt.htm

OncoLink/The University of Pennsylvania Cancer Center Resource
http://cancer.med.upenn.edu/

Newsgroups
- sci.med.diseases.cancer
- alt.support.cancer
- alt.support.cancer.prostate
- alt.support.cancer.testicular

American Heart Association
http://www.amhrt.org

Heart and Stroke Foundation of Canada
http://www.hsf.ca/

The Heart: An Online Exploration
http://www.fi.edu/biosci/heart.html

Cut to the Heart
http://www.pbs.org/wgbh/pages/nova/heart/

Newsgroups
- sci.med.cardiology
- alt.support.heart

Drug Use, Misuse, and Abuse

Alcoholics Anonymous
http://www.alcoholics-anonymous.org

National Institute on Alcohol Abuse and Alcoholism
http://www.niaaa.nih.gov/

National Association for Children of Alcoholics
http://www.health.org/nacoa/

Web of Addictions
http://www.well.com/user/woa/

Al-Anon/Alateen
http://solar.rtd..utk.edu/~al-anon/

Habitsmart
http://www.cts.com/crash/habtsmrt/

Newsgroups
- alt.recovery
- clari.news.alcohol

National Institute on Drug Abuse
http://www.nida.nih.gov

Higher Education Center for Alcohol and Other Drug Prevention
http://www.edc.org/hec/

Cocaine Anonymous World Services
http://www.ca.org/

Narcotics Anonymous
http://www.na.org/index.htm

National Organization for the Reform of Marijuana Laws
http://www.natlnorml.org/

CDC's Tobacco Information and Prevention Sourcepage
http://www.cdc.gov/tobacco/

Prevention Online
http://www.health.org/

NicNet: Nicotine and Tobacco Network
http://www.acsc.arizona.edu/nicnet/

Tobacco Control Resource Center
http://www.tobacco.neu.edu/

The Quitnet
http://www.quitnet.org/

Smokescreen Tobacco Central Network
http://www.Smokescreen.org

Newsgroups
- alt.support.stop-smoking
- alt.support.non-smokers
- alt.support.non-smokers.moderated
- clari.news.smoking
- sci.med.cannabis
- alt.support.recovery.na
- alt.drugs
- clari.news.drugs
- talk.politics.drugs

Planning for Tomorrow

American Environmental Health Foundation
http://www.aehf.com/

The Envirolink
http://www.envirolink.org/

Environmental Protection Agency
http://www.epa.gov/

Environmental Organization Web Directory
http://www.webdirectory.com

Medscout
http://www.medref.com

MedScape
http://www.medscape.com/

Idea Central Health Policy Page
http://epn.org/idea/health.html

The Alternative Medicine Homepage
http://www.pitt.edu/~cbw/altm.html

Caregiver Survival Resources
http://www.caregiver911.com/

Administration on Aging
http://www.aoa.dhhs.gov/

The Alzheimer's Page
http://www.biostat.wustl.edu/alzheimer/

The National Council on the Aging
http://www.ncoa.org/

University of Texas Medical Branch Center on Aging
http://sagesite.utmb.edu/

Choice in Dying
http://www.choices.org/

The Compassionate Friends
http://www.compassionatefriends.org

Hospice Hands
http://hospice-cares.com/

Newsgroups
- clari.news.aging
- alt.support.alzheimers
- bionet.neuroscience.amyloid
- alt.support.grief
- soc.support.pregnancy.loss

EMERGENCY!

By definition, an emergency is a situation in which you have to think and act fast. Start by assessing the circumstances. Shout for help if you're in a public place. Look for any possible dangers to you or the victim, such as a live electrical wire or a fire. Seek medical assistance as quickly as possible. Dial 911, the operator, or a local emergency phone number, and keep it near every phone in your house. Don't attempt rescue techniques, such as cardiopulmonary resuscitation (CPR), unless you are trained. If you have a car, be sure you know the shortest route from your home to the nearest 24-hour hospital emergency department.

Supplies

Every home should have a kit of basic first aid supplies kept in a convenient location out of the reach of children. Stock it with the following:

- Bandages
- Sterile gauze pads and bandages
- Adhesive tape
- Scissors
- Cotton balls or absorbent cotton
- Cotton swabs
- Thermometer
- Syrup of ipecac to induce vomiting
- Antibiotic ointments
- Sharp needle
- Safety pins
- Calamine lotion

Keep a similar kit in your car or boat. You might want to add some extra items from your home, such as a flashlight, soap, blanket, paper cups, and any special equipment that a family member with a chronic illness may need.

Bleeding

Blood loss is frightening and dangerous. Direct pressure stops external bleeding. Since internal bleeding can also be life-threatening, you must be aware of the warning signs.

For an Open Wound

1. Apply direct pressure over the site of the wound. Cover the entire wound.

2. Use sterile gauze, a sanitary napkin, a clean towel, sheet, or handkerchief or, if necessary, your washed bare hand. Ice or cold water in a pad will help stop bleeding and decrease swelling.

3. Apply firm, steady pressure for five to fifteen minutes. Most wounds stop bleeding within a few minutes.

4. If the wound is on a foot, hand, leg, or arm, use gravity to help slow the flow of blood. Elevate the limb so that it is higher than the victim's heart.

5. If the bleeding doesn't stop, press harder.

6. Seek medical attention if the bleeding was caused by a serious injury, if stitches will be needed to keep the wound closed, or if the victim has not had a tetanus booster within the last ten years.

For Internal Bleeding

1. Suspect internal bleeding if a person coughs up blood, vomits red or brown material that looks like coffee grounds, passes blood in urine or stool, or has black, tarlike bowel movements.

2. Do not let the victim take any medication or fluids by mouth until seen by a doctor, because surgery may be necessary.

3. Have the victim lie flat. Cover him or her lightly.

4. Seek immediate medical attention.

For a Bloody Nose

1. Have the victim sit down, leaning slightly forward so the blood does not run down his or her throat. The person should spit out any blood in his or her mouth.

2. Use the thumb and forefingers to pinch the nose. If the victim can do the pinching, apply a cold compress to the nose and surrounding area.

3. Apply pressure for ten minutes without interruption.

4. If pinching does not work, gently pack the nostril with gauze or a clean strip of cloth. Do not use absorbent cotton, which will stick. Let the ends hang out so you can remove the packing easily later. Pinch the nose, with the packing in place, for five minutes.

5. If a foreign object is in the nose, do not attempt to remove it. Ask the person to blow gently. If that does not work, seek medical attention.

6. The nose should not be blown or irritated for several hours after a nosebleed stops.

Breathing Problems

If a person appears to be unconscious, approach carefully. The victim may be in contact with electrical current. If so, make sure the electricity is shut off before touching the victim. The first function you should check is respiration. Tap or shake the victim's shoulder gently, shouting, "Are you all right?" Look for any signs of breathing: Can you hear breath sounds? Can you feel breath on your cheek? If the person is breathing, do not perform mouth-to-mouth resuscitation.

If you aren't certain if the victim is breathing, or if there are no signs of breath, follow these steps:

1. Lay the person on his or her back on the floor or ground. Roll the victim over if necessary, being careful to turn the head with the remainder of the body as a unit to avoid possible neck injury. Loosen any tight clothing around the neck or chest.

2. Check for any foreign material in the mouth or throat and remove it quickly.

3. Open the airway by tilting the head back and lifting the chin up.

4. Pinch the nostrils shut with your thumb and index finger.

5. Take a deep breath, open your mouth wide and place it securely over the victim's, and give two slow breaths, each lasting 1 to 10 seconds. Remove your mouth, turn your head, and check to see if the victim's chest rises and falls. If you hear air escaping from the victim's mouth and see

the chest fall, you know that you are getting air into the lungs.

6. Repeat once every five seconds (twelve breaths per minute) until professional help takes over, or the victim begins breathing on his or her own. It may take several hours to revive someone. If you stop, the victim may not be able to breathe on his or her own. Once the person does begin to breathe independently, always get professional help.

7. If air doesn't seem to be entering the chest, or the chest doesn't fall between breaths, tilt the head further back. If that doesn't work, follow the directions for choking emergencies later in this section.

8. If the victim is a child, do not pinch the nose shut. Cover both the mouth and nose with your mouth, and place your free hand very lightly on the child's chest. Use small puffs of air rather than big breaths. Feel the chest inflate as you blow, and listen for exhaled air. Repeat once every three seconds (twenty breaths per minute).

Broken Bones

If you suspect that a person has broken a leg, do not move him or her unless there is immediate danger.

1. Check for signs of breathing. If there is none or breathing is very weak, administer mouth-to-mouth resuscitation.

2. If the person is bleeding, apply direct pressure on the site of the wound.

3. Try to keep the victim warm and calm.

4. Do not try to push a broken bone back into place if it is sticking out of the skin. You can apply a moist dressing to prevent it from drying out.

5. Do not try to straighten out a fracture.

6. Do not allow the victim to walk.

7. Splint unstable fractures to prevent painful motion.

Burns

1. If fire caused the burn, cool the affected area with water to stop the burning process.

2. Remove the victim's garments and jewelry and cover him or her with clean sheets or towels.

3. Call for help immediately.

4. If chemicals caused the burn, wash the affected area with cool water for at least twenty minutes. Chemical burns of the eye require immediate medical attention after flushing with water for twenty minutes.

Choking

A person with anything stuck in the throat and blocking the airway can stop breathing, lose consciousness, and die within four to six minutes. A universal signal of distress because of choking is clasping the throat with one or both hands. Other signs are an inability to talk and noisy, difficult breathing. You need to take immediate action, but *NEVER* slap the victim's back. This could make the obstruction worse.

If the victim can speak, cough, or breathe, do not interfere. Coughing alone may dislodge the foreign object. if the choking continues without lessening, call for medical help.

If the victim cannot speak, cough, or breathe but is conscious, use the Heimlich maneuver, as follows

1. Stand behind the victim (who may be seated or standing) and wrap your arms around his or her waist.

2. Make a fist with one hand and place the thumb side of your fist against the victim's abdomen, just above the navel. Grasp your fist with your other hand and press into his or her abdomen with a quick, upward thrust. Do not exert any pressure against the rib cage with your forearms.

3. Repeat this procedure until the victim is no longer choking or loses consciousness.

4. If the person is lying facedown, roll the victim over. Facing the person, kneel with your legs astride his or her hips. Put the heel of one hand below the rib cage and place your other hand on top. Press into the abdomen with a quick, upward thrust. Repeat thrusts as needed.

5. If you start choking when you're by yourself, place your fist below your rib cage and above your navel. Grasp this fist with your other hand and press into your abdomen with a quick, upward thrust. You also can lean over a fixed, horizontal object, such as a table edge or chair back, and press your upper abdomen against it with a quick, upward thrust. Repeat as needed until you dislodge the object.

If the Victim Is Unconscious

1. Place him or her on the ground and give mouth-to-mouth resuscitation as described earlier.

2. If the victim does not start breathing and air does not seem to be going into his or her lungs, roll the victim onto his or her back and give one or more manual thrusts: Place one of your hands on top of the other with the heel of the bottom hand in the middle of the abdomen, slightly above the navel and below the rib cage. Press into the abdomen with a quick, upward thrust. Do not push to either side. Repeat 6 to 10 times as needed.

3. Clear the airway. Hold the victim's mouth open with one hand and use your thumb to depress the tongue. Make a hook with the index finger of your other hand and, using a gentle, sweeping motion, reach into the victim's throat and feel for a swallowed foreign object in the airway.

4. Repeat the following steps in this sequence:

   –00 Six to ten abdominal thrusts
   • Probe in mouth
   • Try to inflate lungs
   • Repeat

5. If the victim suddenly seems okay, but no foreign material has been removed, take him or her directly to the hospital. A foreign object, such as a fish or chicken bone or other jagged object, could do internal damage as it passes through the victim's system.

If the Victim Is a Child

1. If the child is coughing, do nothing. The coughing alone may dislodge the object.

2. If the airway is blocked and the child is panicky and fighting for breath, do *NOT* probe the airway with your fingers to clear an unseen foreign object. You might push the material back into the airway, worsening the obstruction.

3. For an infant younger than a year, hang the child over your arm so that the head is lower than the trunk. Using the heel of your hand, administer four firm blows high on the back between the shoulder blades. For a bigger child, follow the same procedure, but invert the child over your knee rather than your arm.

4. After four back blows, perform four chest thrusts (the Heimlich maneuver as described above).

Drowning

A person can die of drowning four to six minutes after breathing stops. Although prevention is the wisest course, follow these steps in case of a drowning emergency:

1. Get the victim out of the water fast. Be extremely cautious, because a drowning person may panic and grasp at a rescuer, endangering that individual as well. If possible, push a branch or pole within the victim's reach.

2. If the victim is unconscious, use a flotation device if at all possible. Carefully place the person on the device. Once out of the water, place the victim on his or her back.

3. If the victim is not breathing, start mouth-to-mouth resuscitation Continue until the person can breathe unassisted or help arrives. (Note that it may take an hour or two for a drowning victim to resume independent breathing.) Do not leave the victim alone for any reason.

4. Once the person is breathing without assistance, even if he or she is still coughing, you need only stay nearby until professional help arrives.

Electrical Shock

1. If you suspect that an electrical shock has knocked a person unconscious,

approach very carefully. Do not touch the victim unless the electricity has been turned off.

2. Shut off the power at the plug, circuit breaker, or fuse box. Simply shutting off an appliance does not remove the shock hazard. Use a dry stick to move a wire or downed power line from the victim. Keep in mind that you also are in danger until the power is off.

3. If the person's breathing is weak or has stopped, follow the steps for mouth-to-mouth resuscitation.

4. Even if the victim returns to consciousness, call for medical help. While waiting, cover the victim with a blanket or coat to keep him or her warm. Place a blanket underneath the body if the surface is cold. Be sure the person lies flat if conscious, with legs raised. If the victim is unconscious, place him or her on one side, with a pillow supporting the head. Do not give the victim anything to eat or drink.

5. Electrical burns can extend deep into the tissue, even when they appear minor. Do not put butter, household remedies, or sprays on burns without a doctor's instruction. Do not use ice or cold water on an electrical burn that is more than two inches across.

Heart Attack

Chest pain can be caused by indigestion, strained muscles, or lung infections. The warning signs of a heart attack are:

- Intense pain that lasts for more than two minutes, produces a tight or crushing feeling, is centered in the chest, or spreads to the neck, jaw, shoulder, or arm
- Shortness of breath that is worse when the person lies flat and improves when the person sits
- Heavy sweating
- Nausea or vomiting
- Irregular pulse
- Pale or bluish skin or lips
- Weakness
- Severe anxiety, feeling of doom

If an individual develops these symptoms:

1. Call for emergency medical help immediately.

2. Have the person sit up or lie in a semi-reclining position. Loosen tight clothing. Keep him or her comfortably warm.

3. If the person loses consciousness, turn on his or her back and check for breathing and pulse. If vomiting occurs, turn the victim's head to one side and clean the mouth.

4. If the person has medicine for angina pectoris (chest pain) and is conscious, help him or her take it.

5. If the person is unconscious, and you are trained to perform cardiopulmonary resuscitation (CPR), check for a pulse at the wrist or neck. If there is none, begin CPR in conjunction with mouth-to-mouth resuscitation. Do not attempt CPR unless you are trained. It is not a technique you can learn from a book.

Poisoning

Many common household substances, including glue, aspirin, bleaches, and paint, can be poisonous. Make sure you know the emergency numbers for the Poison Control Center and Fire Department Rescue Squad. Keep them near your telephone. Be prepared to provide the following information:

- The kind of substance swallowed and how much was swallowed
- If a child or adult swallowed the substance
- Symptoms
- Whether or not vomiting has occurred
- Whether you gave the person anything to drink
- How much time it will take to get to an emergency room

The Poison Control Center or rescue team will tell you whether or not to induce vomiting or neutralize a swallowed poison. Here are some additional guidelines:

1. Always assume the worst if a small child has swallowed or might have swallowed something poisonous. Call the local Poison Control Center or emergency number (911 in many

areas). Keep the suspected item or container with you to answer questions.

2. Do not give any medications unless a physician or the Poison Control Center instructs you to do so.

3. Do not follow the directions for neutralizing poisons on the container unless a doctor or the Poison Control Center confirms that they are appropriate measures to take.

4. If the child is conscious, give moderate doses of water to dilute the poison.

5. If a poisoning victim is unconscious, make sure he or she is breathing. If not, give mouth-to-mouth resuscitation. Do not give anything by mouth or attempt to stimulate the person. Call for emergency help immediately.

6. If the person is vomiting, make sure he or she is in a position in which he or she cannot choke on what is brought up.

7. While vomiting is the fastest way to expel swallowed poisons from the body, never try to induce vomiting if the person has swallowed any acid or alkaline substance, which can cause burns of the face, mouth, and throat (examples include ammonia, bleach, dishwasher detergent, drain and toilet cleaners, lye, oven cleaners, or rust removers), or petroleum-like products, which produce dangerous fumes that can be inhaled during vomiting (examples include floor polish, furniture wax, gasoline, kerosene, lighter fluid, turpentine, and paint thinner).

A CONSUMER'S GUIDE TO MEDICAL TESTS

✔ **What They Tell the Doctor**

✔ **How Often You Need Them**

✔ **What to Do About Abnormal Results**

*D*o you wonder what the doctor sees when he looks into your eyes with that little light, or what it means when your blood or urine test is normal? In this section we cover some of the most common tests your doctor does, what they tell, and how often they should be done.

General Information

- Always ask your doctor what tests are being done, why they are being ordered, what they involve, and what the results mean.
- No test is foolproof. If a result is unexpected, whether normal or abnormal, your doctor should repeat the test before making any decisions.
- Modern X-ray machines expose you to a minuscule amount of radiation. Nevertheless, be sure to tell the physician or X-ray technician if there is even a chance you may be pregnant.
- Often a doctor orders a test because that is the only way to prove you do *not* have a disease.

Allergy Skin Testing

- Skin testing is still the most reliable method.
- The physician either pricks your skin twenty to forty or more times to introduce a tiny bit of potentially allergic material or injects a small amount.
- Children who are frightened by multiple needle sticks and are unlikely to sit still for as long as necessary may have blood (RAST) tests instead.

What results mean

If you develop redness or a hivelike bump around an area, you are probably allergic to the injected substance. Sometimes you can avoid the offending material, but things like pollen and dust are everywhere. Your allergist may recommend desensitizing shots to reduce your reaction. Note that the results of skin tests won't be reliable if you take antihistamines within 48 hours of the test.

How often to be tested

Skin tests are necessary only if you cannot get allergy relief from other measures such as over-the-counter medications, reducing mold and dust in the house, and staying away from animals.

Blood-Pressure Reading

- High blood pressure, a major cause of stroke and heart attacks, usually causes no symptoms.
- The upper number in a reading—the systolic—refers to peak amount of pressure generated when your heart pumps blood, the lower number—the diastolic—measures the least amount of pressure.

What results mean

Most doctors today think the lower the pressure the better, which means a reading of 120/80 or less. Because the mere anxiety of having your blood pressure taken can cause a mild elevation, your doctor will want to repeat an abnormal test, ideally on a different day, before diagnosing high blood pressure.

How often to be tested

Everyone—no matter how healthy—should have a blood-pressure reading taken at least once a year, more often if you have high blood pressure

Blood Tests

- Blood may be taken from either a finger prick or, more commonly, a vein in your arm.
- See below for information on cholesterol testing, which is also done from a blood sample.

Complete Blood Count (CBC)

This is the most commonly performed of all blood tests.

What results mean

A *low red-cell count*, called anemia, can be caused by something as simple as too little iron in your diet, as complex as an abnormality in your digestion, or as serious as a bone marrow problem or silent bleeding. Iron deficiency is the most frequent cause, with women who menstruate and limit their intake of red meat at the greatest risk. If your doctor diagnoses this problem, ask about making dietary changes as well as taking iron supplements.

A high white-cell count, a measure of the body's defenses against infection, usually indicates some kind of infection. Depending on the type of cell that predominates, your doctor may be able to identify whether you have a bacterial or viral infection.

Platelets, the first participants in blood clotting, may be decreased because of a viral infection, abnormal bleeding, or for no identifiable reason.

Chemistry Panels (Chem 12 or 18, SMA 12 or 24)

Kidney, bone, liver, pancreas, prostate, and some glandular functions are screened by these tests.

What results mean

An abnormality may signal a problem that needs treatment. Because accuracy decreases when many tests are run together, any specific abnormal test should be repeated, especially if unexpected.

CAT (Computerized Axial Tomography) Scan

- A CAT scan is 100 times more sensitive than an X-ray.

- You lie as motionless as possible in a large tube while an X ray beam travels 360 degrees around you. The test takes about an hour.

What results mean

The test can help diagnose such conditions as tumors, blood clots, cysts, and bleeding in the brain as well as in various other organs.

Cholesterol Test

- Anyone can have a high cholesterol level, but you are more apt to be at risk if there is a family history of early heart attacks, strokes, or high cholesterol tests.

- Your doctor will look at not only total cholesterol but also the levels of high-density lipoprotein (HUL), the "good" cholesterol that prevents cholesterol from sticking to your blood vessels, and low-density lipoprotein (LDL), the "bad" cholesterol that does the reverse.

What results mean

Experts today think optimum cholesterol levels are below 200 mg/ml of blood. The following chart shows the risk by age of various cholesterol levels.

Cholesterol Risk Chart

Age	Moderate Risk	High Risk
20–29	200–220 mg/ml	Over 220
30–39	220–240	Over 240
Over 40	240–260	Over 260

Persistently high cholesterol values will prompt your doctor to advise dietary and lifestyle changes—less fat intake, more exercise—and perhaps medication. This will particularly be the case if LDL levels also are high (less than 130 mg/ml is considered desirable, 130–159 is borderline risk, and over 160 is high risk).

How often to be tested

If your cholesterol level is under 200 and your LDL level is under 130, repeat the test every five years. if your test is borderline, repeat it annually. (Note that the test should be taken when you have not eaten for at least twelve hours.)

If you have a family history of cholesterol problems, have your children tested annually from age 2; if you don't, have them tested around age 10 and every few years thereafter. Children under 2 should not be given a low-cholesterol diet; they need extra fat to make brain tissue and hormones for growth.

Fundoscopy

- The doctor looks into your eye with a little light.

What results mean

The beginnings of cataracts may be visible, as well as irregularities in the blood vessels that indicate damage from high cholesterol (fatty deposits in the blood vessels), high blood pressure (narrowing and notching), diabetes, or other diseases. If the optic nerve is swollen, there may be excess pressure inside your skull.

What your doctor *cannot* see are the early signs of glaucoma, which can lead to blindness if not treated. Over age 20, have a pressure check for glaucoma from an opthalmologist or optometrist every three years—or every year if you have a family history of glaucoma.

Heart Tests

- The following tests are listed from the simplest through the most complicated.

- Also see listings for blood pressure readlings, cholesterol tests, and pulse.

Electrocardiogram (EKG, ECG)

- A machine amplifies the electrical signals from your heart and records them on paper.

What results mean

An EKG can detect such things as an enlarged heart, abnormal levels of potassium or calcium, disease of the small vessels of the heart, and where an abnormal heart rhythm originates. It is a nonspecific test, however, and more advanced studies should be done if serious disease is suspected.

Echocardiogram

This is a painless test in which sound waves are used to produce a picture of the heart in action on a TV-type screen.

What results mean

The test investigates the size of the heart chambers, the thickness of the walls, how the four heart valves are working, and the condition of the membrane surrounding the heart. Mitral valve prolapse, a common minor abnormality, often shows up on this test, as well as more serious problems.

Stress Test

Your heart rate, blood pressure, and EKG are constantly monitored as you exercise on a treadmill that goes faster and faster with a steeper and steeper incline. This test—also called an exercise tolerance test or treadmill test—should be performed in the presence of a cardiologist and in or near a hospital in case the strain causes heart problems that need emergency treatment. The test should be stopped immediately if you experience any lightheadedness, chest pain, nausea, or palpitations.

What results mean

The changes that an increasing strain on the heart causes can tell your doctor if you are at risk of a heart attack. This is because a blockage in the coronary arteries—the blood vessels that feed your heart muscle—may show up only during exercise.

Angiography

A dye is injected into various arteries, and X rays are taken.

What results mean

The doctor can detect blockages in the blood vessels that can lead to heart attack or stroke, as well as aneurysms (weakened spots in the blood-vessel walls). The test carries some risk of causing stroke.

Kidney Tests

- The tests noted here involve taking X rays. In addition, ultrasound (similar to an echocardiogram) can be used to outline the kidneys.

Intravenous Pyelogram (IVP)

After an iodine-containing substance is injected into a vein, X rays are taken at five-minute intervals to show the outlines of the kidney, ureter, and bladder.

What results mean

Tumors, kidney stones, and swelling of the kidney tissue can be seen, as well as blockage to urine flow or a mass that may be pressing on the kidney. A kidney that is not functioning will not appear on the X ray, and one in an abnormal position can be found.

Voiding Cystourethrogram (VCUG)

A technician will fill your bladder with a dye injected through a catheter and take X rays while you urinate.

What results mean

If you have recurrent urinary-tract infections, the test will show if there is a significant backup of urine from the bladder into the ureter, in which case daily antibiotics may be needed to prevent infection. Investigating recurrent urinary tract infections is particularly important for children.

Magnetic Resonance Imaging (MRI)

- MRI uses no radiation but produces pictures of the brain that are much more detailed than those of a CAT scan.

What results mean

In addition to locating bleeding or tumors, as a CAT scan does, the test picks up subtle signs such as those of Parkinson's disease and multiple sclero-sis in the brain or a herniated disc in the spinal column.

Mammography

- Only a small amount of radiation is used to take the mammogram. You usually stand up and put your breast on a photographic plate where it is compressed with a plastic shield or balloonlike device. It shouldn't hurt. If your breasts are tender at certain times in your menstrual cycle, schedule your mammogram when they are least sensitive.
- Mammograms can detect breast abnormalities at easily treated stages before you can feel them, but they are not foolproof. Examine your breasts monthly.

What results mean

Mammograms can detect cysts, abscesses, and tumors. Whether a mass is benign or malignant is hard to tell in the early stages, so abnormalities usually need to be biopsied or removed totally to determine treatment.

How often to be tested

Although there is controversy over the benefits of mammography for women under 50, many experts still recommend having a first mammogram between ages 35 and 40, followed by one every two years between 40 and 50, and yearly thereafter. If your mother or sister has had breast cancer, consult your doctor for an appropriate schedule. And if you have a lump, pain, or nipple discharge, have a mammogram right away, no matter what your age.

You also should have a breast examination by a doctor at least every three years between ages 20 and 40, and every year after 40.

Pap Smear

- A routine part of every gynecological examination.
- Your doctor takes a painless swab from the cervix and vaginal walls and sends it to a lab for analysis.

What results mean

Pap smears can detect not only cervical cancer but also inflammation and many infections, minor and more serious; they also provide important information about the state of your female hormones. A normal test is termed class 1, and abnormal results are graded by degree into four classifications, with only the most severe—a class V test—signifying outright cancer. Treatment depends on the diagnosis and may range from doing nothing for a minor inflammation to, in rare cases, a hysterectomy for cancer. Because the error rate of Pap smears is high, the doctor should always repeat an abnormal test.

How often to be tested

Women who are on birth control pills and are sexually active should have a Pap smear every six months; other women should be checked every year,

Physical Examination

- The routine physical exam generally includes a pulse and blood-pressure reading, measure of height and weight, blood tests (including a cholesterol test), fundoscopy, and sometimes other tests as well, such as a stool test for blood.

What results mean

A physical exam serves as a general measure of health and sometimes picks up early signs of disease.

How often to have a physical exam

Most doctors no longer recommend yearly physicals for everybody. A good schedule to follow instead is to have a complete checkup every four or five years under age 40, every three years between 40 and 50, every two years between 50 and 60, and every year after that. At any age, you should have more frequent examinations if you have chronic medical problems such as diabetes or high blood pressure, are obese, or smoke cigarettes.

Pulse

- To take your own pulse, press two fingertips over the artery in your wrist, just below the base of the thumb. Count the beats in 20 seconds, then multiply by 3.

What results mean

The normal pulse rate—the speed at

which your heart pumps blood—is 60–80 beats a minute; it should be regular, without skipped or extra beats. Abnormal rates can be due to thyroid problems (too high causes a fast rate, too low a slow one), heart problems, anxiety (even the stress of a physical exam), or weakness from an illness such as the flu or other problems.

The character of your pulse is also important. A discrepancy between the strength of the pulse on one side of the neck and the other may mean you are in danger of a stroke. A pulse that is abnormally strong and bounding can signal a problem with a heart valve. if the pulse is weak, you may have blockages in your blood vessels from diabetes, atherosclerosis (hardening of the arteries), or a variety of other disorders.

Stomach and Intestinal Tests

- Though most of these tests are uncomfortable, they generally are not painful.

Barium Enema

Barium, a radioactive material, is instilled in your large intestine through a tube inserted into your anus. Because barium is constipating, drink fluids afterward. Don't be alarmed if you have white stools for a day or two.

What results mean

The doctor will be able to see tumors or polyps, any obstructions, and other abnormalities.

Gastroscopy and Proctoscopy

In gastroscopy, for which you will be sedated, the doctor looks into the stomach with a flexible tube that goes through your mouth. The procedure is essentially the same for protoscopy, except that the doctor looks into your large intestine through a tube inserted into your anus.

What results mean

Your doctor can see where bleeding comes from, remove a polyp, or biopsy a mass.

Upper GI Series

You will be asked to down a drink of barium so that X rays can be taken of the esophagus, stomach, duodenum, and sometimes the small intestine.

What results mean

Your doctor can diagnose swallowing disorders, hiatus hernias, ulcers, tumors, and some inflammations of the stomach and small bowel.

Stool Test for Occult Blood

A small sample of stool that remains on the doctor's glove after a rectal exam or that is collected by you at home is tested for blood that is invisible to the eye.

What results mean

This test is done routinely as part of a regular checkup to detect the earliest sign of cancer of the colon. it is also part of an investigation of anemia or abdominal pain. If your test is positive, tell your doctor if you recently ate radishes, turnips, or red meat, took large doses of vitamin C or iron pills, or had a nosebleed. All of these things can produce misleading results.

Urinalysis

- Urine can tell about the health not only of the kidneys but also of other organ systems.

What results mean

Specific gravity is the degree to which your urine is concentrated or diluted. If it is persistently too dilute, your doctor may ask for a first morning sample to see how well your kidneys concentrate your urine overnight. Urine that is too concentrated may indicate poor fluid intake, decreased kidney function, or dehydration from vomiting and diarrhea.

pH or acidity or alkalinity is useful information when there is a history or possibility of kidney stones, urinary-tract infection, or kidney disease.

Glucose or sugar in the urine may mean you have diabetes. You will need a blood test to confirm the diagnosis, as some families filter sugar easily through their kidneys but do not have any disease. Inflammation of the pancreas and

thyroid problems also may cause sugar in the urine.

Blood in the urine may mean infection, a stone, or an inflammation of the kidney. Excessive exertion such as running sometimes causes some blood to leak into the urine; this usually disappears after resting.

Protein molecules are large and under normal conditions should not filter into the urine. However, they may appear in small amounts in the urine after strenuous exercise or an illness, especially one with a fever. In large amounts, protein in the urine warrants a search for an underlying kidney problem.

Nitrites, substances produced when bacteria multiply, may be the earliest or only sign of an infection.

White blood cells may be present because of a urinary-tract or vaginal infection.

X Ray

- The simple X ray is a nonspecific test that is being replaced more and more by CAT scans, magnetic resonance imaging, and other tests.

What results mean

An X ray can detect such things as an enlarged heart, a broken bone, a sinus infection, or pneumonia.

COUNTING YOUR CALORIES AND FAT

Total calorie values for each item in this table were rounded to the nearest 5 calories (calories from fat and fat grams were not). The portion sizes are given in common household units and in grams. The portion size shown may not be the amount that you eat. If you choose larger or smaller portions than listed, increase or decrease the calorie and fat counts accordingly. Check nutrition labels on foods for additional information, including saturated fat, cholesterol, and sodium content.

Breads, Cereals, and Other Grain Products

BREADS	CALORIES	FAT GRAMS	CALORIES FROM FAT
Bagel			
plain, 1, 3-1/2 inch diameter	195	1	10
oat bran, 1, 3-1/2 inch	180	1	8
poppy seed, 1, Sara Lee	190	1	9
Cracked-wheat bread, 1, 25g slice	65	1	9
French bread, 1, 25g slice	70	1	7
Pita bread			
white, 1, 6-1/2 inch diameter	165		6
whole wheat, 1, 6-1/2 inch diameter	170		15
Pumpernickel, 1, 32g slice	80	1	9
Raisin, 1, 26g slice	70	1	10
Rye, 1, 32g slice	85	1	10
White			
regular, 1, 25g slice	65	1	8
Wonder bread light, 2 slices, 45g	80	1	9
Whole wheat			
regular, 1, 25g slice	70	1	11
Wonder bread, 2 slices, 45g	80	<1	14

ROLLS			
Croissant, prepared w/butter, 1, 57g	230	12	108
Dinner, 1, 28g	85	2	19
Frankfurter or hamburger, 1, 43g	125	2	20
French, 1, 38g	105	2	15
Hard, 1 3-1/2 inch, 57g	165	2	22

QUICK BREADS, BISCUITS, MUFFINS, BREAKFAST PASTRIES			
Biscuit			
plain, 2-1/2 in diameter, 60g	210	10	88
from dry mix, 3 inch diameter, 57g	190	7	62
from refrig. dough, 2-1/2 diam., 27g	95	4	36
Banana bread, 1 slice, 60g	195	57	
Coffee cake			
cinnamon w/crumb topping, 63g	265	15	132
butter streusel, Sara Lee, 41g	160	7	63
Danish			
cheese, Sara Lee, individual, 36g	130	8	72
cheese-filled, Entenmann's, fat-free 54g	130	0	0
Doughnuts			
plain cake, 1, 47g	200	11	97
glazed, 1, 45g	190	10	93
English muffin, plain, 1, 57g	135	1	9
Muffin			
blueberry, 2-1/2 inch, 1, 57g	160	4	33
bran w/raisins, Dunkin' Donuts 1, 104g	310	9	81

	CALORIES	FAT GRAMS	CALORIES FROM FAT
Pancake			
plain, from dry mix, 1, 56g	200	1	9
plain, frozen Aunt Jemima, 3, 114g	185	2	22
Waffle			
plain, 7 inch diameter, 75g	220	11	95
blueberry, frozen, Eggo, 2, 78g	220	8	72

BREAKFAST CEREAL			
All-Bran, 1/2 cup, 30g	80	1	9
Bran flakes, 3/4 cup, 28g	100	1	9
Cheerios, 1-1/4 cup, 28g	110	2	18
Corn flakes, 1 cup, 30g	110	0	0
Cream of Wheat			
regular or instant, cooked, 2/3 cup, 168g	100	0	0
instant, cooked, 2/3 cup, 161g	100	<1	0
mix'n eat, 1 pkg., 28g	100	0	0
Frosted Flakes, 3/4 cup, 30g	120	0	0
Frosted Mini-Wheats, 1 cup, 55g	190	1	9
Grape-Nut Flakes, 1 cup, 28g	100	1	9
Granola, date nut, Erewhon, 1/4 cup, 28g	130	6	50
Oatmeal			
reg., quick, or instant, cooked, 1 cup, 234g	145	2	21
cinnamon & spice, Instant , 1 pkg., 46g	170	2	18
Raisin bran, 1 cup, 55g	170	1	9
Rice Chex, 1 cup, 31g	120	0	0
Rice Krispies, 1-1/4 cup, 30g	110	0	0
Shredded wheat, Quaker	220	2	14
Special K, 1 cup, 30g	110	0	0
Total, 1 cup, 28g	100	1	9
Wheaties, 1 cup, 28g	100	1	9

PASTA AND RICE			
Macaroni			
cooked, plain, 1/2 cup, 65g	95	<1	3
spinach, cooked, Ronzoni, 1/2 cup, 67g	105	<1	4
Pasta,			
fresh, cooked, plain, 1 cup, 170g	225	2	16
homemade w/egg, cooked, 1 cup, 170g	220	3	27
Ravioli, cheese, cooked, Contadina, 1/3 container, 190g	270	11	99
Rice, cooked, 1/2 cup			
Brown, medium grain, 98g	110	1	7
White, glutinous, 120g	115	<1	2
White, long grain instant, 82g	80	<1	1
White, medium grain, 93g	120	<1	2
Wild rice, 82g	85	<1	3
Spaghetti, cooked, plain, 1 cup, 140g	155	<1	4

CRACKERS			
Cheez-it, Sunshine, 24 crackers, 32g	140	8	72
Finn-Crisp dark, 3 crackers, 15g	60	0	0
Matzo, plain, 1 (28g)	110	<1	4
Ritz, Nabisco, 4 crackers, 14g	70	4	36
Saltine, 10 crackers, 28g	120	4	36
Soup or oyster, 4 crackers, 14g	70	4	36
Triscuit, Nabisco, 6 crackers, 28g	120	4	36

Fruits

FRUITS			
(calories in cooked and canned fruit include both fruit and liquid)			
Apple, raw, sliced, 1/2 cup, 55g	30	<1	2

A16

	CALORIES	FAT GRAMS	CALORIES FROM FAT
Applesauce, 1/2 cup			
sweetened, 128g	95	<1	2
unsweetened, 122g	50	<1	1
Apricots			
canned, heavy syrup, 3 halves, 85g	70	<1	1
canned, light syrup pack, 3 halves, 85g	55	<1	0
dried, cooked without sugar, 1/2 cup, 125g	105	<1	2
raw, 4 halves, 78g	35	<1	3
Avocados			
California, 3 inch, 1/2, 86g	155	15	135
Florida, 3-5/8 inch, 1/2, 152g	170	13	121
Banana, medium, 114g	105	1	5
Blueberries, 1/2 cup			
frozen, unsweetened, 78g	40	<1	4
frozen, sweetened, 115g	95	1	5
raw, 72g	40	<1	3
Cherries, 1/2 cup			
raw, sweet, 72g	50	1	6
sweet, frozen, sweetened, 130g	115	<1	2
sour red, frozen, unsweetened, 78g	35	<1	3
Cranberry sauce, sweetened, 1/4 cup, 70g	110	0	0
Dates, dried, 10, 83g	230	<1	3
Fruit cocktail, canned, 1/2 cup			
juice pack, 124g	55	<1	0
heavy syrup, 128g	95	<1	1
Grapefruit, raw, 3-3/4 inch, 1/2, 118g	40	<1	1
Melon, honeydew, cubed, 1/2 cup, 85g	30	<1	1
Oranges, 1/2 cup			
Mandarin, canned, light syrup, 122g	80	0	0
raw, sections, 90g	40	<1	1
Peaches			
Canned, in juice, 1/2 cup, 77g	55	0	0
canned, in light syrup, 1/2 cup, 77g	70	<1	1
Pears			
Canned, in light syrup, 1 half, 77g	35	<1	1
Dried, without added sugar, 1/2 cup, 128g	165	<1	4
Pineapple			
Canned. juice pack, 1/2 cup, 125g	75	<1	1
Raw, diced, 1/2 cup, 78g	40	<1	3
Plums			
canned, juice pack, 3, 95g	55	<1	0
raw, 2-1/8 inch diameter, 66g	35	<1	4
Prunes			
dried, cooked, without sugar, 1/2 cup, 106g	115	<1	2
dried, uncooked, 10, 84g	200	<1	4
Raisins, seedless, 1/4 cup, 41g	125	<1	2
Raspberries, 1/2 cup			
frozen, unsweetened, 125g	61	1	6
raw, 62g	30	<1	3
Rhubarb, cooked, sweetened, 1/2 cup, 120g	140	<1	1
Tangerines, sections, 1/2 cup, 98g	45	<1	2
Watermelon, 10 inches x 1 inch, 480g	155	2	19
JUICES			
Apple juice or cider, 1 cup, 249g	120	0	0
Apricot nectar, canned, 3/4 cup, 188g	105	<1	2
Cranberry juice cocktail, 3/4 cup, 190g	110	<1	2
Grape juice			
bottled, 3/4 cup, 188g	110	0	0
from frozen concentrate, 3/4 cup, 188g	96	<1	2
Grapefruit			
Lemonade, 3/4 cup			
homemade, prepared w/sugar, 186g	90	0	0
from frozen concentrate, 186g	75	<1	0

	CALORIES	FAT GRAMS	CALORIES FROM FAT
Orange juice, 3/4 cup			
fresh, 186g	85	<1	3
from frozen concentrate, 187g	85	<1	1
Pineapple juice, canned, 3/4 cup, 188g	105	<1	1
Prune juice, canned, 3/4 cup, 192g	135	<1	1
Snapple, 1 bottle			
Dixie peach, 295g	140	0	0
Lemonade, 240g	110	0	0
Passion supreme, 309g	160	0	0
Pink grapefruit cocktail, 249g	120	0	0
V-8 juice, canned, 3/4 cup, 182g	35	0	0
VEGETABLE			
Alfalfa sprouts, raw, 1 cup, 33g	10	<1	2
Artichoke, cooked, medium, 120g	60	<1	2
Asparagus, 1/2 cup			
canned, drained, 120g	25	1	7
cooked, drained, 90g	20	<1	3
Bean sprouts, Mung, raw, 1/2 cup, 52g	15	<1	1
Beet greens, cooked, drained, 1/2 cup, 72g	20	<1	1
Beets, 1/2 cup			
canned, sliced, drained, 85g	25	<1	1
cooked, sliced, drained, 85g	35	<1	1
Broccoli, 1/2 cup			
frozen florets, cooked, 71g	20	0	0
raw, chopped, 44g	10	<1	1
Brussels sprouts, cooked, drained, 1/2 cup, 78g	30	<1	4
Cabbage, 1/2 cup			
Chinese bok-choy, shredded, raw, 35g	5	<1	1
shredded, raw, 35g	10	<1	1
shredded, cooked, drained, 75g	15	<1	3
Carrots			
frozen, sliced, cooked, drained, 1/2 cup, 73g	25	<1	1
raw, 7-1/1 inches x 1-1/8 inch, 72g	30	<1	1
Cauliflower, 1/2 cup			
frozen, cooked, drained, 90g	15	<1	2
raw, 1 inch pieces, 50g	10	<1	1
Celery, raw			
cooked, drained, 1/2 cup, 75g	15	<1	1
raw, 7-1/2 in x 1-1/4 inch, 40g	5	<1	1
Corn, cooked			
canned, yellow, cream style, 1/2 cup, 128g	90	1	5
canned, solids & liquid, 1/2 cup, 128g	80	1	5
frozen, white, cooked, drained, 1/2 cup, 82g	65	<1	1
on the cob, drained, 1 ear, 140g	85	1	9
Cucumber, raw, sliced, 1/2 cup, 52g	10	<1	1
Eggplant			
cooked, drained, 1 inch pieces, 1/2 cup, 48g	15	<1	1
in tomato sauce, 1 cup, 231g	75	<1	3
Green beans, 1/2 cup			
canned, drained, 68g	25	0	0
cooked, drained, 62g	20	<1	2
frozen, French style 85g	25	0	0
raw, snap, 55g	15	<1	1
Kale, cooked, drained, 1/2 cup, 65g	20	<1	2
Lettuce			
Iceberg, 1/4 of a 6-inch head, 135g	20	<1	2
looseleaf, shredded, 1/2 cup, 28g	5	<1	1
Romaine, shredded, 1/2 cup, 28g	5	<1	4
Lima beans, cooked, drained, 1/2 cup, 85g	105	<1	2
Mushrooms			
canned, pieces, drained, 1/2 cup, 78g	20	<1	2
raw, whole, 1, 18g	5	<1	1
Shiitake, cooked, 1/2 cup, 73g	40	<1	1
Onions			
canned, solids & liquid, 1 inch, 63g	10	<1	1
raw, chopped, 1/2 cup, 80g	30	<1	1
Peas, green, 1/2 cup			

	CALORIES	FAT GRAMS	CALORIES FROM FAT
frozen, cooked, drained, 80g	60	<1	2
raw, 72g	50	<1	3
Peppers, sweet, red or green, 1/2 cup			
cooked, drained, 68g	20	<1	1
raw, 50g	15	<1	1
Potatoes			
baked, w/skin, 4-3/4 inch x 2-1/3 inch, 156g	220	<1	2
boiled, no skin, 2-1/2 inch diameter, 135g	115	<1	1
hash browns, Ore-Ida frozen, 1 patty, 85g	70	<1	0
mashed, w/whole milk, 1/2 cup, 105g	80	1	6
scalloped, frozen, Stouffer's, 1/2 pkg., 165g	135	6	52
Tater Tots, frozen, Ore-Ida, 1-1/4 cup, 85g	160	7	63
Spinach, 1/2 cup			
frozen, cooked, drained, 95g	25	<1	2
raw, chopped, 28g	5	<1	1
Squash, 1/2 cup			
Summer, cooked, drained, 90g	20	<1	3
Winter, baked cubes, 102g	40	1	6
Sweet potatoes			
baked in skin, 5 inches x 2 inches, 114g	115	<1	1
canned, mashed, 128g	130	<1	2
Tomato sauce, canned, 1/2 cup, 122g	35	<1	2
Tomatoes, 1/2 cup			
canned, stewed, 103	35	0	0
raw, chopped, 90g	20	<1	3
Turnip greens, cooked, drained, 1/2 cup, 72g	15	<1	2
Turnips, cooked, mashed, 1/2 cup, 115g	20	<1	1

Meat, Poultry, Fish, and Alternates

(Serving sizes are cooked, edible parts.)

BEEF

	CALORIES	FAT GRAMS	CALORIES FROM FAT
Beef liver, 3 oz, 85g			
braised	135	4	37
pan-fried	185	7	61
Corned beef, canned, 1 oz, 28g	70	4	38
Ground beef, broiled, medium, 3 oz, 85g			
extra lean	220	14	125
ground chuck	230	16	141
regular	245	18	158
Roast beef, 3 oz, 85g			
bottom round, lean & fat	160	6	56
eye of round, lean & fat	195	11	98
pot roast, lean & fat	280	20	182
rib, lean & fat	300	24	216
tip round, lean & fat	160	7	60
Sirloin, broiled, lean & fat, 30 oz, 85g	165	6	55
Veal, loin, lean only, roasted, 30z, 85g	150	6	53

LAMB

	CALORIES	FAT GRAMS	CALORIES FROM FAT
Ground lamb, broiled, 3 oz, 85g	240	17	150
Leg of lamb, lean & fat, roasted, 3 oz, 85g	250	18	158
Shoulder chop, lean & fat, braised, 3 oz, 85g	295	20	185

PORK

	CALORIES	FAT GRAMS	CALORIES FROM FAT
Bacon, thick, broiled, 1 slice, 10g	55	4	40
Bacon, Canadian, grilled, 1 slice, 23g	45	2	18
Ham			
center slice, 3 oz, 85g	170	11	99
canned, lean, 3 oz, 85g	100	4	35
canned, regular, 30 oz, 85g	190	13	116
Pork chop, loin, broiled, 3 oz, 85g	205	11	100
Pork loin ribs, braised, 3 oz, 85g	250	18	165
Pork roast, center loin, 3 oz, 85g	200	11	103
Pork roast, sirloin, 3 oz, 85g	175	8	72

	CALORIES	FAT GRAMS	CALORIES FROM FAT
Pork shoulder, roasted, 3 oz, 85	245	20	180

SAUSAGE AND LUNCHEON MEATS

	CALORIES	FAT GRAMS	CALORIES FROM FAT
Bologna, 1 slice, 28g			
beef & pork	90	8	72
turkey	55	4	40
Braunschweiger, 1 slice, 18g	65	6	52
Chicken breast			
Oscar Mayer, roasted, 1 slice, 28g	25	<1	3
Healthy Choice, roasted, 3 slices, 28g	30	<1	4
Ham, boiled, 1 slice, 21g	20	1	9
Salami			
beef, 1 slice, 23g	60	5	43
turkey, 10% fat, 1 oz, 28g	45	3	24
Sausage, summer, beef, 1 slice, 23g	70	6	54
Turkey			
Oscar Mayer, roasted, 1 slice, 28g	25	1	7
Oscar Mayer, fat free, smoked, 4 slices, 52g	40	<1	3

POULTRY

	CALORIES	FAT GRAMS	CALORIES FROM FAT
Chicken breast, 1/2 breast			
boneless, w/out skin, roasted, 86g	140	3	28
boneless, w/skin, flour fried, 98g	220	9	78
Chicken drumstick, 1			
w/out skin, roasted, 72g	75	2	22
w/skin, roasted, 81g	110	6	52
Chicken liver, simmered, 1/2 cup, 70g	110	4	34
Chicken, thigh, 1			
w/out skin, roasted, 71g	110	6	51
w/skin, roasted, 81g	155	10	86
Turkey, ground, cooked, 1 patty, 82g	195	11	97
Turkey, roasted			
dark meat w/out skin, diced, 1/2 cup, 64g	120	5	42
dark meat w/skin, 3 oz, 85g	190	10	88
light meat w/out skin diced, 1/2 cup, 64g	100	2	19
light meat w/skin, 3 oz, 85g	170	7	64
Turkey liver, simmered, 1/2 cup, 70g	120	4	38

FISH AND SHELLFISH

	CALORIES	FAT GRAMS	CALORIES FROM FAT
Anchovies, canned in oil, drained, 5, 20g	45	2	17
Clams, canned, drained, 1/2 cup, 80g	120	2	14
Fish fillets			
breaded, frozen, 2, 99g	280	19	171
breaded, Healthy Choice, 1, 99g	160	5	45
Flounder, cooked, dry heat, 3 oz, 85g	100	1	12
Halibut, cooked, dry heat, 3 0z, 85g	120	2	22
Salmon 3 oz, 85g			
Chinook, cooked, dry heat	195	11	102
Chum, cooked, dry heat	130	4	37
Coho, cooked, moist heat	155	6	57
Sardines, Atlantic, canned in oil, drained solids, 2, 24g	50	3	25
Sea Bass, cooked, dry heat, 3 oz, 85g	105	2	20
Shrimp, cooked			
breaded & fried, 4, 30g	75	4	33
moist heat, large, 4, 22g	20	<1	2
Tuna, light, canned in water, 1/2 cup, 74g	85	1	5

EGGS

	CALORIES	FAT GRAMS	CALORIES FROM FAT
Fried, whole, 1, 46g	90	7	62
Hard-cooked, whole, 1, 50g	80	5	48
Poached, whole, 1, 50g	75	5	45
Scrambled, w/marg. & whole milk, 1, 64g	105	8	7
Soft-boiled, whole, 1, 50g	80	6	50
Whites, raw, 1, 33g	15	0	0

BEANS AND PEAS

	CALORIES	FAT GRAMS	CALORIES FROM FAT
Baked beans, canned			
pork & beans, tomato sauce, 1/2 cup, 114g	100	1	13
w/pork, molasses & sugar, 1/2 cup, 126g	190	6	58

	CALORIES	FAT GRAMS	CALORIES FROM FAT
Black-eyed peas, 1/2 cup			
canned, solids & liquid, 120g	90	1	6
cooked, drained, 1/2 cup, 82g	80	<1	3
Chickpeas (garbanzos), canned, 1/2 cup, 120g	145	1	12
Black beans, cooked, 1/2 cup, 86g	115	<1	4
Kidney beans, cooked, 1/2 cup, 88g	110	<1	4
Lima beans, cooked, drained, 1/2 cup, 85g	105	<1	2
Navy beans, cooked, 1/2 cup, 91g	130	1	5
Refried beans, canned, 1/2 cup, 126g	135	1	12

NUTS AND SEEDS

	CALORIES	FAT GRAMS	CALORIES FROM FAT
Almonds, unblanched			
dried, 3 Tbs., 28g	165	15	133
dry roasted, 3 Tbs., 26g	150	13	119
Cashews, dry roasted, 3 Tbs., 28g	165	13	118
Coconut, dried, sweetened, flaked, 2 Tbs., 9g	45	3	27
Peanut butter, 2 Tbs., 32g	190	14	126
Peanuts, roasted			
dry roasted, 3 Tbs., 28g	165	14	125
honey roasted, 3 Tbs., 28g	170	14	126
Pecans, dried, 1/2 cup, 28g	190	19	173
Pine nuts, dried, 1 Tbs., 10g	50	5	46
Pistachios, dry roasted, 3 Tbs., 28g	170	15	135
Sesame seeds			
Tahini, raw kernels, 1 Tbs., 15g	85	7	65
dried, kernels, 1 Tbs., 8g	45	4	39
Sunflower seeds, dry roasted, 3 Tbs., 28g	165	14	127
Walnuts, dried, 1/4 cup, 28g	180	18	158

MEAT SUBSTITUTES

	CALORIES	FAT GRAMS	CALORIES FROM FAT
Burger, vegetarian			
Vege burger, Natural Touch, 1, 64g	140	6	54
Veggie Sizzler, nonfat, Soy Boy, 1, 85g	90	0	0
Hot dog, Not Dogs, 1, 43g	105	5	45
Tofu			
fried, 2-3/4 x 1 x 1/2 inch, 29g	80	6	53
regular, 1/2 cup, 124g	95	6	53

Dairy Products

CHEESE

	CALORIES	FAT GRAMS	CALORIES FROM FAT
American, light, 1 slice, 28g	70	4	36
Blue, crumbled (not packed) 1/4 cup, 34g	120	10	87
Brie, 1 oz, 28g	95	8	70
Cheddar			
1-inch cube, 17g	70	6	51
light, 1 slice, 28g	70	4	36
Colby, 1oz, 28g	110	9	79
Cottage cheese, 1/2 cup			
creamed, large curd, 113g	115	5	46
dry curd, 73g	60	<1	3
lowfat, 1% fat, 113g	80	1	10
Cream cheese, 2 Tbs..			
light, Philadelphia brand, 28g	60	5	45
regular, 30g	105	10	94
whipped, Philadelphia brand, 28g	100	10	90
Feta, 1 oz, 28g	75	6	54
Mozzarella, 1 oz, 28g			
regular	80	6	54
part skim	70	4	40
Parmesan, grated, 1 Tbs.., 5g	25	2	14
Swiss			
1-inch cube, 15g	55	4	37

	CALORIES	FAT GRAMS	CALORIES FROM FAT
light, 1 slice, 28g	70	3	27

CREAM

	CALORIES	FAT GRAMS	CALORIES FROM FAT
Half & half, 1 Tbs., 15g	20	2	16
Heavy, whipping, 1 Tbs., 15g	50	6	48
Sour cream			
cultured, 2 Tbs., 24g	50	5	45
light, 50% less fat, 2 Tbs., 30g	40	2	22
Whipped cream, pressurized, 1 Tbs., 3g	10	1	6

IMITATION CREAM PRODUCTS

	CALORIES	FAT GRAMS	CALORIES FROM FAT
Coffee creamers			
non-dairy, liquid, Coffee Rich, 1 Tbs., 14g	25	1	13
non-dairy, liquid, Int'l Delight, 1 Tbs., 15g	45	2	14
Sour cream			
imitation, cultured, nondairy, 2 Tbs., 28g	60	5	49
imitation, non-butterfat, 2 Tbs., 24g	45	4	36
powdered, Coffee-Mate, 1 tsp., 2 g	10	1	6
Whipped topping			
non-dairy, pressurized, 2 Tbs., 9g	25	2	19
non-dairy, frozen, Cool Whip, 1 Tbs., 4g	10	1	7

MILK

	CALORIES	FAT GRAMS	CALORIES FROM FAT
Buttermilk, 1% fat, 1 cup, 245g	100	2	19
Chocolate milk, 1 cup, 250g			
lowfat, 1% fat	160	2	22
whole,	210	8	76
Condensed, sweetened, 2 Tbs., 38g	125	3	30
Evaporated, canned, 2 tbs., 32g			
lowfat	30	1	5
skim	25	<1	1
whole	40	2	21
Lowfat, 1% fat, 1 cup, 244g	100	3	23
Skim, 1 cup, 245g	85	<1	4
Whole, 3.3% fat, 1 cup, 244g	150	8	73

YOGURT

	CALORIES	FAT GRAMS	CALORIES FROM FAT
Fruit flavors, custard, Yoplait, 1 cont., 170g	190	4	36
Fruit-on-the-bottom, lowfat, 1 cont., 226g	230	3	27
Plain, 1 cont., 226g			
lowfat	145	4	32
nonfat	125	<1	4

Soups

CANNED SOUPS

(Canned, condensed soups are prepared with water, unless otherwise noted.)

	CALORIES	FAT GRAMS	CALORIES FROM FAT
Bean & ham, Healthy Choice, 1/2 can, 228g	220	4	36
Beef broth, ready-to-serve, 1 cup, 240g	15	1	5
Black bean, Health Valley, 1 cup, 240g	110	0	0
Chicken broth, ready-to-serve, 1/2 can, 249g	30	3	27
Chicken noodle, Campbell's, 1 cup, 226g	60	2	18
Chicken rice, 1 cup, 241g	60	2	17
Clam chowder, New England			
frozen, Stouffer's, 1 cup, 227g	180	9	81
prepared w/skim milk, 1 cup, 233g	100	2	18
prepared w/water, Campbell's, 1 cup, 244g	80	2	20
Cream of Chicken, 1 cup, 244g	110	7	62
Cream of mushroom, 1 cup			
prepared w/water, 244g	130	9	81
prepared w/whole milk, 248g	205	14	122
Minestrone			
prepared w/water, 1 cup, 241g	80	3	23
ready-to-serve, Hain, 1/2 can, 270g	160	3	27
Tomato, 1 cup			
prepared w/water, 244g	85	2	17

	CALORIES	FAT GRAMS	CALORIES FROM FAT
prepared w/whole milk, 248g	160	6	54
Vegetable			
prepared w/water, 1 cup, 241g	90	1	9
ready-to-serve, Pritikin, 1/2 can, 209g	70	0	0
DRIED OR DEHYDRATED SOUPS			
Black bean, Nile Spice, 1 container, 309g	180	1	5
Chicken vegetable, 1 cup, 251g	50	1	7
Cream of chicken, 1 cup, 261g	105	5	48
Mushroom, 1 cup, 253g	95	1	44
Onion, 1 pkg., 7g	20	<1	4
Split pea, 1 cup, 271g	135	2	14
Tomato, 1 cup, 265g	105	2	22

Desserts, Snack Foods, and Candy

	CALORIES	FAT GRAMS	CALORIES FROM FAT
CAKES			
Angel food, 1/12 of 10 inch tube, 50g	130	<1	1
Boston Cream Pie, 1/6 of 20 oz, 92g	230	8	70
Carrot cake, Sara Lee, snack size, 1, 52g	180	7	63
Cheesecake, plain, 1/6 of 17 oz, 80g	255	18	160
Cupcake, 1			
chocolate, Hostess, 46g	170	5	45
yellow, w/icing, 36g	130	4	34
Devil's food, w/icing, 1/6 of 9 inch, 69g	235	8	72
Fruitcake, 1 slice, 34g	140	4	35
Pound cake, Sara Lee, 1/10 of cake, 30g	130	7	63
Yellow cake, w/icing, 1/8 of 8 oz, 64g	240	9	84
COOKIES AND BARS			
Brownies, chocolate			
frozen, Weight-Watchers, 1, 36g	100	3	27
from mix, 2 inch square, 33g	140	7	59
Chocolate chip			
Chips Ahoy!, 3, 32g	160	8	72
refrigerated, Pillsbury, 2, 31g	140	7	59
Creme sandwich, Nabisco, 2, 28g	140	6	54
Fig bar, 2, 31g	110	2	21
Gingersnaps, Sunshine, 6, 28g	120	4	36
Graham crackers, 4, 1-1/2 squares, 28g	120	2	18
Oatmeal raisin, Barbara's, 2, 38g	160	7	63
Oreo, Nabisco, 2, 28g	100	4	36
Shortbread, 1-5/8 inch square, 4, 32g	160	8	69
Vanilla wafers, Nabisco, 7, 28g	120	4	36
PIES			
Apple, 1/8 of 9 inch pie, 155g	410	19	175
Blueberry, 1/8 of 9 inch, 147g	360	17	157
Cherry, 1/8 of 9 inch pie, 180g	485	22	198
Chocolate cream, 1/8 of 9 inch, 142g	400	23	206
Custard, 1/8 of 9 inch, 127g	260	11	102
Lemon meringue, 1/8 of 9 inch, 127g	360	16	147
Pumpkin, 1/8 of 9 inch, 155g	315	14	130
OTHER DESSERTS			
Custard, baked, 1/2 cup, 141g	150	7	60
Frozen yogurt, vanilla, 1/2 cup			
Haagen-Dazs, 98g	160	2	22
Yoplait, soft, 72g	90	3	27
Gelatin, Jell-O, 1/2 cup, 140g	80	0	0
Ice cream, vanilla, 1/2 cup			
regular, 10% fat, 66g	135	7	65

	CALORIES	FAT GRAMS	CALORIES FROM FAT
Haagen-Dazs, 106g	260	17	153
Ice cream, chocolate, 1/2 cup			
regular, 10% fat, 66g	145	7	65
Haagen-Dazs, 106g	270	17	153
Ice milk sandwich, Weight Watchers, 78g	160	4	36
Juice bars			
Strawberry, Fruit'n Juice, Dole, 74g	70	0	0
Strawberry, Welch's, 85g	80	0	0
Puddings, from mix, prepared w/2% milk			
butterscotch, 1/2 cup, 148g	150	2	20
chocolate, 1/2 cup, 147g	150	2	20
tapioca, 1/2 cup, 141g	145	2	22
vanilla, 1/2 cup, 144g	140	2	20
Sherbet, 1/2 cup, 87g	135	2	17
SNACK FOODS			
Corn chips, 3/4 cup, 28g	155	9	85
Crackers (see Crackers)			
Nuts (see Nuts and Seeds)			
Popcorn			
air-popped, 1 cup, 8g	30	<1	3
microwave, natural flavor, 1 cup, 8g	35	2	18
Potato chips, 1 cup, 28g	150	10	90
Pretzels			
Dutch, twisted, 2-3/4 inch, 2, 32g	120	1	10
Sticks, 2-1/2 x 1/8 inch, 60, 30g	115	1	9
Twists, thin, Rold Gold, 10, 28g	110	1	9
CANDY			
Caramel, plain, 3/4 inch, 8g	30	1	6
Fudge, chocolate, 1 cu inch, 17g	65	1	13
Gum drops, 8, 28g	110	0	0
Hard candy, 5, 28g	105	0	0
Jellybeans, 10 large or 26 small, 28g	105	<1	1
Hershey's Kisses, 6, 28g	150	9	81
Lollipops, 1, 28g	110	0	0

Beverages

(Milk and juices are in Dairy Products and Fruits sections.)

	CALORIES	FAT GRAMS	CALORIES FROM FAT
CARBONATED SODAS			
Cola, 1-1/2 cup, 370g	150	<1	0
Diet cola, w/aspartame, 1-1/2 cup, 355g	4	0	0
Gingerale, 1-12 cup, 366g	125	0	0
Grape soda, 1-12/ cup, 372g	160	0	0
Lemon-lime, 1-1/2 cup, 368g	145	0	0
Orange soda, 1-12/ cup, 372g	180	0	0
Root beer, 1-12/ cup, 370g	150	0	0
COFFEE AND TEA			
Coffee			
brewed, 1 cup, 235g	5	<1	0
brewed, decaffeinated, 1 cup, 240g	3	0	0
instant, 1 cup, 240g	5	0	0
Tea, brewed, 1 cup 237g	2	<1	0
Tea, brewed herb, unflavored, 1 cup, 236g	2	<1	0
Tea, iced, instant, lemon flavored			
sweetened w/aspartame, 1 cup, 259g	2	0	0
sweetened w/sugar, made w/4 tsp., 23g	85	<1	0
ALCOHOLIC BEVERAGES			
Beer, 1-1/2 cup, 355g			
light	100	0	0
regular	145	0	0
nonalcoholic	50	0	0

	CALORIES	FAT GRAMS	CALORIES FROM FAT
Gin, Rum, Whiskey, or Vodka, 80-proof, 1 jigger, 42g	95	0	0
Wine, 1 glass			
red, 147g	105	0	0
white, 147g	100	0	0
Wine cooler, 1 glass, 360g	175	<1	0
Wine, dessert, 1 glass			
dry, 59g	75	0	0
sweet, 59g	90	0	0

Fats, Oils, and Condiments

FATS AND OILS

	CALORIES	FAT GRAMS	CALORIES FROM FAT
Butter			
regular or unsalted, 1 tsp., 5g	35	4	37
whipped, 1 Tbs., 11g	80	9	80
Margarine			
spread, tub, 1 Tbs., 14g	75	9	75
stick, 1 Tbs., 14g	100	11	100
Oil			
corn, 1 Tbs., 14g	120	14	122
olive, 1 Tbs., 14g	120	14	122
vegetable spray, 1-1/4 seconds, 1g	5	1	5
Salad dressing			
blue cheese, 1 Tbs., 15g	75	8	72
French, 1 Tbs., 16g	65	6	57
French, low calorie, 1 Tbs., 16g	20	1	9
Italian, 1 Tbs., 15g	70	7	64
Italian, low calorie, 1 Tbs., 16g	15	1	12
mayonnaise-like, 1 Tbs., 15g	55	5	43
thousand island, 1 Tbs., 16g	60	6	50

CONDIMENTS

	CALORIES	FAT GRAMS	CALORIES FROM FAT
Barbecue sauce, 1 Tbs., 15g	15	<1	3
Catsup, 1 Tbs., 15g	15	<1	0
Gravy, canned			
au jus, 1/4 cup, 60g	10	<1	1
beef, 1/4 cup, 58g	30	1	12
chicken, 1/4 cup, 60g	45	3	30
turkey, 1/4 cup, 60g	30	1	11
Horseradish, prepared, 1 tsp., 5g	2	<1	0
Mustard, prepared, 1 tsp., 5g	4	<1	2
Olives			
black, canned, small, 3, 10g	10	1	9
green, medium, 4, 13g	15	2	14
green, stuffed, 10, 34g	35	4	34
Pickles			
dill, kosher spears, 1, 28g	5	0	0
sweet, gherkins, small, 2-1.2 inches, 2, 30g	40	<1	0
Relish, sweet pickle, 2 Tbs., 30g	40	<1	1
Soy sauce, tamari, 1 Tbs., 18g	10	<1	0
Tartar sauce, 1 Tbs., 14g	75	8	68

SUGAR, JAMS, AND JELLIES

	CALORIES	FAT GRAMS	CALORIES FROM FAT
Chocolate syrup			
fudge-type, 2 Tbs., 42g	145	6	51
thin-type, 2 Tbs., 38g	82	<1	3
Honey, 1 Tbs., 21g	65	0	0
Jams and preserves, 1 Tbs., 20g	50	<1	0
Jellies, 1 Tbs., 19g	50	<1	0
Maple syrup, 2 Tbs., 40g	105	<1	1
Sugar			
brown, unpacked, 1 cup, 145g	545	0	0
white, granulated, 1 tsp., 4g	15	0	0

Fast Foods

BURGERS AND SANDWICHES

	CALORIES	FAT GRAMS	CALORIES FROM FAT
Burger King			
Big Fish	700	41	370
Broiler Chicken	550	29	260
Double Cheeseburger with Bacon	640	39	350
Hamburger	330	15	140
Whopper	640	39	350
McDonald's			
Big Mac	530	28	250
Filet-O-Fish	360	16	150
Hamburger	270	10	90
MacLean Deluxe	350	12	110
McChicken	570	30	270
McGrilled Chicken	510	30	270
Wendy's			
Big Bacon Classic	610	33	290
Chicken Club	500	23	200
Grilled Chicken Sandwich	310	8	70
Hamburger, with everything	420	20	180

SALADS, FRIES, AND MISCELLANEOUS

(Salad values are given for salads without dressing.)

	CALORIES	FAT GRAMS	CALORIES FROM FAT
Burger King			
Broiled Chicken Salad	200	10	90
French fries, medium	370	20	180
Garden Salad	100	5	45
Salad dressing, 30g, thousand island	140	12	110
Salad dressing, 30g, ranch	180	19	170
Salad dressing, 30g, reduced calorie Italian	15	<1	5
McDonald's			
Chef Salad	210	11	100
Fajita Chicken Salad	160	6	60
French fries, large	450	22	200
French fries, small	210	10	90
Salad dressing, 1 pkg., blue cheese	190	17	150
Salad dressing, 1 pkg., lite vinaigrette	50	2	20
Salad dressing, 1 pkg., ranch	180	19	170
Pizza Hut			
Breadsticks, 5	770	25	223
Buffalo wings, 12	565	35	310
Cheese pizza, 1/8 of med., thin crust	205	8	75
Cheese pizza, 1/8 of med., pan pizza	260	11	98
Pepperoni pizza, 1/8 of med., thin crust	215	10	69
Veggie Lover's, 1/8 of med., thin crust	185	7	61
Wendy's			
Baked potato, plain	310	0	0
Baked potato w/chili and cheese	620	24	220
Baked potato w/sour cream and chives	380	6	60
Deluxe Garden Salad	110	6	50
Salad dressing, 2 Tbs., blue cheese	170	19	170
Salad dressing, 2 Tbs., fat-free French	30	0	0
Salad dressing, 2 Tbs., ranch	90	10	90

DESSERTS

	CALORIES	FAT GRAMS	CALORIES FROM FAT
Burger King			
Dutch apple pie	300	15	140
McDonald's			
Baked apple pie	260	13	120
Cookies	260	9	80
Pizza Hut			
Dessert pizza, 1/8 of med.	245	5	46
Wendy's			
Chocolate chip cookies, 1, 57g	270	11	100

YOUR HEALTH DIRECTORY

*I*n *An Invitation to Health,* I emphasize that you shoulder a great deal of responsibility for your health and the quality of your life. Given the complexity of our minds and bodies and the many social and environmental factors that affect us, this responsibility can be a very heavy burden. But your load can be made lighter if you know where to turn for health information, services, and support.

In this directory, you will find over 100 health-related topics and about 250 resources, including addresses, phone numbers, and websites for government agencies, community organizations, professional associations, recovery groups, and Internet sources. Many of these organizations and groups have toll-free 800 or 888 phone numbers, and an increasing number of them have websites (one caution: as you may have experienced, website addresses—like street addresses and phone numbers—do change on occasion). Much of the material available from these groups is free.

Also included in Your Health Directory are clearinghouses and information centers that are especially rich sources of health knowledge. Their main purpose is to collect, help manage, and disseminate information. Clearinghouses often perform other services as well, such as creating original publications and providing tailored responses to individual requests. These organizations also may provide referrals to other groups that can help you.

Many of the groups listed here have local offices or chapters. You can call, write, or visit the websites of these organizations to find out if there is a branch in your vicinity, or you can check your local telephone directory.

The purpose of this directory is to help you be in control of your health. If you know where to turn for answers to your questions and if you know what choices you have, you may find that you have more control over your life.

General Information Resources

Agency for Health Care Policy Research
2101 E. Jefferson Street, Suite 501
Rockville, MD 20852
(301) 594-1360

Go Ask Alice
http://www.columbia.edu/cu/health-wise/all.html

Internet Grateful Med
National Library of Medicine
(offers assisted searching in online databases of the NLM)
8600 Rockville Pike
Bethesda, MD 20894
(800) 638-8480
(301) 402-1076
http://igm.nlm.nih.gov

National Center for Health Statistics (NCHS)
(produces vital statistics and health statistics for the United States)
Data Dissemination Branch
6525 Belcrest Road, Room 1064
Hyattsville, MD 20782
(301) 436-8500
http://www.cdc.gov/nchswww/

ODPHP National Health Information Center
P.O. Box 1133
Washington, D.C. 20013-1133
(301) 565-4167
(800) 336-4797
http://odphp.oash.dhhs.gov

National Institutes of Health (NIH)
9000 Rockville Pike
Bethesda, MD 20892
(301) 496-4000
http://www.nih.gov

New York Online Access to Health
http://www.noah.cuny.edu

Tel-Med Health Information Service
(provides taped messages on health concerns) See white pages of telephone directory for listing

Yahoo Health Directory
http://www.yahoo.com/health

Resources By Topic

Abortion

National Abortion Federation
(provides information about abortion and referral for abortion services)
(202) 667-5881
(800) 772-9100
http://www.prochoice.org

Accident Prevention

Centers for Disease Control and Prevention
1600 Clifton Road N.E.
Atlanta, GA 30333
(404) 639-3311
http://www.cdc.gov

National Safety Council
1121 Spring Lake Drive
Itasca, IL 60143-3201
(630) 775-2056
(800) 621-7619
http://www.nsc.org

Adoption

Adoptees' Liberty Movement Association (ALMA) Society
(provides assistance for adopted children to locate natural parents and for natural parents to locate relinquished children)
P.O. Box 727
Radio City Station
New York, NY 10101-0727
(212) 581-1568
http://www.almanet.com

AASK (Adopt a Special Kid)
(provides assistance to families who adopt older and handicapped children)
1025 N. Reynolds Road
Toledo, OH 43615
(419) 534-3350
http://www.aask.org

Aging

American Association of Retired Persons
601 E Street N.W.
Washington, D.C. 20049
(800) 424-3410
(202) 434-2277
http://www.aarp.org

Gray Panthers
2025 Pennsylvania Avenue, N.W.
Suite 821
Washington, D.C. 20006
(800) 280-5362
(202) 466-3132

AIDS (Acquired Immunodeficiency Syndrome)

Gay Men's Health Crisis
119 West 24th Street
New York, NY 10011
(212) 807-6664
http://www.gmhc.org

National AIDS Hotline
(800) 342-2437

San Francisco AIDS Foundation
P.O. Box 426182
San Francisco, CA 94162-6182
(415) 487-3000
http://www.sfaf.org

Alcohol Abuse and Alcoholism

Al-Anon and Alateen
(support groups for friends and relatives of alcoholics)
1600 Corporate Landing Parkway
Virginia Beach, VA 23454
(757) 563-1600
http://www.al-anon-alateen.org
See white pages of telephone directory for listing of local chapter

Alcohol Hotline
(800) ALCOHOL

Alcoholics Anonymous
P.O. Box 459
Grand Central Station
New York, NY 10163
(212) 870-3400
http://www.alcoholics-anonymous.org
See white pages of telephone directory for listing of local chapter

National Association of Children of Alcoholics
11426 Rockville Pike
Suite 100
Rockville, MD 20852
(888) 55-4COAS
(301) 468-0985
http://www.health.org/nacoa

National Clearinghouse for Alcohol and Drug Information
P.O. Box 2345
Rockville, MD 20847-2345
(800) 729-6686
(301) 468-2600
http://www.health.org/index.htm

National Institute on Alcohol Abuse and Alcoholism
6000 Executive Boulevard
Willco Building
Bethesda, MD 20892-7003
(301) 443-3860
http://www.niaaa.nih.gov

Women for Sobriety, Inc.
(support groups for women with drinking problems)
P.O. Box 618
Quakertown, PA 18951-0618
(800) 333-1606
(215) 536-8026
http://www.womenforsobriety.org/

Alzheimer's Disease

Alzheimer's Association
919 N. Michigan Avenue
Suite 1000
Chicago, IL 60611
(800) 272-3900
(312) 335-8700

Arthritis

Arthritis Foundation
1330 West Peachtree Street
Atlanta, GA 30309
(800) 283-7800
(404) 872-7100
http://www.arthritis.org

Asthma

Asthma and Allergy Foundation of America
1125 15th Street N.W.
Suite 502
Washington, D.C. 20005
(800) 7-ASTHMA
(202) 466-7643
http://www.aafa.org/home.html

Lung Line
National Jewish Center for Immunology and Respiratory Medicine
(information and referral service)
1400 Jackson Street
Denver, CO 80206
(800) 222-5864
(303) 388-4461
http://www.njc.org/Markethtml/Lungline.html

Attention Deficit Disorder

National Attention Deficit Disorder Association (National ADDA)
P.O. Box 972
Mentor, OH 44061-0972
(800) 487-2282
http://www.add.org

Children and Adults with Attention Deficit Disorder (CHADD)
499 N.W. 70th Avenue
Suite 101
Plantation, FL 33317
(305) 587-3700

Learning Disabilities Association (LDA)
4156 Library Road
Pittsburgh, PA 15234
(412) 341-1515
http://www.ldanatl.org

Automobile Safety

American Automobile Association (AAA)
1000 AAA Drive
Heathrow, FL 37246
(407) 444-7000
http://www.aaa.com

See also white or yellow pages of telephone directory for listing of local chapter

Insurance Institute for Highway Safety
1005 North Glebe Road
Suite 800
Arlington, VA 22201
(703) 247-1500

National Highway Traffic Safety Association
Office of Publications
400 7th Street S.W.
Room 6123
Washington, D.C. 20590
(202) 366-2587
http://www.nhtsa.dot.gov

Auto Safety Hotline
(for consumer complaints about auto safety and child safety seats, and requests for information on recalls)
(800) 424-9393

Birth Control and Family Planning

Advocates for Youth
(offers programs aimed at reducing teenage pregnancy)
1025 Vermont Avenue N.W.
Suite 200
Washington, D.C. 20005
(202) 347-5700
http://www.advocatesforyouth.org

American College of Obstetricians and Gynecologists
(provides literature and contraceptive information)
409 12th Street S.W.
Washington, D.C. 20024
(202) 638-5577
http://www.acog.com

Association for Voluntary Surgical Contraception (AVSC)
(provides information and referrals to individuals concerning tubal ligation or vasectomy)
79 Madison Avenue
7th Floor
New York, NY 10016-7802
(212) 561-8000

Planned Parenthood Federation of America (PPFA)
810 Seventh Avenue
New York, NY 10019
(212) 541-7800
http://www.plannedparenthood.org

See also white or yellow pages of telephone directory for listing of local chapter

Birth Defects

Cystic Fibrosis Foundation (CFF)
6931 Arlington Road
Bethesda, MD 20814
(800) FIGHT-CF
(301) 951-4422
http://www.cff.org

March of Dimes Birth Defects Foundation
1275 Mamaroneck Avenue
White Plains, NY 10605
(888) 663-4637
(914) 428-7100
http://www.modimes.org

Blindness

American Foundation for the Blind
1 Penn Plaza
Suite 300
New York, NY 10001
(800) AFB-LINE
(212) 502-7600
http://www.afb.org

National Federation for the Blind
1800 Johnson Street
Baltimore, MD 21230
(800) 638-7518
(410) 659-9314
http://www.nfb.org

National Library Service for the Blind and Physically Handicapped
Library of Congress
1291 Taylor Street, N.W.
Washington, D.C. 20542
(800) 424-8567
(202) 707-5100
http://www.loc.gov/nls

Blood Banks

American Red Cross
431 18th Street N.W.
Washington, D.C. 20006
(202) 737-8300
http://www.redcross.org

See also white or yellow pages of telephone directory for listing of local chapter

Brain

Brain Research Foundation
208 S. LaSalle Street
Suite 1426
Chicago, IL 60604
(312) 782-4311

Breast Cancer

Reach to Recovery
(support program for women who have undergone mastectomies as a result of breast cancer)
American Cancer Society
1599 Clifton Road N.E.
Atlanta, GA 30329-4251
(800) ACS-2345
(404) 320-3333

Burn Injuries

National Burn Victim Foundation
246-A Madisonville Road
P.O. Box 409
Basking Ridge, NJ 07920
(201) 676-7700
http://www.nbvf.org

Phoenix Society for Burn Victims
(self-help organization for burn victims and their families)

11 Rust Hill Road
Levittown, PA 19056
(800) 888-BURN
(215) 946-BURN
http://www.firealert.com/phoenix.htm

Cancer

American Cancer Society
1599 Clifton Road N.E.
Atlanta, GA 30329
(800) 227-2345
(404) 320-3333
http://www.cancer.org

Cancer Information Service
National Cancer Institute
9000 Rockville Pike
Building 31, Room 10A16
Bethesda, MD 20892-0001
(800) 4-CANCER
(301) 496-4000
http://www.nci.nih.gov/hpage/cis.htm

Leukemia Society of America, Inc.
600 Third Avenue
New York, NY 10011
(800) 955-4LSA
(212) 573-8484
http://www.leukemia.org

National Coalition for Cancer Survivorship
1010 Wayne Avenue
Suite 505
Silver Spring, MD 20910
(301) 650-8868
http://www.cansearch.org

National Council on Independent Living
2111 Wilson Boulevard, Suite 405
Arlington, VA 22201
(703) 525-3406

R. A. Bloch Cancer Foundation (Cancer Connection)
(support group that matches cancer patients with volunteers who are cured, in remission, or being treated for the same type of cancer)
4435 Main Street
Suite 500
Kansas City, MO 64111
(800) 433-0464
(816) 932-8453
http://www.blochcancer.org

Child Abuse

National Center for Assault Prevention
(provides services to children, ado-

lescents, mentally retarded adults, and elderly)
606 Delsea Drive
Sewell, NJ 08080
(800) 258-3189
(609) 582-7000
http://www.ncap.org

National Child Abuse Hotline
(800) 422-4453

National Committee for the Prevention of Child Abuse
(provides literature on child abuse prevention programs)
200 S. Michigan Avenue
17th Floor
Chicago, IL 60604
(312) 663-3520
http://childabuse.org

Parents Anonymous
(self-help group for abusive parents)
675 W. Foothill Blvd., Suite 220
Claremont, CA 91711-3475
(909) 621-6184
http://www.parentsanonymous-natl.org

Childbirth

American College of Nurse-Midwives
(RNs who provide services through the maternity cycle)
818 Connecticut Avenue N.W.
Suite 900
Washington, D.C. 20006
(202) 728-9860

American College of Obstetricians and Gynecologists
409 12th Street S.W.
P.O. Box 96920
Washington, D.C. 20090
(202) 638-5577
http://www.acog.com

Lamaze International
1200 19th Street N.W.
Suite 300
Washington, D.C. 20036-2422
(800) 368-4404
(202) 857-1128
http://www.lamaze-childbirth.com

International Childbirth Education Association
P.O. Box 20048
Minneapolis, MN 55420
(612) 854-8660
http://www.icea.org

National Association of Parents and Professionals for Safe Alternatives in Childbirth
(provides information and support for alternatives in birth experiences)
Route 1, Box 646
Marble Hill, MO 63764
(314) 238-2010

Parent Care
(resource for parents of premature and high-risk infants)
9041 Colgate Street
Indianapolis, IN 46268-1210
(317) 872-9913

Child Health and Development

National Center for Education in Maternal and Child Health
2000 15th Street, N.
Suite 701
Arlington, VA 22201
(703) 524-7802

National Institute of Child Health and Human Development
31 Center Drive, MSC-2425
Building 31/2A32
Bethesda, MD 20892-2425
(301) 496-5133
http://www.nih.gov/nichd

Chiropractic

American Chiropractic Association
1701 Clarendon Boulevard
Arlington, VA 22209
(800) 986-INFO
(703) 276-8800
http://www.amerchiro.org

Consumer Information

Consumer Information Catalog
(catalog of publications developed by federal agencies for consumers)
Department WWW
Pueblo, CO 81009
http://www.pueblo.gsa.gov

Consumer Information Center
(distributes publications developed by federal agencies for consumers)
18 F Street N.W.
Washington, D.C. 20405
(202) 501-1794

Consumer Product Safety Commission
Office of Information Services
(800) 638-2772
(301) 504-0000
http://www.cpsc.gov

Consumers Union of the United States
(tests quality and safety of consumer products; publishes *Consumer Reports* magazine)
101 Truman Avenue
Yonkers, NY 10703
(914) 378-2000
http://www.consumerreports.org

Council of Better Business Bureaus (CBBB)
4200 Wilson Boulevard
Suite 800
Arlington, VA 22203
(703) 276-0100
http://www.bbb.org

See also white or yellow pages of telephone directory for listing of local chapter

Food and Drug Administration (FDA)
Office of Consumer Affairs
Consumer Inquiries
5600 Fishers Lane (HFE-88)
Rockville, MD 20857
(301) 827-4420
http://www.fda.gov

Crime Victims

Crisis Prevention Institute, Inc.
(offers programs on non-violent physical crisis interventions)
3315-K N. 124th Street
Brookfield, WI 53005
(800) 558-8976
(414) 783-5787

National Association for Crime Victims Rights (NACVR)
P.O. Box 16161
Portland, OR 97216
(503) 252-9012

Death and Grieving

SHARE
(support group for parents who have suffered loss of newborn baby)
c/o St. John's Hospital
800 E. Carpenter Street
Springfield, IL 62729
(217) 544-6464

Dental Health

American Dental Association (ADA)
211 E. Chicago Avenue
Chicago, IL 60611
(312) 440-2500
http://www.ada.org

National Institute of Dental Research
Office of Communication
9000 Rockville Pike
Building 31, Room 2C35
Bethesda, MD 20892
(301) 496-4261
http://www.nidr.nih.gov

Depressive Disorders

Depressives Anonymous: Recovery from Depression (DARFD)
329 East 62nd Street
New York, NY 10021
(212) 689-2600

National Depressive and Manic Depressive Association (NDMDA)
730 N. Franklin
Suite 501
Chicago, IL 60610
(312) 642-0049
(800) 826-3632
http://www.ndmda.org

DES (Diethylstibestrol)

DES Action, USA
(support group for persons exposed to DES)
1615 Broadway, Suite 510
Oakland, CA 94612
(510) 465-4011
http://www.desaction.org

Diabetes

American Diabetes Association
National Center
1660 Duke Street
Alexandria, VA 22314
(800) ADA-DISC
(703) 549-1500
http://www.diabetes.org

Juvenile Diabetes Foundation International (JDFI)
120 Wall Street
New York, NY 10005-4001
(800) JDF-CURE
(212) 785-9500
http://www.jdfcure.org

National Diabetes Information Clearinghouse
1 Information Way
Bethesda, MD 20892-3560
(301) 654-3327
http://www.niddk.nih.gov

Digestive Diseases

National Digestive Diseases Information
Clearinghouse (NDDIC)
Box NDDIC
9000 Rockville Pike
Bethesda, MD 20892
(301) 654-3810

Domestic Violence

Batterers Anonymous
(self-help group designed to rehabilitate men who abuse women)
1850 N. Riverside Avenue, Suite 220
Rialto, CA 92376
(909) 355-1100

National Coalition Against Domestic Violence (NCADV)
P.O. Box 18749
Denver, CO 80218
(303) 839-1852

National Domestic Violence Hotline
(800) 799-SAFE

National Network to End Domestic Violence
701 Pennsylvania N.W.
Suite 900
Washington, D.C. 20004
(202) 347-9520

Down Syndrome

National Association for Down Syndrome (NADS)
P.O. Box 4542
Oak Brook, IL 60522-4542
(708) 325-9112
http://www.nads.org

National Down Syndrome Society (NDSS)
666 Broadway, 8th Floor
New York, NY 10012-2317
(800) 221-4602
(212) 460-9330
http://www.ndss.org

Drug Abuse

Cocaine Anonymous World Services
P.O. Box 2000
Los Angeles, CA 90049
(800) 347-8998
(310) 559-5833
http://www.ca.org

Narcotics Anonymous (NA)
(support group for recovering recent
narcotics addicts)
P.O. Box 999
Van Nuys, CA 91409
(818) 773-9999
http://www.na.org

*See also white or yellow pages of tele-
phone directory for listing of local
chapter*

National Cocaine Hotline
(800) COCAINE

**National Institute on Drug Abuse
Helpline**
(800) 662-4357
http://nida.nih.gov

**National Parents Resource Institute
for Drug Education (PRIDE)**
3610 Dekalb Technology Parkway
Atlanta, GA 30340
(770) 458-9900
http://www.prideusa.org

Substance Abuse Prevention
Alcohol, Drug Abuse, and Mental
Health Administration
5600 Fishers Lane
Rockwall 11 Building
Rockville, MD 20852
(301) 443-0365

Drunk Driving Groups

Mothers Against Drunk Driving
511 E. John Carpenter Freeway
Suite 700
Irving, TX 75062
(800) GET-MADD
(214) 744-6233
http://www.madd.org

*See also white pages of telephone
directory for listing of local chapter*

Remove Intoxicated Drivers (RID)
P.O. Box 520
Schenectady, NY 12301
(518) 372-0034
(518) 393-HELP

**Students Against Drunk Driving
(SADD)**
200 Pleasant Street
Marlboro, MA 01752
(508) 481-3568

Eating Disorders

**American Anorexia/Bulimia
Association (AA/BA)**
(self-help group that provides information and referrals to physicians
and therapists)
165 West 46th Street, #1108
New York, NY 10036
(212) 575-6200
http://members.aol.com/amanbu/

**Anorexia Nervosa and Related
Eating Disorders (ANRED)**
(provides information and referrals
for people with eating disorders)
P.O. Box 5102
Eugene, OR 97405
(541) 344-1144
http://www.anred.com

Environment

**Environmental Protection Agency
(EPA)**
Public Information Center
PM 211-B
401 M Street S.W.
Washington, D.C. 20460
(202) 260-2080
http://www.epa.gov

Greenpeace, USA
1436 U Street N.W.
Washington, D.C. 20009
(800) 326-0959
(202) 462-1177
http://www.greenpeaceusa.org

Natural Resources Defense Council
40 West 20th Street
New York, NY 10011
(212) 727-2700
http://www.nrdc.org

Sierra Club
85 2nd Street, 2nd Floor
San Francisco, CA 94105
(415) 977-5500
http://www.sierraclub.org

World Wildlife Fund
1250 24th Street N.W.
Washington, D.C. 20037
(202) 293-4800
http://www.wwfus.org

Epilepsy

Epilepsy Foundation of America
4351 Garden City Drive
Landover, MD 20785-2267
(800) EFA-1000
(301) 459-3700
http://www.efa.org

Gay and Lesbian Organizations and Services

Human Rights Campaign
1101 14th Street N.W.
Washington, D.C. 20005
(202) 628-4160
http://www.hrc.org

**National Gay and Lesbian Task
Force (NGLTF)**
2320 17th Street N.W.
Washington, D.C. 20009
(202) 332-6483
http://www.ngltf.org

**Parents, Family, and Friends of
Lesbians and Gays (P-FLAG)**
1101 14th Street N.W.
Washington, D.C. 20005
(202) 638-4200
http://www.pflag.org

Handicapped and Disabled

**American Alliance for Health,
Physical Education, Recreation,
and Dance (AAHPERD)**
(provides information about recreation and fitness opportunities for
the handicapped)
1900 Association Drive
Reston, VA 20191
(703) 476-3400
http://www.aahperd.org

**National Council on Independent
Living**
2111 Wilson Boulevard, Suite 405
Arlington, VA 22201
(703) 525-3406

**National Library Service for the
Blind and Physically Handicapped**
Library of Congress
1291 Taylor Street, N.W.
Washington, D.C. 20542
(800) 424-8567
(202) 707-5100
http://www.loc.gov/nls

Special Olympics International (SOI)
1325 G Street N.W.
Suite 500
Washington, D.C. 20005
(202) 628-3630
http://www.specialolympics.org

Hazardous Waste

Environmental Protection Agency (EPA)
Public Information Center
PM 211-B
401 M Street S.W.
Washington, D.C. 20460
(202) 260-2080
http://www.epa.gov

Hazardous Waste Hotline Information
(800) 424-9346

Health Care

American Association for Therapeutic Humor (AATH)
(publishes a newsletter and sponsors seminars for people in the helping professions)
222 S. Merimac Street
Suite 303
St. Louis, MO 63105
(314) 863-6232
http://ideanurse.com/aath

American Medical Association
515 N. State Street
Chicago, IL 60610
(312) 464-5000
http://www.ama-assn.org

American Nurses Association
600 Maryland Avenue S.W.
Washington, D.C. 20024-2571
(800) 274-4ANA
(202) 651-7000
http://www.nursingworld.org

Medical Self-Care Magazine
P.O. Box 717
Inverness, CA 94937

Health Education

Center for Health Promotion and Education
Centers for Disease Control and Prevention
Mail Stop A34
1600 Clifton Road, N.E.
Atlanta, GA 30333
(404) 639-3534

Hearing Impairment

American Society for Deaf Children
(resource group for parents of hard of hearing and deaf children)
2848 Arden Way
Suite 210
Sacramento, CA 95825
(800) 942-ASDC
(916) 482-0120

Better Hearing Institute (BHI)
(provides educational and resource materials on deafness)
Box 1840
Washington, D.C. 20013
(800) EAR-WELL
(703) 642-0580
http://www.betterhearing.org

Heart Disease

American Heart Association (AHA)
7272 Greenville Avenue
Dallas, TX 75231
(800) 242-8721
(214) 373-6300
http://www.amheart.org

National Heart, Lung, and Blood Institute
(provides information on cardiovascular risk factors and disease)
4733 Bethesda Avenue, Suite 530
Bethesda, MD 20814
(301) 951-3260
http://www.nhlbi.nih.gov/nhlbi/nlhbi.htm

Holistic Medicine

American Holistic Medical Association (NHMA)
6728 Old McLean Village Drive
McLean, VA 22101
(703) 556-8729
http://www.ahmaholistic.com

Homeopathy

National Center for Homeopathy (NCH)
801 N. Fairfax Street, Suite 306
Alexandria, VA 22314
(703) 548-7790
http://www.healthworld.com/nch

Hospice

National Hospice Organization
1901 N. Moore Street, Suite 901
Arlington, VA 22209
(703) 243-5900
http://nho.org

Immunization

National Center for Prevention Services
Centers for Disease Control
1600 Clifton Road, N.E.
Atlanta, GA 30333
(404) 332-4559

Infant Care

American Red Cross
431 18th Street N.W.
Washington, D.C. 20006
(202) 737-8300
http://www.redcross.org

LaLeche League International
(provides information and support to women interested in breast-feeding)
1400 N. Meacham Road
Schaumburg, IL 60173
(800) LA-LECHE
(847) 519-7730
http://www.lalecheleague.org

Infectious Diseases

Centers for Disease Control and Prevention
1600 Clifton Road, N.E.
Atlanta, GA 30333
(404) 639-3534
http://www.cdc.gov

Infertility

Resolve, Inc.
(offers counseling, information, and support to people with problems of infertility)
1310 Broadway
Somerville, MA 02144-1779
(617) 623-0744
http://www.resolve.org

In-Vitro Fertilization
Eastern Virginia Medical School
Howard and Georgeanna Jones Institute
for Reproductive Medicine
601 Colley Avenue
Norfolk, VA 23507
(804) 446-8948

Inherited Diseases

Alliance of Genetic Support Groups
(provides information about inherited diseases; publishes a directory of genetic counseling services)
  35 Wisconsin Circle
  Suite 440
  Chevy Chase, MD 20815
  (800) 336-GENE

Kidney Disease

American Kidney Fund (AKF)
(provides information on financial aid to patients, organ transplants, and kidney-related diseases)
  6110 Executive Boulevard
  Suite 1010
  Rockville, MD 20852
  (800) 638-8299
  (301) 881-3052
  http://www.akfinc.org

American Association of Kidney Patients (AAKP)
  100 S. Ashley Dr.
  Suite 280
  Tampa, FL 33602-5346
  (800) 749-2257
  http://www.aakp.org/aakpteam.html

National Kidney Foundation (NKF)
  30 East 33rd Street
  Suite 1100
  New York, NY 10016
  (800) 622-9010
  (212) 889-2210
  http://www.kidney.org

Learning Disorders

Learning Disabilities Association of America (LDA)
  4156 Library Road
  Pittsburgh, PA 15234
  (412) 341-1515

Liver Disease

American Liver Foundation (ALF)
  1425 Pompton Avenue
  Cedar Grove, NJ 07009
  (800) 465-4837

Lung Disease

American Lung Association (ALA)
  1740 Broadway
  New York, NY 10019
  (800) LUNG-USA
  (212) 315-8700
  http://www.lungusa.org

NHLBI Educational Program Information Center
(provides information on cardiovascular risk factors)
  P.O. Box 30105
  Bethesda, MD 20824
  (301) 951-3260

National Jewish Center for Immunology and Respiratory Medicine
  1400 Jackson Street
  Denver, CO 80206
  (303) 388-4461

Lupus Erythematosus

Lupus Foundation of America (LPA)
  1300 Picard Drive
  Suite 200
  Rockville, MD 20850-4303
  (301) 670-9292
  (800) 558-0121
  http://www.lupus.org/lupus/index.html

Marriage and Family

Women Work! The National Network for Women's Employment
(national advocacy group for women over 35 who have lost their primary means of support through death, divorce, or disabling of spouse)
  1625 K Street N.W.
  Suite 300
  Washington, D.C. 20006
  (202) 467-6346

Family Service of America
  1701 K Street N.W.
  Suite 200
  Washington, D.C. 20006
  (202) 223-3447
  http://www.fsanet.org/main/

Stepfamily Association of America
(provides information and publishes quarterly newsletter)
  650 J Street, Suite 205
  Lincoln, NE 68508
  (402) 477-7837
  (800) 735-0329
  http://www.stepfam.org

Medical Information

Medic Alert Foundation
(provides those with medical problems bracelets or neck chains with special emblems to alert medical or law enforcement personnel)
  2323 Colorado Avenue
  Turlock, CA 95382
  (800) 825-3785

Medications (Prescriptions and Over-the-Counter)

Food and Drug Administration (FDA)
  Office of Consumer Affairs Public Inquiries
  5600 Fishers Lane (HFE-88)
  Rockville, MD 20857
  (301) 443-3170
  http://www.fda.gov

Mental Health

American Psychiatric Association
  1400 K Street N.W.
  Washington, D.C. 20005
  (202) 682-6000
  http://www.psych.org

American Psychological Association
  750 First Street N.E.
  Washington, D.C. 20002
  (202) 336-5500
  http://www.apa.org

National Alliance for the Mentally Ill (NAMI)
(self-help advocacy organization for persons with schizophrenia and depressive disorders and their families)
  200 N. Glebe Road
  No. 1015
  Arlington, VA 22201
  (800) 950-NAMI
  (703) 524-7600

National Institute of Mental Health
  Information Resources and Inquiries Branch
  5600 Fishers Lane
  Room 15C05
  Rockville, MD 20857
  (301) 443-4515

National Mental Health Association (NMHA)
  1021 Prince Street
  Alexandria, VA 22314-2971
  (800) 969-NMHA
  (703) 684-7722
  http://www.nmha.org

Recovery, Inc.
(self-help group for former mental patients)

Association of Nervous and Former
Mental Patients
802 N. Dearborn Street
Chicago, IL 60610
(312) 337-5661

Mental Retardation

**Association for Retarded Citizens
(ARC)**
500 E. Border Street
Suite 300
Arlington, TX 76010
(817) 261-6003
http://www.thearc.org

Missing and Runaway Children

Child Find of America
(800) I-AM-LOST

**National Center for Missing and
Exploited Children (NCMEC)**
2101 Wilson Boulevard, Suite 550
Arlington, VA 22201
(703) 235-9000
(800) 843-5678
http://www.missingkids.org

Runaway Hotline
(800) 231-6946

Neurological Disorders

**National Institute of Neurological
and Communicative Disorders and
Stroke**
National Institutes of Health
9000 Rockville Pike
Bethesda, MD 20205
(301) 496-4000

Nutrition

American Dietetic Association
216 West Jackson Boulevard
Chicago, IL 60606-6995
(312) 899-0040
http://www.eatright.org

**American Institute of Nutrition
(AIN)**
9650 Rockville Pike
Bethesda, MD 20814-3990
(301) 530-7050

Food and Drug Administration (FDA)
Office of Consumer Affairs
Public Inquiries

5600 Fishers Lane (HFE-88)
Rockville, MD 20857
(301) 443-3170
http://www.fda.gov

Food and Nutrition Board
Institute of Medicine
2101 Constitution Avenue N.W.
Washington, D.C. 20418
(202) 334-1732

**Food and Nutrition Information
Center**
National Agricultural Library
Room 304
10301 Baltimore Avenue
Baltimore, MD 20705
(301) 504-5719
http://nalusda.gov/fnic/

Occupational Safety and Health

**Clearinghouse for Occupational
Safety and Health Centers for
Disease Control**
National Institute for Occupational
Safety and Health
5600 Fishers Lane
Rockville, MD 20857
(202) 472-7134

Organ Donations

The Living Bank (TLB)
(provides information and acts as
registry and referral service for people wanting to donate organs for
research or transplantation)
P.O. Box 6725
Houston, TX 77265
(800) 528-2971
in Texas (713) 961-9431

Osteopathic Medicine

**American Osteopathic Association
(AOA)**
142 East Ontario Street
Chicago, IL 60611
(312) 280-5800
(800) 621-1773
http://www.am-osteo-assn.org

Parent Support Groups

**National Organization of Mothers
with Twin Clubs (NOMOTC)**
P.O. Box 23188
Albuquerque, NM 87192-1188
(505) 275-0955

Parents Anonymous
(self-help group for abusive parents)
675 W. Foothill Boulevard
Suite 220
Claremont, CA 91711-3416
(909) 621-6184

Parents Without Partners, Inc.
401 N. Michigan Avenue
Chicago, IL 60611
(312) 644-6610
http://www.parentswithoutpartners.org

Pesticides

**National Pesticides
Telecommunications Network**
Agricultural Chemistry Extension
Oregon State University
333 Weniger Hall
Corvallis, OR 97331
(800) 858-7378

Phobias

**Anxiety Disorders Association of
American (ADAA)**
(provides information about phobias
and referrals to therapists and support groups)
11900 Parklawn Drive
Suite 100
Rockville, MD 20852
(301) 231-9350
http://www.adaa.org

TERRAP Programs
(headquarters for national network of
treatment clinics for agoraphobia)
932 Evelyn Street
Menlo Park, CA 94025
(415) 327-1312
(800) 2-PHOBIA

Physical Fitness

*See local yellow and white pages of
telephone directory for listing of local
health clubs and YMCAs, YWCAs, and
Jewish Community Centers*

**Cooper Institute for Aerobics
Research**
12330 Preston Road
Dallas, TX 75230
(214) 701-8001

**President's Council on Physical
Fitness and Sports**
701 Pennsylvania Avenue N.W.
Suite 250
Washington, D.C. 20004
(202) 272-3430

Women's Sports Foundation
Eisenhower Park
East Meadow, NY 11554
(516) 542-4700
(800) 227-3988
http://www.lifetimetv.com/WoSport/

Poisoning

See emergency numbers listed in the front of your local phone directory

National Poison Hotline
(800) 962-1253

Pregnancy

National Center for Education in Maternal and Child Health
2000 15th Street N.
Suite 701
Arlington, VA 22201-2617
(703) 524-7802

Product Safety

Consumer Product Safety Commission
Washington, D.C. 20207
(800) 638-CPSC
http://www.cpsc.gov

Radiation Control and Safety

Center for Devices and Radiological Health
Office of Consumer Affairs
5600 Fishers Lane HFC-210
Rockville, MD 20857
(301) 443-4190
http://www.fda.gov/cdrh/index.html

National Institute of Environmental Health Sciences
P.O. Box 12233
Research Triangle Park, NC 27709
(919) 541-3345
http://www.niehs.nih.gov

Rape

See white pages of telephone directory for listing of local rape crisis and counseling centers

National Clearinghouse on Marital and Date Rape
(for-profit referral service)
2325 Oak Street
Berkeley, CA 94708
(510) 524-1582
http://members.aol.com/ncmdr/index.html

National Coalition Against Sexual Assault
912 N. 2nd Street
Harrisburg, PA 17102
(717) 232-6745
http://www.achiever.com/freehmpg.ncas/

Reye's Syndrome

National Reye's Syndrome Foundation
426 North Lewis
Bryan, OH 43506
(419) 636-2679
(800) 233-7393

Self-Care/Self-Help

National Self-Help Clearinghouse (NSHC)
(provides information about self-help groups)
25 West 43rd Street
Room 620
New York, NY 10036
(212) 354-8525

United Way of America
701 N. Fairfax Street
Alexandria, VA 22314
(703) 836-7100
http://www.unitedway.org

Sex Education

American Association of Sex Educators, Counselors, and Therapists (AASECT)
435 North Michigan Avenue
Suite 1717
Chicago, IL 60611
(312) 644-0828
http://www.aasect.org

Advocates for Youth
(develops programs and material to educate youth on sex and sexual responsibility)
1025 Vermont Avenue, N.W. Suite 200
Washington, D.C. 20005
(202) 347-5700

Planned Parenthood Federation of America (PPFA)
810 Seventh Avenue
New York, NY 10019
(212) 541-7800
http://www.plannedparenthood.org

Sex Information and Education Council of the U.S. (SIECUS)
(maintains an information clearinghouse on all aspects of human sexuality)
130 West 42nd Street
Suite 350
New York, NY 10036
(212) 819-9770
http://www.siecus.org

Sexual Abuse and Assault

National Center for Assault Prevention
(provides services to children, adolescents, mentally retarded adults, and elderly)
606 Delsea Drive
Sewell, NJ 08080
(609) 582-7000
(800) 258-3189

National Committee for Prevention of Child Abuse
332 S. Michigan Avenue
Suite 1600
Chicago, IL 60604
(312) 663-3520

Parents United International
(support group for individuals—and their families—who have experienced molestation as children)
615 15th Street
Modesto, CA 95354-2510
(408) 453-7616

Sexual Difficulties

Impotence Institute of America
(provides information on causes and treatment of impotence)
119 S. Ruth Street
Maryville, TN 37803
(423) 983-6092

Sexually Transmitted Diseases

Centers for Disease Control and Prevention
1600 Clifton Road, N.E.
Atlanta, GA 30333
(404) 639-3311
http://www.cdc.gov

Herpes Resource Center
American Social Health Association
P.O. Box 13827
Research Triangle Park, NC 27709
(919) 361-8488
http://www.ashastd.org/herpes/hrc.
html

National STD Hotline
(800) 227-8922

Sickle Cell Disease

Center for Sickle Cell Disease
Howard University
2121 Georgia Avenue N.W.
Washington, D.C. 20059
(202) 806-7930

Sickle Cell Disease Association of America
200 Corporate Pointe, Suite 495
Culver City, CA 90230
(310) 216-6363
(800) 421-8453

Skin Disease

National Psoriasis Foundation
6600 S.W. 92nd Avenue, Suite 300
Portland, OR 97223
(503) 244-7404
http://www.psoriasis.org

Sleep and Sleep Disorders

American Narcolepsy Association
1255 Post Street
Suite 404
San Francisco, CA 94109
(415) 788-4793

American Sleep Disorders Association
6301 Bandel Road
Suite 101
Rochester, MN 55901
(507) 287-6006
http://www.asda.org

Better Sleep Council
333 Commerce Street
Alexandria, VA 22314
(703) 683-8371

Smoking and Tobacco

Action on Smoking and Health (ASH)
(provides information on non-smokers' rights and related subjects)
2013 H Street N.W.
Washington, D.C. 20006
(202) 659-4310
http://ash.org

American Cancer Society
(provides information about quitting smoking and smoking cessation programs)
1599 Clifton Road, N.E.
Atlanta, GA 30329
(800) 227-2345
http://www.cancer.org

American Heart Association
(provides information about quitting smoking and smoking cessation programs)
7272 Greenville Avenue
Dallas, TX 75321
(800) 242-8721
(214) 373-6300
http://www.amhrt.org

American Lung Association
(provides information about quitting smoking and smoking cessation programs)
1740 Broadway
New York, NY 10019
(800) LUNG-USA
(212) 315-8700
http://www.lungusa.org

Americans for Nonsmokers' Rights
2530 San Pablo Avenue
Suite J
Berkeley, CA 94702
(510) 841-3032
http://www.no-smoke.org

Stress Reduction

Association for Applied Psychophysiology and Biofeedback (AABP)
10200 W. 44th Avenue
Suite 304
Wheat Ridge, CO 80033
(800) 477-8892
(303) 422-8436

Stroke

Council on Stroke
American Heart Association
7320 Greenville Avenue
Dallas, TX 75321
(214) 373-6300

National Institute of Neurological and Communicative Disorders and Stroke
National Institutes of Health
9000 Rockville Pike
Bethesda, MD 20892
(301) 496-4000

Stuttering

National Center for Stuttering
200 East 33rd Street
New York, NY 10016
(800) 221-2483
(212) 532-1460
http://www.stuttering.com

Sudden Infant Death Syndrome (SIDS)

SIDS Alliance
(provides information and referrals for families who have lost an infant because of SIDS)
1314 Bedford Avenue
Suite 210
Baltimore, MD 21208
(800) 221-7437
(410) 653-8226

Suicide Prevention

American Association of Suicidology (AAS)
4201 Connecticut Avenue N.W.
Suite 310
Washington, D.C. 20008
(202) 237-2280
http://www.cyberpsych.org/aas/index.
htm

National Runaway Switchboard
3080 N. Lincoln Avenue
Chicago, IL 60657
(800) 621-4000
(773) 880-9860
http://www.nrscrisisline.org/

Suicide Prevention Hotline
(800) 827-7571

Surgery

**National Second Surgical Opinion
Program**
(800) 638-6833
in Maryland (800) 492-6603

Terminal Illness

**Choices in Dying—The National
Council for the Right to Die (CID)**
(promotes research on death and
dying and works for the right of
terminally ill persons to refuse extraordinary life-prolonging measures)
200 Varick Street, 10th Floor
New York, NY 10014-4810
(800) 989-1011
(212) 366-5540

**Make-a-Wish Foundation of
America (MAWFA)**
(dedicated to granting the special
wishes of terminally ill children)
100 W. Clarendon Avenue

Suite 2200
Phoenix, AZ 85013
(800) 722-9474
(602) 279-9474
http://www.wish.org

Make Today Count (MTC)
(self-help group for persons with
terminal illness)
1235 E. Cherokee Street
Springfield, MO 65804
(800) 432-2273
(417) 885-3324

Weight Control

Overeaters Anonymous (OA)
6075 Zenith Court, N.E.
Rio Rancho, NM 87124-6424
(505) 891-2664

Take Off Pounds Sensibly (TOPS)
P.O. Box 07360
4575 S. Fifth Street
Milwaukee, WI 53207-0360
(800) 932-8677
(414) 482-4620

Weight Watchers International
175 Crossways Park West
Woodbury, NY 11797

(516) 949-0400
http://www.weight-watchers.com

Wellness

Wellness Associates
(publishes The Wellness Inventory)
121489 Orr Springs Road
Ukiah, CA 95482
(707) 937-2331

Women's Health

**Boston Women's Health Book
Collective**
(authors of *The New Our Bodies,
Ourselves*, a well-known book on
women's health)
240A Elm Street
Somerville, MA 02144
(617) 625-0271

**National Women's Health Network
(NWHN)**
514 10th Street N.W.
Suite 400
Washington, D.C. 20004
(202) 347-1140

Text and Photography Credits

This page constitutes an extension of the copyright page. We have made every effort to trace the ownership of all copyrighted material and to secure permission from copyright holders. In the event of any question arising as to the use of any material, we will be pleased to make the necessary corrections in future printings. Thanks are due to the following authors, publishers, and agents for permission to use the material indicated.

Photo Credits

Pulsepoints Photo: Randy M. Ury/The Stock Market
Spotlight on Diversity Photo: Rob Lewine/The Stock Market

Chapter 1

p.   1   Mathias Oppersdorff/Photo Researchers, Inc.
p.   5   Yvonne Hemsey/Gamma Liaison
p.   6   Courtesy National Heart, Lung and Blood Institute
p.   9   Carl J. Single, Syracuse Newspapers/The Image Works
p. 12   Courtesy of Centers for Disease Control
          Robert Aschenbrenner/Stock, Boston
p. 13   David Young-Wolff/PhotoEdit

Chapter 2

p. 16   Andy Sacks/Tony Stone Images
p. 20   Goldberg/Monkmeyer Press
p. 21   Forsyth/Monkmeyer Press
          Bernard Wolf/Monkmeyer Press
p. 22   Bruce Ayres/Tony Stone Images
p. 24   James Schnepf/Liaison International

Chapter 3

p. 31   Lori Adamski Peek/Tony Stone Images
p. 32   Myrleen Ferguson Cate/PhotoEdit
p. 33   Bob Schatz/Liaison International
p. 35   Ronnie Kaufman/The Stock Market
p. 36   Michael Greenlar/The Image Works
p. 38   Bruce Ayers/Tony Stone Images
p. 39   Brent Peterson/The Stock Market
p. 41   Paul Avis/Liaison International
p. 44   Ed Malles/Liaison International
p. 46   Dr. R. Nesse/Andrew Sacks

Chapter 4

p. 51   Alan Becker/The Image Bank, Copyright 1998
p. 52   Gary Conner/PhotoEdit
          John P. Kelly/The Image Bank, Copyright 1998
          Tom & Dee Ann McCarthy/PhotoEdit
p. 55   Randy M. Ury/The Stock Market
p. 57   © David Madison 1998
p. 61   The Stock Market

Chapter 5

p. 68   Gabriel M. Covian/The Image Bank, Copyright 1998
p. 71   Bob Daemmrich Photos/The Image Works
p. 80   Mark C. Burnett/Stock, Boston
          Medical Images, Inc.
p. 82   Felicia Martinez/PhotoEdit
          Montaine/Monkmeyer Press
p. 84   Marc Alcarez/The Picture Cube

Chapter 6

p. 89   Network Productions/The Image Works
p. 96   Collins/Monkmeyer Press
p. 98   David Young-Wolff/PhotoEdit
p. 102   Ronnie Kaufman/The Stock Market
          Thomas R. Stewart/The Stock Market

Chapter 7

p. 107   Bruce Ayers/Tony Stone Images
p. 110   Jeff Greenberg/PhotoEdit
p. 115   Courtesy of Posmentier Graphics
p. 124   Deborah Davis/PhotoEdit
p. 129   T. Petillot/Explorer/Photo Researchers, Inc.

Chapter 8

p. 134   Bill Bachmann/The Image Works
p. 140   © Joel Gordon 1988
p. 142   © Joel Gordon 1990
          © Joel Gordon 1990
p. 143   © Joel Gordon 1995
p. 144   © Joel Gordon 1988
p. 145   © Joel Gordon 1988
p. 146   © Joel Gordon 1988
p. 151   Tim Hermetz/Gamma Liaison
p. 153   Petit Format/Nestle/Science Source/Photo Researchers, Inc.
p. 156   David Austen/Tony Stone Images

Chapter 9

p. 163   Steven Peters/Tony Stone Images
p. 172   Scott Camazine/Photo Researchers, Inc.
p. 176   Rhoda Sidney/Stock, Boston
p. 178   From Morse S.A., Moreland A.A., Holmes K.K.: Atlas of Sexually Transmitted Diseases and AIDS, Second Edition, 1996, Mosby-Wolfe. By permission of Mosby International, Ltd.
p. 179   (a) St. Bartholomew's Hospital/Science Photo Library/Photo Researchers, Inc.
          (b) Biophoto Associates/Photo Researchers, Inc.
p. 180   Marazzi/Science Photo Library/Photo Researchers, Inc.
p. 181   E. Gray/Science Photo Library/Photo Researchers, Inc.

Chapter 10

p. 190   Al Bello/Tony Stone Images
p. 195   Will & Deni McIntyre/Photo Researchers, Inc.
p. 197   Cabisco/Visuals Unlimited
          Sloop-Ober/Visuals Unlimited
p. 199   Bruce Ayres/Tony Stone Images

Text Credits

Glossary

abscess A localized accumulation of pus and disintegrating tissue.

absorption The passage of substances into or across membranes or tissues.

abstinence Voluntary refrainment from sexual intercourse.

acid rain Rain with a high concentration of acids produced by air pollutants emitted during the combustion of fossil fuels and the smelting of ores; damages plant and animal life and buildings.

acquired immunodeficiency syndrome (AIDS) The final stages of HIV infection, characterized by a variety of severe illnesses and decreased levels of certain immune cells.

acupuncture A Chinese medical practice of puncturing the body with needles inserted at specific points to relieve pain or cure disease.

acute injuries Physical injuries, such as sprains, bruises, and pulled muscles, which result from sudden traumas, such as falls or collisions.

adaptive response The body's attempt to reestablish homeostasis or stability.

addiction A behavioral pattern characterized by compulsion, loss of control, and continued repetition of a behavior or activity in spite of adverse consequences.

additive Characterized by a combined effect that is equal to the sum of the individual effects.

additives Substances added to foods to enhance certain qualities, such as appearance, taste, or freshness.

adjustment disorder An extraordinary response to a stressful event or situation.

adoption The legal process for becoming the parent to a child of other biological parents.

advance directives Documents that specify an individual's preferences regarding treatment in a medical crisis.

aerobic circuit training Combining aerobic and strength exercises to build both cardiovascular fitness and muscular strength and endurance.

aerobic exercise Physical activity in which sufficient or excess oxygen is continually supplied to the body.

after-intercourse methods Treatments, such as large doses of oral contraceptives, menstrual extraction, or dilation and curettage, given after unprotected intercourse to prevent pregnancy.

ageism A form of discrimination based on myths about aging and the elderly.

aging The characteristic pattern of normal life changes that occur as an individual gets older.

alcohol abuse Continued use of alcohol despite awareness of social, occupational, psychological, or physical problems related to its use, or use of alcohol in dangerous ways or situations, such as before driving.

alcohol dependence Development of a strong craving for alcohol due to the pleasurable feelings or relief of stress or anxiety produced by drinking.

alcoholism A chronic, progressive, potentially fatal disease characterized by impaired control of drinking, a preoccupation with alcohol, continued use of alcohol despite adverse consequences, and distorted thinking, most notably denial.

allergy A hypersensitivity to a particular substance in one's environment or diet.

altruism Acts of helping or giving to others without thought of self-benefit.

Alzheimer's disease A progressive deterioration of intellectual powers due to physiological changes within the brain; symptoms include diminishing ability to concentrate and reason, disorientation, depression, apathy, and paranoia.

amenorrhea The absence or suppression of menstruation.

amino acids Organic compounds containing nitrogen, carbon, hydrogen, and oxygen; the essential building blocks of proteins.

amnion The innermost membrane of the sac enclosing the embryo or fetus.

amphetamine Any of a class of stimulants that trigger the release of epinephrine, which stimulates the central nervous system; users experience a state of hyper-alertness and energy, followed by a crash as the drug wears off.

anabolic steroids Drugs derived from testosterone and approved for medical use, but often used by athletes to increase their musculature and weight.

anaerobic exercise Physical activity in which the body develops an oxygen deficit.

androgynous Not tied to traditional gender roles, as in a marriage.

androgyny The expression of both masculine and feminine traits.

anemia A condition characterized by a marked reduction in the number of circulating red blood cells or in hemoglobin, the oxygen-carrying component of red blood cells.

angina pectoris A severe, suffocating chest pain caused by a brief lack of oxygen to the heart.

angioplasty Surgical repair of an obstructed artery by passing a balloon catheter through the blood vessel to the area of disease and then inflating the catheter to compress the plaque against the vessel wall.

anorexia nervosa A psychological disorder in which refusal to eat and/or an extreme loss of appetite leads to malnutrition, severe weight loss, and possibly death.

antagonistic Opposing or counteracting.

antibiotics Substances produced by microorganisms, or synthetic agents, that are toxic to other types of microorganisms; in dilute solutions, used to treat infectious diseases.

antidepressant A drug used primarily to treat symptoms of depression.

antioxidants Substances that prevent the damaging effects of oxidation in cells.

antiviral drug A substance that decreases the severity and duration of a viral infection if taken prior to or soon after onset of the infection.

anxiety A feeling of apprehension and dread, with or without a known cause; may range from mild to severe and may be accompanied by physical symptoms.

anxiety disorders A group of psychological disorders involving episodes of apprehension, tension, or uneasiness, stemming from the anticipation of danger and sometimes accompanied by physical symptoms, which cause significant distress and impairment to an individual.

aorta The main artery of the body, arising from the left ventricle of the heart.

appetite A desire for food, stimulated by anticipated hunger, physiological changes within the brain and body, the availability of food, and other environmental and psychological factors.

arrhythmia Any irregularity in the rhythm of the heartbeat.

arteriosclerosis Any of a number of chronic diseases characterized by degeneration of the arteries and hardening and thickening of arterial walls.

arthritis Inflammation of the joints.

artificial insemination The introduction of viable sperm into the vagina by artificial means for the purpose of inducing conception.

assertive Behaving in a confident manner to make your needs and desires clear to others in a nonhostile way.

asthma A disease or allergic response characterized by bronchial spasms and difficult breathing.

atherosclerosis A form of arteriosclerosis in which fatty substances (plaque) are deposited on the inner walls of arteries.

atrial fibrillation A condition characterized by an irregular, abnormally rapid heartbeat.

atrium (plural atria) Either of the two upper chambers of the heart, which receive blood from the veins.

attention deficit/hyperactivity disorder (ADHD) A spectrum of difficulties in controlling motion and sustaining attention, including hyperactivity, impulsivity, and distractibility.

autoimmune Resulting from the attack on body tissue by an immune system that fails to recognize the tissue as self.

autonomy The ability to draw on internal resources; independence from familial and societal influences.

autoscopy The sensation of one's self being outside its body, often experienced by individuals in near-death medical crises.

aversion therapy A treatment that attempts to help a person overcome a dependence or bad habit by making the person feel disgusted or repulsed by that habit.

axon The long fiber that conducts impulses from the neuron's nucleus to its dendrites.

axon terminal The ending of an axon, from which impulses are transmitted to a dendrite of another neuron.

ayurveda A traditional Indian medical treatment involving meditation, exercise, herbal medications, and nutrition.

bacteria (singular, bacterium) One-celled microscopic organisms; the most plentiful pathogens.

bacterial vaginosis A vaginal infection caused by overgrowth and depletion of various microorganisms living in the vagina, resulting in a malodorous white or gray vaginal discharge.

barbiturates Antianxiety drugs that depress the central nervous system, reduce activity and induce relaxation, drowsiness, or sleep; often prescribed to relieve tension and treat epileptic seizures or as a general anesthetic.

barrier contraceptives Birth-control devices that block the meeting of egg and sperm, either by physical barriers, such as condoms, diaphragms, or cervical caps, or by chemical barriers, such as spermicide, or both.

basal body temperature The body temperature upon waking, before any activity.

basal metabolic rate (BMR) The number of calories required to sustain the body at rest.

behavior therapy Psychotherapy that emphasizes application of the principles of learning to substitute desirable responses and behavior patterns for undesirable ones.

benign hypertrophy Enlargement of the prostate gland, resulting in a pinching of the urethra.

benzodiazepines Antianxiety drugs that depress the central nervous system, reduce activity and induce relaxation, drowsiness, or sleep; often prescribed to relieve tension, muscular strain, sleep problems, anxiety, and panic attacks; also used as an anesthetic and in the treatment of alcohol withdrawal.

binge eating The rapid consumption of an abnormally large amount of food in a relatively short time.

biofeedback A technique of becoming aware, with the aid of external monitoring devices, of internal physiological activities in order to develop the capability of altering them.

bipolar disorder Severe depression alternating with periods of manic activity and elation.

bisexual Sexually oriented toward both sexes.

blended family A family formed when one or both of the partners bring children from a previous union to the new marriage.

blood-alcohol concentration (BAC) The amount of alcohol in the blood, expressed as a percentage.

body mass index (BMI) The percentage of fat in one's body.

bone-marrow transplantation A cancer treatment involving high doses of radiation or chemotherapy during which the marrow is destroyed and then replaced with healthy bone marrow.

botulism Possibly fatal food poisoning, caused by a type of bacterium, which grows and produces its toxin in the absence of air and is found in improperly canned food.

bradycardia An abnormally slow heart rate, under 60 beats per minute.

breech birth A birth in which the infant's buttocks or feet pass through the birth canal first.

bulimia nervosa Episodic binge eating, often followed by forced vomiting or laxative abuse, and accompanied by a persistent preoccupation with body shape and weight.

burnout A state of physical, emotional, and mental exhaustion resulting from constant or repeated emotional pressure.

caesarean delivery The surgical procedure in which an infant is delivered through an incision made in the abdominal wall and uterus.

calorie The amount of energy required to raise the temperature of 1 gram of water by 1 Celsius. In everyday usage related to the energy content of foods and the energy expended in activities, a calorie is actually the equivalent of a thousand such calories, or a Kilocalorie.

candidiasis An infection of the yeast Candida albicans, commonly occurring in the vagina, vulva, penis, and mouth and causing burning, itching, and a whitish discharge.

capillary A minute blood vessel that connects an artery to a vein.

carbohydrates Organic compounds, such as starches, sugars, and glycogen, that are composed of carbon, hydrogen, and oxygen, and are sources of bodily energy.

carbon monoxide A colorless, odorless gas produced by the burning of gasoline or tobacco; displaces oxygen in the hemoglobin molecules of red blood cells.

carcinogen A substance that produces cancerous cells or enhances their development and growth.

cardiopulmonary resuscitation (CPR) A method of artificial stimulation of the heart and lungs; a combination of mouth-to-mouth breathing and chest compression.

cardiovascular fitness The ability of the heart and blood vessels to circulate blood through the body efficiently.

celibacy Abstention from sexual activity; can be partial or complete, permanent or temporary.

cell-mediated The portion of the immune response that protects against parasites, fungi, cancer cells, and foreign tissue, primarily by means of T cells, or lymphocytes.

certified social worker A person who has completed a two-year graduate program in counseling people with mental problems.

cervical cap A thimble-sized rubber or plastic cap that is inserted into the vagina to fit over the cervix and prevent the passage of sperm into the uterus during sexual intercourse; used with a spermicidal foam or jelly, it serves as both a chemical and a physical barrier to sperm.

cervix The narrow, lower end of the uterus that opens into the vagina.

chanchroid A soft, painful sore or localized infection usually acquired through sexual contact.

chemoprevention The use of natural or synthetic substances to reduce the risk of developing cancer.

chiropractic A method of treating disease, primarily through manipulating the bones and joints to restore normal nerve function.

chlamydial infections A sexually transmitted disease caused by the bacterium Chlamydia trachomatis, often asymptomatic in women, but sometimes characterized by urinary pain; if undetected and untreated, may result in pelvic inflammatory disease (PID).

chlorinated hydrocarbons Highly toxic pesticides, such as DDT and chlordane, that are extremely resistant to breakdown; may cause cancer, birth defects, neurological disorders, and damage to wildlife and the environment.

cholesterol An organic substance found in animal fats; linked to cardiovascular disease, particularly atherosclerosis.

chronic fatigue syndrome (CFS) A cluster of symptoms whose cause is not yet known; a primary symptom is debilitating fatigue.

chronic obstructive lung disease (COLD) Any one of several lung diseases characterized by obstruction of breathing, including emphysema and chronic bronchitis.

circumcision The surgical removal of the foreskin of the penis.

cirrhosis A chronic disease, especially of the liver, characterized by a degeneration of cells and excessive scarring.

clinical practice guidelines Recommendations used by physicians to determine appropriate health care for specific conditions.

clitoris A small erectile structure on the female, corresponding to the penis on the male.

cocaine A white crystalline powder extracted from the leaves of the coca plant which stimulates the central nervous system and produces a brief period of euphoria followed by a depression.

codependence An emotional and psychological behavioral pattern in which the spouses, partners, parents, children, and friends of individuals with addictive behaviors allow or enable their loved ones to continue their self-destructive habits.

cognitive therapy A technique used to identify an individual's beliefs and attitudes, recognize negative thought patterns, and educate in alternative ways of thinking.

cohabitation Two people living together as a couple, without official ties such as marriage.

coitus interruptus The removal of the penis from the vagina before ejaculation.

colpotomy Surgical sterilization by cutting or blocking the fallopian tubes through an incision made in the wall of the vagina.

coma A state of total unconsciousness.

companion-oriented marriage A marital relationship in which the partners share interests, activities, and domestic responsibilities.

complementary proteins Incomplete proteins that, when combined, provide all the amino acids essential for protein synthesis.

complete proteins Proteins that contain all the amino acids needed by the body for growth and maintenance.

complex carbohydrates Starches, including cereals, fruits, and vegetables.

conception The merging of a sperm and an ovum.

conditioning The gradual building up of the body to enhance one or more of the three main components of physical fitness: flexibility, cardiovascular or aerobic fitness, and muscular strength and endurance.

condom A latex sheath worn over the penis during sexual acts to prevent conception and/or the transmission of disease; some condoms contain a spermicidal lubricant.

congestive heart failure Inability of the heart to pump at normal capacity, resulting in decreased blood flow throughout the body, collection of blood fluids in the lungs, and pulmonary congestion.

constant-dose combination pill An oral contraceptive that releases synthetic estrogen and progestin at constant levels throughout the menstrual cycle.

contraception The prevention of conception; birth control.

coping mechanism Any of several conscious and unconscious mental processes that enable a person to cope with a difficult situation or problem; usually healthier, more mature, and more effective than a defense mechanism.

coronary angiography A diagnostic test in which a thin tube is threaded through the blood vessels of the heart, a dye is injected, and X rays are taken to detect blockage of the arteries.

coronary bypass Surgical correction of a blockage in a coronary artery by grafting an artery from the patient's leg or chest wall onto the damaged artery to detour blood around the blockage.

corpus luteum A yellowish mass of tissue that is formed, immediately after ovulation, from the remaining cells of the follicle; it secretes estrogen and progesterone for the remainder of the menstrual cycle.

Cowpers glands Two small glands that discharge into the male urethra; also called bulbourethral glands.

crib death The unexplained death of an apparently healthy baby under one year of age during sleep; also called sudden infant death syndrome (SIDS).

cross-training Alternating two or more different types of fitness activities.

crucifers Plants, including broccoli, cabbage, and cauliflower, that contain large amounts of fiber, proteins, and indoles.

culture The set of shared attitudes, values, goals, and practices of a group that are internalized by an individual within the group.

cunnilingus Sexual stimulation of a woman's genitals by means of oral manipulation.

cystitis Inflammation of the urinary bladder.

decibel (dB) A unit for measuring the intensity of sounds.

deleriants Chemicals, such as solvents, aerosols, glue, cleaning fluids, petroleum products, and some anesthetics, that produce vapors with psychoactive effects when inhaled.

delirium tremens (DTs) The delusions, hallucinations, and agitated behavior following withdrawal from long-term chronic alcohol abuse.

dementia Deterioration of mental capability.

dendrites Branching fibers of a neuron that receive impulses from axon terminals of other neurons and conduct these impulses toward the nucleus.

depression In general, feelings of unhappiness and despair; as a mental illness, also characterized by an inability to function normally

depressive disorders A group of psychological disorders involving pervasive and sustained depression.

dermatitis Any inflammation of the skin.

designer drugs Illegally manufactured psychoactive drugs that have dangerous physical and psychological effects.

detoxification The supervised removal of a poisonous or harmful substance (such as a drug) from the body; a therapy for alcoholics in which they are denied alcohol in a controlled environment.

diabetes mellitus A disease in which the inadequate production of insulin leads to failure of the body tissues to break down carbohydrates at a normal rate.

diagnostic-related group (DRG) A category of conditions requiring hospitalization for which the cost of care has been determined prior to a clients hospitalization.

diaphragm A bowl-like rubber cup with a flexible rim that is inserted into the vagina to cover the cervix and prevent the passage of sperm into the uterus during sexual intercourse; used with a spermicidal foam or jelly, it serves as both a chemical and a physical barrier to sperm.

diastole The period between contractions in the cardiac cycle, during which the heart relaxes and dilates as it fills with blood.

digestion The process of chemically and mechanically breaking down foods into compounds capable of being absorbed by body cells.

dilation and evacuation (D and E) A medical procedure in which the contents of the uterus are removed through the use of instruments.

dioxins A family of chemicals used in industry; some forms are believed to be extremely toxic.

distress A negative stress stage that may result in illness.

do-not-resuscitate (DNR) A directive expressing an individual's preference that resuscitation efforts not be made during a medical crisis.

drug Any substance, other than food, that when taken, affects bodily functions and structures.

drug abuse The excessive use of a drug in a manner inconsistent with accepted medical practice.

drug misuse The use of a drug for a purpose (or person) other than that for which it was medically intended.

dyathanasia The act of permitting death by the removal or ending of any extraordinary efforts to sustain life; passive euthanasia.

dysfunctional Characterized by negative and destructive patterns of behavior between partners or between parents and children.

dysmenorrhea Painful menstruation.

dyspareunia A sexual difficulty in which a woman experiences pain during sexual intercourse.

dysthymia Frequent, prolonged mild depression.

eating disorders Bizarre, often dangerous patterns of food consumption, including anorexia nervosa, bulimia nervosa, and bulimarexia.

e coli *Escherichia coli*, a bacteria often spread through undercooked or inadequately washed foods.

ecosystem A community of organisms sharing a physical and chemical environment and interacting with each other.

ectopic pregnancy A pregnancy in which the fertilized egg has implanted itself outside the uterine cavity, usually in the fallopian tube.

ejaculation The expulsion of semen from the penis.

ejaculatory duct The canal connecting the seminal vesicles and vas deferens.

electrocardiogram (ECG, EKG) A graphic record of the electric current associated with heartbeats.

electromagnetic fields (EMFs) The invisible electric and magnetic fields generated by an electrically charged conductor.

embryo An organism in its early stage of development; in humans, the embryonic period lasts from about the second to the eighth week of pregnancy.

emotional health The ability to express and acknowledge one's feelings and moods.

emotional intelligence A term used by some psychologists to evaluate the capacity of people to understand themselves and relate well with others.

endocrine system The group of ductless glands that produce hormones and secrete them directly into the blood for transport to target organs.

endometrium The mucous membrane lining the uterus.

endorphins Mood-elevating, pain-killing chemicals produced by the brain.

endurance The ability to withstand the stress of continued physical exertion.

enkephalins Naturally occurring opioids that the body uses to relieve pain and stress.

environmental tobacco smoke Secondhand cigarette smoke; the third leading preventable cause of death.

epididymis That portion of the male duct system in which sperm mature.

epidural block An injection of anesthesia into the membrane surrounding the spinal cord to numb the lower body during labor and childbirth.

epilepsy A variety of neurological disorders characterized by sudden attacks (seizures) of violent muscle contractions and unconsciousness.

erogenous Sexually sensitive.

estrogen The female sex hormone that stimulates female secondary sex characteristics.

ethyl alcohol The intoxicating agent in alcoholic beverages; also called ethanol.

eustress Positive stress, which stimulates a person to function properly.

euthanasia Any method of painlessly causing death for a terminally ill person.

failure rate The number of pregnancies that occur per year for every 100 women using a particular method of birth control.

fallopian tubes The pair of channels that transport ova from the ovaries to the uterus; the usual site of fertilization.

false negative A diagnostic test result that falsely indicates the absence of a particular condition.

false positive A diagnostic test result that falsely indicates the presence of a particular condition.

family A group of people united by marriage, blood, or adoption, residing in the same household, maintaining a common culture, and interacting with one another on the basis of their roles within the group.

fat-soluble vitamins Vitamins absorbed through the intestinal membranes, with the aid of fats in the diet or bile from the liver, and stored in the body.

fellatio Sexual stimulation of a man's genitals by means of oral manipulation.

fertilization The fusion of the sperm and egg nuclei.

fetal alcohol effects (FAE) Milder forms of FAS, including low birth weight, irritability as newborns, and permanent mental impairment as a result of the mother's alcohol consumption during pregnancy.

fetal alcohol syndrome (FAS) A cluster of physical and mental defects in the newborn, including low birth weight, smaller-than-normal head circumference, intrauterine growth retardation, and permanent mental impairment-caused by the mother's alcohol consumption during pregnancy.

fetus The human organism developing in the uterus from the ninth week until birth.

fiber Indigestible materials in food that lower blood cholesterol or facilitate digestion and elimination.

flap surgery Surgical removal of diseased tissue and bone from under the gums of the teeth.

flexibility The range of motion allowed by one's joints; determined by the length of muscles, tendons, and ligaments attached to the joints.

food allergies Hypersensitivities to particular foods.

food toxicologists Specialists who detect toxins in food and treat the conditions toxins produce.

frostbite The freezing or partial freezing of skin and tissue just below the skin, or even muscle and bone; more severe than frostnip.

frostnip Sudden blanching or lightening of the skin on hands, feet, and face, resulting from exposure to high wind speeds and low temperatures.

fungi (singular, fungus) Organisms that reproduce by means of spores.

gallstones Clumps of solid material, usually cholesterol, that form in bile stored in the gallbladder.

gamma globulin The antibody-containing portion of the blood fluid (plasma).

gender Maleness or femaleness, as determined by a combination of anatomical and physiological factors, psychological factors, and learned behaviors.

gene therapy A cancer treatment involving the insertion of genes into a patient.

general adaptation syndrome (GAS) The sequenced physiological response to a stressful situation; consists of three stages: alarm, resistance, and exhaustion.

generalized anxiety disorder (GAD) An anxiety disorder characterized as chronic distress.

generic Refers to products without trade names that are equivalent to other products protected by trademark registration.

gerontologist A specialist in the interdisciplinary field that studies aging.

gingivitis Inflammation of the gums.

glia Support cells for neurons in the brain and spinal cord that separate the brain from the bloodstream, assist in the growth of neurons, speed transmission of nerve impulses, and eliminate damaged neurons.

gonadotropins Gonad-stimulating hormones produced by the pituitary gland.

gonads The primary reproductive organs in a man (testes) or woman (ovaries).

gonorrhea A sexually transmitted disease caused by the bacterium *Neisseria gonorrhoeae*; symptoms include discharge from the penis; women are generally asymptomatic.

greenhouse effect An environmental phenomenon in which the buildup of carbon dioxide and other greenhouse gases leads to warming of the planet.

guided imagery An approach to stress control, self-healing, or motivating life changes by means of visualizing oneself in the state of calmness, wellness, or change.

gum disease Inflammation of the gum and bones that hold teeth in place.

hallucinogen A drug that causes hallucinations.

hashish A concentrated form of a drug, derived from the cannabis plant, containing the psychoactive ingredient TCH, which causes a sense of euphoria when inhaled or eaten.

health A state of complete well-being, including physical, psychological, spiritual, social, intellectual, and environmental components.

health maintenance organization (HMO) An organization that provides health services on a fixed-contract basis.

health promotion An educational and informational process in which people are helped to change attitudes and behaviors in an effort to improve their health.

heat cramps Painful muscle spasms caused by vigorous exercise accompanied by heavy sweating in the heat.

heat exhaustion Faintness, rapid heart beat, low blood pressure, an ashen appearance, cold and clammy skin, and nausea, resulting from prolonged sweating with inadequate fluid replacement.

heat stress Physical response to prolonged exposure to high temperature; occurs simultaneously with or after heat cramps.

heat stroke A medical emergency consisting of a fever of at least 105°F, hot dry skin, rapid heartbeat, rapid and shallow breathing, and elevated or lowered blood pressure, caused by the breakdown of the body's cooling mechanism.

helminth A parasitic roundworm or flatworm.

hemoglobin The oxygen-transporting component of red blood cells; composed of heme and globin.

hepatitis An inflammation and/or infection of the liver caused by a virus, often accompanied by jaundice.

herbal medicine An ancient form of medical treatment using substances derived from trees, flowers, ferns, seaweeds, and lichens to treat disease.

herbology The practice of herbal medicine.

hernia The abnormal protrusion of an organ or body part through the tissues of the walls containing it.

herpes simplex A condition caused by one of the herpes viruses and characterized by lesions of the skin or mucous membranes; herpes virus type 2 is sexually transmitted, and causes genital blisters or sores.

hertz A unit for measuring the frequency of sound waves.

heterosexual Primary sexual orientation toward members of the other sex.

holographic will A will wholly in the handwriting of its author.

home health care Provision of medical services and equipment to patients in the home to restore or maintain comfort, function, and health.

homeopathy A system of medical practice that treats a disease by administering dosages of substances that would in healthy persons produce symptoms similar to those of the disease.

homeostasis The body's natural state of balance or stability.

homosexual Primary sexual orientation toward members of the same sex.

hormones Substances released in the blood that regulate specific bodily functions.

hormone replacement therapy (HRT) The use of supplemental hormones during and after menopause.

hospice A homelike health-care facility or program committed to supportive care for terminally ill people.

host A person or population that contracts one or more pathogenic agents in an environment.

hostile or offensive environment A workplace made hostile, abusive, or unbearable by persistent inappropriate behaviors of coworkers or supervisors.

human immunodeficiency virus (HIV) A type of virus that causes a spectrum of health problems, ranging from a symptomless infection to changes in the immune system, to the development of life-threatening diseases because of impaired immunity.

human papilloma virus (HPV) A pathogen that causes genital warts and increases the risk of cervical cancer.

humoral A portion of the immune response that provides lifelong protection against bacterial or viral infections, such as mumps, by means of antibodies whose production is triggered by the release of antigens upon first exposure to the infectious agent.

hunger The physiological drive to consume food.

hydrostatic weighing The weighing of a person in water to distinguish buoyant fat from denser muscle.

hypertension High blood pressure occurring when the blood exerts excessive pressure against the arterial walls.

hypothermia An abnormally low body temperature; if not treated appropriately, coma or death could result.

hysterectomy The surgical removal of the uterus.

hysterotomy A procedure in which the uterus is surgically opened and the fetus inside it removed.

immune deficiency Partial or complete inability of the immune system to respond to pathogens.

immunity Protection from infectious diseases.

implantation The embedding of the fertilized ovum in the uterine lining.

impotence A sexual difficulty in which a man is unable to achieve or maintain an erection.

incest Sexual relations between two individuals too closely related to contract a legal marriage.

incomplete proteins Proteins that lack one or more of the amino acids essential for protein synthesis.

incubation period The time between when a pathogen enters the body and the first symptom.

indemnity A form of insurance that pays a major portion of medical expenses after a deductible amount is paid by the insured person.

indoles Naturally occurring chemicals found in foods such as winter squash, carrots, and crucifers; may help lower cancer risk.

induced abortion A procedure to remove the uterine contents after pregnancy has occurred.

infertility The inability to conceive a child.

infiltration A gradual penetration or invasion.

inflammation A localized response by the body to tissue injury, characterized by swelling and the dilation of the blood vessels.

inflammatory bowel disease (IBD) A digestive disease that causes frequent and intense diarrhea, abdominal pain, gas, fever, and rectal bleeding; Crohns disease is an inflammation anywhere in the digestive tract, and ulcerative colitis causes severe ulcers in the inner lining of the colon and rectum.

informed consent Permission (to undergo or receive a medical procedure or treatment) given voluntarily, with full knowledge and understanding of the procedure or treatment and its consequences.

influenza Any number of a type of fairly common, highly contagious viral diseases.

inhalants Substances that produce vapors having psychoactive effects when sniffed.

intercourse Sexual stimulation by means of entry of the penis into the vagina; coitus.

interpersonal therapy (IPT) A technique used to develop communication skills and relationships.

intimacy A state of closeness between two people, characterized by the desire and ability to share one's innermost thoughts and feelings with each other either verbally or nonverbally.

intoxication Maladaptive behavioral, psychological, and physiologic changes that occur as a result of substance abuse.

intramuscular Into or within a muscle.

intrauterine device (IUD) A device inserted into the uterus through the cervix to prevent pregnancy by interfering with implantation.

intravenous Into a vein.

ionizing radiation A form of energy emitted from atoms as they undergo internal change.

irradiation Exposure to or treatment by some form of radiation.

irritable bowel syndrome A digestive disease caused by intestinal spasms, resulting in frequent need to defecate, nausea, cramping, pain, gas and a continual sensation of rectal fullness.

isokinetic Having the same force; exercise with specialized equipment that provides resistance equal to the force applied by the user throughout the entire range of motion.

isometric Of the same length; exercise in which muscles increase their tension without shortening in length, such as when pushing an immovable object.

isotonic Having the same tension or tone; exercise requiring the repetition of an action that creates tension, such as weight lifting or calisthenics.

kidney stones Formations of calcium salts or minerals that form in the kidneys; may be passed out of the body in urine, surgically removed, or decomposed by high-frequency sound waves.

labia majora The fleshy outer folds that border the female genital area.

labia minora The fleshy inner folds that border the female genital area.

labor The process leading up to birth: effacement and dilation of the cervix; the movement of the baby into and through the birth canal, accompanied by strong contractions; and contraction of the uterus and expulsion of the placenta after the birth.

lacto-vegetarians People who eat dairy products as well as fruits and vegetables (but not meat, poultry, or fish).

Lamaze method A method of childbirth preparation taught to expectant parents to help the woman cope with the discomfort of labor; combines breathing and psychological techniques.

laparoscopy A surgical sterilization procedure in which the fallopian tubes are observed with a laparoscope inserted through a small incision, and then cut or blocked.

laparotomy A surgical sterilization procedure in which the fallopian tubes are cut or blocked through an incision made in the abdomen.

licensed clinical social worker (LCSW). See certified social worker.

lifestyle An individual's way of life, as indicated and expressed by one's daily practices, interests, possessions, and so on.

lipoprotein A compound in blood that is made up of proteins and fat; a high-density lipoprotein (HDL) picks up excess cholesterol in the blood; a low-density lipoprotein (LDL) carries more cholesterol and deposits it on the walls of arteries.

living will A written statement providing instructions for the use of life-sustaining procedures in the event of terminal illness or injury.

lochia The vaginal discharge of blood, mucus, and uterine tissue that occurs after birth.

locus of control An individual's belief about the source of power and influence over one's life.

lumpectomy The surgical removal of a breast tumor and its surrounding tissue.

Lyme disease A disease caused by a bacterium carried by a tick; it may cause heart arrhythmias, neurological problems, and arthritis symptoms.

lymph nodes Small tissue masses in which some immune cells are stored.

mainstream smoke The smoke inhaled directly by smoking a cigarette.

mainstreaming The placement of disabled students into regular school classes with specialized attention given in the classroom or in separate sessions.

major depression Sadness that does not end.

male pattern baldness The loss of hair at the vertex, or top, of the head.

malpractice The failure of a doctor or other health-care professionals to provide appropriate and skillful medical or surgical treatment.

mammography X-ray examination of the breasts for early detection of cancer.

managed care Health-care services and reimbursement predetermined by third-party insurers.

marijuana The drug derived from the cannabis plant, containing the psychoactive ingredient THC, which causes a mild sense of euphoria when inhaled or eaten.

marriage and family therapist A psychiatrist, psychologist, or social worker who specializes in marriage and family counseling.

mastectomy The surgical removal of an entire breast.

masturbation Manual (or nonmanual) self-stimulation of the genitals, often resulting in orgasm.

medical history The health-related information collected during the interview of a client by a health-care professional.

meditation A group of approaches that use quiet sitting, breathing techniques, and/or chanting to relax, improve concentration, and become attuned to one's inner self.

menarche The onset of menstruation at puberty.

menopause The complete cessation of ovulation and menstruation for twelve consecutive months.

menstruation Discharge of blood from the vagina as a result of the shedding of the uterine lining at the end of the menstrual cycle.

mental disorder Behavioral or psychological syndrome associated with distress or disability or with a significantly increased risk of suffering death, pain, disability, or loss of freedom.

mental health The ability to perceive reality as it is, to respond to its challenges, and to develop rational strategies for living.

meta-analysis Summarization and review of research in a particular area to evaluate the results of several large clinical trials in a uniform manner.

metastasize To spread to other parts of the body via the bloodstream or lymphatic system.

microwaves Extremely high frequency electromagnetic waves that increase the rate at which molecules vibrate, thereby generating heat.

migraine headache Severe headache resulting from the constriction, then dilation of blood vessels within the brain; sometimes accompanied by vomiting and nausea.

mindfulness A method of stress reduction that involves experiencing the physical and mental sensations of the present moment.

minerals Naturally occurring inorganic substances, small amounts of some being essential in metabolism and nutrition.

minilaparotomy A surgical sterilization procedure in which the fallopian tubes are cut or sealed by electrical coagulation through a small incision just above the pubic hairline.

minipill An oral contraceptive containing a small amount of progestin and no estrogen, which prevents contraception by making the mucus in the cervix so thick that sperm cannot enter the uterus.

miscarriage A pregnancy that terminates before the twentieth week of gestation; also called spontaneous abortion.

mononucleosis An infectious viral disease characterized by an excess of white blood cells in the blood, fever, bodily discomfort, a sore throat, and kidney and liver complications.

mons pubis The rounded, fleshy area over the junction of the female pubic bones.

mood A sustained emotional state that colors one's view of the world for hours or days.

moral The internal standard of right and wrong by which one makes judgments and decisions.

multiphasic pill An oral contraceptive that releases different levels of estrogen and progestin to mimic the hormonal fluctuations of the natural menstrual cycle.

mutagen An agent that causes alterations in the genetic material of living cells.

mutation A change in the genetic material of a cell or cells that is brought about by radiation, chemicals, or natural causes.

myocardial infarction (MI) A condition characterized by the dying of tissue areas in the myocardium, caused by interruption of the blood supply to those areas; the medical name for a heart attack.

near-death experiences See autoscopy.

negligence The failure to act in a way that a reasonable person would act.

neoplasm Any tumor, whether benign or malignant.

nephrosis A cluster of symptoms indicating chronic damage to the kidneys.

neuron The basic working unit of the brain, which transmits information from the senses to the brain and from the brain to specific body parts; each nerve cell consists of an axon, an axon terminal, and dendrites.

neuropsychiatry The study of the brain and mind.

neurotransmitters Chemicals released by neurons that stimulate or inhibit the action of other neurons.

nicotine The addictive substance in tobacco; one of the most toxic of all poisons.

nocturnal emissions Ejaculations while dreaming; wet dreams.

noncompliance Failure to take a prescription drug according to the doctor's instructions.

nongonococcal urethritis (NGU) Inflammation of the urethra caused by organisms other than the gonococcus bacterium.

nonopioids Chemically synthesized drugs that have sleep-inducing and pain-relieving properties similar to those of opium and its derivatives.

norms The unwritten rules regarding behavior and conduct expected or accepted by a group.

nucleus The central part of a cell, contained in the cell body of a neuron.

nutrients Elements in food that the body cannot produce on its own, which are essential for growth, repair, and energy.

nutrition The science devoted to the study of dietary needs for food and the effects of food on organisms.

obesity The excessive accumulation of fat in the body; a condition of being 20% or more above the ideal weight for a person of that height and gender.

obsessive-compulsive disorder (OCD) An anxiety disorder characterized by obsessions and/or compulsions that impair one's ability to function and form relationships.

oncogene A gene that, when activated by radiation or a virus, may cause a normal cell to become cancerous.

opioids Drugs that have sleep-inducing and pain-relieving properties, including opium and its derivatives and nonopioid, synthetic drugs.

optimism The tendency to seek out, remember, and expect pleasurable experiences.

oral contraceptives Preparations of synthetic hormones that inhibit ovulation; also referred to as birth control pills or simply the pill.

organic phosphates Toxic pesticides that may cause cancer, birth defects, neurological disorders, and damage to wildlife and the environment.

organic Term designating food produced with, or production based on the use of, fertilizer originating from plants or animals, without the use of pesticides or chemically formulated fertilizers.

orgasm A series of contractions of the pelvic muscles occurring at the peak of sexual arousal.

osteoporosis A condition common in older people in which the bones become increasingly soft and porous, making them susceptible to injury.

outcomes The ultimate impacts of particular treatments or absence of treatment.

ovary The female sex organ that produces egg cells, estrogen, and progesterone.

over-the-counter (OTC) drugs Medications that can be obtained legally without a prescription from a medical professional.

overloading Method of physical training involving increasing the number of repetitions or the amount of resistance gradually to work the muscle to temporary fatigue.

overtrain Working muscles too intensely or too frequently, resulting in persistent muscle soreness, injuries, unintended weight loss, nervousness, and an inability to relax.

overuse injuries Physical injuries to joints or muscles, such as strains, fractures, and tendinitis, which result from overdoing a repetitive activity.

ovo-lacto-vegetarians People who eat eggs, dairy products, and fruits and vegetables (but not meat, poultry, or fish).

ovulation The release of a mature ovum from an ovary approximately 14 days prior to the onset of menstruation.

ovulation method A method of birth control based on the observation of changes in the consistency of the mucus in the vagina to predict ovulation.

ovum (plural, **ova**) The female gamete (egg cell).

ozone layer An upper layer of the earth's atmosphere that protects the earth from harmful ultraviolet radiation from the sun.

panic attack A short episode characterized by physical sensations of light-headedness, dizziness, hyperventilation, and numbness of extremities, accompanied by an inexplicable terror, usually of a physical disaster such as death.

panic disorder An anxiety disorder in which the apprehension or experience of recurring panic attacks is so intense that normal functioning is impaired.

Pap smear A test in which cells removed from the cervix are examined under a microscope for signs of cancer; also called a Pap test.

pathogen A microorganism that produces disease.

PCP (phencyclidine) A synthetic psychoactive substance that produces effects similar to other psychoactive drugs when swallowed, smoked, sniffed, or injected, but may also trigger unpredictable behavioral changes.

pedophilia Sexual contact between an adult and an unrelated child.

pelvic inflammatory disease (PID) An inflammation of the internal female genital tract, characterized by abdominal pain, fever, and tenderness of the cervix.

penis The male organ of sex and urination.

percutaneous transluminal coronary angioplasty (PTCA) A procedure for unclogging arteries; also called balloon angioplasty.

perimenopause The period from a woman's first irregular cycles to her last menstruation.

perinatology The medical specialty concerned with the diagnosis and treatment of pregnant women with high-risk conditions and their fetuses.

perineum The area between the anus and vagina in the female and between the anus and scrotum in the male.

periodentitis Severe gum disease in which the tooth root becomes infected.

persistent vegetative state A state of being awake and capable of reacting to physical stimuli, such as light, while being unaware of pain or other environmental stimuli.

personality disorder An inflexible, maladaptive pattern of behavior that impairs an individual's ability to function.

phobia An anxiety disorder marked by an inordinate fear of an object, a class of objects, or a situation, resulting in extreme avoidance behaviors.

physical dependence The physiological attachment to, and need for, a drug.

physical fitness The ability to respond to routine physical demands, with enough reserve energy to cope with a sudden challenge.

phytochemicals Chemicals such as indoles, coumarins, and capsaicin, which exist naturally in plants and have disease-fighting properties.

placenta An organ that develops after implantation and to which the embryo attaches, via the umbilical cord, for nourishment and waste removal.

plaque The sludgelike substance that builds up on the inner walls of arteries.

pneumonia An inflammation of the lungs caused by infection or irritants.

pollutant A substance or agent in the environment, usually the by-product of human industry or activity, that is injurious to human, animal, or plant life.

pollution The presence of pollutants in the environment.

polyabuse The misuse or abuse of more than one drug.

polychlorinated biphenyls (PCBs) A family of chemical compounds, ranging from light, oily fluids to greasy or waxy substances, that have been widely used as industrial coolants and lubricants and in the manufacture of plastics, paints, and varnishes; a possible human carcinogen.

postpartum depression The emotional downswing that occurs after having a baby due to hormonal changes, physical exhaustion, and psychological pressures.

posttraumatic stress disorder (PTSD) The repeated reliving of a trauma through nightmares or recollection.

potentiating Making more effective or powerful.

preconception care Health care to prepare for pregnancy.

precycling The use of products that are packaged in recycled or recyclable material.

preferred provider organization (PPO) A group of physicians contracted to provide health care to members at a discounted price.

premature ejaculation A sexual difficulty in which a man ejaculates so rapidly that his partner's satisfaction is impaired.

premature labor Labor that occurs after the twentieth week but before the thirty-seventh week of pregnancy.

premenstrual dysphoric disorder (PMDD) A disorder that causes symptoms of psychological depression during the last week of the menstrual cycle.

premenstrual syndrome (PMS) A disorder that causes physical discomfort and psychological distress prior to a woman's menstrual period.

prevention Information and support offered to help healthy people identify their health risks, reduce stressors, prevent potential medical problems, and enhance their well-being.

primary care Ambulatory or outpatient care provided by a physician in an office, emergency room, or clinic.

progesterone The female sex hormone that stimulates the uterus, preparing it for the arrival of a fertilized egg.

progestin-only pill See minipill.

progressive relaxation A method of reducing muscle tension by contracting, then relaxing certain areas of the body.

promotion The process of enabling people to improve and increase control over their health in order to achieve a state of optimal health.

proof The alcoholic strength of a distilled spirit, expressed as twice the percentage of alcohol present.

prostate gland A structure surrounding the male urethra that produces a secretion that helps liquefy the semen from the testes.

prostatitis Inflammation of the prostate gland.

protection Measures that an individual can take when participating in risky behavior to prevent injury or unwanted risks.

protein A substance that is basically a compound of amino acids; one of the essential nutrients.

protozoa Microscopic animals made up of one cell or a group of similar cells.

psoriasis A chronic skin disorder caused by stress, skin damage, or illness and resulting in scaly, deep-pink, raised patches on the skin.

psychiatric drugs Medications that regulate a person's mental, emotional, and physical functions to facilitate normal functioning.

psychiatric nurse A nurse with special training and experience in mental health care.

psychiatrists Licensed medical doctors with additional training in psychotherapy, psychopharmacology, and treatment of mental disorders.

psychoactive Mood-altering.

psychodynamic Interpreting behaviors in terms of early experiences and unconscious influences.

psychological dependence The emotional or mental attachment to the use of a drug.

psychologists Mental health care professionals who have completed doctoral or graduate programs in psychology and are trained in a variety of psychotherapeutic techniques, but who are not medically trained and do not prescribe medications.

psychoneuroimmunology A scientific field that explores the relationships between and among the mind, the central nervous system, and the immune system.

psychoprophylaxis See Lamaze method.

psychotherapy Treatment designed to produce a response by psychological rather than physical means, such as suggestion, persuasion, reassurance, and support.

psychotropic Mind-affecting.

pyelonephritis Inflammation of the kidney.

quackery Medical fakery; unproven practices claiming to cure diseases or solve health problems.

quadrantectomy The surgical removal of a large portion of the breast and surrounding lymph glands.

quid pro quo A form of harassment in which a person in power or authority makes unwanted sexual advances as a condition for receiving a job, promotion, or favor.

rape Sexual penetration of a female or a male by means of intimidation, force, or fraud.

rapid-eye-movement (REM) sleep Regularly occurring periods of sleep during which the most active dreaming takes place.

receptors Molecules on the surface of neurons on which neurotransmitters bind after their release from other neurons.

recycling The processing or reuse of manufactured materials to reduce consumption of raw materials.

refractory period The period of time following orgasm during which the male cannot experience another orgasm.

rehabilitation medicine The use of surgical procedures, medication, and physical therapy to improve the condition of patients with disabling conditions such as blindness, deafness, and arthritis.

reinforcements Rewards or punishments for a behavior that will increase or decrease one's likelihood of repeating the behaviors.

relapse prevention An alcohol recovery treatment method that focuses on social skills training to develop ways of preventing or minimizing a relapse.

rep (or repetition) In weight training, a single performance of a movement or exercise.

repetitive motion injury (RMI) Inflammation of or damage to a part of the body due to repetition of the same movements.

rescue marriage A marital relationship in which one partner has had a traumatic childhood and views marriage as a way of healing the past.

resting heart rate The number of heartbeats per minute during inactivity.

reuptake Reabsorption by the originating cell of neurotransmitters that have not connected with receptors and have been left in synapses.

rhythm method A birth-control method in which sexual intercourse is avoided during those days of the menstrual cycle in which fertilization is most likely to occur.

romantic marriage A marital relationship in which sexual passion never fades.

rubella An infectious disease that may cause birth defects if contracted by a pregnant woman; also called German measles.

satiety A feeling of fullness after eating.

saturated fat A chemical term indicating that a fat molecule contains as many hydrogen atoms as its carbon skeleton can hold. These fats are normally solid at room temperature.

schizophrenia A general term for a group of mental disorders with characteristic psychotic symptoms, such as delusions, hallucinations, and disordered thought patterns during the active phase of the illness, and a duration of at least six months.

scrotum The external sac or pouch that holds the testes.

seasonal affective disorder (SAD) An annual rhythm of depression that appears to be linked to seasonal variations in light.

secondary sex characteristics Physical changes associated with maleness or femaleness, induced by the sex hormones.

self-actualization A state of wellness and fulfillment that can be achieved once certain human needs are satisfied; living to one's full potential.

self-efficacy Belief in one's ability to accomplish a goal or change a behavior.

self-esteem Confidence and satisfaction in oneself.

self-talk Repetition of positive messages about one's self-worth to learn more optimistic patterns of thought, feeling, and behavior.

semen The viscous whitish fluid that is the complete male ejaculate; a combination of sperm and secretions from the prostate gland, seminal vesicles, and other glands.

seminal vesicles Glands in the male reproductive system that produce the major portion of the fluid of semen.

set A person's expectations or preconceptions about a situation or experience; mind-set.

set-point theory The proposition that every person has an unconscious control system for keeping body fat (and therefore weight) at a predetermined level, or set point.

sets In weight training, the number of repetitions of the same movement or exercise.

sex Maleness or femaleness, resulting from genetic, structural, and functional factors.

sexual addiction A preoccupation with sex so intense and chronic that an individual cannot have a normal sexual relationship with a spouse or lover; sexual compulsion.

sexual coercion Sexual activity forced upon a person by the exertion of psychological pressure by another person.

sexual compulsion See sexual addiction.

sexuality The behaviors, instincts, and attitudes associated with being sexual.

sexually transmitted diseases (STDs) Any of a number of diseases that are acquired through sexual contact.

sexual orientation Sexual attraction to (and behavior with) individuals of one's own sex, the other sex, or both.

sidestream smoke The smoke emitted by a burning cigarette and breathed by everyone in a closed room, including the smoker; contains more tar and nicotine than mainstream smoke.

simple carbohydrates Sugars; like all carbohydrates, they provide the body with glucose.

skin calipers An instrument used to pinch skin folds at the arms, waist, and back to determine the percentage of body fat.

smog A grayish or brownish fog caused by the presence of smoke and/or chemical pollutants in the air.

social isolation A feeling of unconnectedness with others caused by and reinforced by infrequency of social contacts.

social phobia A severe form of social anxiety marked by extreme fears and avoidance of social situations.

sperm The male gamete produced by the testes and transported outside the body through ejaculation.

spermatogenesis The process by which sperm cells are produced.

spinal block An injection of anesthesia directly into the spinal cord to numb the lower body during labor and childbirth.

spiritual health The ability to identify one's basic purpose in life and to achieve one's full potential; the sense of connectedness to a greater power.

sterilization A surgical procedure to end a person's reproductive capability.

stimulant An agent, such as a drug, that temporarily relieves drowsiness, helps in the performance of repetitive tasks, and improves capacity for work.

strength Physical power; the maximum weight one can lift, push, or press in one effort.

stress The nonspecific response of the body to any demands made upon it; may be characterized by muscle tension and acute anxiety, or may be a positive force for action.

stressor Specific or nonspecific agents or situations that cause the stress response in a body.

stroke A cerebrovascular event in which the blood supply to a portion of the brain is blocked.

subcutaneous Under the skin.

suction curettage A procedure in which the contents of the uterus are removed by means of suction and scraping.

sudden infant death syndrome (SIDS) See crib death.

synapse A specialized site at which electrical impulses are transmitted from the axon terminal of one neuron to a dendrite of another.

synergistic Characterized by a combined effect that is greater than the sum of the individual effects.

syphilis A sexually transmitted disease caused by the bacterium *Treponema pallidum*, and characterized by early sores, a latent period, and a final period of life-threatening symptoms including brain damage and heart failure.

systemic disease A pathologic condition that spreads throughout the body.

systole The contraction phase of the cardiac cycle.

tachycardia An abnormally rapid heart rate, over 100 beats per minute.

tar A thick, sticky dark fluid produced by the burning of tobacco, made up of several hundred different chemicals, many of them poisonous, some of them carcinogenic.

target heart rate Sixty to eighty-five percent of the maximum heart rate; the heart rate at which one derives maximum cardiovascular benefit from aerobic exercise.

teratogen Any agent that causes spontaneous abortion or defects or malformations in a fetus.

terminal illness An illness in which death is inevitable.

testes (singular, testis) The male sex organs that produce sperm and testosterone.

testosterone The male sex hormone that stimulates male secondary sex characteristics.

thallium scintigraphy A diagnostic test in which radioactive isotopes are injected into the bloodstream, and images of the rays emitted by the isotopes are captured and then translated into images of the heart as it pumps.

thanatology The discipline of humanitarian care-giving for critically ill patients and their grieving family members and friends.

toxicity Poisonousness; the dosage level at which a drug becomes poisonous to the body, causing either temporary or permanent damage.

toxic shock syndrome (TSS) A disease characterized by fever, vomiting, diarrhea, and often shock, caused by a bacteria that releases toxic waste products into the bloodstream.

traditional marriage A marital relationship in which the roles of the partners are distinct; defined by gender-based cultural norms and expectations.

transcendence The sense of passing into a foreign region or dimension, often experienced by a person near death.

trans fats Fats formed when liquid vegetable oils are processed to make table spreads or cooking fats, and also found in dairy and beef products; considered to be especially dangerous dietary fats.

transgendered Having a gender identity opposite ones biological sex; transsexual.

transient ischemic attack (TIA) A cerebrovascular event in which the blood supply to a portion of the brain is blocked temporarily; repeated attacks are predictors of more severe strokes.

trichomoniasis An infection of the protozoa *Trichomonas vaginalis*; females experience vaginal burning, itching, and discharge, but male carriers may be asymptomatic.

triglyceride A blood fat that flows through the blood after meals and is linked to increased risk of coronary artery disease.

tubal ligation The suturing or tying shut of the fallopian tubes to prevent pregnancy.

tubal occlusion The blocking of the fallopian tubes to prevent pregnancy.

tuberculosis A highly infectious bacterial disease that primarily affects the lungs and is often fatal.

twelve-step programs Self-help group programs based on the principles of Alcoholics Anonymous.

ulcer A lesion in, or an erosion of, the mucous membrane of an organ.

unsaturated fat A chemical term indicating that a fat molecule contains fewer hydrogen atoms than its carbon skeleton can hold. These fats are normally liquid at room temperature.

urethra The canal through which urine from the bladder leaves the body; in the male, also serves as the channel for seminal fluid.

urethral opening The outer opening of the thin tube that carries urine from the bladder.

urethritis Infection of the urethra.

uterus The female organ that houses the developing fetus until birth.

vagina The canal leading from the exterior opening in the female genital area to the uterus.

vaginal contraceptive film (VCF) A small dissolvable sheet saturated with spermicide that can be inserted into the vagina and placed over the cervix.

vaginal spermicide A substance that kills or neutralizes sperm, inserted into the vagina in the form of a foam, cream, jelly, or suppository.

vaginismus A sexual difficulty in which a woman experiences painful spasms of the vagina during sexual intercourse.

values The criteria by which one makes choices about one's thoughts and actions and goals and ideals.

vas deferens Two tubes that carry sperm from the epididymis into the urethra.

vasectomy A surgical sterilization procedure in which each vas deferens is cut and tied shut to stop the passage of sperm to the urethra for ejaculation.

vector A biological or physical vehicle that carries the agent of infection to the host.

vegans People who eat only plant foods.

ventricle Either of the two lower chambers of the heart, which pump blood out of the heart and into the arteries.

video display terminal (VDT) A screen or monitor that emits electromagnetic fields from all sides; these fields may lead to increased reproductive problems, miscarriages, low birth weights, and cataracts.

virus A submicroscopic infectious agent; the most primitive form of life.

visualization An approach to stress control, self-healing, or motivating life changes by means of guided, or directed, imagery.

vital signs Measurements of physiological functioning; specifically, temperature, blood pressure, pulse rate, and respiration rate.

vitamins Organic substances that are needed in very small amounts by the body and carry out a variety of functions in metabolism and nutrition.

wellness A state of optimal health.

withdrawal Development of symptoms that cause significant psychological and physical distress when an individual reduces or stops drug use.

zero population growth (ZPG) The state at which the number of births equals the number of deaths.

zygote A fertilized egg.

Index